Renal Disease Progression and Management

Role of Vasoactive Agents, Cytokines, Lipids and Nutrition

Renal Disease Progression and Management

Role of Vasoactive Agents, Cytokines, Lipids and Nutrition

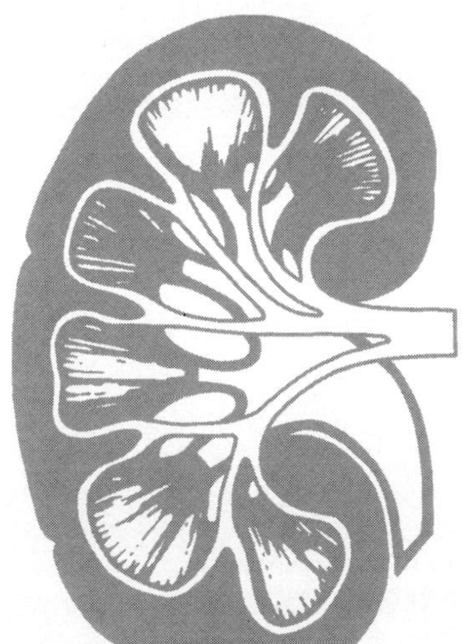

Editors - **Morrell M. Avram and Saulo Klahr**

W. B. Saunders Company • A Division of Harcourt Brace & Company

W.B. SAUNDERS COMPANY
A Division of
Harcourt Brace & Company

The Curtis Center
Independence Square West
Philadelphia, Pennsylvania 19106-3399

Library of Congress Card Number 95-71697

Renal Disease Progression and Management
Role of Vasoactive Agents, Cytokines, Lipids and Nutrition

ISBN 0-7216-3833-3

Printed in the United States of America.

Last digit is the print number: 9 8 7 6 5 4 3 2 1

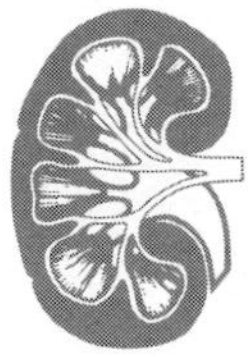

Senior Contributors

Gerald B. Appel, M.D.
Professor of Clinical Medicine
Columbia University School of Medicine
Director of Clinical Nephrology
Columbia Presbyterian Medical Center
New York, New York

Morrell Michael Avram, M.D.
Professor of Medicine
Chief, Division of Nephrology
The Long Island College Hospital
Brooklyn, New York

Jonas Bergström, M.D.
Director and Professor, Institute of Renal Medicine
Huddinge University Hospital
Karolinska Institute, Stockholm, Sweden

Staffan Bjork, M.D.
Department of Nephrology
Sahlgrenska Hospital
Goteborg, Sweden

Wayne Border, M.D.
Chief, Division of Nephrology
University of Utah Medical Center
Salt Lake City, Utah

Barry M. Brenner, M.D.
Samuel A. Levine Professor of Medicine
Director - Renal Division, Harvard Medical School
Brigham & Women's Hospital
Boston, Massachusetts

Hans R. Brunner, M.D.
Professor of Medicine
Head, Hypertension Division, University Hospital
Lausanne, Switzerland

Giuseppe D'Amico, M.D.
Director and Professor, Divisione di Nefrologia
Ospedale San Carlo Borromeo
University of Milano
Milan, Italy

Dick de Zeeuw, M.D.
Professor, Department of Medicine
State University Hospital
Groningen, The Netherlands

Jonathan R. Diamond, M.D.
Professor of Medicine
Penn State College of Medicine
The Milton S. Hershey Medical Center
Hershey, Pennsylvania

Eli A. Friedman, M.D.
Distinguished Teaching Professor
Chief, Division of Renal Diseases
SUNY - Health Science Center at Brooklyn
Brooklyn, New York

Bruce R. Gordon, M.D.
Associate Professor of Medicine, The Rogosin Institute
New York Hospital Cornell Medical Center
New York, New York

Raymond M. Hakim, M.D., Ph.D.
Professor of Medicine, Department of Medicine
Division of Nephrology
Vanderbilt University Medical Center
Nashville, Tennessee

Thomas Hostetter, M.D.
Professor of Medicine
Director, Division of Renal Diseases
University of Minnesota Hospital
Minneapolis, Minnesota

D. Roger Illingworth, M.D., Ph.D.
Professor of Medicine
Division of Endocrinology, Diabetes and Clinical Nutrition
Oregon Health Sciences University
Portland, Oregon

Claude Jacobs, M.D.
Chief, Service de Néphrologie
Hôpital de la Pitié
Paris, France

George A. Kaysen, M.D., Ph.D.
Professor of Medicine
Chief, Division of Nephrology
University of California, Davis
Sacramento, California

William F. Keane, M.D.
Professor of Medicine and Chairman
Department of Medicine
Division of Nephrology, University of Minnesota
Hennepin County Medical Center
Minneapolis, Minnesota

Saulo Klahr, M.D.
Simon Professor of Medicine
Co-Chairman, Department of Medicine
Washington University School of Medicine
Physician-in-Chief, The Jewish Hospital of St. Louis
St. Louis, Missouri

Joel D. Kopple, M.D.
Chief, Division of Nephrology & Hypertension
Professor of Medicine, UCLA School of Medicine
Torrance, California

Andrew S. Levey, M.D.
Associate Professor of Medicine
Tufts University School of Medicine
Director, Nephrology Clinical Research Unit
Associate Director, Renal Transplantation Program
New England Medical Center
Boston, Massachusetts

Edmund G. Lowrie, M.D.
President, National Medical Care, Inc.
Waltham, Massachusetts

Shaul G. Massry, M.D.
Bernard J. Hanley Professor of Medicine
Chief, Division of Nephrology
University of Southern California
Los Angeles, California

William E. Mitch, M.D.
E. Garland Herndon Professor of Medicine
Director, Renal Division
Emory University School of Medicine
Department of Medicine
Atlanta, Georgia

Neal Mittman, M.D.
Associate Professor of Clinical Medicine
Associate Director, Division of Nephrology
The Long Island College Hospital
Brooklyn, New York

Carl Erik Mogensen, M.D.
Professor of Medicine
Medical Department M
Second University Clinic of Internal Medicine
Kommunehospitalet
Aarhus, Denmark

Joel Neugarten, M.D., J.D.
Associate Professor of Medicine
Albert Einstein School of Medicine
Associate Director, Renal Division
Montefiore Medical Center
Bronx, New York

Hans-Henrik Parving, M.D.
Chief Physician and Director
Steno Diabetes Center
Gentofte, Denmark

Jerome G. Porush, M.D.
Professor of Medicine
Chief, Division of Nephrology and Hypertension
The Brookdale Hospital Medical Center
SUNY - Health Science Center at Brooklyn
Brooklyn, New York

Detlef Schlondorff, M.D.
Chief, Division of Nephrology
Professor of Medicine
Albert Einstein College of Medicine
Bronx, New York

W. Gordon Walker, M.D.
Division of Nephrology
Professor of Medicine
Johns Hopkins University School of Medicine
Baltimore, Maryland

Contents

HYPERTENSION AND PROGRESSION OF RENAL DISEASE

INTERVENTIONS AFFECTING PROGRESSION OF RENAL DISEASE

CYTOKINES AND VASOACTIVE AGENTS IN RENAL DISEASE

LIPIDS AND RENAL DISEASE

DYSLIPIDEMIA AND PROTEINURIA

UREMIA AND RENAL REPLACEMENT THERAPY

This book is dedicated to Maria for 40 years of happiness and joy.

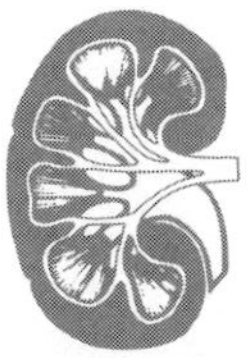

Preface

Over the past decade, there has been a profusion of interest in the pathophysiology of progressive renal disease. The complex web of interconnecting influences is beginning to unfold in tiny increments. Maladaptive hemodynamic changes, interacting and counteracting endocrine and autocrine influences, as well as the ubiquitous monocytic infiltration of the glomerulus and interstitium with consequent synthesis and release of vasoactive agents, proinflammatory cytokines, and growth factors have all been recognized as major factors in progressive renal injury.

More than a decade ago, Brenner and associates proposed the relationship between glomerular hemodynamics, hyperfiltration, and progressive glomerular sclerosis. Inexorable progression is often seen after the initial injury is no longer evident, suggesting a final common pathway. Since that time, substantial volumes of research have detailed the beneficial effects of hemodynamic manipulations, especially through inhibition of the renin-angiotensin system, but also through dietary protein restriction. Many investigators, initially in laboratory animals but more recently in human models of glomerular injury (especially diabetic nephropathy), have documented beneficial antiproteinuric effects as well as stabilization of renal function with short- and long-term intervention.

Recently, the prominent role of the tubulointerstitium in progressive renal injury, including glomerulopathies, has been increasingly recognized. The prognostic importance of tubulointerstitial fibrosis in glomerular diseases has long been noted, but pathogenetic mechanisms linking interstitial mononuclear recruitment, fibroblast proliferation, and cytokine-mediated injury to immunologic renal destruction are now becoming clear.

Cytokines regulate the basic processes of cell homeostasis and tissue repair in all organs. Border and colleagues present compelling evidence that expression of a cytokine, transforming growth factor-β (TGF-β), can mediate accumulation of extracellular matrix, ultimately resulting in glomerular fibrosis that can be attenuated pharmacologically. Klahr and associates elegantly illustrate the complex interactions of various factors in renal injury by demonstrating the importance of angiotensin II in tubulointerstitial fibrosis following ureteral obstruction, using angiotensin II inhibition or receptor blockade to ameliorate mononuclear infiltration, reduce matrix accumulation, and lessen expression of TGF-β and type IV collagen.

Remarkable advances have been made in understanding the role of dyslipidemic injury in the initiation and progression of renal diseases. Hyperlipidemia as a consequence of persistent proteinuria has long been recognized. The potential toxicity of dyslipidemia to the renal circulation as atherosclerosis is easily envisioned, but lipoprotein toxicity to the glomerulus and the final pathway to glomerulosclerosis has only recently been supported. Dietary and pharmacologic manipulation of dyslipidemia in patients with nephrotic syndrome and in patients on renal replacement therapy is a relatively recent area of investigation and debate.

Dietary restrictions in the face of progressive renal failure present a clinical paradox. Whereas protein restriction, and possibly control of dyslipidemia, may retard the progression of renal protein restriction, protein-calorie malnutrition is highly prevalent in patients maintained on renal replacement therapy and has been recognized as an important factor in the excessive morbidity and mortality in these patients. Pathophysiologic mechanisms implicating treatment modalities as well as the uremic state have been elucidated, and the use of risk profiles that permit early identification of high-risk patients may allow early intervention to lessen catabolism and improve nutrition.

This book, comprised of selected manuscripts presented at two international symposia held at the Avram Center for Kidney Diseases of The Long Island College Hospital in Brooklyn, NY, offers current insights into the progression of renal disease and the efficacy of various interventions, as well as the management of uremia and its consequences. The editors believe that these excellent contributions will be of great interest to physicians who treat patients with renal disease and may stimulate new investigations of the factors contributing to progressive renal failure.

Morrell M. Avram, MD
Brooklyn, NY
Saulo Klahr, MD
St Louis, MO

HYPERTENSION AND PROGRESSION OF RENAL DISEASES

Introduction

It is estimated that in 30% of patients reaching end-stage renal disease (ESRD), hypertension is the underlying cause. The association between malignant hypertension and the development of renal disease has been recognized since the turn of the century. However, the effects of less severe forms of hypertension on the development of renal disease and its progression have been documented only recently.

Walker addresses hypertension-related renal injury. He reports that analysis of the Multiple Risk Factor Intervention Trial data yields information of importance in developing strategies for reducing the incidence of ESRD. Control of diastolic blood pressure below 95 mm Hg appears to preserve renal function in non-black patients. At the same time, the apparent exemption of blacks from this renal protective effect of blood pressure control identifies an area in which additional studies are badly needed. The failure to find an association between lipids and declining renal function does not exclude a role for lipids, but it does suggest that blood pressure control is more likely to yield earlier evidence of renal protection in essential hypertension. In a similar fashion, the observation that blood pressure and angiotensin-aldosterone levels are the two most important predictors of declining renal function in diabetics indicates that adequate blood pressure control is at least as important as maintaining angiotensin-aldosterone levels in diabetic nephropathy. The independent effect identified for angiotensin and aldosterone raises the possibility that not all drug regimens are equally effective in protecting the kidney.

More than 10 years ago, Brenner and associates, on the basis of studies in animal models, proposed that maladaptive glomerular hemodynamic changes modulate the inexorable progression of renal disease. Mackenzie and Brenner, in a review, extend the hypothesis, originally set forth by Brenner and colleagues in 1988, that an inverse relationship exists between total nephron number and the risk of developing arterial hypertension. They argue that low birth-weight and ''programmed deficits'' in nephron number at birth are determinants of essential hypertension in later life.

The report by Levey addresses the effectiveness of therapy in clinical trials, emphasizing that progressive renal disease requires a detailed effort to measure outcome. The author emphasizes that each measurement of renal function, glomerular filtration rate, creatinine clearance, and serum creatinine concentration, has both limitations and strengths based on practical, technical, and physiologic considerations that may affect and influence the statistical analysis.

Hypertension-Related Renal Injury: A Major Contributor to End-Stage Renal Disease

W. Gordon Walker, MD

● The US Renal Data System Annual Report reveals that 57% of new cases of end-stage renal disease are attributed to hypertensive nephropathy and diabetic nephropathy. Analyses of the data on serum creatinine from the Multiple Risk Factor Intervention Trial confirms that one in 20 of the hypertensive men exhibits a rate of decline in renal function that equals or exceeds 3% per year, the rate of loss being greater in older men, black men, and men with higher baseline blood pressure. Effective blood pressure treatment with maintenance of diastolic blood pressure below 95 mm Hg protected renal function in non-blacks but not in blacks, despite comparable blood pressure reduction in blacks. A longitudinal study of a diabetic cohort (n = 131) revealed that hypertension, plasma angiotensin II, and aldosterone are independent predictors of accelerated loss of renal function in diabetic nephropathy, possibly aggravated by diuretic usage as part of the antihypertensive regimen in diabetic nephropathy. No significant loss of renal function could be documented in those individuals whose blood pressure was adequately controlled (systolic blood pressure, <140 mm Hg). These findings provide emphasis for the importance of adequate blood pressure control in both essential hypertension and hypertension associated with diabetes mellitus. They also provide support for the proposal that careful blood pressure control offers promise for reducing the incidence of end-stage renal disease in both hypertensive nephropathy and diabetic nephropathy.

INDEX WORDS: Hypertension; diabetes mellitus; end-stage renal disease; reciprocal creatinine; renal function; cholesterol; angiotensin II; aldosterone; prevention.

CLINICAL nephrology has focused, perhaps disproportionately, on dialysis, including techniques for its improvement and problems of preterminal uremia, and on the clinical complications of maintenance dialysis. Egger et al's[1] report on the national incidence of specific diseases responsible for end-stage renal disease (ESRD) requiring maintenance dialysis has re-emphasized the importance of epidemiology in the study of ESRD. Any effective strategy for preventing or reducing the incidence of ESRD must begin with prevalence and incidence data on ESRD and the specific diseases contributing to the ESRD population.

THE PREVALENCE AND INCIDENCE OF CAUSES OF END-STAGE RENAL DISEASE

Hypertension and diabetes were listed as the most common diagnoses causing ESRD in the Health Care Financing Administration's medical database.[1] This pattern has been repeatedly confirmed in the annual reports of the US Renal Data System, which was established to "collect and analyze information on the incidence, prevalence, morbidity and mortality of end-stage renal disease (ESRD) in the United States."[2]

Table 1 summarizes the annual incidence data of ESRD by diagnostic category for the 5 years between 1984 and 1988.[2] Diabetes-related ESRD has increased 50% during the 5 years shown in Table 1 and cases due to hypertensive nephropathy have increased 40%, together accounting for three quarters of the total increase in annual incidence during this period. In contrast, the incidence of ESRD related to glomerulonephritis and polycystic kidney disease has remained virtually unchanged. More importantly, diabetes and hypertension now account for over half (57%) of new cases of ESRD annually.[2] This increasing incidence in both hypertensive nephropathy and diabetic nephropathy and the magnitude of their combined presentation make it readily apparent that these trends must be reversed if a significant reduction in overall ESRD incidence is to be achieved.

There are nevertheless uncertainties associated with these data: (1) How reliable is the diagnosis of hypertensive nephropathy? If correct, does it reflect contributions from the large group of mild to moderate hypertensives in the United States or is it a reflection of some complicating event in the course of the disease, such as renovascular hypertension? (2) What are the relative contributions of insulin-dependent type 1 and non–insulin-dependent type 2 diabetes mellitus and what are the factors responsible for increasing the risk of renal failure within diabetes? (3) What is the

Supported in part by USPHS Grants No. HL3303, HL20455, RR00722, RR00035, and DK 39885; The Irving Blum Memorial Fund; The Singley-Welty Diabetes Research Fund; and the Endowment Fund of the Good Samaritan Hospital.

Table 1. Incidence (in Millions) of Reported End-Stage Renal Disease Therapy by Diagnosis (1984 to 1988)

	1984 (%)	1985 (%)	1986 (%)	1987 (%)	1988 (%)
Diabetes	30 (26.8)	34 (27.9)	38 (29.2)	42 (30)	45 (30.6)
Hypertension	28 (25)	31 (25.4)	33 (25.4)	36 (25.7)	39 (26.5)
Glomerulonephritis	18 (16)	19 (14.7)	19 (14.6)	20 (14.3)	20 (13.6)
Cystic disease	4 (3.6)	5 (4)	5 (3.8)	5 (3.6)	5 (3.4)
Total crude rate	112 (100)	122 (100)	130 (100)	140 (100)	147 (100)

Note. The rates are crude rates unadjusted for age, race, and sex. The figures in parentheses are percentages of total crude death rate. The data reported here have been supplied by the United States Renal Data System. The interpretation and reporting of these data are the responsibility of the author and in no way should be seen as an official policy or interpretation of the US Renal Data System.

extent of corroborating evidence that can be found in other studies to support the US Renal Data System findings? And, perhaps most importantly, (4) What are the mechanism(s) of renal injury that lead to ESRD?

The relative contributions of hypertension, hyperlipidemia, protein intake, and perhaps genetic factors in determining both the initiation and rate of progression of renal damage are important issues that bear directly on intervention and prevention strategies. This presentation focuses on some aspects of these questions and the extent to which relevant clinical information is available.

HYPERTENSIVE NEPHROPATHY AS A CAUSE OF END-STAGE RENAL DISEASE

Bright's original report associating small scarred kidneys with abnormally thickened arteries implied an association between arterial hypertension and progressive kidney damage long before any means of clinical measurement of arterial blood pressure was available.[3] Nearly a century passed before documentation of the association between the pathologic entity nephrosclerosis as postmortem and the pre-existence of sustained elevation of blood pressure provided clinical pathologic correlation that clearly established this association. The evolution of our understanding of this relationship of nephrosclerosis with arterial hypertension and renal functional impairment has been summarized in the excellent review by Luke,[4] who also called attention to significant racial differences and raised the question whether the renal architecture among blacks differs in some way that increases the risk of damage from elevated blood pressure. Luke also offered the alternate proposal that these changes identified in the kidney and its circulation in blacks may account for the increased prevalence of high blood pressure in blacks.

The question whether mild to moderate hypertension[5] is associated with progressive renal damage has remained unanswered and received little attention prior to Egger et al's report.[1] Paradoxically, this increase in ESRD attributed to hypertensive nephropathy is coeval with a significant decrease in mortality associated with both myocardial infarction and stroke.[6] Since this decline in mortality has been attributed in significant part to more effective treatment of hypertension, the increase in hypertension-related ESRD must be reconciled with the declining incidence of mortality due to myocardial infarction and stroke. It thus becomes critical to ascertain whether significant progressive renal damage can be documented among patients with mild to moderate hypertension.

We have recently reported[7] on changes in renal function in a subset of the Multiple Risk Factor Intervention Trial (MRFIT), which provides at least a partial answer to this question. Of the 12,866 MRFIT participants, 5,524 had a baseline diastolic blood pressure of 90 mm Hg or greater and were receiving no antihypertensive medication at the time of enrollment in the MRFIT study. The average age of this group was 46.5 $\pm$ 5.9 (SD) years. The average blood pressure at entry was 143/97 mm Hg and the average serum creatinine 1.1 $\pm$ 0.14 mg/dL. In both the special intervention and usual care groups in this subset, mean diastolic blood pressures decreased to levels below 90 mm Hg at the second anniversary following enrollment and the mean serum creatinine decreased in both groups. All individuals had serum creatinine measurements at each anniversary of enrollment; hence, reciprocal creatinine slope, $\Delta(1/Cr)/\Delta(t)$, determined for each participant was used to evaluate individual changes in renal function. A slope of −0.03 or less was exhibited by 5.6% of this subset, representing loss of renal function of 3% per year or greater. This rate of decline was greater in older individuals, in those with higher systolic blood pressure at entry, and in blacks. No evidence for an association between declining renal function and either high-density lipoprotein or low-protein lipoprotein cholesterol could be identified.

Most importantly there were significant differences demonstrable between blacks and non-blacks in the study and there was also an identifiable and quite significant difference in response to therapy. These findings assume particular importance in light of the much higher incidence of hypertension-related ESRD reported among blacks.[2]

Among non-blacks, those individuals whose average diastolic blood pressure was maintained below 95 mm Hg during the period of follow-up exhibited a mean value for reciprocal creatinine slope that was positive (+0.0012 dL/mg/yr) while those individuals whose diastolic blood pressure remained ≥95 mm Hg had a mean value that was negative (−0.0013, $P < 0.007$ for difference). This is consistent with significant protection of renal function with effective treatment of blood pressure that maintains diastolic pressure below 95 mm Hg in non-blacks.[7] In contrast, blacks failed to show any evidence of response to therapy (blacks < 95 mm Hg = −0.0023 ± 0.001 *v* blacks ≥ 95 mm Hg = −0.0013 ± 0.0025; $P > 0.5$). Within the special intervention group, this continued decline was demonstrable in both groups of blacks, despite the fact that antihypertensive treatment resulted in a lowering of blood pressure that was identical with that seen in non-blacks in the special intervention group.

Although it must be emphasized that MRFIT was not designed primarily as a study to evaluate the effect of adequate blood pressure treatment on renal function, the sample size and study duration were nevertheless such that the differences are highly significant and lend support to Luke's proposal that there is a greater risk of hypertension-related renal damage in blacks.[4,7,8] The MRFIT data indicate that this is not readily eliminated by effective blood pressure control. Whether this difference reflects a differing response to drugs and an inherent genetic difference or implies that differing levels of blood pressure control may be needed for blacks remains to be determined. Alternately, it could reflect a more severe nature of the disease in blacks that requires longer to control even though blood pressure control is adequate.

A rate of decline of 3% per year or greater, if persistent, will result in virtually total loss of renal function within 25 to 30 years. Given the average age of 46 years for this MRFIT cohort, development of ESRD would be likely for those individuals in whom this rate of decline continues to age 70 years. The US Renal Data System data reveal that the average age of dialysis entrants with the diagnosis of hypertensive nephropathy is 67 years, a figure that agrees well with the MRFIT analysis. Moreover, the 5.6% of MRFIT participants in this high-risk category could, if representative of the US hypertensive population, identify a population at risk that is more than adequate to account for the annual incidence of hypertension-related ESRD.[7] Given the indication of benefit conferred by adequate treatment (diastolic blood pressure, <95 mm Hg), this post hoc analysis of the MRFIT data strongly suggests that this residual risk may reflect inadequate blood pressure control. Confirmation requires an appropriately designed prospective trial and represents an urgent need.

The failure of blacks to respond to adequate blood pressure control is cause for concern. It may well be the principal reason for the significantly greater incidence (2.8:1) of hypertension-related ESRD observed in blacks.[2] The recent MRFIT data analysis underscores the urgent need to address this problem.

THE ROLE OF HYPERTENSION IN DIABETIC NEPHROPATHY

Although diabetic nephropathy as a major contributor to ESRD was not anticipated in the Report of the Committee on Chronic Kidney Disease,[9] its emergence as the major cause of ESRD among new dialysis entrants has focused attention on this clinical entity. It has long been recognized that more than one third of insulin-dependent diabetes patients (type I or juvenile diabetes) progress to renal failure,[10] but the magnitude of the contribution of non–insulin-dependent diabetes (type II) remains to be defined accurately. Early data from the Health Care Financing Administration did not distinguish between type I and type II diabetes. Subsequently, reports indicate that more than 80% of the diabetic constituency of the ESRD population in some dialysis units represents renal failure in type II diabetes.[11,12] Much more information is needed about the development and progression of nephropathy in type II diabetes mellitus.

We previously reported on a prospective observational study of a cohort of diabetic subjects and on factors influencing the rate of progression of diabetic nephropathy.[13-15] The cohort consisted of both insulin-dependent and non–insulin-dependent diabetes (total cohort, 131: 47 insulin-dependent and 84 non–insulin-dependent) and the report covered the first 3.5 years of observation. The report documented a more significant and progressive increase in serum creatinine in individuals whose systolic blood pressure remained elevated above 140 mm Hg while on therapy. In contrast, individuals whose blood pressure was maintained below this level showed no significant deterioration in renal function. This appeared to be true for both insulin-dependent and non–insulin-dependent diabetes. Comparison of the hypertensive and normotensive groups reveal that no significant difference in age, duration of diabetes, or baseline renal function could account for the difference. It was concluded on the basis of this initial analysis of the data that persistent elevation of the blood pressure adds significantly to the risk of progressive renal damage in both insulin-dependent and non–insulin-dependent diabetes.

The study has been continued with semiannual observations on some of the participants spanning a period of 8 years. Table 2 contains an update of some of the findings, which includes this extended period of observation. Methodology and basis for classification have been previously described.[13-15] Reciprocal creatinine slope ($\Delta(1/Cr)/\Delta(t)$) has been used as the indicator of change in renal function. Table 2 compares the reciprocal creatinine slope between the normotensive and hypertensive groups for the entire cohort and also for the insulin-dependent and non–insulin-dependent subsets. Baseline data and mean follow-up values are also presented for angiotensin II, aldosterone, and systolic and diastolic blood pressures. The rate of increase in albumin excretion, which was available on only part of the cohort, is also incorporated in Table 2 for those individuals who had repeated observations on microalbuminuria that spanned a period of more than 1 year. Sequential data were available on 77 of the cohort of 131.

Statistical comparison of reciprocal creatinine slope confirmed the previous observation that serum creatinine increased more rapidly in the hypertensive group. For the total cohort, the difference in mean reciprocal creatinine slope was significant with renal function in the hypertensive subset declining more rapidly ($P < 0.001$). When insulin-dependent and non–insulin-dependent diabetic patients were examined separately, this difference was demonstrable in both groups ($P < 0.01$ and $P < 0.007$, respectively).

Table 2 also contains mean values and standard errors for important covariates that were associated with declining renal function, divided according to follow-up systolic blood pressure. For the entire cohort, the hypertensive group exhibited significantly higher levels of circulating angiotensin II and aldosterone. Although data on microalbuminuria are incomplete, no difference was demonstrable in the average level of baseline microalbuminuria, but the rate of increase was significantly greater for individuals with persistent hypertension. The classification of blood pressure for analysis was based on mean follow-up systolic blood pressure; however, a significant difference was demonstrable for diastolic blood pressure in the persistently hypertensive cohort ($P < 0.001$) even though mean values for diastolic blood pressure in both groups were within the range ordinarily considered to be normal.

Table 3 presents the bivariate correlations for reciprocal creatinine slope and the covariates of interest. The upper triangle contains the individual (bivariate) correlation coefficients and the lower triangle contains the corresponding significance levels. Declining renal function is significantly associated with mean follow-up systolic blood pressure ($P < 0.01$). Equally importantly, hypertension in the diabetic patient correlates with both mean angiotensin II and the mean levels of plasma aldosterone during follow-

Table 2. Baseline and Follow-up Data on Longitudinal Study Cohort of Diabetes Mellitus

Mean Follow-up Systolic Blood Pressure	Total Diabetic Cohort		IDDM		NIDDM	
	≤140 mm Hg	>140 mm Hg	≤140 mm Hg	>140 mm Hg	≤140 mm Hg	>140 mm Hg
Plasma angiotensin II (pg/mL)						
Baseline	8.40 ± 1.0	9.42 ± 1.2	7.3 ± 1	14.1 ± 3.8	9.7 ± 1.1	8.4 ± 1.2
Mean follow-up	7.94 ± 0.56	10.0 ± 0.73	7.2 ± 0.65	11.5 ± 1.6	8.4 ± 0.9	9.6 ± 0.8
Plasma aldosterone (ng/dL)						
Baseline	10.1 ± 1.4	13.6 ± 1.43	8.0 ± 2	13.6 ± 2.9	12.3 ± 1.9	13.6 ± 1.6
Mean follow-up	6.4 ± 0.9	8.5 ± 1.0	4.8 ± 0.8	9.7 ± 3.3	8.0 ± 1.6	8.2 ± 0.95
Microalbuminuria*						
Baseline rate of increase (μg/24 hr)	136 ± 64	108 ± 50	206 ± 106	154 ± 48	69 ± 40	111 ± 62
During follow-up (μg/d/mo)	+27 ± 22	+250 ± 82	7 ± 13.9	184 ± 100	47 ± 41	152 ± 68
Systolic blood pressure (mm Hg)						
Baseline	127.4 ± 1.6	168.3 ± 2.3	123 ± 2.2	164 ± 5.9	133 ± 2.3	169.6 ± 2.4
Mean follow-up	125.2 ± 1.3	163.7 ± 1.7	120.1 ± 1.9	158.3 ± 4.4	129.9 ± 1.3	165.03 ± 1.9
Diastolic blood pressure (mm Hg)						
Baseline	73.5 ± 1.1	86.5 ± 1.2	70.4 ± 1.6	82.5 ± 3.2	76.4 ± 1.4	87.5 ± 1.3
Mean follow-up	72.3 ± 0.9	84.7 ± 1.1	70.7 ± 1.3	85.1 ± 2.5	73.7 ± 1.3	84.5 ± 1.25
Δ(1/Cr)/Δ(t) (mg/dL/mo)	−0.001 ± 0.002	−.0105 ± 0.003	−.0017 ± 0.002	−.0051 ± 0.002	−.0014 ± 0.003	−.0018 ± 0.004

Abbreviations: IDDM, insulin-dependent diabetes mellitus; NIDDM, non–insulin-dependent diabetes mellitus.
* Data available for only 77 of 139 patients.

up. The associations identified in Table 3 establish a significant relationship between the level of blood pressure during follow-up and both declining renal function (Δ(1/Cr)/Δ(t) and changes in proteinuria. When mean values for β_2-microglobulin are used as an indicator of renal impairment (instead of reciprocal creatinine slope), the same associations emerge. Thus, in this cohort the level of blood pressure is an important predictor of the state of renal function with evidence of significant involvement of the renin angiotensin-aldosterone system. In contrast, it was not possible to identify similar associations for either fasting blood sugar or glycosylated hemoglobin. The significant association between mean angiotensin II and mean cholesterol and triglyceride during follow-up is an interesting finding, but its significance remains to be determined.

Multiple linear regression analysis of reciprocal creatinine slope and the covariates presented in Table 2 identified follow-up systolic blood pressure ($P < 0.006$), hyperangiotensinemia, and hyperaldosteronemia ($P < 0.02$) as independent predictors of more rapidly declining renal function after control of other covariates. In contrast, neither age, race, duration of diabetes, mean fasting blood glucose during follow-up, nor mean cholesterol level during follow-up were significant when blood pressure, angiotensin II, and aldosterone were controlled for.

Our preliminary report on this cohort noted an association between diuretic therapy and increased risk of progressive decline in renal function[15] among individuals whose blood pressure was not adequately controlled. This association has been re-examined after longer follow-up and results are summarized here because of the therapeutic implications. Since non–insulin-dependent and insulin-dependent diabetes mellitus patients tended to exhibit the same sort of behavior and identified the same significant covariates, the entire cohort has been used for this analysis; the numbers involved in the insulin-dependent patients were insufficient to provide reasonable power for separate analyses of the two diabetes type.

Table 4 presents information on three categories of patients: normotensive individuals who have never received diuretic therapy, individuals on maintenance diuretic therapy whose average

Table 3. Bivariate Correlations Between Variables of Interest in Longitudinal Study Cohort of Diabetes Mellitus

	$\Delta(1/Cr)/\Delta(t)$	Mean Follow-up Systolic Blood Pressure	Mean Follow-up Angiotensin II	Mean Follow-up Aldosterone	Rate of Increase of μAlb	Mean Follow-up β_2-Microglobulin	Mean Follow-up Cholesterol	Mean Follow-up Triglycerides	Mean Follow-up Fasting Blood Sugar
$\Delta(1/Cr)/\Delta(t)$		−0.23	−0.18	−0.29	−0.51	−0.19	+0.05	+0.02	−0.14
Mean Follow-up systolic blood pressure	0.01		+0.22	+0.23	+0.39	+0.46	+0.25	+0.11	+0.08
Mean angiotensin II	0.06	0.04		+0.16	+0.20	+0.15	+0.37	+0.24	+0.13
Mean aldosterone	0.002	0.01	0.09		−0.03	−0.11	+0.08	+0.01	+0.08
Rate of increase albumin	0.001	0.006	0.10	NS		+0.45	−0.15	−0.06	+0.24
β_2-Microglobulin	0.003	0.0005	NS	NS	0.001		+0.07	+0.06	+0.08
Cholesterol	NS	0.004	0.0005	NS	NS	NS		+0.39	+0.04
Triglycerides	NS	NS	0.007	NS	NS	NS	0.0005		−0.04
Mean fasting blood sugar	NS	NS	NS	NS	0.04	NS	NS	NS	

Note. The upper triangle contains the correlation coefficient between pairs of variables as indicated; the lower triangle contains the significance level for the indicated pair.

Abbreviations: μAlb, microalbuminuria; NS, not significant.

blood pressure during follow-up exceeded 140 mm Hg (ie, diuretic therapy with inadequate blood pressure control), and the group of persistently hypertensive patients whose treatment did not include diuretic therapy. Renal function declined more rapidly among the persistently hypertensive patients who were receiving diuretics; indeed, only this group exhibited a significant rate of decline. The slight differences in average systolic blood pressure during follow-up in these two groups did not differ significantly ($P > 0.15$). The follow-up mean values for fasting blood sugar did not differ between the two groups, nor were differences identifiable between age, follow-up diastolic blood pressure, duration of diabetes, or glycosylated hemoglobin.

Table 4. Diuretic Effects on Hypertensive Diabetics

	N	$\Delta(1/Cr)\Delta(t)$	Baseline Serum Creatinine (mg/dL)	Follow-up Systolic Blood Pressure (mm Hg)	Follow-up Angiotensin II (pg/mL)	Follow-up Serum Cholesterol (mg/dL)	Follow-up Mean Fasting Blood Sugar (mg/dL)
Normal blood pressure, no diuretic therapy	45	+0.00065 ± 0.0020	0.91 ± 0.025	122.4 ± 1.5	7.3 ± 0.57	221.2 ± 6.3	204.6 ± 10
High systolic blood pressure (>140 mm Hg), diuretic therapy	48	−0.01582 ± 0.00410	1.24 ± 0.100	165.8 ± 2.3	11.3 ± 0.85	257.1 ± 8.5	222.1 ± 10.8
High systolic blood pressure (>140 mm Hg), no diuretic therapy	23	−0.00011 ± 0.0041	0.94 ± 0.040	160.2 ± 3.0	7.8 ± 0.86	231.1 ± 8.8	214.8 ± 13.2
Probability		0.002	0.002	0.001	0.001	0.002	>0.3

The mean level for follow-up cholesterol, however, was higher than that exhibited in the hypertensive group receiving no diuretic therapy ($P < 0.045$). The baseline serum creatinine was slightly higher for the persistently hypertensive patients who were receiving diuretics at the time of entry into the study ($P < 0.04$). The mean follow-up angiotensin II level was significantly more elevated for the hypertensive patients receiving diuretics ($P = 0.001$). Not shown in Table 4, but exhibiting a similar pattern, is aldosterone ($P < 0.002$). Of particular interest was the fact that multivariate analysis revealed that elevated levels of angiotensin II and aldosterone were significant predictors of a more accelerated decline in renal function, even after controlling for the presence of diuretics.

The persistently hypertensive group receiving diuretic therapy was the only group at significant risk for progressive deterioration of renal function during follow-up. This increase in risk associated with diuretic usage occurred in the absence of a demonstrable difference between age, blood pressure levels, or duration of diabetes for the two persistently hypertensive groups. Although the creatinine at entry was slightly higher in the diuretic group, the mean value is still within the normal range at the time of entry and this hardly seems an adequate explanation for the more rapid decline in renal function. In fact, the fourth subset of the cohort, those individuals whose blood pressure was successfully treated with a regimen that included diuretics, responded adequately to treatment ($\Delta(1/Cr)/\Delta(t) = -0.0039 \pm 0.0036$), with a mean reciprocal creatinine slope that did not differ from zero or from the other two nondiuretic groups in the cohort. It did, however, differ significantly from the persistently hypertensive subset whose regimen for blood pressure treatment included diuretics ($P < 0.03$), apparently signifying a beneficial therapeutic effect when diuretics are used, provided adequate control of blood pressure is achieved. Of particular importance was the fact that the persistently hypertensive group receiving diuretic therapy did not differ in any other significant respect from the hypertensive group whose regimen did not include diuretics in any other significant respect. Ages were virtually identical. Thus, except for the modest differences in baseline creatinines between the two hypertensive groups, the only significant differences were the follow-up levels of angiotensin II and aldosterone and a marginally significant difference in serum cholesterol.

The major results of this longitudinal observation study point to high blood pressure and relative excess of angiotensin II and aldosterone as the primary predictors of accelerated decline in renal function in diabetic nephropathy. The fact that this decline is exhibited by those persistently hypertensive patients whose antihypertensive regimen includes diuretics raises concern about the safety of diuretic usage, particularly when therapy fails to control the blood pressure adequately. While the apparent potential hazard of diuretic usage can only be confirmed by a properly designed randomized prospective trial, until this issue is resolved, prudence dictates that diuretics should be used with caution and only in conjunction with agents that suppress the renin angiotensin system. The data further indicate that the currently accepted goal of 90 to 95 mm Hg (diastolic) as the targeted treatment goal is not adequate for the diabetic patient with hypertension, but that a treatment goal of 140/85 mm Hg or less appears necessary for renal protection.

DISCUSSION

Both the MRFIT study and the Longitudinal Diabetic Study have identified highly significant associations between blood pressure and the rate of loss of renal function, creating a presumption of a causal role for hypertension. The fundamental pathogenetic mechanism underlying this progressive damage in diabetes and in essential hypertension remains to be established with certainty.

Experimental evidence associating glomerular hyperperfusion with progressive injury is impressive and has been reviewed earlier in this symposium.[16] Glomerular hyperfiltration is a commonly observed finding in early diabetic nephropathy.[17,18] It remains to be shown, however, that progressive renal damage is limited exclusively to those individuals who early exhibit significant and sustained glomerular hyperfiltration. The situation with regard to non–insulin-dependent diabetes mellitus is even much less satisfactory. Information documenting hyperfiltration in early type II diabetes is scant at best.

It should be pointed out, however, that hyperfiltration can be markedly aggravated by angiotensin II because of its effect on the efferent arteriole of the glomerulus.[19] The documentation presented in the preceding section that associates the highest levels of angiotensin II with progressive renal damage is certainly consistent with such a mechanism. The experimental studies of DeClue et al[20] that document the particular hazard of angiotensin excess in the presence of a surfeit of sodium in accentuating hypertension may be uniquely applicable to the diabetic patients because of their greater tendency to retain sodium.[21] In these individuals the combined excess of angiotensin II and aldosterone coupled with persistent hypertension in diabetic patients could set the stage for direct vascular toxicity as well as for aggravation of any pre-existing glomerular hyperfiltration. The potential for a directly toxic effect of angiotensin II resulting from its demonstrated mitogenic activity has been discussed elsewhere in this symposium.[22]

The documentation of extensive benefits accruing from control of blood pressure by means of diuretic therapy in the MRFIT and Hypertension Detection and Follow-up Program studies as well as others,[23-25] plus the wide variation in cost of effective antihypertensive therapy make it imperative that apparent deleterious effects described above are well-documented before a recommendation against the use of diuretics is made. The possible interpretation that the group receiving diuretic therapy in the diabetes study represented individuals with pre-existing, albeit slight, evidence of renal impairment and thus responding differently to therapy is at variance with the MRFIT and Hypertension Detection and Follow-up Program data, in which benefit has been shown.[23,25,26]

The demonstration that excess fat or cholesterol intake is associated with aggravation of renal damage and progressive renal impairment in experimental animals is of potential therapeutic importance. Documentation of a similar association in human renal disease is scant. The possibility must be considered, of course, that the observation times in the present studies were too short to identify such an association. The more recent association reported between lipoprotein(a) and coronary artery disease raises the further question of whether this agent may also play a role in the accelerated nephrosclerosis of diabetes.[27] It was not possible to identify a statistical association between the level of cholesterol and evidence of progressive renal damage in either the present diabetes cohort or the MRFIT participants, even though the levels of serum cholesterol were higher in hypertensives, and particularly higher in the hypertensive group receiving diuretic therapy. Such an association between severity of proteinuria and elevated cholesterol has been documented in a cross-sectional study of the natives of Nauru.[28] The data presented in the present study do indicate that persistent hypertension and abnormalities (excess) of the renin angiotensin-aldosterone system are much more important determinants of the rate of progression of renal damage. The association between cho-lesterol and increased vascular morbidity and mortality in diabetes has been well established,[27-29] but its role in progressive renal disease in humans requires further study.

It seems unlikely that factors known to be responsible for accelerating renal damage in the presence of pre-existing and marked reduction in renal function[30-32] play any substantial role in this early blood pressure-related decline in renal function. The role of other humoral agents and autocoids may be much more important in the production of structural vascular changes that lead to altered hemodynamics and reduction in renal function. Both tissue culture studies and some in vivo experimental studies have produced evidence that growth factors, angiotensin II, endothelin somatostatin, eicosanoids, and numerous other agents may be responsible for the smooth muscle cell proliferation that is thought to underlie the structural change and vascular damage leading to the increased morbidity and mortality associated with this disease.[33-35] These promising studies may produce tools that will facilitate inquiry into the underlying mechanisms of hypertension-related renal damage and identify new therapeutic approaches, but at present information is lacking on their importance in and specific contributions to hypertension-related vascular and end-organ damage. Association of the type reported here between progressive decline of renal function and angiotensin II and aldosterone represents a first step in establishing such information.

Evidence obtained from the MRFIT and from a longitudinal study of both type I and type II diabetics thus indicates that hypertension and relative excesses of angiotensin and aldosterone are significant covariates of this increased rate of loss of renal function and may play a causal role. Assignment of causality to these significant covariates must await appropriately designed and randomized clinical trials. The magnitude of this problem both as an increasing public health issue and as a major element of the increasing cost attendant on providing adequate care of patients with renal failure make it imperative that such studies be given a high priority. Such important issues as racial differences in risk factors and severity of risk, goal blood pressure necessary for renal protection and whether this is different in diabetic and hypertensive patients, and the stage in the evolution of the disease at which intervention should be focused are all important issues that must be addressed early in any intervention effort.

ADDENDUM

Two additional studies have been published[36,37] that address the role of blood pressure control in patients with diabetic renal disease[36] and patients with a variety of chronic renal diseases.[37] In addition, a meta-regression analysis of the effect of antihypertensive therapy on the kidney in patients with diabetes has been published.[38]

ACKNOWLEDGMENT

The continuing assistance of J. Hermann and S. Manson is gratefully acknowledged.

REFERENCES

1. Eggers PW, Connerton R, McMullan M: The Medicare experience with end-stage renal disease: Trends in incidence, prevalence, and survival. Health Care Financ Rev 5:69-88, 1984

2. US Renal Data System, USRDS 1990 Annual Report. The National Institutes of Health. National Institute of Diabetes and Digestive and Kidney Disease, Bethesda, MD, August 1990

3. Bright R: Cases and observations, illustrative of renal disease accompanied with secretion of albuminous urine. Guy's Hosp Rep 1:338-400, 1836

4. Luke RG: Nephrosclerosis, in Schrier RW, Gottschalk CW (eds): Diseases of the Kidney. Boston, MA, Little, Brown, 1988, pp 1573-1595

5. Furburg C, Cutler J: Diuretic agents vs beta blockers: Comparison of effects on mortality of stroke, coronary events. Hypertension 13:I57-I67, 1989 (suppl)

6. National High Blood Pressure Education Program (NHBPEP) Working Group Report on Hypertension and Chronic Renal Failure. US Department of Health and Human Services, Public Health Service, National Institutes of Health, National Heart, Lung and Blood Institute, NIH Publication No. 90-3032, August 1990

7. Walker WG, Neaton JD, Cutler JA, Neuwirth R, Cohen JD for the MRFIT Research Group: Renal function change in hypertensive members of the Multiple Risk Factor Intervention Trial: Racial and treatment effects. JAMA 268:3085-3091, 1992

8. Rostand SG, Brown G, Kirk KA, Rutsky EA, Dustan HP: Renal insufficiency in treated essential hypertension. N Engl J Med 320:684-688, 1989

9. Report of the Committee on Chronic Kidney Disease. Gottschalk CW, Chairman. Washington, DC, Government Printing Office Document #933-491, 1967

10. Krolewski AS, Canessa M, Warram JH, Laffel LMB, Christlieb AR, Knowler WC, Rand LI: Predisposition to hypertension and susceptibility to renal disease in insulin-dependent diabetes mellitus. N Engl J Med 318:140-145, 1988

11. Cowie CC, Port FK, Wolfe RA, Savage PJ, Moll PP, Hawthorne VM: Disparities in incidence of diabetic end-stage renal disease according to race and type of diabetes. N Engl J Med 321:1074-1079, 1989

12. Gimenez L, Briefel G, Zachary J, Walker WG: Relative contribution of type I and type II diabetics to the chronic dialysis population. Kidney Int 35:226, 1989 (abstr)

13. Walker WG, Hermann J, Murphy R, Patz A: Elevated BP and angiotensin II are associated with accelerated loss of renal function in diabetic nephropathy. Trans Am Clin Climatol Assoc 97:94-104, 1985

14. Walker WG, Hermann J, Murphy RP, Russell RP: Prospective study of the impact of hypertension upon kidney function in diabetes mellitus. Nephron 55:21-26, 1990 (suppl 1)

15. Walker WG, Hermann J, Yin DP, Murphy RP, Patz A: Diuretics accelerate diabetic nephropathy in hypertensive insulin-dependent and non–insulin-dependent subjects. Trans Assoc Am Physicians 100:305-315, 1987

16. Neuringer JR, Brenner BM: Hemodynamic theory of progressive renal disease: A 10-year update in brief review. Am J Kidney Dis 22:98-104, 1993

17. Ditzel J, Schwartz M: Abnormally increased glomerular filtration rate in short-term insulin-treated diabetic subjects. Diabetes 16:264-267, 1967

18. Mogensen CE, Anderson MJF: Increased kidney size and glomerular filtration rate in early juvenile diabetes. Diabetes 22:706-712, 1973

19. Bender W, LaFrance N, Walker WG: The mechanism of acute deterioration of renal function in patients with renovascular hypertension following inhibition of angiotensin converting enzyme. Hypertension 6:I193-I197, 1984 (suppl 1)

20. DeClue JW, Guyton AC, Cowley AW, Coleman TG, Norman RA, McCaa RE: Subpressor angiotensin infusion, renal sodium handling, and salt-induced hypertension in the dog. Circ Res 43:503-512, 1978

21. Weidmann P, Ferrari P: Central role of sodium in hypertension in diabetic subjects. Diabetes Care 14:220-232, 1991

22. Smith LJ, Rosenberg ME, Hostetter TH: Effect of angiotensin II blockade on dietary protein-induced renal growth. Am J Kidney Dis 22:120-127, 1993

23. Multiple Risk Factor Intervention Trial Research Group: Multiple Risk Factor Intervention Trial: Risk factor changes and mortality results. JAMA 248:1465-1477, 1982

24. Cutler JA, Neaton JD, Hulley SB, Kuller L, Paul O, Stamler J for the MRFIT Research Group: Coronary heart disease and all-causes mortality in the Multiple Risk Factor Intervention Trial: Subgroup findings and comparisons with other trials. Prev Med 14:293-311, 1985

25. Hypertension Detection and Follow-up Program Cooperative Group: Five-year findings of the Hypertension Detection and Follow-up Program. II. Mortality by race-sex and age. JAMA 242:3572-3577, 1979

26. Walker WG, Ford CE, Cutler JA, Shulman NB for the HDFP Research Group: Change in renal function during treatment in the Hypertension Detection and Follow-up Program (HDFP). Am J Hypertens 5:58a, 1992

27. Guillausseau P-J, Peynet J, Chanson P, Legrand A, Altman JJ, Poupon J, NGuyen M, Rousselet F, Lubetzhi J: Lipoprotein(a) in diabetic patients with and without chronic renal failure. Diabetes Care 15:976-979, 1992

28. Prior IAM, Beaglehole R, Davidson F, Salmond CE: The relationships of diabetes, blood lipids, and uric acid levels in Polynesians. Adv Metab Disord 9:242-261, 1978

29. Medalie J, Papier CM, Goldbourt MA, Herman JB: Major factors in the development of diabetes mellitus in 10,000 men. Arch Intern Med 135:811-817, 1975

30. Gimenez L, Walker WG, Tew WP, Hermann JA: Prevention of phosphate-induced progression of uremic in rats by 3-phosphocitric acid. Kidney Int 22:36-41, 1982

31. Walser M, Mitch WE, Collier VU: Calcium and phosphorus in chronic renal failure during nutritional therapy, in Berlyne GM (ed): Contributions to Nephrology. Basel, Switzerland, Karger S, 1980, pp 92-102

32. Tew WP, Malis CD, Lehninger AL, Walker WG, Howard JE: Inhibition of PTH induced nephrocalcinosis by phosphocitrate, in Smith LH, Robertson WG, Finlayson B (eds): Urolithiasis: Clinical and Basic Research. New York, NY, Plenum, 1981

33. Fine LG, Hammerman MK, Abboud HE: Evolving role of growth factors to acute and chronic disease. J Am Soc Nephrol 2:1163-1170, 1992

34. Johnson RJ, Alpers CE, Yoshimura A, Lombardi D, Pritzl P, Floege J, Schwartz SM: Renal injury from angiotensin II-mediated hypertension. Hypertension 19:464-474, 1992

35. Jackson CL, Schwartz SM: Pharmacology of smooth muscle cell replication. Hypertension 20:713-736, 1992

36. Lewis EJ, Hunsicker LG, Bain RP, Rohde RD, and the Collaborative Study Group: The effect of angiotensin-converting enzyme inhibition on diabetic nephropathy. N Engl J Med 329:1456-1462, 1993

37. Klahr S, Levey AS, Beck GJ, Caggiula AW, Hunsicker L, Kusek JW, Striker G, and the Modification of Diet in Renal Disease Study Group: The effects of dietary protein restriction and blood-pressure control on the progression of chronic renal disease. N Engl J Med 330:877-884, 1994

38. Kasiske BL, Kalil RS, Ma JZ, Liao M, Keane WF: Effect of antihypertensive therapy on the kidney in patients with diabetes: A meta-regression analysis. Ann Intern Med 118:129-138, 1993

Fewer Nephrons at Birth: A Missing Link in the Etiology of Essential Hypertension?

Harald S. Mackenzie, MB, MRCP(UK), and Barry M. Brenner, MD

● In 1988, Brenner et al advanced the hypothesis that the nephron endowment at birth is inversely related to the risk of developing essential hypertension in later life (Am J Hypertens 1:335-347, 1988). This novel perspective on the origins of essential hypertension was taken from the viewpoint that the development and maintenance of hypertension must involve a renal factor favoring sodium retention, thereby preventing pressure-induced natriuresis from restoring blood pressure toward normal levels. Since nephron numbers in the normal population range from 300,000 to 1,100,000 or more, it was reasoned that a congenital deficit in nephron endowment itself could be the renal risk factor for hypertension: demographic groups in whom hypertension is unusually prevalent tend to have smaller kidneys, implying fewer nephrons, and some inbred hypertensive rat strains have, on average, fewer nephrons than their respective normotensive controls. We argue that recent independent observations in humans relating low birth weight to both increased risk of hypertension in later life and the formation of fewer nephrons at birth lend strong support to the nephron number hypothesis. Moreover, independent experimental studies in rodents suggest that maternal protein intake during gestation is directly related to the numbers of nephrons formed and that when protein intake is restricted, the offspring develop hypertension in maturity. The concept that nephron numbers may be programmed during gestation, as these observations imply, is discussed in relation to the potential advantages and disadvantages of such a mechanism for the next generation; parallels are drawn with the relationship of low birth weight to pancreatic beta cell development and maturity-onset diabetes. We suggest that the programming of fewer nephrons at birth may provide a fitting and overlooked explanation for the eventual development of hypertension in those of low birth weight, especially in cases in which type II diabetes coexists.

INDEX WORDS: Hypertension; etiology; epidemiology; intrauterine growth retardation; low birth weight; nephron number; thrifty genotype; diabetes; syndrome X.

WHILE the etiology of essential hypertension remains enigmatic, recent reports that low birth weight infants have a higher incidence of hypertension and cardiovascular disease in later life[1,2] have stimulated speculation into the mechanism underlying this relationship and its relevance to the origins of essential hypertension. Current discussions of the fetal origins of essential hypertension have addressed the roles of growth and growth factors in children and adults[3,4] and maternal nutrition during gestation[2] as etiologic factors. In addition, the kidney is usually acknowledged to contribute to the development and persistence of essential hypertension by preventing pressure natriuresis, which otherwise would be expected to restore blood pressure toward normotensive levels.[5] We suggest that, particularly in the case of essential hypertension associated with low birth weight, the nature of this renal defect is best accounted for by a deficiency of nephrons at birth, since it appears that fewer nephrons are formed when fetal nutrition is compromised, eg, in low birth weight infants.

This review extends the hypothesis originally set forth by Brenner et al in 1988[6] that an inverse relationship exists between total nephron number and the risk of developing arterial hypertension. We argue that deficiencies in total nephron complement at birth may represent an important and overlooked link between the kidney and essential hypertension; new data concerning programming of nephron number in utero are discussed which, in our view, strongly support the contention that nephron number at birth is a determinant of blood pressure in later life.

THE KIDNEY AND BLOOD PRESSURE

It has been evident for well over half a century that the kidney and hypertension are closely associated.[7-9] The notion that the kidney plays a role in blood pressure regulation also is well established. Ledingham and Cohen[10] demonstrated the importance of intravascular volume and cardiac output in determining blood pressure; Borst and Borst-de Geuss,[11] discussing hypertension from a similar perspective, reasoned that susceptibility to hypertension must involve renal sodium avidity. Guyton et al later argued the primacy of the kidney in the long-term determination of blood pressure by virtue of its regulation of intravascular fluid volume.[12] Their view of the kidney as the ultimate regulator of long-term arterial pressure, and therefore invariably implicated in the pathogenesis and maintenance of hypertension, has since gained widespread support from a growing body of experimental evidence and clinical observations. Cross-transplantation experiments between hypertensive and normotensive rat strains, for example, suggest that hypertension is determined by characteristics of the donor kidney rather than by the milieu of the recipient[13,14]; similar conclusions have been drawn from observations that the hypertension in human renal transplant recipients is related to the blood pressure of the donor or the presence of hypertensive risk factors in the donor prior to transplantation[15] rather than to the pre-existence of hypertension in the recipient.[16]

NEPHRON SUPPLY AND BLOOD PRESSURE

Based on these foundations the hypothesis was advanced that the total nephron supply is an independent factor that determines susceptibility of individuals or populations to develop hypertension under similar environmental conditions.[6] It was reasoned that deficiencies in the total nephron supply, by limiting total renal excretory capacity and thereby influencing the point at which steady-state conditions between arterial pressure and sodium excretion are achieved, could profoundly affect long-term blood pressure regulation. When renal mass is greatly reduced, as in the case of extensive experimental ablation of the kidney in rodents, blood pressure increases in the systemic arterial circulation and in the glomerular capillaries, thus increasing glomerular filtration rate and promoting fluid excretion.[17] However, sustained elevations in glomerular capillary hydraulic pressure are associated with the development of focal and segmental glomerular sclerosis leading to further loss of nephrons and a self-perpetuating vicious cycle of hypertension and progressive glomerular injury.[18,19] Proteinuria and glomerulosclerosis also have been observed in humans following surgical resection of more than two thirds of the total renal mass for neoplastic disease or trauma.[20] An increased incidence of hypertension has been reported from some, although not all, long-term follow-up studies of kidney donors,[21-24] and the incidence of hypertension may be found to increase further in these cohorts as the number of years from the time of their kidney donation increases.

The relevance of nephron supply to blood pressure is not altogether surprising in such gross examples of renal mass reduction or in the severe depletion of intact nephrons occurring in advanced chronic renal failure, in which global inadequacy of kidney function is evident. However, hypertension and glomerulosclerosis also have been observed in individuals in whom innate deficits in nephron number of lesser severity exist, arguing (1) that nephron deficits of lesser severity than 5/6 ablation cause hypertension and (2) that although renin production from ischemic renal parenchyma at the margins of the surgical scar or infarct may be a contributing factor, it is clearly not the sole mechanism of hypertension in experimental renal mass reduction. Individuals born with deficits of nephron number (ie, congenital oligomeganephronia) develop glomerulosclerosis and end-stage renal disease during adolescence.[25-27] Preliminary observations suggest that mice with heterozygous expression of a genetic defect, characterized by a congenital shortfall in nephron number of approximately 50%, also develop hypertension and glomerulosclerosis in maturity. Experimental manipulations in pregnant rats that result in offspring with fewer nephrons also appear to lead to the development of hypertension in maturity[28] (vide infra). Together these observations support the assertion that extrinsic injury to the renal parenchyma is not a prerequisite for development of hypertension; rather, the cycle of hypertension, renal injury, and hypertensive glomerulosclerosis may have its origins in an inadequate endowment of nephron numbers at birth.

VARIABILITY IN NEPHRON SUPPLY

The total number of nephrons in humans, which follows a gaussian distribution in the normal population, is defined at birth, after which no new nephrons are formed. The variation in nephron complement in the normal population would, at first sight, seem too subtle by comparison to the above-mentioned cases to contribute significantly to the development of hypertension. Recent advances in the methodology for determining glomerular (and therefore nephron) number have, however, revealed that the total nephron complement in the human kidney varies markedly among otherwise normal individuals, ranging from as low as 300,000 to 1,100,000 or more.[29-31] Moreover, it has been determined that the absolute number of nephrons in the human apparently averages closer to 600,000 rather than the "million" usually cited in textbooks.[31] Together these data indicate that the spread of nephron number is broader than often appreciated; indeed, few examples of other anthropometric characteristics reveal such extensive variation within the so-called normal population. It therefore has been suggested that those individuals at the lower end of the nephron number distribution may be prone to developing essential hypertension, whereas those at the upper end may be relatively protected from the development of this phenotypic characteristic.

Thus, deficiencies in total nephron supply could conceivably impinge at two stages in the natural history of untreated hypertension: first, in its initiation (eg, by restricting sodium excretion and favoring the development of hypertension on salt-replete diet) and second, by placing the individual at an advanced starting point along the final common pathway of nephron loss in chronic renal failure, a course invariably accompanied by arterial hypertension.

Although a moderate deficiency in nephrons alone might not be expected to result in hypertension, several lines of data suggest that those individuals with a relatively deficient nephron endowment at birth are predisposed to developing hypertension when subjected to dietary or other stresses. Several demographic groups in whom hypertension is unusually prevalent may have relatively fewer nephrons or a smaller kidney to body size ratio, the latter also implying fewer nephrons per kidney,[31] than the general population. For example, the incidence of hypertension is high in Japan,[32,33] and autopsy studies demonstrate that on average the Japanese population has smaller kidneys in comparison to white populations.[34] Hypertension also occurs with greater frequency and severity in Americans of African descent.[35] In general, black subjects have smaller kidneys, attain higher blood pressures in response to sodium loading, and display a reduced capacity to excrete a sodium load.[36] It has been suggested that this feature may relate to the natural selection, over 100,000 or more generations, of traits favorable to existence in tropical or subtropical Africa.[37]

Interestingly, the spontaneously hypertensive rat and the Milan hypertensive rat, rodent models of hypertension produced by selective inbreeding, also are characterized by nephron counts 10% to 20% below those of their respective normotensive controls.[6] The PVG strain, on the other hand, which exhibits resistance to the development of experimental hypertension, has relatively greater numbers of nephrons.[6]

DETERMINANTS OF NEPHRON NUMBER

Genetic factors initially had been expected to account for much of the normal distribution of nephron numbers in the population. As both hypertension[38] and the tendency to retain sodium after acute salt loading[39,40] are heritable traits, genetically determined differences in nephron numbers have been proposed to account for both characteristics.[6] Recent evidence, however, suggests that the number of nephrons at birth also may be affected by conditions in utero. Low birth weight resulting from intrauterine growth retardation in humans has been shown to be associated with deficiencies in nephron number of up to 20%, even in pregnancies that went to term.[41,42] Experimentally, deficits in nephron number also can be induced in the offspring of rats by producing ischemia of the maternal uterine horn, by treating pregnant rats with aminoglycoside,[43] or by placing them on diets deficient in protein, provided that the protein content is approximately 8% or less, compared with the 20% protein content of standard laboratory rodent chow.[44] At the other end of the spectrum, the offspring of female mice either fed diets high in protein during pregnancy or uninephrectomized prior to mating have been reported to have kidneys with supernumerary nephrons providing greater renal reserve than controls.[45]

LOW BIRTH WEIGHT, NEPHRON NUMBERS, AND HYPERTENSION

The observation that low birth weight is associated with higher blood pressures in later life[46] and possibly in infancy[47] and childhood has added a new and provocative dimension to the nephron number hypothesis. Given the association between low birth weight and fewer nephrons discussed above, it is naturally tempting to speculate that the origins of hypertension in adults who were of low birth weight lie in a deficient endowment of nephrons secondary to intrauterine growth retardation.[48] Studies of salt sensitivity in these specific groups, or other data that could provide surrogate evidence of decreased renal excretory capacity, have not yet been reported. Nevertheless, we believe that the synthesis of several recent observations provides strong support for this hypothesis. Modest reductions in nephron number in rats, induced by gentamicin administration during gestation, have been shown to be associated with glomerulosclerosis in maturity[49]; confirmation of an additional association with hypertension awaits further studies. In addition to several reports of associations between low birth weight and hypertension in human populations (for a recent summary, see ref 48), a similar finding has been reported recently in the offspring of rats fed a low-protein diet during pregnancy.[28] Maternal dietary protein restriction of 6% was found to be associated with a mean systolic blood pressure of 159 mm Hg in offspring at 9 weeks compared with 137 mm Hg at 9 weeks in offspring of rats fed normal protein intake.

If nephron numbers are programmable in utero, as the above data suggest, with the potential for remote adverse consequences, such as hypertension and accelerated glomerulosclerosis, what are the advantages of such a mechanism of adaptation to environmental change, passed on as a legacy to the next generation?

THE THRIFTY GENOTYPE HYPOTHESIS

Some insights into the potential advantages of programming nephron number may be derived from considering the concepts underlying the ''thrifty genotype hypothesis'' for diabetes mellitus. Neel originally postulated that the diabetic trait was a legacy from millennia of human existence as hunter–gatherers.[50] The capacity to use energy with maximum economy would confer an advantage on those individuals having both a lower resting metabolic rate and a higher capacity to convert large amounts of ingested nutrients into adipose tissue when meat, usually scarce, was in brief abundance, ie, after a big game kill. The mechanism postulated to achieve this maximal utilization of energy was a ''quick insulin trigger'' on pancreatic β-cells, capable of providing sufficient insulin to move large amounts of absorbed glucose intracellularly. This would, in turn, stimulate fatty acid synthesis and other anabolic metabolic pathways, thereby minimizing loss of energy through glycosuria and maximizing energy storage for intervening periods of ''gathering'' while in pursuit of the next big game kill. The persistence of such heritable traits through a process of natural selection, while of benefit to humans in primitive or largely vegetarian agrarian habitat, would be out of place in affluent modern conditions in which food is in continual abundance and protein and energy intakes are sustained at much higher levels. The metabolic consequences of inheriting the thrifty genotype under such circumstances, Neel argued, would be overstimulation of the pancreatic islet cells, hyperinsulinemia, insulin resistance, renewed β-cell stimulation, and eventual ''exhaustion'' of islets, resulting in diabetes. In such terms he offered an explanation for the persistence of the diabetic trait as an enduring human characteristic, rather than being bred out through natural selection. Although revised to address non–insulin-dependent diabetes specifically,[51] the ''thrifty genotype hypothesis'' has been viewed with skepticism for numerous reasons, such as the controversial nature of data supporting the notion that obese individuals have lower metabolic rates than nonobese individuals.[52-54] Nevertheless, it provides a useful model for considering the high rates of diabetes in cultures undergoing rapid introduction to modern ''Western'' culture and environment. The notion of fewer β-cells hyperfunctioning to meet increased insulin demands when faced with overnutrition leading to β-cell dropout and eventual failure of insulin production also bears striking resemblance to the proposed cycle of nephron hyperfunction and obsolescence linking dietary factors with the progressive nature of renal disease.[55]

With regard to the thrifty genotype hypothesis as a conceptual paradigm for the persistence of hypertension, one must consider the potential for increased blood pressure to be a favorable trait. It has been suggested that a greater capacity to increase blood pressure provided an advantage in the ''flight and fight' response and therefore its persistence through natural selection.[56] Alternatively, Lever and Harrap have suggested that blood pressure and growth are inextricably linked[3] and that increased blood pressure may be required to sustain growth, given the close relationship between growth and blood pressure during the adolescent growth spurt.

THE THRIFTY PHENOTYPE AND HYPERTENSION

Similarities between nephron supply and blood pressure and β-cell endowment and diabetes may extend beyond the conceptual level. An association has been reported between low birth weight and increased risk of non–insulin-dependent diabetes,[57,58] giving rise to the ''thrifty phenotype hypothesis.''[59] Moreover, it appears that the number of pancreatic β-cells, as with the number of nephrons, may also be determined by maternal nutritional factors in utero.[59,60] These latter observations also imply that genetic differences alone need not explain differences in glucose tolerance among peoples greatly differing in their diet, levels of physical activity, and culture, and may, in part, provide an explanation for the frequency of the ''thrifty'' phenotype despite the complexities and unresolved issues concerning its putative genetic basis.[61,62]

If programmed undercapacities of nephrons and β cells are considered together, a coherent teleologic argument is suggested. In times of famine, reducing overcapacity both of nephrons and pancreatic islet cells would represent an integrated metabolic adjustment favoring ready availability of energy sources to meet metabolic needs on the one hand, and the achievement of electrolyte conservation at minimal renal energy expenditure, by reducing redundancy, on the other. Conversely, in times of plenty, appropriate programming would endow the kidney with greater reserves of nephrons to meet greater excretory demands and the pancreas with a greater capacity to secrete insulin, thereby shifting metabolism towards synthesis, growth, and energy storage. The major disadvantage of such a homeostatic strategy is the ease by which it could be rendered maladaptive by extreme changes in the availability of food occurring within a generation. Under such circumstances, in which the programming of, for example, fewer pancreatic β cells and fewer nephrons is rendered inappropriate, then it may be anticipated that glomerular hyperfiltration, hyperinsulinemia, hypertension, diabetes, hyperlipidemia, and glomerulosclerosis could all follow. According to this line of reasoning, if increased nutrition were to persist over one or two generations, a decrease in the incidence of diabetes would be predicted, as appropriately programmed individuals from later generations matured. Such a pattern has been reported for the incidence of diabetes in Micronesian Nauruans,[63] a finding consistent with the thrifty phenotype hypothesis.[59,64] Does appropriate programming of nephron numbers, by analogy, explain the decreasing incidence of hypertension[65] in Japan?

NEPHRON NUMBERS: THE MISSING RENAL FACTOR?

Barker et al suggested that low birth weight may be so closely associated with non–insulin-dependent diabetes that the so-called syndrome X should be renamed ''small baby syndrome'' from their observation that an inverse relationship exists between birth weight and the incidence of syndrome X.[2] We propose that programmed deficits in nephron numbers could represent the renal factor promoting hypertension in the syndrome they describe. Lever and Harrap[3] suggested that hypertension may represent an overall disorder of growth itself with origins in childhood, due to overexpression of a hypothetical master gene possibly stimulated during neonatal catch-up growth in response to low birth weight. The resulting stimulus leads to increased vascular smooth muscle cell growth and increased peripheral vascular resistance. Whereas these investigators suggest that the renal factor in hypertension may be increased renal vascular resistance, we propose that a deficit in nephron numbers provides a compelling alternative or additional explanation. Weder and Schork[4] modified and extended Lever and Harrap's theories, postulating that blood pressure increases in parallel with growth specifically to match renal function to the increased demands of greater body mass. By addressing the normal discrepancies in organ growth rates (allometry) that occur, they suggest that when kidney growth lags behind somatic growth, sodium retention is favored and blood pressure increases, thereby predisposing to hypertension in later life.[4] This may be of particular relevance to low birth weight, since in neonates catch-up in blood pressure seems to outstrip catch-up in growth.[47] Weder and Schork did not specify the nature of the deficit associated with renal growth lag[4]: we submit that a reduced nephron complement, either genetically determined or acquired in utero, provides a fitting explanation.

CONCLUSIONS AND FUTURE DIRECTIONS

Particularly in the case of hypertension associated with low birth weight, we believe that a strong argument may be made for programmed reductions in nephron supply accounting for the renal defect that permits the development and maintenance of elevated blood pressure. Further experimental studies are required to confirm this view. The extent to which the normal distribution of nephron numbers follows the normal distribution of blood pressure in the general population awaits autopsy studies in which total nephron number is determined by up-to-date counting methods in subjects for whom a detailed record of blood pressure measurements are available. While full discussions of the implied coupling of pancreatic β cell and renal function suggested by the apparent similarities between programming of nephron and β-cell number, and of hyperinsulinemia,[3,66] insulin resistance,[67] and their respective roles in hypertension,[3] lies beyond the scope of this review, these issues are intriguing and also merit further study.

REFERENCES

1. Barker DJP, Bull AR, Osmond C, Simmonds SJ: Fetal and placental size and risk of hypertension in later life. BMJ 301:259-262, 1990
2. Barker DJ, Hales CN, Fall CH, Osmond C, Phipps K, Clark PM: Type 2 (non–insulin-dependent) diabetes mellitus, hypertension and hyperlipidaemia (syndrome X): Relation to reduced fetal growth. Diabetologia 36:62-67, 1993
3. Lever AF, Harrap SB: Essential hypertension: A disorder of growth with origins in childhood? J Hypertens 10:101-120, 1992
4. Weder AB, Schork NJ: Adaptation, allometry, and hypertension. Hypertension 24:145-156, 1994
5. Luke RG: Essential hypertension: A renal disease? Hypertension 21:380-390, 1993
6. Brenner BM, Garcia DL, Anderson S: Glomeruli and blood pressure. Less of one, more the other? Am J Hypertens 1:335-347, 1988
7. Bright R: Tabular view of morbid appearances in 100 cases connected with albuminous urine. Guy's Hosp Rep 1:380-410, 1836
8. Goldblatt H, Lynch J, Hanzal RF, Summerville W: Studies on experimental hypertension: I. The production of persistent elevation of systolic blood pressure by means of renal ischemia. J Exp Med 59:347-379, 1934
9. Wilson C, Byrom FB: Renal changes in malignant hypertension. Lancet 1:136-139, 1939
10. Ledingham JM, Cohen RD: The role of the heart in the pathogenesis of renal hypertension. Lancet 2:979-981, 1963
11. Borst JGG, Borst-de Geus A: Hypertension explained by Starling's theory of circulatory hemodynamics. Lancet 1:677-682, 1963
12. Guyton AC, Coleman TG, Cowley AVJ, Scheel KW, Manning RDJ, Norman RAJ: Arterial pressure regulation. Overriding dominance of the kidneys in long-term regulation and in hypertension. Am J Med 52:584-594, 1972
13. Bianchi G, Fox U, Di FG, Giovanetti AM, Pagetti D: Blood pressure changes produced by kidney cross-transplantation between spontaneously hypertensive rats and normotensive rats. Clin Sci Mol Med 47:435-448, 1974
14. Dahl LK, Heine M, Thompson K: Genetic influence of the kidneys on blood pressure. Evidence from chronic renal homografts in rats with opposite predispositions to hypertension. Circ Res 40:94-101, 1974
15. Guidi E, Bianchi G, Rivolta E: Hypertension in man with a kidney transplant: Role of familial versus other factors. Nephron 41:14-21, 1985
16. Curtis JJ, Luke RG, Dustan HP, Kashgarian M, Whelchel JD, Jones P, Diethelm AG: Remission of essential hypertension after renal transplantation. N Engl J Med 309:1009-1015, 1983
17. Brenner BM: Nephron adaptation to renal injury or ablation. Am J Physiol 249:F374-389, 1985
18. Hostetter TH, Olson JL, Rennke HG, Venkatachalam MA, Brenner BM: Hyperfiltration in remnant nephrons: A potentially adverse response to renal ablation. Am J Physiol 241:F85-F93, 1981
19. Rennke HG, Klein PS: Pathogenesis and significance of nonprimary focal and segmental glomerulosclerosis. Am J Kidney Dis 13:443-456, 1989
20. Novick AC, Gephardt G, Guz B, Steinmuller D, Tubbs RR: Long-term follow-up after partial removal of a solitary kidney. N Engl J Med 325:1058-1062, 1991
21. Watnick TJ, Jenkins RR, Rackoff P, Baumgarten A, Bia MJ: Microalbuminuria and hypertension in long-term renal donors. Transplant 45:59-65, 1988
22. Torres VE, Offord KP, Anderson CF, Velosa JA, Frohnhert PP, Donadio JV Jr, Wilson DM: Blood pressure determinants in living-related renal allograft donors and their recipients. Kidney Int 1987;31:1383-1390.
23. Rugiu C, Oldrizzi L, Lupo A, Valvo E, Loschiavo C, Tessitore N, Gammaro L, Ortaldo V, Fabris A, Panzetta G, Maschio G: Clinical features of patients with solitary kidneys. Nephron 43:10-15, 1986
24. Hakim RM, Goldszer RC, Brenner BM: Hypertension and proteinuria: Long-term sequelae of uninephrectomy in humans. Kidney Int 25:930-936, 1984

25. Fetterman GH, Habib R: Congenital bilateral oligonephronic renal hypoplasia with hypertrophy of nephrons (oligomeganephronie). Am J Clin Pathol 52:199-120, 1969

26. Carter JE, Lirenman DS: Bilateral renal hypoplasia with oligomeganephronia. Oligomeganephronic renal hypoplasia. Am J Dis Child 120:537-542, 1970

27. McGraw M, Poucell S, Sweet J, Baumal R: The significance of focal segmental glomerulosclerosis in oligomeganephronia. Int J Pediatr Nephrol 5:67-72, 1984

28. Langley SC, Jackson AA: Increased systolic blood pressure in adult rats induced by fetal exposure to maternal low protein diets. Clin Sci 86:217-222, 1994

29. Moore RA: The total number of glomeruli in the normal human kidney. Anat Rec 48:153-168, 1931

30. Dunnill MS, Halley W: Some observations on the quantitative anatomy of the kidney. J Pathol 110:113-121, 1973

31. Nyengaard JR, Bendtsen TF: Glomerular number and size in relation to age, kidney weight, and body surface in normal man. Anat Rec 232:194-201, 1992

32. Takahashi E, Sasaki N, Takeda J, Ito H: The geographic distribution of cerebral hemorrhage and hypertension in Japan. Hum Biol 29:139-166, 1957

33. Kikkawa R, Araki S, Haneda M, Kajiwara N, Hidaka H, Shigeta Y: Hypertension and the development of complications in patients with non–insulin dependent diabetes mellitus in Japan. J Am Soc Nephrol 3:S120-125, 1992

34. Tauchi H, Tsuboi K, Okutomi J: Age changes in the human kidney of different races. Gerontologia 17:87-97, 1971

35. Final Report of the Subcommittee on Definition and Prevalence of the 1984 Joint National Committee: Hypertension prevalence and the state of awareness, treatment and control in the United States. Hypertension 7:457-468, 1985

36. Luft FC, Rankin LI, Bloch R: Cardiovascular and humoral responses to extremes of sodium intake in normal black and white men. Circulation 60:697-706, 1979

37. Helmer OM: Hormonal and biochemical factors controlling blood pressure, in (eds): Les Concepts de Claude Barnard sur le Milieu Interieur. Paris, France, Librairies de l'Academie de Medecine, 1967, pp 115-128

38. Deutscher S, Epstein FH, Kjelsberg MO: Familial aggregation of factors associated with coronary heart disease. Circulation 33:911-924, 1966

39. Grim CE, Luft FC, Miller JZ, Brown PL, Gannon MA, Weinberger MH: Effects of sodium loading and depletion in normotensive first-degree relatives of essential hypertensives. J Lab Clin Med 94:764-771, 1979

40. Falkener B, Onesti G, Hayes P: The role of sodium in essential hypertension in genetically in genetically hypertensive adolescents, in Onesti G, Kim KE (eds): Hypertension in the Young and the Old. New York, NY, Grune & Stratton, 1981, pp 29-35

41. Hinchliffe SA, Howard CV, Lynch MR, Sargent PH, Judd BA, van VD: Renal developmental arrest in sudden infant death syndrome. Pediatr Pathol 13:333-343, 1993

42. Hinchliffe SA, Lynch MR, Sargent PH, Howard CV, Van VD: The effect of intrauterine growth retardation on the development of renal nephrons. Br J Obstet Gynecol 99:296-301, 1992

43. Gilbert T, Lelièvre-Pégorier M, Merlet-Bénichou C: Immediate and long-term renal effects of fetal exposure to gentamicin. Pediatr Nephrol 4:445-450, 1990

44. Merlet-Bénichou C, Gilbert T, Muffat-Joly M, Lelièvre-Pégorier M, Leroy B: Intrauterine growth retardation leads to a permanent nephron deficit in the rat. Pediatr Nephrol 8:175-180, 1994

45. Aberbukh Z, Weissgarten J, Berman S, Cohn M, Chaim S, Horne T, Golik A, Cohen N, Modai D: Effect of dietary manipulations on glomerular filtration rate of mice offspring of nephrectomized mothers. Am J Nephrol 13:190-193, 1993

46. Barker DJP, Osmond C, Golding J, Kuh D, Wadsworth MEJ: Growth in utero, blood pressure in childhood and adult life, and mortality from cardiovascular disease. BMJ 298:564-567, 1989

47. Levine RS, Hennekens CH, Jesse MJ: Blood pressure in prospective population based cohort of newborn and infant twins. BMJ 308:298-302, 1994

48. Brenner BM, Chertow GM: Congenital oligonephropathy and the etiology of adult hypertension and progressive renal injury. Am J Kidney Dis 23:171-175, 1994

49. Gilbert T, Lelievre PM, Merlet BC: Long-term effects of mild oligonephronia induced in utero by gentamicin in the rat. Pediatr Res 30:450-456, 1991

50. Neel JV: Diabetes mellitus: A ''thrifty'' genotype rendered detrimental by ''progress.'' Am J Hum Genet 14:353-362, 1962

51. Neel JV: The thrifty genotype revisited, in Köbberling JR, Tattersall R (eds): The Genetics of Diabetes Mellitus. London, UK, Academic Press, 1982, pp 283-293

52. Garrow JS, Webster J: Are pre-obese people energy thrifty? Lancet 1:670-671, 1985

53. Garrow J: The thrifty genotype and non–insulin dependent diabetes. BMJ 306:933-934, 1993

54. Ravussin E: Energy metabolism in obesity. Studies in the Pima Indians. Diabetes Care 16:232-238, 1993

55. Brenner BM, Meyer TW, Hostetter TH: Dietary protein intake and the progressive nature of kidney disease: The role of hemodynamically mediated glomerular injury in the pathogenesis of progressive glomerular sclerosis in aging, renal ablation, and intrinsic renal disease. N Engl J Med 307:652-659, 1982

56. Julius S, Jamerson K: Sympathetics, insulin resistance and coronary risk in hypertension—The chicken-and-egg question. J Hypertens 12:495-502, 1994

57. Hales CN, Barker DJ, Clark PM, Cox LJ, Fall C, Osmond C, Winter PD: Fetal and infant growth and impaired glucose tolerance at age 64. BMJ 303:1019-1022, 1991

58. McCance DR, Pettitt DJ, Hanson RL, Jacobsson LT, Knowler WC, Bennett PH: Birth weight and non–insulin dependent diabetes: Thrifty genotype, thrifty phenotype, or surviving small baby genotype? BMJ 308:942-945, 1994

59. Hales CN, Barker DJ: Type 2 (non–insulin-dependent) diabetes mellitus: The thrifty phenotype hypothesis. Diabetologia 35:595-601, 1992

60. Snoeck A, Remacle C, Reusens B, Hoet JJ: Effect of a low protein diet during pregnancy on the fetal rat endocrine pancreas. Biol Neonate 57:107-118, 1990

61. Dowse G, Zimmet P: The thrifty genotype in non–insulin dependent diabetes. BMJ 306:532-533, 1993

62. Turner RC, Levy JC, Clark A: Complex genetics of type 2 diabetes: Thrifty genes and previously neutral polymorphisms. Q J Med 86:413-417, 1993

63. Dowse GK, Zimmet PZ, Finch CF, Collins VR: Decline in incidence of epidemic glucose intolerance in Nauruans: Implications for the "thrifty genotype." Am J Epidemiol 133:1093-1104, 1991

64. Cruikshank K: The thrifty genotype and non–insulin dependent diabetes. BMJ 306:934, 1994 (letter)

65. Ueshima H, Tatara K, Asakura S, Okamoto M: Declining trends in blood pressure level and the prevalence of hypertension, and changes in related factors in Japan, 1956-1980. J Chronic Dis 40:137-147, 1987

66. Collins VR, Dowse GK, Finch CF, Zimmet PZ: An inconsistent relationship between insulin and blood pressure in three Pacific island populations. J Clin Epidemiol 43:1369-1378, 1990

67. Zimmet PZ: Hyperinsulinemia—How innocent a bystander? Diabetes Care 3:56-70, 1993

Assessing the Effectiveness of Therapy to Prevent the Progression of Renal Disease

Andrew S. Levey, MD

● Most studies of progressive renal disease assess the effectiveness of therapy from sequential measurements of renal excretory function, such as glomerular filtration rate, creatinine clearance, and serum creatinine concentration. This review summarizes the strengths and limitations of these measurements and proposes guidelines for selecting the outcome measure in clinical trials. In addition, this review examines certain issues related to the design and interpretation of studies on the progression of renal disease. Although this work primarily addresses issues relevant to clinical trials, the principles involved are relevant to the assessment of renal function in clinical settings as well.

INDEX WORDS: Renal function; clinical trials; progression of renal disease.

THE SUCCESS of a variety of therapies to slow the progression of experimentally induced renal disease in animals has stimulated a large number of clinical trials in humans. In this review, I will discuss the general topic of assessing the effectiveness of therapy in clinical trials. This topic is important because one cannot even begin planning for a clinical trial without knowledge of the characteristics of the measure used to assess the effect of therapy, and because some clinical trials may have come to erroneous conclusions as a result of the outcome measure that was selected. The goals of this discussion are (1) to review the basics of the design of clinical trials, as related to assessing therapies to slow the progression of renal disease and (2) to review the strengths and limitations of possible outcome measures to assess the effectiveness of therapy.

BASICS OF CLINICAL TRIALS

Relation of Variability and Hypothesized Effect of Therapy to Sample Size

As in all scientific inquiry, the first step in planning a clinical trial is to state the hypothesis. This statement must include not only the therapeutic intervention to be studied, but also the measure of outcome by which the effect of therapy is to be assessed. In estimating the number of subjects to include in the trial, knowledge of the characteristics of the outcome measure is essential.[1] In particular, one must be able to estimate the outcome in the control group, the variability in outcome in the control group, and the variability in outcome in the experimental group (usually assumed to be equal to variability in control group). In addition, one must hypothesize the magnitude of the change in outcome in the experimental group. In the example of clinical trials to determine the effect of therapy on the progression of renal disease, one must estimate the mean rates of progression in the control group and the experimental group and the variability in rates of progression among patients in both groups. As shown in Table 1, these factors determine sample size, and therefore cost.[2] If the variability among patients is small and if the hypothesized difference is large, the effect of therapy can be detected with a small number of patients. However, if the variability is large, or if the hypothesized difference is small, a large number of patients is required. Consequently, one cannot even begin to perform a clinical trial without first having estimated these factors. This demonstrates the need for preliminary data, and in some cases a pilot study, before embarking on a controlled trial.

Sensitivity and Specificity of the Outcome Measure

In principle, the study outcome should be both sensitive to study interventions and specific for them. In practice, however, the study outcomes that are available to assess the progression of renal disease are neither sensitive nor specific. Although renal pathology is generally accepted as providing the most sensitive and specific information for the diagnosis of renal disease, not enough is known about the rate and variability of the evolution of structural changes during the progression of most renal diseases in humans. In addition, the risk of repeated renal biopsy to obtain serial pathologic information is prohibitive in most cases. Thus few clinical trials use changes in renal structure as an outcome measure. We know more about the evolution of changes in renal function. However, changes in function generally do not occur until changes in structure are large, and many factors, other than progression of underlying disease, can affect renal function. Thus, functional changes are less sensitive and less specific indicators of progression. Nonetheless, if these other factors affect renal function in both the control and the experimental group to the same extent, their effects may not obscure the effect of the therapy. If they affect the two groups differentially, however, then they cause bias towards finding that one of the two groups is affected more, irrespective of the effect of therapy. Some examples of bias and ways to overcome bias are shown in Table 2.

Errors in Interpretation of Clinical Trials

Two types of errors may occur in the interpretation of clinical trials. A type 1 (alpha) error is defined as finding an effect where none exists. Explanations for type 1 errors include bias in favor of a better outcome in the experimental group and chance (luck). The *P* value for the comparison of the outcome measure between the control and experimental group reflects the probability of such an error. Traditionally, a *P* value less than 0.05, indicating a probability of a type 1 error of less than 5 in 100, is taken as evidence of a ''significant'' effect of therapy. Nonetheless, in all clinical trials, whether the effect of therapy is significant or not, there is the possibility of a type 1 error. This justifies undertaking secondary analyses, and sometimes additional clinical trials, to confirm positive results.

A type 2 (beta) error is defined as overlooking an effect of the intervention. Explanations for type 2 errors include bias in favor of a better outcome in the control group, inadequate sample size, too few bad outcomes in the control group, or excess variability. The probability of a type 2 error is reflected in the ''power'' of the clinical trial, with power = 1 − beta. Traditionally, power $\geq$0.80 is considered adequate. For clinical trialsin which preliminary data suggest a negative result, however, more rigorous study conditions are required, and power $\geq$0.90 is preferable. Recently, some investigators have used meta-analysis and cumulative meta-analysis to combine results from different clinical trials to increase sample size and power.[3] If properly conducted, these analyses can allow the benefits of therapeutic interventions to be discovered earlier. Meta-analysis can be misleading, however, because of ''publication bias,'' that is, the greater enthusiasm for investigators to report positive outcomes and for editors to accept reports of positive studies for publication.

Table 1. Effect of Variability and Hypothesized Difference in Mean Rates of Progression in Two Groups on Sample Size Requirement to Detect the Hypothesized Difference

	Hypothesized Difference in Mean Rates of Progression Between Two Groups		
	10%	20%	50%
CV (%)	Sample Size* Needed to Detect a Significant Difference Between Two Groups*		
15	80	20	<10
25	200	40	10
50	600	300	30

* Sample size is the total number of patients, divided into two equal groups, that must be included in a clinical trial to detect an hypothesized difference in the mean rates of progression between the groups. CV is the coefficient of variation in rate of progression among patients included in the trial (assumed to be equal in both groups). Calculations are performed for an alpha error of 0.05 (two-sided) and a beta error of 0.20 (one-sided).

Used with permission from *Kidney International,* volume 38, page 170, 1990.[2]

Table 2. Examples of Bias and Ways to Overcome Bias in Clinical Trials

Potential Bias	Way to Overcome Bias
Bias in comparability of the control and experimental group.	Random assignment to control and experimental therapy.
Bias in performance of measurements.	Same protocol and schedule of measurements in each group.
Bias in patient and physician interpretation of events during study.	Blinding of treatment and outcome measurements, if possible.
Bias in interactions between therapy and study outcome.	Knowledge of effects of therapy on outcome measurement.

OUTCOME MEASUREMENTS TO ASSESS THE EFFECT OF THERAPY IN CLINICAL TRIALS

An exhaustive review of assessment of renal function and structure is beyond the scope of this article and can be found elsewhere.[4] In the following discussions selected information related to the assessment of renal excretory function that is relevant to clinical trials will be briefly reviewed.

Glomerular Filtration Rate

The traditional method for measuring glomerular filtration rate (GFR), the renal clearance of inulin during a continuous infusion of inulin, has largely been supplanted by alternative methods using a bolus infusion and alternative filtration markers chelated to radioisotopes. The accuracy and precision of estimates of GFR obtained from these alternative measurements, compared with the traditional method of inulin clearance, are acceptable, and radiation exposure from a single examination is minimal.[5] Although many radioisotope-labeled filtration markers have been studied, only ^{125}I-iothalamate, ^{99m}Tc-DTPA, and ^{51}Cr-EDTA have been used extensively. The physical half-life of ^{125}I-iothalamate is long (60 days), making it ideal for use in a multicenter clinical trial with a central laboratory. The principal drawback is its high cost and short shelf-life (45 days). On the other hand, ^{99m}Tc-DTPA is inexpensive, but its short half-life (6 hours) requires on-site preparation, quality control, and counting, which are undesirable for a multicenter trial. Although widely used in Europe, ^{51}Cr-EDTA is not available in the United States.

The use of ^{125}I-iothalamate in multicenter clinical trials has been evaluated in 2,250 patients enrolled in the Modification of Diet in Renal Disease (MDRD) Study and the Diabetes Control and Complications Trial. The median intratest coefficient of variation (CV; defined as the standard deviation divided by the mean of the GFRs of the four clearance periods during the test) was 9.4% and 11.7%, respectively, in these two trials, indicating acceptable technical performance.[6] Nonetheless, technical limitations remain. The clearance procedure requires patient preparation. The time of day, relation to meals and medications, and posture during the test must be standardized. A negative onsite pregnancy test in women with child-bearing potential is also required. A technician must be available for several hours to obtain serum and urine specimens. Radiation exposure, although low, may be of concern to some patients.

Table 3. Factors Potentially Affecting Glomerular Filtration Rate in Clinical Trials of Progressive Renal Disease

Progression or remission of renal disease
Diurnal variation
Relationship to meals
Habitual protein intake
Blood glucose control (in diabetic patients)
Level of arterial blood pressure
Class of antihypertensive agents
Marked surfeit or deficit of extracellular fluid volume
Pregnancy
Reduction in renal mass

The major limitations to using changes in GFR as an outcome measurement in clinical trials, however, relate to factors other than technical limitations in performing the measurements. First, a decline in GFR may not be a sensitive test of progressive renal injury. The earliest stages of glomerular disease appear to be associated with alterations in structure and permeability to macromolecules. In diabetic nephropathy, increased albumin excretion signals the presence of structural damage before a decline in GFR.[7] Other investigators have also demonstrated progression of renal injury in systemic lupus erythematosus, assessed from structural changes, that was not reflected by changes in GFR.[8] Second, a decline in GFR may not be a specific test of progression of renal disease. Table 3 lists factors in addition to progressive renal injury that may influence GFR. Particularly important in clinical trials are the effect of the level of arterial blood pressure, class of antihypertensive agents, blood glucose control in diabetes, and habitual protein intake.[9-11] Third, as discussed in more detail below, there are general limitations in using the rate of change of any outcome measurement.

Creatinine Clearance

Advantages to using endogenous creatinine as a filtration marker include its simplicity and widespread acceptance over 50 years. The major limitation, however, is the tubular secretion of creatinine, which is highly variable among individuals and over time and which may lead to inaccurate prediction of GFR from creatinine clearance (C_{cr}). In one representative study using simultaneous measurements of the clearance of creatinine and ^{125}I-iothalamate during a 4-hour renal clearance procedure among subjects with a wide range of renal function, the correlation between C_{cr} and GFR was excellent ($r = 0.90$).[12] The correlation was lower ($r = 0.70$), however, using the more traditional method of determining C_{cr} from a 24-hour urine collection and a single measurement of serum creatinine concentration (P_{cr}). Moreover, the strength of these correlations derived, in part, from the wide range of renal function in the patients included in the study. In study populations with a more narrow range of renal function, one would expect weaker correlations. This is particularly important in clinical trials in which it is desirable that patients have uniform characteristics at entry, including a narrow range of GFR.

Variability in tubular secretion in creatinine is especially large in patients with GFR in the range of 40 to 80 mL/min/1.73 m^2.[13] Hence, the relationship between C_{cr} and GFR is least predictable when the impairment in renal function is mild to moderate. In one representative study, the sensitivity of a reduction in C_{cr} in detecting a reduction in GFR was only 75%.[13] Similarly, creatinine secretion is too variable over time within individuals to permit accurate prediction of changes in GFR from a single measurement of GFR and sequential measurements of C_{cr}.[14] Consequently, over relatively short intervals of follow-up, the correlation of the rates of change in GFR and C_{cr} is weak.[15,16] In the feasibility phase of the MDRD Study, the mean correlations between the rate of change in C_{cr}, determined from 24-hour creatinine clearances, and GFR, determined from ^{125}I-iothalamate clearance, over approximately 1 year were only 0.56 and 0.50, respectively, in subjects with an initial GFR of 25 to 56 mL/min/1.73 m^2 (Study A) and 7.5 to 24 mL/min/1.73 m^2 (Study B).[15]

Other limitations of using C_{cr} as an outcome measurement include the well-known difficulty of assuring completeness of 24-hour urine collections, method-dependent differences among serum creatinine assays, imprecision in all assays at low values for serum creatinine, and the effect of meat meals on serum creatinine concentration.[11,17] Overall, despite the limitations discussed above, creatinine clearance could be a useful outcome measurement in a clinical trial if the following conditions apply: the range of renal function among study participants is wide; the decline in renal function during the study is large; the therapy being studied does not affect the tubular secretion of creatinine; the clearance is measured during a 4-hour renal clearance procedure, under standard conditions, as is recommended for GFR measurements; and serum and urine creatinine are measured in a central laboratory.

Serum Creatinine and Reciprocal Serum Creatinine

In clinical practice, the P_{cr} is traditionally interpreted as an index of GFR. However, as described in detail elsewhere,[2,17] GFR is only one of many factors that affect P_{cr}. First, a wide range of technical factors affect the measurement of P_{cr}. Most important is the effect of different analytic methods on P_{cr}. As a result, the reference range for P_{cr} in laboratories differs according to the analytic method and, in my experience, values for P_{cr} in a single patient may differ by 0.5 mg/dL in different laboratories. Second, physiologic and metabolic factors that affect P_{cr} include the tubular secretion of creatinine (as discussed above), the effect of muscle mass and protein intake on creatinine generation, and the effect of impaired renal function on extrarenal metabolism of creatinine. As a result, an elevated P_{cr} is not a sensitive indicator of a decline in GFR[13] and the rates of decline in reciprocal serum creatinine ($1/P_{cr}$) and GFR may be only weakly correlated.[18,19] Thus, stability of serum creatinine over relatively short intervals should not be taken as a sign that renal disease has not progressed. Nonetheless, an elevation in P_{cr} is a specific test for decreased GFR[13] and, in principle, a substantial further increase in P_{cr} from an elevated initial value is likely to be highly specific for a further decline in GFR. Based on this rationale, many clinical trials have used an increase in serum creatinine as an outcome measurement. This strategy is sound only if the increase in P_{cr} is large; the therapy under study does not affect creatinine secretion, generation, extrarenal metabolism, or analytical measurement; and serum creatinine is measured in a central laboratory.

Table 4. Clinical Conditions That Cause Errors in the Estimation of Glomerular Filtration Rate From Measurement of Serum Creatinine

Condition	Effect On C_{cr}	Effect On P_{cr}	Comment
Plasma ketosis	None	Increase	Ketones react in the picric acid assay for creatinine.
Therapy with certain cephalosporins or fluctyosine	None	Increase	These compounds react in the picric acid and iminohydrolase assays for creatinine, respectively.
Therapy with cimetidine or trimethoprim	Decrease	Increase	These drugs inhibit tubular secretion of creatinine.
Ingesting cooked meat	Increase	Increase	Produce a transient increase in GFR and creatinine generation.
Restriction of dietary protein	Decrease	Decrease	Produce a sustained decrease in GFR and creatinine generation.
Vigorous prolonged exercise	None	Increase	May increase muscle creatinine generation.
Muscle wasting	None	Decrease	Decrease in muscle creatinine generation.
Muscle growth	None	Increase	Increase in muscle creatinine generation.

Abbreviations: C_{cr}, creatinine clearance; P_{cr}, serum creatinine.

The limitations in assessing GFR from the P_{cr} are important in clinical practice, as well as in clinical trials. Table 4 summarizes clinical conditions that may cause errors in the estimation of GFR from serum creatinine.

LIMITATIONS IN USING THE RATE OF PROGRESSION AS A MEASUREMENT OF OUTCOME

Irrespective of the parameter of renal structure or function that is measured in a clinical trial, there are limitations in assessing the rate of change as the outcome measurement. These include the assumption of a constant rate of progression, the large variability among patients in rates of progression, the imprecision in estimating the rate, and the interpretation of changes in the rate.

Assumption of a Constant Rate of Progression

A large number of studies have reported the patterns and rates of decline in renal function in patients with progressive renal disease. In general, the rate of decline in renal function in individual patients appeared to be relatively constant over 2 to 4 years, with the mean rates of decline in the range of 0.3 to 1.0 mL/min/mo for GFR and C_{cr} and 0.003 to 0.01 dL/mg/mo for $1/P_{cr}$.[20,21] At these rates of progression, it would take 5 to 15 years for GFR or C_{cr} to decline from 75 mL/min/1.73 m^2 to approximately 15 mL/min/1.73 m^2 or for serum creatinine to increase from 1.2 mg/dL to approximately 4.5 mg/dL. Thus, the pace of progression is generally slow, and whether the rate of decline in renal function is truly constant over the long course of renal disease is uncertain. Hence, it is not certain that differences among individuals in the rate of decline in GFR observed during the course of a clinical trial will be reflected in differences in the interval until the onset of renal failure. Validation of the rate of decline in GFR as a measurement of outcome requires long-term studies that demonstrate this relationship.

Variability in Rates of Progression

In the above-mentioned studies, variability in rates of progression was typically large, with the interpatient CV ranging from 50% to greater than 100%. In addition, the patients in these studies were selected because they had already demonstrated progressive renal insufficiency. The true variability of rates of progression is unknown, but it is likely to be greater among the overall population of patients with renal disease. In clinical trials, it may not be possible to include an extended period of observation prior to enrollment to exclude patients with more slowly progressing or nonprogressing renal disease. Rather, patients are generally selected because they demonstrate impaired renal function, and it is assumed that renal function will continue to worsen during the trial. Thus, the rates of progression in clinical trials may be even more variable and slower on average.

The relationship of rate and variability in rates of progression to the level of renal function has not been studied extensively. In the feasibility phase of the MDRD Study, the mean rate of decline in GFR was slower and the variability among patients in rates of decline was significantly greater in patients with higher baseline renal function. The mean and standard deviation were −0.31 mL/min/1.73 m^2/mo and 0.62 mL/min/1.73 m^2/mo, respectively (CV = 200%), among patients with higher initial GFR (Study A), and −0.36 mL/min/1.73 m^2/mo and 0.39 mL/min/1.73 m^2/mo, respectively (CV = 108%), among patients with lower initial GFR (Study B).[15] Thus, clinical trials in which the rate of decline in GFR is used as the measurement of outcome may require a very large number of patients if patients with only moderately impaired or normal GFR are included.

Imprecision in Estimating the Rate of Progression

Because the pace of renal disease is slow, patients must be observed for a long interval to precisely assess the rate of progression. In the feasibility study for the MDRD Study, in which the mean duration of follow-up was 14 months, the precision of the estimate of the rate of decline in renal function improved with increasing duration of follow-up.[22] Table 5 shows the steady decline in the median value and 95% confidence interval for the standard deviation of the estimate of the individual rates of decline in GFR. Similar relationships were observed for the rates of decline in C_{cr} and $1/P_{cr}$. It is also important to note that the estimates of the rate of decline were less precise among patients with higher initial GFR (Study A), in whom the median standard deviation of the estimate of the rate of decline was approximately the same value as the mean rate of decline in the study cohort. Thus, it is necessary for a long follow-up interval in clinical trials in which the rate of decline in renal function is used as the outcome measurement.

Interpretation of Changes in the Rate of Progression

In many studies, changes in the rate of decline in renal function during the interval of follow-up have been attributed to the therapeutic interventions under investigation. This interpretation, however, does not take account of the possibility of spontaneous changes in the rate or the possibility of changes in the rate due to regression to the mean.

To determine whether spontaneous changes occur in the rate of decline in renal function, we analyzed data from 77 patients from our hospital or reported in the literature in whom the rate of decline in $1/P_{cr}$ was apparently constant (correlation of $1/P_{cr}$ *v* time greater than 0.84) using a method of linear regression analysis to search for changes in the rate of decline or "breakpoints."[23] We found statistically significant changes in the rate in one third to one half of patients. Because the changes in rate were not obviously associated with therapeutic interventions or associated medical conditions, we concluded that they occurred spontaneously. The mean value for serum creatinine at the time of the change in rate was 5.3 mg/dL and the mean absolute value of the magnitude of the change in rate was 0.007 dL/mg/mo. These values are similar to those reported in clinical trials in which the change in rate was attributed to a therapeutic intervention. Interestingly, the rate of decline significantly more often became less negative, suggesting that the decline

Table 5. Effect of Duration of Follow-up on the Precision of the Estimate of the Rate of Decline in Glomerular Filtration Rate in the Modification of Diet in Renal Disease Feasibility Study

		GFR Slope Standard Deviation*	
No. of Months of Follow-up	N	Median	95% CI
Study A			
6	14	0.61	0.13, 1.13
9	14	0.40	0.17, 0.57
12	14	0.33	0.17, 0.39
Study B			
6	34	0.22	0.13, 0.35
9	34	0.18	0.11, 0.25
12	34	0.13	0.10, 0.16

Abbreviation: CI, confidence interval.

* Slope of GFR is measured in mL/min/1.73 m^2/mo.

Adapted and reprinted with permission from Modification of Diet in Renal Disease (MDRD) Study Group (prepared by Levey AS, Gassman JJ, Hall PM, Walker WG): Assessing the progression of renal disease in clinical studies: Effects of duration of follow-up and regression to the mean. J Am Soc Nephrol 1:1087-1094, 1991.[22]

Table 6. Effect of Regression to the Mean on the Rate of Decline in Renal Function in the Modification of Diet in Renal Disease Feasibility Study

	Study A (N = 28)	Study B (N = 63)	Overall (N = 91)
Screening slope (dL/mg/mo)	−0.0078	−0.0062	−0.0066
Observed follow-up slope (dL/mg/mo)	−0.0035	−0.0052	−0.0047
Predicted follow-up slope (dL/mg/mo)	−0.0063	−0.0049	−0.0053
Observed slope − screening slope (dL/mg/mo)	0.0043	0.0010	0.0019
Predicted slope − screening slope (dL/mg/mo)	0.0015	0.0013	0.0013
(Predicted slope − screening slope)/ (observed slope − screening slope) × 100%	34.9	130.0	68.4

Data are presented as means.

Reprinted with permission from Modification of Diet in Renal Disease (MDRD) Study Group (prepared by Levey AS, Gassman JJ, Hall PM, Walker WG): Assessing the progression of renal disease in clinical studies: Effects of duration of follow-up and regression to the mean. J Am Soc Nephrol 1:1087-1094, 1991.[22]

in $1/P_{cr}$ actually slows rather than remains constant over time.

The effect of regression to the mean on the rate of decline in $1/P_{cr}$ was investigated in the feasibility phase of the MDRD Study (Table 6).[22] Because patients were selected for entry into the MDRD Study only if the decline in $1/P_{cr}$ during screening was less than or equal to a defined value (−0.003 dL/mg/mo), we anticipated that the rate of decline might increase (become less negative) during follow-up because of regression to the mean. We compared the observed changes in rate from screening to follow-up to changes predicted simply from regression to the mean. In patients with higher initial GFR (Study A), the expected difference in rate was 34.9% of the observed difference; hence, 34.9% of the change in rate could be attributed to regression to the mean. In patients with lower initial GFR (Study B), the expected difference exceeded the observed difference; hence, all the change in rate could be attributed to regression to the mean.

The occurrence of spontaneous changes in the rate of decline in $1/P_{cr}$ and changes in the rate due to regression to the mean argue strongly against using the patient as his or her own control in assessing the effect of therapy on the rate of decline in $1/P_{cr}$. Attributing changes in the rate of decline in $1/P_{cr}$ to the effect of therapy requires comparison to a control group that did not receive the therapy. Although these studies examined the rate of decline in $1/P_{cr}$, their conclusions apply equally to the rate of change of C_{cr}, GFR, or any other parameter of renal function or structure.

RECOMMENDATIONS

Current data demonstrate that GFR can be measured accurately and precisely in clinical trials by clearance of radioisotope-labeled filtration markers. However, because of technical limitations and high cost, other filtration markers are being investigated. In some circumstances, measurements of creatinine clearance or serum creatinine are acceptable for estimation of GFR. However, because of factors that influence these determinations other than GFR, it is wise also to include measurements of GFR, perhaps at reduced frequency, to validate the findings. In addition, the measurement of other renal functions, such as permeability to macromolecules (albumin, protein, and dextrans), and renal structure need to be evaluated in progressive renal diseases to establish their role as possible outcome measurements in clinical trials.

Issues related to study design are also of critical importance. Randomized trials with a concurrent control group are necessary to avoid bias. Cross-over design studies, in which patients serve as their own controls, comparing the rate of progression in one time interval to the rate in a later time interval, have serious limitations. Because of the slow pace of renal disease, clinical trials must be of long duration, and because of the large variability in rates of progression, many patients will be required. Thus, multicenter collaboration will be necessary, and expenses will be large. A national agenda is required to prioritize the many suggestions for clinical trials and to direct funding for them. Possibly, the use of meta-analysis and cumulative meta-analysis may increase efficiency in the clinical investigation of progressive renal disease.

ACKNOWLEDGMENT

The author is grateful to Lee Hebert, MD, for his careful review of the manuscript and thoughtful suggestions.

REFERENCES

1. Friedman LM, Furberg CD, DeMets DL. Fundamentals of Clinical Trials. Boston, MA, John Wright, 1981
2. Levey AS: Nephrology forum: Measurement of renal function in chronic renal disease. Kidney Int 38:167-184, 1990
3. Lau J, Antman EM, Jimenez-Silva J, Kupelnick B, Mosteller F, Chalmers TC: Cumulative meta-analysis of therapeutic trials for myocardial infarction. N Engl J Med 327:248-254, 1992
4. Levey AS, Madaio MP, Perrone RD: Laboratory assessment of renal disease: Clearance, urinalysis and renal biopsy, in Brenner BM, Rector FC, Jr (eds): The Kidney (ed 4). Philadelphia, PA, Saunders, 1991, pp 919-968
5. Levey AS: Use of glomerular filtration rate measurements to assess the progression of renal disease. Semin Nephrol 9:370-379, 1989
6. Levey AS, Schluchter MD, Cleary PA, Teschan PE, Lorenz RA, Molitch ME, Mitch WE, Siebert C, Hall PM, Steffes MW, MDRD Study, DCCT: GFR measurements in clinical trials. J Am Soc Nephrol 2:239, 1991 (abstr)
7. Mauer SM, Steffes MW, Ellis EN, Sutherland DER, Brown DM, Goetz FC: Structural-functional relationships in diabetic nephropathy. J Clin Invest 74:1143-1155, 1984
8. Chagnac A, Kiberd BA, Farinas MC, Strober S, Sibley RK, Hoppe R, Myers BD: Outcome of acute glomerular injury in proliferative lupus nephritis. J Clin Invest 84:922-930, 1989
9. Bank N: Mechanisms of diabetic hyperfiltration. Kidney Int 40:792-807, 1991
10. Keane WF, Anderson S, Aurell M, de Zeeuw D, Narins RG, Povar G: Angiotensin converting enzyme inhibitors and progressive renal insufficiency. Ann Intern Med 111:503-516, 1989
11. King AJ, Levey AS: Dietary protein and renal function. J Am Soc Nephrol 3:1723-1737, 1993
12. Lemann J, Bidani AK, Bain RP, Lewis EJ, Rohde RD: Collaborative Study Group of Angiotensin Converting Enzyme Inhibition in Diabetic Nephropathy: Use of the serum creatinine to estimate glomerular filtration rate in health and diabetic nephropathy. Am J Kidney Dis 16:236-243, 1990
13. Shemesh O, Golbetz H, Kriss JP, Myers BD: Limitations of creatinine as a filtration marker in glomerulopathic patients. Kidney Int 28:830-838, 1985
14. Petri M, Bockenstedt L, Colman J, Whiting-O'Keefe Q, Fitz G, Sebastian A, Hellmann D: Serial assessment of glomerular filtration rate in lupus nephropathy. Kidney Int 34:832-839, 1988
15. Modification of Diet in Renal Disease Study Group: The Modification of Diet in Renal Disease (MDRD) Study: Design, methods and results from the feasibility study. Am J Kidney Dis 20:18-33, 1992
16. Walser M, Drew HH, LaFrance ND: Creatinine measurements often yield false estimates of progression in chronic renal failure. Kidney Int 34:412-418, 1988
17. Perrone RD, Madias NE, Levey AS: Serum creatinine as an index of renal function: New insights into old concepts. Clin Chem 38:1933-1953, 1992
18. Modification of Diet in Renal Disease Study Group (prepared by Levey AS, Berg RL, Gassman JJ, Hall PM, Walker WG): Creatinine filtration, secretion and excretion during progressive renal disease. Kidney Int 36:S73-S80, 1989
19. Walser M, Drew HH, LaFrance ND: Reciprocal creatinine slopes often give erroneous estimates of progression of chronic renal failure. Kidney Int 36:S81-S85, 1989
20. Levey AS, Perrone RD, Madias NE: Serum creatinine and renal function. Ann Rev Med 39:469-490, 1988
21. Walser M: Progression of chronic renal failure in man. Kidney Int 37:1195-1210, 1990
22. Modification of Diet in Renal Disease (MDRD) Study Group (prepared by Levey AS, Gassman JJ, Hall PM, Walker WG): Assessing the progression of renal disease in clinical studies: Effects of duration of follow-up and regression to the mean. J Am Soc Nephrol 1:1087-1094, 1991
23. Shah BV, Levey AS: Spontaneous changes in the rate of decline in reciprocal serum creatinine: Errors in predicting the progression of renal disease from extrapolation of the slope. J Am Soc Nephrol 2:1186-1191, 1992

INTERVENTIONS AFFECTING PROGRESSION OF RENAL DISEASE

Introduction

It is a widely held belief that once chronic renal insufficiency is established, renal disease is almost always progressive, leading ultimately to end-stage renal disease (ESRD) if the patients survive long enough. Understanding the mechanisms responsible for the progression of chronic renal disease has resulted in the rational use of strategies to slow or halt the loss of renal function.

A decade ago, Brenner and associates proposed, on the basis of studies in animals, that maladaptive glomerular hemodynamic changes exert a major influence on the factors that initiate and modulate the progression of renal disease. Neuringer and Brenner, in a brief review, present a 10-year update of the hemodynamic theory of progressive renal disease. This review describes the relationship between hyperfiltration, glomerular hypertension, progression of renal injury, diabetic nephropathy, and the key role played by dietary protein restriction and antihypertensive therapy.

Klahr outlines evidence suggesting that protein intake conditions the activity of the renin-angiotensin system and the renal production and excretion of eicosanoids. Increased renin production in response to high-protein intake may account for the increased synthesis of angiotensin II. In turn, angiotensin activates phospholipases in cell membranes, leading to an increased release of arachidonic acid, the precursor of eicosanoids. Angiotensin II directly or indirectly increases the activity of cyclooxygenase, the rate-limiting enzyme in the synthesis of prostanoids and thromboxane A_2. The beneficial effects of low-protein diets on the progression of renal disease may be mediated in part by decreased activity of the renin-angiotensin system.

Smith et al report new data showing that during high-protein feeding, renin gene transcripts and circulating renal renin appear to be increased along with renal growth. They report the effect of angiotensin II inhibition on dietary protein-induced tubular, glomerular, and whole kidney growth in the normal adult rat.

Parving et al report two 10-year prospective studies in hypertensive insulin-dependent diabetic patients with diabetic nephropathy, finding that long-term treatment with angiotensin-converting enzyme inhibitors combined with diuretics protects renal function and enhances survival in this population.

Mogensen et al describe the reproducibility of glomerular filtration rate measurements in diabetic patients. Additionally, they review previous studies on the course of diabetic renal disease and its relationship to abnormal albuminuria. Finally, the beneficial effects of blood pressure control on the progression of diabetic renal disease are emphasized.

Gransvoort et al report that ACE inhibitors are effective in lowering urinary protein excretion in proteinuric patients with renal disease. The long-term benefit of such a treatment is as yet unknown, but the authors argue that the benefits may be dual. First, the lowering of proteinuria may relieve symptoms associated with the nephrotic syndrome. Second, the reduction in protein loss may protect the kidney against progressive loss of renal function. During a 2-year follow-up of proteinuric patients with renal disease, ACE inhibition resulted in a sustained reduction of proteinuria, an increase in serum albumin, and a decrease in serum cholesterol. In addition, the investigators found that the estimated degree of renal function decline correlated with the degree of the initial antiproteinuric effect of the ACE inhibitor: the greater the initial antiproteinuric effect, the less steep the slope of renal function loss.

Burnier et al report on the acute renal tubular effects of two angiotensin II receptor antagonists, losartan and irbesartan, in normotensive volunteers. Both induced natriuresis, greater during salt depletion, with decreased distal sodium reabsorption.

Friedman et al report the favorable impact of erythropoietin on three anemic nephropathic diabetic patients with retinopathy and macular edema, suggesting that an increased cell mass might ameliorate tissue and cellular hypoxia by increasing oxygen transporting capacity.

Hemodynamic Theory of Progressive Renal Disease: A 10-Year Update in Brief Review

Julia R. Neuringer, MD, and Barry M. Brenner, MD

● Experimental studies have suggested that glomerular hypertension is ultimately damaging to the kidney. Prevention of glomerular hypertension by dietary protein restriction or antihypertensive therapy lessens glomerular injury in several experimental models of chronic renal disease. Glomerular hypertension and hyperfiltration also occur in humans with diabetes mellitus, solitary or remnant kidneys, and various forms of acquired renal disease. Clinical studies are beginning to show that dietary protein restriction and antihypertensive therapy may slow progression in these disorders. Large multicenter trials are currently under way to better define the effects of these therapeutic maneuvers on the progression of chronic renal disease.

INDEX WORDS: Kidney; glomerulus; hyperfiltration; chronic renal failure; glomerular hypertension; dietary protein restriction; antihypertensive therapy; diabetic nephropathy.

CHRONIC renal insufficiency in humans is characterized by progression to end-stage renal failure, often despite resolution of the initial disease process.[1,2] A decade ago, Brenner and colleagues proposed, on the basis of studies in animals, that maladaptive glomerular hemodynamic changes exert a major influence on the factors that initiate and modulate the process of disease progression.[3,4] These hemodynamic changes lead to glomerular hyperfiltration, which occurs both experimentally and clinically in several disease states as well as in response to a reduction in functional nephron number, whether induced genetically, surgically, or by acquired renal disease. The elevated single nephron glomerular filtration rate (SNGFR) common to these pathophysiologic conditions is usually caused by increases in the glomerular capillary plasma flow rate (Q_A) and mean glomerular capillary hydraulic pressure ($\bar{P}_{GC}$), which in turn are due to adaptive reductions in preglomerular and postglomerular arteriolar resistances.

Progressional glomerular sclerosis and proteinuria eventually occur in most experimental models of renal disease characterized by glomerular hyperfiltration and hypertension. Systemic hypertension often is also present, as in extreme renal ablation,[4] bilateral renal infarction,[5] post-salt hypertension,[6,7] two-kidney one-clip Goldblatt hypertension,[8,9] desoxycorticosterone (DOCA)-salt hypertension,[10] and the Fawn-hooded rat,[11] a strain congenitally predisposed to chronic renal failure. Systemic hypertension is not required for the development of glomerular capillary hyperfiltration and hypertension, however, since in diabetic rats a pathologic reduction in afferent arteriolar resistance (R_A) not only increases Q_A but allows a greater fraction of the systemic blood pressure to be transmitted into the glomerular capillary network, thereby raising $\bar{P}_{GC}$ despite normal renal perfusion pressure.[12,13]

LESS GLOMERULAR HYPERTENSION MEANS LESS GLOMERULAR INJURY

Amelioration of glomerular capillary hyperfiltration and hypertension by therapeutic maneuvers invariably lessens renal injury. For example, through several possible mechanisms,[3,14,15] dietary protein restriction limits the adaptive increases in SNGFR and $\bar{P}_{GC}$ that occur in various models of experimental renal disease.[4,10,16-20] Systemic blood pressure tends not to decline with protein restriction, yet glomerular injury is consistently ameliorated compared with control animals on normal[4,10,16-18] or high[18,19,21] protein diets, once again emphasizing the importance of glomerular rather than systemic hemodynamics in the development of glomerular injury. Dietary protein restriction also has been shown to preserve renal function[17] and limit structural injury, even when instituted in the setting of established renal injury,[18] a finding perhaps more relevant to the management of human renal disease.

Antihypertensive drug therapy also slows the progression of experimental renal disease. The importance of single nephron rather than systemic hemodynamics is again evident in that agents which lower systemic blood pressure without improving glomerular hemodynamics do not usually ameliorate glomerular injury. Studies have also revealed that glomerular capillary hypertension, rather than hyperperfusion or hyperfiltration, is in fact the most critical determinant of glomerular cell injury. Anderson et al[22,23] and

Lafayette et al[24] treated partially nephrectomized rats with either the angiotensin-converting enzyme (ACE) inhibitor enalapril or with "triple therapy," a combination of reserpine, hydralazine, and hydrochlorothiazide. Both approaches ameliorated systemic hypertension. Triple therapy, having no effect on glomerular flows and pressures, did not protect against glomerular injury. Enalapril preserved normal glomerular capillary pressure and ameliorated proteinuria and glomerulosclerosis, however, despite the fact that glomerular capillary hyperperfusion and hyperfiltration persisted. An angiotensin II receptor antagonist afforded the same protective effect as enalapril.[24] Other investigators,[13,17,18,25-31] using other experimental models[13,25-28,30,31] as well as other therapeutic maneuvers to reduce $\bar{P}_{GC}$,[17,29,30] have obtained similar results. Thus, if glomerular capillary hypertension is controlled, glomerular injury may be prevented or greatly reduced.

The most thoroughly studied antihypertensive regimens in models of progression are triple therapy, ACE inhibitors, and calcium antagonists. Their effects on progression have been reviewed in detail elsewhere.[32-35] A few important points deserve mention here. Although glomerular hemodynamics were not assessed in many studies, the data available tend to support a critical role for glomerular capillary hypertension in the development of renal structural injury. For instance, triple therapy, which may[25,36,37] or may not[23,27,38] afford renal protection, rarely does so unless glomerular capillary hypertension is controlled.[23,25,27,36,38] Similarly, ACE inhibitors, which protect in most models of experimental renal disease,[13,18,22-28,31,39,40] rarely[39] limit glomerular injury without also reducing $\bar{P}_{GC}$. Thus, when glomerular capillary hypertension is ameliorated, irrespective of the therapeutic maneuver used, glomerular structural injury is reduced or even prevented. Conversely, factors that induce or aggravate glomerular capillary hypertension, including dietary protein[19,20] or cholesterol[41] supplementation, superimposed clip hypertension,[42] erythropoietin administration,[29] or uninephrectomy,[16] invariably augment glomerular injury.

Nonhemodynamic processes may also contribute to the progression of chronic renal disease.[43] Thus, lipid-lowering agents,[44] heparin,[45] and dietary sodium restriction[46-48] limit glomerular injury without controlling glomerular cap-illary hypertension in the uninephrectomized spontaneously hypertensive rat (SHR)[46] and in rats with subtotal nephrectomy,[44,45,47,48] presumably by limiting glomerular lipid deposition, intravascular thrombosis, compensatory growth, or capillary wall tension. Vasoactive substances themselves also may have effects on clotting and cell growth, and thus might contribute to progression in both hemodynamic and nonhemodynamic ways. Whether the beneficial effects of nifedipine in rats with DOCA-salt hypertension[49] or subtotal nephrectomy,[40] in which injury but not glomerular hypertension is ameliorated, are due to these or other as yet unidentified protective mechanisms remains to be determined.

The converse may also be true, namely, that glomerular injury develops or worsens in the absence of absolute or relative glomerular capillary hypertension. In this regard, dietary protein supplementation tends to accelerate glomerular injury in uninephrectomized rats in the setting of normal glomerular capillary pressures.[50] Similarly, glomerular injury develops in rats with adriamycin or puromycin nephrosis in the absence of glomerular capillary hypertension,[39] although in other studies elevated glomerular capillary pressures were observed in these same experimental models.[51-53] Moreover, control of glomerular hypertension by ACE inhibition ameliorates[53] or at least delays the development of glomerular injury in these rats,[52] due possibly to a salutary effect of the ACE inhibitor on glomerular barrier function[31] in these models of massive proteinuria[54] in addition to their beneficial hemodynamic effects.

Whether abnormal glomerular hemodynamics are the sole or principal factors in the pathogenesis and progression of diabetic glomerulopathy also has been the subject of intense interest in the past decade.[13,20,27,28,55-60] Unfortunately, it is difficult to compare many of these studies due to differences in experimental design, including rat strain, the definition of tissue injury (mesangial expansion *v* focal glomerulosclerosis) and the degree of glycemic control aimed for and/or achieved in the experimental animals. The latter point is particularly important since the degree of glycemic control critically affects glomerular hemodynamics. When hyperglycemia is moderate,[12,13,20,27,28,57] glomerular capillary hyperfiltration and hypertension develop. With more severe hyperglycemia, glomerular capillary pressure may be normal[12,58,59] or even reduced,[60,61] in association with reductions in SNGFR.[12,60,61] Thus, differences in metabolic control most likely account for the fact that glomerular hypertension was present in some diabetic animals but not in others. It is also likely that the development of glomerular injury in severely hyperglycemic rats, in which glomerular pressures are normal, is mediated at least in part by other (ie, metabolic) factors.

THE ROLE OF ALTERED GLOMERULAR HEMODYNAMICS IN HUMANS

The influence of hyperfiltration, the most readily monitored surrogate of altered glomerular hemodynamics, on renal function in humans has been most thoroughly evaluated in kidney transplant donors and in patients uninephrectomized for acquired renal disease.[62,63] Even after one to two decades, total GFR often averages approximately 70% of prenephrectomy values despite the 50% reduction in renal mass, indicating that the remaining kidney is indeed hyperfiltering. Most studies have shown that in association with this hyperfiltration, the prevalence of hypertension in both groups tends to increase after uninephrectomy,[63] although only in transplant donors is hypertension apt to be more prevalent than in local, control populations. Similarly, the prevalence of proteinuria tends to increase in both groups after uninephrectomy, and in one study of patients nephrectomized for renal disease,[64] proteinuria was shown to increase as a function of time after surgery as well. However, most investigators have not been able to demonstrate that blood pressure, proteinuria, or GFR correlate in any way with time since nephrectomy, or with each other. Most conclude that because values for GFR remain relatively stable over time, hyperfiltration in these uninephrectomized adults must not be adversely affecting the remaining kidney. This conclusion seems premature, however, as the mean duration of follow-up in these patients is usually less than two decades. Experimental data clearly show that although renal insufficiency develops very gradually in uninephrectomized animals, it eventuates much earlier than in two-kidney control patients.[65] It is therefore crucial that renal function in these individuals be followed for several decades before conclusions regarding long-term safety are reached.

Patients with unilateral renal agenesis differ from uninephrectomized adults in that they hyperfilter from birth. After approximately three decades of hyperfiltration they may develop proteinuria, sometimes[66-71] but not always[72,73] in association with the development of hypertension and renal insufficiency. Nevertheless, patients with this disorder who undergo biopsy for proteinuria invariably exhibit the lesions of focal and segmental glomerular sclerosis,[66-68,70,71] the same lesion that develops experimentally in the setting of reduced renal mass. Interestingly, this is also true of patients nephrectomized for unilateral disease who subsequently undergo biopsy for proteinuria.[66,74] Thus, while it is true that most people with unilateral agenesis do not develop progressive renal disease (and that if they do it may be related to other genitourinary abnormalities that may accompany a solitary kidney), it is reasonable to infer that at least in some, longstanding hyperfiltration may contribute to the development of renal injury.

Several reports have examined the development of renal injury in patients who have undergone a greater than a 50% reduction in total renal mass.[75-80] Thirty-six of the reported patients were followed for an average of 12 years and, of these, 30% developed systemic hypertension de novo or required antihypertensive medications to control their blood pressure. A striking 70% of patients in whom 24-hour urinary excretion rates were measured[77-80] developed significant proteinuria. Novick et al[79] demonstrated that, just as in rats with subtotal nephrectomy, the extent of proteinuria correlated directly with the duration of follow-up and inversely with the amount of renal tissue remaining. Furthermore, in four of five patients undergoing biopsy for moderate to severe proteinuria,[77,79] the pathologic lesion found was focal and segmental glomerulosclerosis. Thus, with respect to the development of hypertension, proteinuria, and glomerulosclerosis, the human model of extensive renal ablation accurately resembles its experimental counterpart. Significantly, two of the three patients followed the longest by Novick et al[79] developed end-stage renal disease requiring hemodialysis, suggesting that subtotal nephrectomy in humans may indeed lead to renal insufficiency as well. The theory that solitary kidneys given in the course of renal transplantation ultimately fail due at least in part to nonimmunologic (ie, hemodynamic) factors has recently been postulated. (See ref 81 for a detailed discussion of this issue.)

Hyperfiltration occurs in certain pathophysiologic conditions even when renal mass is intact, as in diabetes mellitus.[82,83] It has been shown that hyperfiltration predicts the subsequent development of nephropathy in patients with type I diabetes,[84-86] independently of the degree of metabolic control,[85] although others have failed to confirm this finding.[87-89] Whereas two studies showed no association between hyperfiltration and the development of proteinuria, they nevertheless demonstrated that the rate of decline of GFR was faster in hyperfiltering patients than in control patients.[88,89] Studies with longer durations of follow-up are needed to clarify the precise role of hyperfiltration in the progression of diabetic renal disease.

THERAPEUTIC OUTCOMES IN HUMAN RENAL DISEASE

Therapies shown to limit glomerular hyperfunction and to ameliorate renal injury in animals have begun to be tested in humans. Dietary protein restriction[90,91] and antihypertensive drug therapy[32,34,35,92] have been the principal therapeutic interventions tested thus far, and preliminary results have been promising. A recent meta-analysis[93,94] of studies of low-protein diets in renal insufficiency, based only on data from prospective, randomized, controlled trials in nondiabetic patients,[95-100] suggests that dietary protein restriction indeed delays the onset of end-stage renal disease. Evidence also suggests that dietary protein restriction retards the progression of diabetic renal disease as well.[101-104] It is anticipated that the Modification of Diet in Renal Disease Study, a large multicenter clinical trial currently under way, will also clarify the roles of dietary protein restriction and aggressive reduction in blood pressure on the rate of progression of chronic renal disease in humans.[105] Of interest in the Modification of Diet in Renal Disease Feasability Study was the finding that the rate of decline of GFR correlated inversely with the long-term average level of mean arterial blood pressure. Since patients were not randomly assigned to blood pressure goals, it was not possible to determine whether a causal relationship existed. However, a substantial amount of clinical evidence[32,34,35,92] suggests that hypertension accelerates and antihypertensive therapy slows[106,107] the progression of chronic renal disease. Whether certain antihypertensive regimens are more beneficial than others in humans remains an important question in need of further study.

REFERENCES

1. Mitch WE, Walser M, Buffington GA, Lemann J, Jr: A simple method for estimating progression of chronic renal failure. Lancet 2:1326-1328, 1976

2. Rutherford WE, Blondin J, Miller JP, Greenwalt AS, Vavra JD: Chronic progressive renal disease: Rate of change of serum creatinine concentration. Kidney Int 11:62-70, 1977

3. Brenner BM, Meyer TW, Hostetter TH: Dietary protein intake and the progressive nature of kidney disease: The role of hemodynamically mediated glomerular injury in the pathogenesis of progressive glomerular sclerosis in aging, renal ablation, and intrinsic renal disease. N Engl J Med 307:652-659, 1982

4. Hostetter TH, Olson JL, Rennke HG, Venkatachalam MA, Brenner BM: Hyperfiltration in remnant nephrons: A potentially adverse response to renal ablation. Am J Physiol 241:F85-F93, 1981

5. Meyer TW, Rennke HG: Progressive glomerular injury after limited renal infarction in the rat. Am J Physiol 254:F856-F862, 1988

6. Azar SA, Johnson MA, Hertel B, Tobian L: Single-nephron pressures, flows, and resistances in hypertensive kidneys with nephrosclerosis. Kidney Int 12:28-40, 1977

7. Azar S, Johnson MA, Iwai J, Bruno L, Tobian L: Single-nephron dynamics in "post-salt" rats with chronic hypertension. J Lab Clin Med 91:156-166, 1978

8. Schwietzer G, Gertz KH: Changes of hemodynamics and glomerular ultrafiltration in renal hypertension of rats. Kidney Int 15:134-143, 1979

9. Wilson C, Byrom FB: The vicious circle in chronic Bright's disease. Experimental evidence from the hypertensive rat. Q J Med 34:65-93, 1941

10. Dworkin LD, Hostetter TH, Rennke HG, Brenner BM: Hemodynamic basis for glomerular injury in rats with desoxycorticosterone-salt hypertension. J Clin Invest 73:1448-1461, 1984

11. Simons JL, Provoost AP, De Keijzer MH, Anderson S, Troy JL, Rennke HG, Brenner BM: Glomerular hypertension predicts focal segmental glomerular sclerosis in Fawn-Hooded rats. J Am Soc Nephrol 2:691, 1991 (abstr)

12. Hostetter TH, Troy JL, Brenner BM: Glomerular hemodynamics in experimental diabetes mellitus. Kidney Int 19:410-415, 1981

13. Zatz R, Dunn BR, Meyer TW, Anderson S, Rennke HG, Brenner BM: Prevention of diabetic glomerulopathy by pharmacological amelioration of glomerular capillary hypertension. J Clin Invest 77:1925-1930, 1986

14. Premen AJ: Potential mechanisms mediating postprandial renal hyperemia and hyperfiltration. FASEB J 2:131-137, 1988

15. King AJ, Troy JL, Anderson S, Neuringer JR, Gunning M, Brenner BM: Nitric oxide: A potential mediator of amino-acid induced renal hyperemia and hyperfiltration. J Am Soc Nephrol 1:1271-1277, 1991

16. Dworkin LD, Feiner HD: Glomerular injury in uninephrectomized spontaneously hypertensive rats. A consequence of glomerular capillary hypertension. J Clin Invest 77:797-809, 1986

17. Nath KA, Kren SM, Hostetter TH: Dietary protein restriction in established renal injury in the rat. J Clin Invest 78:1199-1205, 1986

18. Meyer TW, Anderson S, Rennke HG, Brenner BM: Reversing glomerular hypertension stabilizes established glomerular injury. Kidney Int 31:752-759, 1987

19. Schnermann J, Gokel M, Weber PC, Schubert G, Briggs JP: Tubuloglomerular feedback and glomerular morphology in Goldblatt hypertensive rats on varying protein diets. Kidney Int 29:520-529, 1986

20. Zatz R, Meyer TW, Rennke HG, Brenner BM: Predominance of hemodynamic rather than metabolic factors in the pathogenesis of diabetic glomerulopathy. Proc Natl Acad Sci USA 82:5963-5967, 1985

21. Hostetter TH, Meyer TW, Rennke HG, Brenner BM: Chronic effects of dietary protein in the rat with intact and reduced renal mass. Kidney Int 30:509-517, 1986

22. Anderson S, Meyer TW, Rennke HG, Brenner BM: Control of glomerular hypertension limits glomerular injury in rats with reduced renal mass. J Clin Invest 76:612-619, 1985

23. Anderson SA, Rennke HG, Brenner BM: Therapeutic advantage of converting enzyme inhibitors in arresting progressive renal disease associated with systemic hypertension in the rat. J Clin Invest 77:1993-2000, 1986

24. Lafayette RA, Mayer G, Park SK, Meyer TW: Angiotensin II receptor blockade limits glomerular injury in rats with reduced renal mass. J Clin Invest 90:766-771, 1992

25. Dworkin LD, Grosser M, Feiner HD, Ullian M, Parker M: Renal vascular effects of antihypertensive therapy in uninephrectomized SHR. Kidney Int 35:790-798, 1989

26. Dworkin LD, Feiner HD, Parker M, Tolbert E: Effects of nifedipine and enalapril on glomerular structure and function in uninephrectomized SHR. Kidney Int 39:1112-1117, 1991

27. Anderson S, Rennke HG, Garcia DL, Brenner BM: Short and long term effects of antihypertensive therapy in the diabetic rat. Kidney Int 36:526-536, 1989

28. Anderson S, Rennke HG, Brenner BM: Nifedipine versus fosinopril in uninephrectomized diabetic rats. Kidney Int 41:891-897, 1992

29. Garcia DL, Anderson S, Rennke HG, Brenner BM: Anemia lessens and its prevention with recombinant human erythropoietin worsens glomerular injury and hypertension in rats with reduced renal mass. Proc Natl Acad Sci USA 85:6142-6146, 1988

30. Lafferty HL, Garcia DL, Rennke HG, Troy JL, Anderson S, Brenner BM: Anemia ameliorates progressive renal injury in experimental DOCA-salt hypertension. J Am Soc Nephrol 1:1180-1185, 1991

31. Remuzzi A, Puntorieri S, Battaglia C, Bertani T, Remuzzi G: Angiotensin converting enzyme inhibition ameliorates glomerular filtration of macromolecules and water and lessens glomerular injury in the rat. J Clin Invest 85:541-549, 1990

32. Neuringer JR, Anderson S, Brenner BM: The role of systemic and intraglomerular hypertension in the progression of chronic renal disease, in Mitch WE (ed): The Progressive Nature of Renal Disease (ed 2). New York, NY, Churchill Livingstone, 1992, pp 1-21

33. Bakris GL: Renal effects of calcium antagonists in diabetes mellitus. Am J Hypertens 4:487S-493S, 1991

34. Luft FC, Johnston CI: Are calcium antagonists of value in ameliorating the course of chronic renal disease? Kidney Int 41:S114-S118, 1992 (suppl 36)

35. Brunner HR: ACE inhibitors in renal disease. Kidney Int 42:463-479, 1992

36. Neugarten J, Kaminetsky B, Feiner H, Schacht RG, Liu DT, Baldwin DS: Nephrotoxic serum nephritis with hypertension: Amelioration by antihypertensive therapy. Kidney Int 28:135-139, 1985

37. Azar S, Keane W, Raij L: Antihypertensive therapy in nephritic spontaneously hypertensive rats. Effects on nephron dynamics and morphology. Kidney Int 27:187, 1985 (abstr)

38. Dworkin LD, Feiner HD, Randazzo J: Glomerular hypertension and injury in desoxycorticosterone-salt rats on antihypertensive therapy. Kidney Int 31:718-724, 1987

39. Fogo A, Yoshida Y, Glick AD, Homma T, Ichikawa I: Serial micropuncture analysis of glomerular function in two rat models of glomerular sclerosis. J Clin Invest 82:322-330, 1988

40. Dworkin LD, Parker M, Tolbert E, Feiner H: Nifedipine and enalapril decrease glomerular injury in rats with remnant kidneys by different mechanisms. J Am Soc Nephrol 1:627, 1990 (abstr)

41. Kasiske BL, O'Donnell MP, Schmitz PG, Kim Y, Keane WF: Renal injury of diet-induced hypercholesterolemia in rats. Kidney Int 37:880-891, 1990

42. Tapia E, Gabbai FB, Calleja C, Franco M, Cermeno JL, Bobadilla NA, Perez JM, Alvarado JA, Herrera-Acosta J: Determinants of renal damage in rats with systemic hypertension and partial renal ablation. Kidney Int 38:642-648, 1990

43. Meyer TW, Scholey JW, Brenner BM: Nephron adaptation to renal injury, in Brenner BM, Rector FC, Jr (eds): The Kidney (ed 4). Philadelphia, PA, Saunders, 1991, pp 1871-1908

44. Kasiske BL, O'Donnell MP, Garvis WJ, Keane WF: Pharmacologic treatment of hyperlipidemia reduces glomerular injury in rat 5/6 nephrectomy model of chronic renal failure. Circ Res 62:367-374, 1988

45. Ichikawa I, Yoshida Y, Fogo A, Purkerson M, Klahr S: Effect of heparin on the glomerular structure and function of remnant nephrons. Kidney Int 34:638-644, 1988

46. Benstein JA, Feiner HD, Parker M, Dworkin LD: Superiority of salt restriction over diuretics in reducing renal hypertrophy and injury in uninephrectomized SHR. Am J Physiol 258:F1675-F1681, 1990

47. Lax DS, Benstein JA, Tolbert E, Dworkin LD: Effects of salt restriction on renal growth and glomerular injury in rats with remnant kidneys. Kidney Int 41:1527-1534, 1992

48. Daniels BS, Hostetter TH: Adverse effects of growth in the glomerular microcirculation. Am J Physiol 258:F1409-F1416, 1990

49. Dworkin LD, Levin RI, Benstein JA, Parker M, Ullian ME, Kim Y, Feiner HD: Effects of nifedipine and enalapril on glomerular injury in rats with deoxycorticosterone-salt hypertension. Am J Physiol 259:F598-F604, 1990

50. O'Donnell MP, Kasiske BL, Schmitz PG, Keane WF: High protein intake accelerates glomerulosclerosis independent of effects on glomerular hemodynamics. Kidney Int 37:1263-1269, 1990

51. O'Donnell MP, Michels L, Kasiske B, Raij L, Keane WF: Adriamycin-induced chronic proteinuria: A structural and functional study. J Lab Clin Med 106:62-67, 1985

52. Scholey JW, Miller PL, Rennke HG, Meyer TW: Effect of converting enzyme inhibition on the course of Adriamycin-induced nephropathy. Kidney Int 36:816-822, 1989

53. Anderson S, Diamond JR, Karnovsky MJ, Brenner BM: Mechanisms underlying transition from acute glomerular injury to late glomerular sclerosis in a rat model of nephrotic syndrome. J Clin Invest 82:1757-1768, 1988

54. Remuzzi G, Bertani T: Is glomerulosclerosis a consequence of altered glomerular permeability to macromolecules? Kidney Int 38:384-394, 1990

55. Castellino P, Shohat J, DeFronzo RA: Hyperfiltration and diabetic nephropathy: Is it the beginning? Or is it the end?? Semin Nephrol 10:228-241, 1990

56. O'Donnell MP, Kasiske BL, Keane WF: Glomerular hemodynamic and structural alterations in experimental diabetes mellitus. FASEB J 2:2339-2347, 1988

57. Bank N, Klose R, Aynedjian HS, Nguyen D, Sablay LB: Evidence against increased glomerular pressure initiating diabetic nephropathy. Kidney Int 31:898-905, 1987

58. Mauer SM, Steffes MW, Azar S, Brown DM: Effects of dietary protein content in streptozotocin diabetic rats. Kidney Int 35:48-59, 1989

59. O'Donnell MP, Kasiske BL, Daniels FX, Keane WF: Effects of nephron loss on glomerular hemodynamics and morphology in diabetic rats. Diabetes 35:1011-1015, 1986

60. Michels LD, O'Donnell MP, Keane WF: Glomerular hemodynamic and structural correlations in long-term experimental diabetic rats. J Lab Clin Med 103:840-847, 1984

61. Michels LD, Davidman M, Keane WF: Determinants of glomerular filtration and plasma flow in experimental diabetic rats. J Lab Clin Med 98:869-885, 1981

62. Fotino S: The solitary kidney: A model of chronic hyperfiltration in humans. Am J Kidney Dis 13:88-98, 1989

63. Oldrizzi L, Rugiu C, De Biase V, Maschio G: The solitary kidney: A risky situation for progressive renal damage? Am J Kidney Dis 17:57-61, 1991 (suppl 1)

64. Higashihara E, Horie S, Takeuchi T, Nutahara K, Aso Y: Long-term consequence of nephrectomy. J Urol 143:239-243, 1990

65. Provoost AP, De Keijzer MH, Molenaar JC: Effect of protein intake on lifelong changes in renal function of rats unilaterally nephrectomized at young age. J Lab Clin Med 114:19-26, 1989

66. Gutierrez-Millet V, Nieto J, Praga M, Usera G, Martinez MA, Morales JM: Focal glomerulosclerosis and proteinuria in patients with solitary kidneys. Arch Intern Med 146:705-709, 1986

67. Rugiu C, Oldrizzi L, Lupo A, Valvo E, Loschiavo C, Tessitore N, Gammaro L, Ortalda V, Fabris A, Panzetta G, Maschio G: Clinical features of patients with solitary kidneys. Nephron 43:10-15, 1986

68. Bhathena DB, Julian BA, McMorrow RG, Baehler RW: Focal sclerosis of hypertrophied glomeruli in solitary functioning kidneys of humans. Am J Kidney Dis 5:226-232, 1985

69. Kiprov DD, Colvin RB, McCluskey RT: Focal and segmental glomerulosclerosis and proteinuria associated with unilateral renal agenesis. Lab Invest 46:275-281, 1982

70. Thorner PS, Arbus GS, Celermajer DS, Baumal R: Focal segmental glomerulosclerosis and progressive renal failure associated with a unilateral kidney. Pediatrics 73:806-810, 1984

71. Weinstein T, Zevin D, Gafter U, Ben-Bassat M, Levi J: Proteinuria and chronic renal failure associated with unilateral renal agenesis. Isr J Med Sci 21:919-921, 1985

72. Oberle G, Neumann HPH, Schollmeyer P, Boesken WH, Stahl RAK: Mild proteinuria in patients with unilateral kidney. Klin Wochenschr 63:1048-1051, 1985

73. Schmitz A, Christensen CK, Christensen T, Solling K: No microalbuminuria or other adverse effects of long-standing hyperfiltration in humans with one kidney. Am J Kidney Dis 13:131-136, 1989

74. Zucchelli P, Cagnoli L, Casanova S, Donini U, Pasquali S: Focal glomerulosclerosis in patients with unilateral nephrectomy. Kidney Int 24:649-655, 1983

75. Foster MH, Sant GR, Donohoe JF, Harrington JT: Prolonged survival with a remnant kidney. Am J Kidney Dis 17:261-265, 1991

76. Lhotta K, Eberle H, Konig P, Dittrich P: Renal function after tumor enucleation in a solitary kidney. Am J Kidney Dis 17:266-270, 1991

77. Solomon LR, Mallick NP, Lawler W: Progressive renal failure in a remnant kidney. Br Med J 291:1610-1611, 1985

78. Stahl RAK, Low I, Schoeppe W: Progressive renal failure in a patient after one and two-thirds nephrectomy. Klin Wochenschr 66:508-510, 1988

79. Novick AC, Gephardt G, Guz B, Steinmuller D, Tubbs R: Long-term follow-up after partial removal of a solitary kidney. N Engl J Med 325:1058-1062, 1991

80. Rutsky EA, Dubovsky EV, Kirk K: Long-term follow-up of a human subject with a remnant kidney. Am J Kidney Dis 18:509-513, 1991

81. Brenner BM, Cohen RA, Milford EL: In renal transplantation, one size may not fit all. J Am Soc Nephrol 3:162-169, 1992

82. Mogensen CE, Andersen MJF: Increased kidney size and glomerular filtration rate in early juvenile diabetes. Diabetes 22:706-712, 1973

83. Christiansen JS, Gammelgaard J, Frandsen M, Parving HH: Increased kidney size, glomerular filtration rate and renal plasma flow in short-term insulin-dependent diabetics. Diabetologia 20:451-456, 1991

84. Mogensen CE: Christensen CK: Predicting diabetic nephropathy in insulin-dependent patients. N Engl J Med 311:89-93, 1984

85. Mogensen CE: Early glomerular hyperfiltration in insulin-dependent diabetics and late nephropathy. Scand J Clin Lab Invest 46:201-206, 1986

86. Rudberg S, Persson B, Dahlquist G: Increased glomerular filtration rate as a predictor of diabetic nephropathy—An 8-year prospective study. Kidney Int 41:822-828, 1992

87. Lervang HH, Jensen S, Brochner-Mortensen J, Ditzel J: Early glomerular hyperfiltration and the development of late nephropathy in type I (insulin-dependent) diabetes mellitus. Diabetologia 31:723-729, 1988

88. Jones SL, Wiseman MJ, Viberti GC: Glomerular hyperfiltration as a risk factor for diabetic nephropathy: Five-year report of a prospective study. Diabetologia 34:59-65, 1991

89. Azevedo MJ, Gross JL: Follow-up of glomerular hyperfiltration in normoalbuminuric type I (insulin-dependent) diabetic patients. Diabetologia 34:611, 1991

90. El Nahas AM, Coles GA: Dietary treatment of chronic renal failure: Ten unanswered questions. Lancet 1:597-600, 1986

91. Mitch WE: Dietary protein restriction in chronic renal failure: Nutritional efficacy, compliance, and progression of renal insufficiency. J Am Soc Nephrol 2:823-831, 1991

92. Jerums G, Allen TJ, Tsalamandris C, Cooper ME: Angiotensin converting enzyme inhibition and calcium channel blockade in incipient diabetic nephropathy. Kidney Int 41:904-911, 1992

93. Fouque D, Laville M, Boissel JP, Chifflet R, Labeeuw M, Zech PY: Controlled low protein diets in chronic renal insufficiency: Meta-analysis. Br Med J 304:216-220, 1992

94. Walker JD: Low protein diets in chronic renal insufficiency. Br Med J 304:983, 1992

95. Ihle BU, Becker GJ, Whitworth JA, Charlwood RA, Kincaid-Smith PS: The effect of protein restriction on the progression of renal insufficiency. N Engl J Med 321:1773-1777, 1989

96. Rosman JB, Langer K, Brandl M, Piers-Becht TPM, van der Hem GK, ter Wee PM, Donker AB JM: Protein-restricted diets in chronic renal failure: a four year follow-up shows limited indications. Kidney Int 36:S96-S102, 1989 (Suppl 27)

97. Locatelli F, Alberti D, Graziani G, Buccianti G, Redaelli B, Giangrande A: Prospective, randomised, multicentre trial of effect of protein restriction on progression of chronic renal insufficiency. Lancet 337:1299-304, 1991

98. Gretz N, Strauch M: Low-protein diet and chronic renal failure. Lancet 338:442, 1991

99. Williams PS, Stevens ME, Fass G, Irons L, Bone JM: Failure of dietary protein and phosphate restriction to retard the rate of progression of chronic renal failure: A prospective, randomised, controlled trial. Q J Med 294:837-855, 1991

100. Jungers P, Chaveau PH, Ployard F, Lebkiri B, Ciancioni C, Man NK: Comparison of ketoacids and low protein diet on advanced chronic renal failure progression. Kidney Int 32:S67-S71, 1987 (suppl 22)

101. Zeller K, Whittaker E, Sullivan L, Raskin P, Jacobson HR: Effect of restricting dietary protein on the progression of renal failure in patients with insulin-dependent diabetes mellitus. N Engl J Med 324:78-84, 1991

102. Parving HH: Protein restriction and renal failure in diabetes mellitus. N Engl J Med 324:1743-1744, 1991

103. Walker JD, Bending JJ, Dodds RA, Mattock MB, Murrells TJ, Keen H, Viberti GC: Restriction of dietary protein and progression of renal failure in diabetic nephropathy. Lancet 2:1411-1414, 1989

104. Parving HH: Low-protein diet and progression of renal disease in diabetic nephropathy. Lancet 335:411-412, 1990

105. Modification of Diet in Renal Disease Study Group: The Modification of Diet in Renal Disease Study: Design, methods, and results from the Feasibility Study. Am J Kidney Dis 20:18-33, 1992

106. Brazy PC, Stead WW, Fitzwilliam JF: Progression of renal insufficiency: Role of blood pressure. Kidney Int 35:670-674, 1989

107. Zucchelli P, Zuccala A, Borghi M, Fusaroli M, Sasdelli M, Stallone C, Sanna G, Gaggi R: Long-term comparison between captopril and nifedipine in the progression of renal insufficiency. Kidney Int 42:452-458, 1992

Low-Protein Diets and Angiotensin-Converting Enzyme Inhibition in Progressive Renal Failure

Saulo Klahr, MD

● Both protein restriction and administration of angiotensin-converting enzyme (ACE) inhibitors have been reported to slow the progression of chronic renal failure. Protein intake conditions the activity of the renin-angiotensin system and the renal production and excretion in the urine of eicosanoids. Both dietary protein restriction and ACE inhibitors decrease proteinuria. The effects of ACE inhibitors on the progression of renal disease may be due to hemodynamic effects (lowering of systemic or intraglomerular pressures) or to decreased activity of growth factors as a result of blockade of angiotensin II production.

INDEX WORDS: Renin; angiotensin; eicosanoids; renal disease.

PROTEIN INTAKE AND GLOMERULAR FILTRATION

PROTEIN is an important modulator of glomerular filtration.[1,2] An increase in protein intake augments glomerular filtration rate (GFR) while protein restriction exerts the opposite effect. These effects of protein on GFR have been demonstrated in both humans and experimental animals. An increase in protein intake stimulates the secretion of glucagon, dopamine, vasopressin, eicosanoids, and renin.[2-5] Although the relative role of these hormones in mediating the amino acid or protein-induced increase in GFR is not known, the role of renin-angiotensin system in modulating glomerular hemodynamics is well established.[6]

Protein intake increases single nephron GFR. The mechanism for the increase has been evaluated by examining tubuloglomerular balance in rats with subtotal nephrectomy fed isocaloric diets containing 6% or 40% casein. Rats fed the 40% casein diet required a greater tubular flow rate to initiate a decrease in single nephron GFR. A 40% to 50% decreased sensitivity of the tubuloglomerular feedback mechanism was observed, which led to the conclusion that a high-protein diet causes a failure of the normal mechanisms controlling GFR.[7] The mechanism may be related to changes in angiotensin production or vascular response to its action or to increased reabsorption of sodium and chloride by the loop of Henle. The increased reabsorption of NaCl may be due to marked hypertrophy of the thick ascending limb of Henle in rats fed a high-protein diet.[8] In the last few years, an increasing body of evidence indicates that protein intake may condition the activity of the renin-angiotensin system. At the same time, protein intake can modify the responses of the vascular tree to angiotensin II.[3]

EFFECTS OF PROTEIN INTAKE ON THE RENIN-ANGIOTENSIN SYSTEM AND ON EICOSANOID PRODUCTION

Dietary protein regulates both the synthesis and release of renin.[9] Renal renin mRNA was higher in rats fed a high-protein diet (50%) than in rats fed a standard rat chow (20% protein). On the other hand, a lower protein intake (6% protein) decreased the activity of renal renin mRNA in rats.[9] Rosenberg et al[10] also examined the effects of dietary protein on GFR, renin activity, and excretion of eicosanoids in humans with glomerular disease. The high-protein diet was accompanied by a higher plasma renin activity and an increased excretion of prostaglandin E_2 (PGE_2) and 6-keto prostaglandin $F_{1\alpha}$ ($PGF_{1\alpha}$). These changes were observed in patients with a wide spectrum of severity of disease and in the absence of changes in weight, mean arterial pressure, or serum protein levels. However, the finding of increased prostaglandin excretion in patients ingesting high-protein diets suggests that augmented eicosanoid synthesis may mediate the increased release of renin in such patients. Protein intake conditions eicosanoid synthesis in isolated glomeruli from rats.[11,12] Glomeruli obtained from high-protein–fed rats produced significantly greater amounts of PGE_2, 6-keto $PGF_{1\alpha}$, and thromboxane A_2 under basal conditions than glomeruli obtained from low-protein–fed rats. To investigate the potential role of the renin-angiotensin system in the dietary protein-induced modulation of glomerular eicosanoid production, rats ingesting a high- or low-protein diet were randomized to groups receiving treatment with an angiotensin-converting enzyme (ACE) inhibitor (enalapril) or no therapy. Enalapril attenuated the protein-induced augmentation in glomerular eicosanoid production. This effect occurred only when enalapril was administered in vivo; the active metabolite, enalaprilate, did not alter PGE_2 production by isolated glomeruli when added in vitro. Thus, dietary protein modulates glomerular eicosanoid synthesis in the rat and this effect seems to be mediated by the renin-angiotensin system. Yanagisawa et al[12] also found that after the addition of angiotensin II in vitro there was increased synthesis of eicosanoids. The increment was greater in glomeruli from rats fed a high-protein diet than in glomeruli from rats fed a low-protein diet. To examine the potential mechanisms by which changes in protein intake may modify eicosanoid synthesis we explored the activities of phospholipase A_2 and phospholipase C.[12] There was a significant increase in phosphatidylethanolamine-specific phospholipase activity in glomeruli from rats fed a high-protein diet when compared with glomeruli from rats fed a low-protein diet. In contrast, phosphatidyl-specific phospholipase A_2 activity was significantly decreased in glomeruli from rats fed a high-protein diet. No significant changes in phosphatidyl-inositol bisphosphate (PIP_2) phospholipase C activities were detected between glomeruli of the two dietary groups. The content and activity of cyclooxygenase was significantly greater in glomeruli from rats fed a high-protein diet than in glomeruli from rats fed a low-protein diet. These studies indicate that the greater synthesis of eicosanoids in glomeruli isolated from rats fed a high-protein diet may be mediated by increases in the amount and activity of cyclooxygenase coupled with enhanced activity of phosphoethanolamine-specific phospholipase A_2. The greater release of arachidonic acid due to enhanced activity of phosphoethanolamine-specific phospholipase A_2 and the increased activity of cyclooxygenase would result in increased eicosanoid synthesis. In rats fed a high-protein diet, inhibition of the synthesis of angiotensin II using an ACE inhibitor prevented the increases in the activities of phospholipase A_2 and cyclooxygenase observed in untreated rats. These observations suggest that increased protein intake augments renin-angiotensin production. The increased activity of angiotensin II in turn conditions the production of eicosanoids. Dietary protein intake also modulated glomerular eicosanoid production in three models of experimental renal disease in the rat: streptozotocin-induced diabetes mellitus, Heymann nephritis, and partial renal ablation.[13,14]

Dietary protein has two important effects on the renin-angiotensin system. Plasma renin activity has been found to be directly related to protein intake and the peripheral vascular response to infused angiotensin was attenuated by increased dietary protein.[3] The mechanism of increased plasma renin activity after increased dietary protein was not related to changes in sodium or potassium intake. Since there was an increase in prostaglandin excretion, and since prostaglandins are believed to mediate renin release,[15] it was suggested that increased plasma renin activity may have resulted from an increase in prostaglandin production. It was found that the pressor response to graded doses of angiotensin II was diminished by 30% to 60% in rats fed a high-protein diet.[3] Angiotensin II binding to mesenteric artery smooth muscle did not differ between rats fed a high-protein or a low-protein diet. Interestingly, chronic administration of captopril did not normalize the pressor response in high-protein–fed rats. Urine excretion of PGE_2 and 6-keto $PGF_{1\alpha}$ was markedly increased by the high-protein diet. Acute inhibition of prostaglandin synthesis with meclofenamate restored the pressor response to angiotensin II in rats fed a high-protein diet to levels comparable to those seen in low-protein–fed rats. This suggests that increased synthesis of eicosanoids may attenuate the vascular response to angiotensin II in rats fed a high-protein diet.

EFFECTS OF ANGIOTENSIN-CONVERTING ENZYME INHIBITORS OR PROTEIN INTAKE ON PROTEINURIA AND THE PROGRESSION OF CHRONIC RENAL DISEASE

Substantial evidence indicates that adequate control of hypertension slows the progression of renal disease in humans.[16] Some studies in experimental animals suggest that antihypertensive agents may differ in their protective effects on the kidney, possibly because they differ in their ability to lower intraglomerular capillary pressure. Several reports indicate that in rats with experimental renal disease, ACE inhibitors but not triple therapy (reserpine, hydralazine, and hydrochlorothiazide) lower glomerular hypertension and decrease glomerular sclerosis in the remnant kidney model.[17] Other studies, however, have not found significant differences in the development of sclerosis in rats with experimental renal disease treated with ACE inhibitors or triple therapy. However, the administration of ACE inhibitors has a beneficial effect in several experimental models of renal disease, including subtotal renal ablation, unilateral nephrectomy in spontaneously hypertensive rats, Goldblatt hypertension induced after unilateral nephrectomy, streptozotocin-induced diabetes mellitus, puromycin-induced nephrotic syndrome, and passive Heymann nephritis. The possibility that ACE inhibitors would also be effective in slowing the progression of renal disease in humans has received considerable attention in the last decade. Several studies in patients with diabetic nephropathy have suggested a beneficial effect of ACE inhibitors on the evolution of renal function accompanied by a clear reduction of proteinuria in most patients.[18] In addition, treatment with ACE inhibitors has resulted in a 30% to 50% reduction in proteinuria in patients with several nondiabetic nephropathies.[19-21] However, marked variability in the decrease in proteinuria was observed, and most of these studies were short term. Recently, Praga et al[21] examined the long-term beneficial effect of ACE inhibition in patients with nephrotic-range proteinuria. They followed the course of 46 nondiabetic patients with proteinuria who were treated with captopril for a minimum of 12 months. In the group as a whole, proteinuria decreased approximately 45%, from 6.3 ± 2.5 g/24 hr to 3.9 ± 3.1 g/24 hr. The decrease was greater in patients with reflux nephropathy and in those with reduction of renal mass, inactive crescentic glomerulonephritis, nephrosclerosis, and IgA nephropathy; patients with membranous glomerulonephritis and idiopathic focal glomerulosclerosis had a lesser response. After the 12-month treatment period, the patients were separated into two groups: those who showed a reduction in proteinuria greater than 45% and those with a response lower than 45%. In the group with the greater antiproteinuric response, a change in the progressive decline in GFR was observed, whereas this was not the case in the group that showed the lesser response. There were no differences between these two groups with respect to age, sex, captopril dose, blood pressure, or renal function at the start of treatment. The decrease in proteinuria observed was unrelated to blood pressure changes. Of note is the fact that the patients with the lesser response to captopril were those with a greater decrement in serum proteins, particularly albumin. The investigators concluded that the significant antiproteinuric effect of captopril in patients with nephrotic proteinuria is accompanied by an arrest or slowing of the progression of renal insufficiency.

Since hypertension per se may play a role in proteinuria, the effects of several antihypertensives on proteinuria have been compared. One of the best studies in this area was conducted by Rosenberg and Hostetter,[19] who compared the effects of administration of ACE inhibitors with those of alpha-1 antagonists on proteinuria. The ACE inhibitor enalapril or the alpha-1 antagonist prazosin was administered to 14 patients with established glomerular disease. After a baseline period of 3 weeks, during which patients received their customary antihypertensive agents, there were two 4-week treatment periods, one for each drug; between these intervals were 4 weeks in which patients followed the same drug regimen as in the baseline period. In the treatment periods, the ACE inhibitor or the alpha-1 antagonist was added to the patient's antihypertensive medications. Mean arterial blood pressure decreased similarly with both drugs. Twenty-four–hour urine protein, albumin, and IgG excretion were not significantly different at the end of the treatment course with the ACE inhibitor or the alpha-1 antagonist. However, compared with baseline values, significant decreases in total protein and IgG excretion occurred only with the ACE inhibitor during the treatment period. Albumin excretion decreased with both drugs. The investigators noticed a greater antiproteinuric effect for a given decrease in blood pressure with the ACE inhibitor as compared with the alpha-1 antagonist. Additionally, reduction in proteinuria occurred in a subset of seven patients whose baseline mean arterial pressure was in the normotensive range. These researchers concluded that reductions in blood pressure, even reductions that place it within the accepted normal range, lessen permselectivity defects of the glomerular membrane.

In several studies, a decrease in dietary protein intake has been reported to ameliorate the progression of chronic renal disease. Dietary protein restriction also has been reported to reduce proteinuria in patients with chronic glomerular diseases. Rosenberg et al[10] found that a low-protein diet improved glomerular permselectivity in patients with glomerular disease, as evidenced by a decreased 24-hour urine excretion of total protein, albumin, and IgG and by a decreased fractional clearance of neutral dextrans of molecular radii 48 Å to 56 Å. The mechanisms by which protein intake modifies glomerular permselectivity are not well understood. Don et al[22] evaluated the effects of ACE inhibitors and dietary protein restriction on proteinuria in 12 patients with chronic glomerular disorders. The patients ingested a constant metabolic diet containing 1.6 g protein/kg body weight/d during the 3-week baseline period. They were then randomized either to a group treated with enalapril titrated to reduce arterial pressure by 10 mm Hg or to a group ingesting an isocaloric 0.8 g/kg protein diet. Five patients in each group completed 3 additional weeks of observation during the treatment period. Enalapril decreased urine protein and albumin losses by 26% and 33%, respectively, without affecting creatinine clearance. Albumin synthesis was unchanged and nitrogen balance increased slightly. Dietary protein restriction had no consistent effect on proteinuria or albuminuria, whereas albumin synthesis and nitrogen balance decreased. Both modes of therapy resulted in a modest increase in plasma potassium concentration. The results of this study indicate that treatment with enalapril is effective in reducing albuminuria and proteinuria in patients with chronic glomerular diseases ingesting a high-protein diet. This salutary effect was accompanied by maintenance of the rate of albumin synthesis. In contrast, restriction of dietary protein intake did not significantly decrease urinary protein or albumin excretion, and the rate of albumin synthesis decreased significantly. Although urinary albumin and protein excretion for the group as a whole did not decrease, the individual patient responses were heterogeneous. Of five patients, dietary protein restriction caused a significant reduction in urine protein excretion in two patients and a reduction in urine albumin excretion in one patient. Even in previously reported studies in which dietary protein restriction reduced urine albumin and/or protein losses in the groups as a whole, the individual patient responses were not uniform.[23,24] It would be of interest to examine the combined effects of dietary protein restriction and ACE inhibitors on proteinuria as compared with the effect of each maneuver separately.

Angiotensin-converting enzyme inhibitors have been found to be variably effective in reducing proteinuria, but this reduction usually has been found in combination with a decrease in GFR, systemic blood pressure, or both. Either of these mechanisms could explain a reduction in proteinuria. A decrease in GFR with no change in glomerular basement membrane characteristics would produce a concomitant decrease in protein excretion. Similarly, a reduction in systemic blood pressure may be translated into a direct reduction in intraglomerular pressure and a decrease in GFR. However, there also may be a specific and separate intraglomerular action of ACE inhibitors that could affect glomerular barrier function. In a group of patients with proteinuria due to membranous glomerulonephritis[20] there was a decrease in 24-hour urinary protein excretion, from 10.4 g/d to 5.3 g/d, and fractional clearance of dextrans greater than 4.1 nm decreased on treatment, indicating both a reduction in macromolecules passing through the shunt pathway of the glomerular basement membrane and a possible decrease in ultrafiltration coefficient.[20] There were no significant changes in GFR, effective renal plasma flow, or mean arterial pressure throughout the study. These results suggest an effect of enalapril on proteinuria that may be due to a specific intraglomerular action. Although several investigators have shown an effect of ACE inhibitors on the progression of renal disease, particularly in patients with diabetic nephropathy, Bauer et al,[25] in a randomized, double-blind, placebo-controlled trial designed to evaluate the effects of enalapril in patients with clinical diabetic nephropathy, recently found no beneficial effect. A longitudinal study lasting 18 months examined the effects of enalapril versus placebo on 24-hour urine protein excretion and the rate of progression of renal disease in 33 patients with clinical diabetic nephropathy. Systemic blood pressure was controlled throughout the trial with conventional antihypertensive drugs. Glomerular filtration rate was determined by technetium 99 dTPA and urine protein was monitored at 3-month intervals. In contrast to placebo therapy, enalapril was associated with an initial (40%) and sustained (33%) decrease in urine protein. Patients randomized to either enalapril-treated or placebo-treated groups experienced mean decreases in GFR, from 1.1 mL/s/1.73 m^2 to 0.85 mL/s/1.73 m^2 and from 1.06 mL/s/1.73 m^2 to 0.97 mL/s/1.73 m^2, respectively. Eleven of 18 patients (61%) randomized to the enalapril group and 10 of 15 patients (66%) randomized to the placebo group demonstrated a decrease in GFR. Their rates of progression were −1.18 mL/min/1.73 m^2/mo and −1 mL/min/1.73 m^2/mo, respectively. In the absence of changes in blood pressure, the addition of an ACE inhibitor to the therapeutic regimen of patients with clinical diabetic nephropathy could not be shown to confer a unique renal protective effect. A prolonged decrease in 24-hour protein excretion could not be shown to predict attenuation in the progression of established clinical diabetic nephropathy.

THE POTENTIAL ROLE OF ANGIOTENSIN II AS A GROWTH FACTOR

It has been shown recently that subcutaneous infusion of angiotensin II from mini-osmotic pumps for 10 days in rats produces a slow pressor response and also produces cardiac and vascular hypertrophy.[26] There are two possible interpretations of this finding. First, vascular hypertrophy may be a consequence of the increase in arterial pressure produced by angiotensin II. It is well recognized that increased pressure within a vessel or cardiac chamber produces hypertrophy locally in that vessel or chamber.[27] Alternatively, or in addition, angiotensin II may have an action on the vessel structure independent of its effect on arterial pressure, presumably through its function as a growth factor. Angiotensin II has been found to have growth factor activity when tested in vitro. In culture, vascular smooth muscle cells respond to angiotensin II by increased secretion of growth-promoting proto-oncogenes, c-*fos*, c-*jun*, c-*myc*,[28-30] by mitosis when incubated in the presence of fetal calf serum,[31-32] by increase of cell size and cell protein when the vascular smooth muscle cells are incubated in protein-free medium,[33,34] and by increased synthesis of extracellular matrix proteins.[28] Some of these effects may be indirect, since angiotensin II also stimulates formation of platelet-derived growth factor by cultured cells. It has also been suggested that a common link operative in the action of angiotensin II may relate to insulin-like growth factor-I (IGF-I). Angiotensin II, growth hormone, insulin, and corticotropin stimulate either local production of immunoreactive IGF-1 or expression of the IGF-1 gene. It is known that IGF-1 stimulates growth in vascular smooth muscle cells. Thus, IGF may act as a final common pathway integrating effects of pressures on a variety of growth factors.[35] In view of the role of angiotensin II as a growth factor and its synergism with other growth factors, such as protein and transforming growth factor-β, the possibility exists that the major effect of ACE inhibitors on the progression of renal disease relates to the blockade of the growth effects of angiotensin II.

REFERENCES

1. Ichikawa I, Purkerson ML, Klahr S, Troy JL, Martinez-Maldonado M, Brenner BM: Mechanism of reduced glomerular filtration rate in chronic malnutrition. J Clin Invest 65:982-988, 1980

2. Klahr S: Effect of protein intake on the progression of renal disease. Annu Rev Nutr 9:87-108, 1989

3. Paller MS, Hostetter TH: Dietary protein increases plasma renin and reduces pressor reactivity to angiotensin II. Am J Physiol 251:F34-F39, 1986

4. Williams M, Young JB, Rosa RM, Gunn S, Epstein FH, Landsberg I: Effect of protein ingestion on urinary dopamine excretion. Evidence for the functional importance of renal decarboxylation of circulating 3,4-dihydroxyphenylalanine in man. J Clin Invest 78:1687-1693, 1986

5. Hirschberg R, Kopple JD: Glucagon and prostaglandins are mediators of amino-acid induced rise in renal hemodynamics. Kidney Int 33:1147-1155, 1988

6. Rosivall L, Navar LE: Effects on renal hemodynamics of intra-arterial infusions of angiotensins I and II. Am J Physiol 245:F181-F187, 1983

7. Seney FD, Persson AEG, Wright FS: Modification of tubuloglomerular feedback signal by dietary protein. Am J Physiol 252:F83-F90, 1987

8. Jakobsson B, Bohman SO, Sundelin B, Aperia A: Mitotic response to high protein intake in different renal cell types in weanling rats. Kidney Int 33:662-666, 1988

9. Rosenberg ME, Chmielewski D, Hostetter TH: Effect of dietary protein on rat renin and angiotensinogen gene expression. J Clin Invest 85:1144-1149, 1990

10. Rosenberg ME, Swanson JE, Thomas BL, Hostetter TH: Glomerular and hormonal responses to dietary protein intake in human renal disease. Am J Physiol 253:F1083-F1090, 1987

11. Don BR, Blake S, Hutchison FN, Kaysen GA, Schambelan M: Dietary protein intake modulates glomerular eicosanoid production in the rat. Am J Physiol 256:F711-F718, 1989

12. Yanagisawa H, Morrissey J, Yates J, Hayes C, Klahr

S: Protein increases glomerular eicosanoid production and activity of related enzymes. Kidney Int 41:1000-1007, 1992

13. Stahl RA, Kudelka S, Helmchen U: High protein intake stimulates prostaglandin formation in remnant kidneys. Am J Physiol 252:F1083-F1094, 1987

14. Schambelan M, Blake S, Sraer J, Bens M, Nivez P, Wahbe F: Increased prostaglandin production by glomeruli isolated from rats with streptozotocin-induced diabetes mellitus. J Clin Invest 75:404-412, 1985

15. Oates JA, Whorton AR, Gerkins JF, Branch J, Hollifield W, Frolich JC: The participation of prostglandins in the control of renin release. Fed Proc 38:72-74, 1979

16. Klahr S: The kidney in hypertension—Villain and victim. N Engl J Med 320:731-733, 1989

17. Brenner BM: Nephron adaptation to renal injury or ablation. Am J Physiol 249:F324-F337, 1985

18. Parving HH, Hommel E, Smidt VM: Protection of kidney function and decrease in albuminuria by captopril in insulin-dependent diabetes with nephropathy. Br Med J 297:1086-1092, 1988

19. Rosenberg ME, Hostetter TH: Comparative effects of antihypertensives on proteinuria: Angiotensin-converting enzyme inhibitor versus α_1-antagonist. Am J Kidney Dis 18:472-482, 1991

20. Thomas DM, Hillis AN, Coles GA, Davies M, Williams JD: Enalapril can treat the proteinuria of membranous glomerulonephritis without detriment to systemic or renal hemodynamics. Am J Kidney Dis 18:38-43, 1991

21. Praga M, Hernández E, Montoyo C, Andrés A, Ruilope LM, Rodicio JL: Long-term beneficial effects of angiotensin-converting enzyme inhibition in patients with nephrotic proteinuria. Am J Kidney Dis 20:240-248, 1992

22. Don BR, Kaysen GA, Hutchison FN, Schambelan M: The effect of angiotensin-converting enzyme inhibition and dietary protein restriction in the treatment of proteinuria. Am J Kidney Dis 17:10-17, 1991

23. Peters JP, Bulger HA: The relation of albuminuria to protein requirement in nephritis. Arch Intern Med 37:153-185, 1926

24. Kaysen GA, Gambertoglio J, Jimenez I, Jones H, Hutchison FN: Effect of dietary protein intake on albumin homeostasis in nephrotic patients. Kidney Int 29:572-577, 1986

25. Bauer JH, Reams GP, Hewett J, Klachko D: A randomized, double-blind, placebo-controlled trial to evaluate the effect of enalapril in patients with clinical diabetic nephropathy. Am J Kidney Dis 20:443-457, 1992

26. Lever AF, Lyall F, Morton JJ, Folkow B: Angiotensin II, vascular structure and blood pressure. Kidney Int 41:S-51-S-55, 1992 (Suppl 37)

27. Bund SJ, West KP, Heagerty AM: Effects of protection from pressure on resistance artery morphology and reactivity in spontaneously hypertensive and Wistar Kyoto rats. Circ Res 68:1230-1240, 1991

28. Naftilan AJ, Pratt RE, Dzau VJ: Induction of platelet-derived growth factor A-chain and c-*myc* gene expressions by angiotensin II in cultured rat vascular smooth muscle cells. J Clin Invest 83:1419-1424, 1989

29. Naftilan AJ, Gilliland GK, Eldridge CS, Kraft AS: Induction of the protooncogene c-*jun* by angiotensin II. Mol Cell Biol 10:5536-5540, 1990

30. Taubman MB, Berk BC, Izumo S, Tsuda T, Alexander RW, Nadal-Ginard B: Angiotensin II induces c-*fos* mRNA in aortic smooth muscle. J Biol Chem 264:526-530, 1989

31. Campbell-Boswell M, Robertson AL, Jr: Effects of angiotensin II and vasopressin on human smooth muscle cells in vitro. Exp Mol Pathol 35:265-276, 1981

32. Lyall F, Morton JJ, Lever AF, Cragoe EJ: Angiotensin II activates Na^+/H^+ exchange and stimulates growth in cultured vascular smooth muscle cells. J Hypertension 6 (Suppl 4):S438-S441, 1988

33. Geisterfer AAT, Peach MJ, Owens GK: Angiotensin II induces hypertrophy, not hyperplasia, of cultured rat aortic smooth muscle cells. Circ Res 62:749-756, 1988

34. Berk BC, Vekshtein V, Gordon HM, Tsuda T: Angiotensin II-stimulated protein synthesis in cultured vascular smooth muscle cells. Hypertens 13:305-314, 1989

35. Lever AF, Harrap S: Essential hypertension: A disorder of growth with origins in childhood? J Hypertens 10:101-120, 1992

Effect of Angiotensin II Blockade on Dietary Protein-Induced Renal Growth

Lawrence J. Smith, MD, Mark E. Rosenberg, MD, and Thomas H. Hostetter, MD

● **Dietary protein provokes renal growth and synthesis of renin. Because angiotensin II (AII) has growth-promoting properties, we tested the possibility that protein-induced renal growth depends on angiotensin II. Normal adult male rats placed on a high-protein diet (50%) developed significant renal and glomerular growth over 6 days compared with rats on a low-protein diet (6%). However, neither angiotensin converting enzyme inhibition with enalapril nor angiotensin receptor antagonism with losartan influenced the degree of whole-kidney, cortical tubular, or glomerular growth. Thus, angiotensin II is not a necessary factor in dietary protein-induced renal growth in normal adult rats.**

INDEX WORDS: Renin; angiotensin; dietary protein; renal growth.

DURING high-protein feeding, circulating renin activity and renin gene transcripts in the kidney are increased; coincidentally, marked renal growth occurs.[1-6] Increased dietary protein induces structural changes with glomerular and tubular hypertrophy as well as functional alterations, including increases in blood flow, glomerular filtration rate, acid and urea excretion, and solute transport.[5-7] In addition to the hemodynamic and tubular transport properties of angiotensin II (AII), evolving evidence supports its role as a promoter of renal growth for mesangial and tubular epithelial cells in vitro.[8,9] Furthermore, the frequent association of renal hypertrophy and injury raise the possibility that AII may mediate in part the injurious effects of dietary protein via renal growth.[6,10] In view of these associations between dietary protein, renal growth, and activation of the renin angiotensin system (RAS), we examined the effect of AII inhibition on dietary protein-induced whole-kidney, glomerular, and tubular growth in the normal adult rat in vivo.

METHODS

Three separate studies were conducted with adult male Sprague-Dawley (Charles River Laboratories, Wilmington, MS) rats (250 to 275 g) housed in individual cages with free access to water. Semisynthetic diet composition (Teklad Corp, Madison, WI) consisted of the following: (1) low-protein, 6% protein: casein (68 g/kg), cornstarch (149 g/kg), sucrose (606 g/kg), and corn oil (49 g/kg); and (2) high-protein, 50% protein: casein (570 g/kg), cornstarch (149 g/kg), sucrose (169 g/kg), and corn oil (44 g/kg). Casein and carbohydrate content varied reciprocally to maintain a isocaloric nature and constant dietary fat content was maintained by adjustments in the corn oil component. All diets were modified with the addition of NaCl (8.8 g/kg chow) to achieve a final composition of 1% NaCl as the combination of AII receptor antagonism and the standard high-protein diet, which contained 0.12% NaCl, was associated with hypotension. Systolic blood pressure measurements were obtained during passive restraint using tail cuff pressure tracings from a pressure transducer (Gould Inc, Oxnard, CA) and dual channel chart recorder (Gilson Medical Electronics, Middleton, WI). All results are reported as means ± standard error. Statistical significance was tested by Student's *t*-test for two groups and was defined as $P < 0.05$.

Experiment No. 1

Twelve rats were fed low-protein–containing diets ad libitum for 6 days (equilibration period) with subsequent randomization to two groups receiving strict pair feeding with either low-protein– or high-protein–containing diets for an additional 6 days, at which time the kidneys were removed under methohexital (50 mg/kg) anesthesia. The equilibration period on the low-protein diets was used to assure that rats were accustomed to ingesting the semisynthetic diets as preliminary studies showed that introduction of such diets immediately after standard chow diets often resulted in fasting and erratic intakes for 1 to 3 days. Right kidney weight was measured on freshly harvested, unperfused tissue. Perfusion fixation of the left kidney was accomplished with 1.25% glutaraldehyde in phosphate buffer delivered at aortic perfusion pressure. Coronal sections of the left kidney were prepared with a tissue slicer containing parallel aligned razor blades separated at 2-mm intervals. Alternate slices were placed right side up in cassettes, and histologic specimens were paraffin embedded, sectioned, and stained with hematoxylin-eosin. Glomerular volume was determined by the standardized point-counting method described by Hirose et al[11] at ×193 magnification (Nikon, Inc, Garden City, NY) with a minimum of 60 glomerular profiles counted per kidney by a blinded observer using a patterned stage movement to eliminate bias.

Cortical volume density and proximal tubule volume density were similarly determined by standardized point-counting methods at ×305 magnification.[12] Glomeruli were isolated from the right nonperfused kidney by a serial sieving

Supported by US Public Health Service Grants No. AM-31437 (T.H.H.) and 1229-DKH3075 (M.E.R.) and by a Young Investigator Grant from the National Kidney Foundation (M.E.R.).

technique using 250 × 150 × 75 μm mesh and manually counted under a microscope at ×40 magnification. Glomerular samples, which represented a more than 90% pure glomerular fraction, were homogenized with a Teflon laboratory stirrer (Talboys Engineering Corp, Emerson, NJ) in phosphate-buffered saline solution for measurement of protein and nucleic acid composition. Quantitation of glomerular composition was performed by the Coomasie method (protein), direct UV spectrophotometry (RNA),[13] and indirect colorimetry (DNA).[14] Due to the initially inconsistent fixation quality of the tissue from the first cohort of animals, the identical experimental protocol was repeated in additional animals solely for additional morphometric determinations, and the values for morphometry from the combined cohorts will be presented in the Results.

Experiment No. 2

Twelve rats were fed low-protein–containing diets ad libitum for 6 equilibration days. Randomization to two groups on the sixth day of low-protein feeding coincided with the introduction of the AII receptor antagonist losartan (formerly known as Dup 753) (30 to 40 mg/kg/d) or placebo 24 hours prior to subsequent dietary manipulation. Losartan was delivered in drinking water with adjustment of the drug concentration (125 to 250 mg/L) dictated by water intakes to maintain near constant daily drug dosing. Strict pair feeding with a high-protein diet was maintained between the two groups of animals when placed on the high-protein diet and continued for an additional 6 days, followed by kidney removal, left kidney perfusion fixation, glomerular composition determinations, and morphometric measurements. A separate group of rats prepared in the same fashion was studied to confirm that losartan at this dose did indeed block the hypertensive effect of exogenous AII. Two control rats receiving no losartan had higher basal arterial pressures (measured in the femoral artery) than two rats receiving losartan (110 and 116 mm Hg *v* 78 and 80 mm Hg, respectively) and had much greater increases in pressure with intravenous boluses of AII at three doses: +18 and +15 mm Hg *v* +2 and +3 mm Hg at 0.1 μg/kg, +30 and +26 mm Hg *v* +7 and +7 mm Hg at 0.2 μg/kg; and +70 and +60 mm Hg *v* +9 and +13 mm Hg at 1 μg/kg.

Experiment No. 3

Under the identical design of experiment no. 2, 12 rats were fed low-protein–containing diets ad libitum for 6 equilibration days. Following randomization to two groups, the ACE inhibitor enalapril (6 to 10 mg/kg/d) or placebo was introduced into the drinking water on the sixth day, again providing 24 hours of drug treatment prior to dietary alteration. Drug concentration (25 to 50 mg/L) was again adjusted to changing water intakes to maintain near constant daily dosing. An additional 6 days of strict pair feeding with high-protein diets ensued, followed by organ harvest, perfusion fixation, glomerular composition, and morphometric volume determinations.

RESULTS

Experiment No. 1

General parameters. By design, the rats consumed equal quantities (15.2 g/d) of the high- and low-protein diets during the pair-feeding period (days 7 to 12). Body weights of the low-protein–fed animals were unchanged, from 261 ± 3 g to 258 ± 3 g (P = NS) during this period; however, the body weights of the high-protein–fed animals increased significantly, from 266 ± 4 g to 285 ± 6 g ($P < 0.05$). Systolic blood pressure (SBP) increased somewhat in the low-protein–fed group during the pair-feeding period (low protein: 134 ± 3 mm Hg to 144 ± 5 mm Hg, P = NS; high protein: 134 ± 6 mm Hg to 131 ± 3 mm Hg, final values $P = 0.053$).

Table 1. Effect of Dietary Protein on Renal and Glomerular Growth (Experiment No. 1)

	50% Protein (n = 6)	6% Protein (n = 6)
Kidney weight (g)	1.18 ± 0.04*	0.90 ± 0.02
Kidney weight/body weight (×10^{-3})	4.28 ± 0.11*	3.48 ± 0.11
Glomerular number (×10^3)	23.6 ± 0.7	24.2 ± 1.6
Glomerular volume (μm^3 × 10^3)	662 ± 109*	483 ± 80
Glomerular protein (ng/glomerulus)	60.0 ± 7.3*	36.5 ± 7.2
Glomerular RNA (ng/glomerulus)	2.3 ± 0.2	1.7 ± 0.2
Glomerular DNA (ng/glomerulus)	10.2 ± 1.1	8.0 ± 1.5
Glomerular protein/DNA	5.8 ± 0.2*	4.5 ± 0.3

Note. Values are means ± SEM.
* $P < 0.05$ versus 6% protein.

Whole-kidney, glomerular, and tubular growth parameters. Final right kidney weights in the rats fed high-protein diets were 1.18 ± 0.04 g versus 0.90 ± 0.02 g in the low-protein–fed animals ($P < 0.05$) (Table 1; Fig 1, left). Right kidney weight to body weight ratios in the high- and low-protein–fed rats were 4.28 ± 0.11 10^{-3} and 3.48 ± 0.11 × 10^{-3}, respectively ($P < 0.05$). Thus, 6 days of high-protein feeding induced a 20% to 30% increase in renal mass.

As anticipated, glomerular number was unchanged between the high- and low-protein groups (23.6 ± 0.7 × 10^3 glomeruli/kidney *v* 24.2 ± 1.6 × 10^3 glomeruli/kidney, P = NS). A significant increase in glomerular protein content (60.0 ± 7.3 ng/glomeruli *v* 36.5 ± 7.2 ng/glomeruli, $P < 0.05$) and a numerical but not statistically significant increase in RNA (2.3 ± 0.2 ng/glomeruli *v* 1.7 ± 0.2 ng/glomeruli, P = NS) and

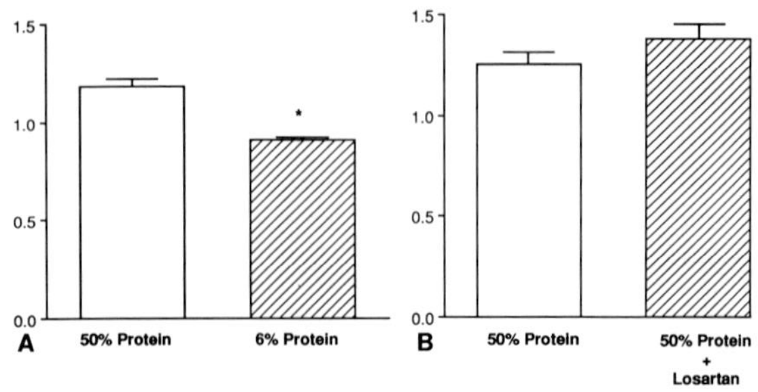

Fig 1. (A) Wet kidney weight on a 50% protein diet was higher than on a 6% diet ($P < 0.05$). (B) Wet kidney weights were no different with and without the AII antagonist losartan on a 50% protein diet.

DNA (10.2 ± 1.1 ng/glomeruli *v* 8.0 ± 1.5 ng/glomeruli, *P* = NS) content occurred with high-protein feeding. Similarly, protein to DNA ratios were significantly greater in the high-protein–fed rats (5.5 ± 0.2 *v* 4.51 ± 0.3, $P < 0.05$), indicating the presence of dietary protein-induced glomerular hypertrophy.

Glomerular volumes were significantly increased by high-protein feeding (662 ± 109 $\mu m^3 \times 10^3$ *v* 483 ± 80 $\mu m^3 \times 10^3$, $P < 0.05$; Fig 2, left panel), confirming the results of prior experiments. Cortical proximal tubular epithelial volume densities were similar (high-protein: 0.50 ± 0.03 *v* low-protein: 0.49 ± 0.01; *P* = NS), indicating proportional growth of the proximal tubule relative to total cortical growth and an increase in absolute proximal epithelial volume. Total cortical volume densities were similarly unchanged (high-protein: 0.86 ± 0.04 *v* low-protein: 0.78 ± 0.03; *P* = NS).

Experiment No. 2

General parameters. Pair feeding assured identical intakes of the high-protein food in both

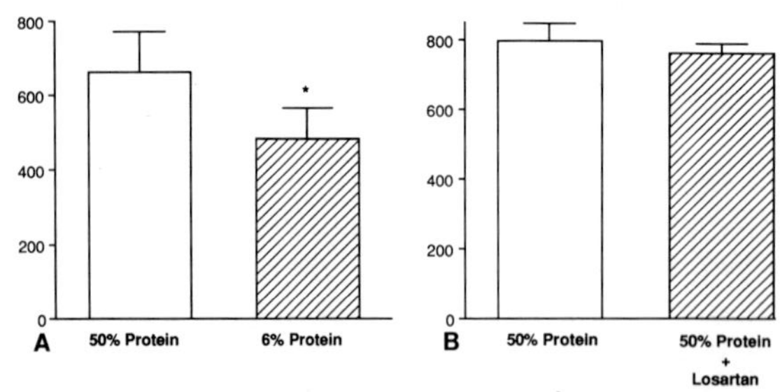

Fig 2. (A) Glomerular volume on a 50% protein diet was higher than on a 6% diet ($P < 0.05$). (B) Glomerular volumes were no different with and without the AII antagonist losartan on a 50% protein diet.

Table 2. Effect of Angiotensin II Receptor Blockade With Losartan on Dietary Protein-Induced Renal and Glomerular Growth (Experiment No. 2)

	Losartan (n = 5)	Control (n = 5)
Kidney weight (g)	1.38 ± 0.07	1.26 ± 0.06
Kidney weight/body weight ($\times 10^{-3}$)	4.88 ± 0.19	4.63 ± 0.21
Glomerular number ($\times 10^3$)	23.6 ± 1.6	25.5 ± 1.9
Glomerular volume ($\mu m^3 \times 10^3$)	758 ± 32	795 ± 53
Glomerular protein (ng/glomerulus)	66.1 ± 4.5	69.1 ± 8.6
Glomerular RNA (ng/glomerulus)	1.9 ± 0.1	1.8 ± 0.1
Glomerular DNA (ng/glomerulus)	12.1 ± 0.5	10.8 ± 1.0
Glomerular protein/DNA	5.5 ± 0.2	6.3 ± 0.4

Note. Values are means ± SEM. No statistical differences were noted.

groups (15.2 ± 0.1 g/d). Body weights increased similarly in both losartan-treated and control rats during high-protein feeding (losartan group: 254 ± 6 g to 283 ± 7 g; control group: 251 ± 7 g to 272 ± 5 g; $P < 0.05$, both groups). Losartan (mean dose, 33 mg/kg/d)-treated animals had a lower average SBP on the final experimental day (losartan group: 96 ± 2 mm Hg *v* control group: 127 ± 9 mm Hg; $P < 0.05$).

Whole-kidney, glomerular, and tubular growth parameters. Final right kidney weights (losartan group: 1.38 ± 0.07 g *v* control group: 1.26 ± 0.06 g; *P* = NS) and right kidney to body weight ratios were not different between the losartan-treated and control rats (4.88 ± 0.19 $\times 10^{-3}$ *v* 4.63 ± 0.21 $\times 10^{-3}$, respectively; *P* = NS) (Table 2; Fig 1, right panel). Glomerular numbers were similar between groups (losartan group: 23.6 ± 1.6 $\times 10^3$ glomeruli/kidney *v* control group: 25.5 ± 1.9 $\times 10^3$ glomeruli/kidney; *P* = NS). One pair of animals was eliminated from all end-point determinations due to excess tubular fragment contamination of the glomerular samples noted during the counting of glomeruli. Glomerular protein content was unaffected by losartan treatment (losartan group: 66.1 ± 4.5 ng/glomeruli *v* control group: 69.1 ± 8.6 ng/glomeruli; *P* = NS). Nucleic acid composition was similarly unaffected (RNA: 1.9 ± 0.1 ng/glomeruli v 1.8 ng/glomeruli, P = NS; DNA: 12.1 $\pm$ 0.5 ng/glomeruli v 10.9 $\pm$ 1.0 ng/glomeruli, P = NS).

Morphometric evaluation of glomerular and cortical proximal tubular compartments demonstrated no effect of losartan on achieved growth. Glomerular volumes were not different between groups (losartan group: 758 $\pm$ 32 $\mu m^3 \times 10^3$ v control group: 795 $\pm$ 53 $\mu m^3 \times 10^3$; P = NS; Fig 2, right), as were cortical proximal tubular epithelial densities (losartan group: 0.49 $\pm$ 0.02 v control group: 0.47 $\pm$ 0.05; P = NS). Total cortical densities were similarly unchanged (losartan group: 0.76 $\pm$ 0.03 v control group: 0.84 $\pm$ 0.03; P = NS). Thus, AII receptor antagonism failed to influence the size of the whole kidney, glomerulus, or cortical proximal tubular epithelium in rats on a high-protein diet.

Experiment No. 3

General parameters. Food intakes for both groups were fixed by pair feeding at the level used in the other two experiments (15.2 $\pm$ 0 g/d). Body weights increased significantly in both enalapril-treated and control groups during high-protein feeding (enalapril group: 259 $\pm$ 5 to 286 $\pm$ 6 g; control group: 261 $\pm$ 4 to 281 $\pm$ 4 g; $P < 0.05$, both groups). Enalapril (mean dose, 8.1 mg/kg/d)-treated animals demonstrated a significant reduction in SBP measured on the final experimental day (enalapril group: 102 $\pm$ 5 mm Hg v control group: 124 $\pm$ 5 mm Hg; $P < 0.05$).

Whole-kidney, glomerular, and tubular growth parameters. Final right kidney weights were no different between groups (enalapril group: 1.25 $\pm$ 0.03; control group: 1.23 $\pm$ 0.03 g; $P < 0.05$) and right kidney to body weight ratios (enalapril group: 4.31 $\pm$ 0.09 $\times 10^3$ v 4.38 $\pm$ 0.10 $\times 10^{-3}$; P = NS) were unchanged by enalapril treatment (Table 3). Glomerular number was similar in both groups (enalapril group: 23.4 $\pm$ 1.4 $\times 10^3$ v control group: 23.5 $\pm$ 0.9 $\times 10^3$). Glomerular protein content (98.2 $\pm$ 9.5 ng/glomeruli v 96.6 $\pm$ 13.0 ng/glomeruli, P = NS), RNA content (1.3 $\pm$ 0.1 ng/glomeruli v 1.7 $\pm$ 0.1 ng/glomeruli; P = NS), and DNA content (11.7 $\pm$ 0.8 ng/glomeruli v 11.7 $\pm$ 1.1 ng/glomeruli; P = NS) were not different between the two groups. Glomerular volume determination similarly revealed no effect of converting enzyme inhibitor (enalapril group: 768 $\pm$ 15 $\mu m^3 \times 10^3$ v control group: 841 $\pm$ 57 $\mu m^3 \times 10^3$; P = NS). Given the absence of an effect on cortical proximal tubular growth of the AII receptor antagonist in experiment no. 2, morphometry of the cortical tubules was not performed in experiment no. 3. Thus, angiotensin-converting enzyme (ACE) inhibition failed to inhibit dietary protein-induced growth of at least the glomerulus and whole kidney.

Table 3. Effect of Angiotensin Converting Enzyme Inhibition With Enalapril on Dietary Protein-Induced Renal and Glomerular Growth (Experiment No. 3)

	Enalapril (n = 6)	Control (n = 6)
Kidney weight (g)	1.25 $\pm$ 0.03	1.23 $\pm$ 0.03
Kidney weight/body weight ($\times 10^{-3}$)	4.31 $\pm$ 0.09	4.38 $\pm$ 0.10
Glomerular number ($\times 10^3$)	23.4 $\pm$ 1.4	23.5 $\pm$ 0.9
Glomerular volume ($\mu m^3 \times 10^3$)	768 $\pm$ 15	841 $\pm$ 57
Glomerular protein (ng/glomerulus)	98.2 $\pm$ 9.5	96.6 $\pm$ 13.0
Glomerular RNA (ng/glomerulus)	1.3 $\pm$ 0.1	1.7 $\pm$ 0.1
Glomerular DNA (ng/glomerulus)	11.6 $\pm$ 0.8	11.9 $\pm$ 1.3
Glomerular protein/DNA	8.3 $\pm$ 0.3	7.9 $\pm$ 0.4

Note. Values are means $\pm$ SEM. No statistical differences were noted.

DISCUSSION

This study aimed to test in vivo the dependence of dietary protein-induced renal growth on AII. The co-existence of rapidly inducible renal growth and the activation of the renin-angiotensin system during high dietary protein intake suggested a possible causal link between the growth and RAS activation. Thus, AII blockade during dietary protein-induced renal growth should permit dissection of an AII-specific renal growth effect. Given the potential difficulty of detecting a large change within low-density anatomic structures (eg, glomerulus) when performing whole-organ measurements (whole kidney weights and composition) we have also attempted a more precise compartmental assessment of renal growth.

As expected, the first experiment demonstrated a sizable effect of high dietary protein intake on whole-kidney, glomerular, and tubular growth. Glomerular growth, evidenced by increases in glomerular volume and protein/glomerulus, appears to be hypertrophic as DNA/glomerulus was not different between groups and protein to DNA ratios were significantly increased in the high-protein–fed group. Cortical proximal tubular hypertrophy paralleled both total cortical and total kidney growth as their fractional volumes remained constant. Treatment with losartan, a type 1 AII receptor antagonist, at vasoactive doses failed to attenuate dietary protein-induced whole-kidney growth (as assessed by kidney weights), suggesting that AII is not a critical factor for the increase in whole organ mass. Examination of the glomerulus and cortical proximal tubule, compartments known to express the greatest density of AII receptors, similarly failed to reveal an AII-dependent growth effect. Further confirmation of the failure of AII blockade to attenuate dietary protein-induced growth derives from the third experiment, as the ACE inhibitor enalapril also caused no modification of whole-kidney or glomerular growth. Thus, it appears that AII is not an essential factor for high-protein–induced renal growth, at least at the levels of kidney structure studied. Of course, it remains possible that isolated microcompartmental effects (for example, within the mesangium, earliest proximal tubule, or vasa recta [sites known to express AII receptors]) occurred in response to AII blockade and exceeded the detection limits of the methods used.

A large number of experiments performed on cultured renal cells in vitro demonstrate growth-promoting actions of AII. In cultured human fetal mesangial cells AII provoked a mitogenic response in a dose-dependent, receptor-mediated fashion, yet the growth effect was largely attenuated in adult phenotype mesangial cells.[8] Both hyperplastic and hypertropic effects have been noted previously in mesangial cells, effects that appear to be dependent on culture media conditions.[15,16] In primary renal rabbit proximal tubular cells, AII potentiates the hypertropic response to epidermal growth factor, although no hypertrophic or hyperplastic effect of AII alone was demonstrated.[17] Furthermore, Wolf and Nielson, in a differentiated mouse proximal tubular cell line, have demonstrated a hypertrophic effect of AII within a narrow but physiologically meaningful concentration range with coincident protooncogene activation.[9] Of note, this growth-promoting effect seemed dependent on relatively high glucose concentrations in the medium.[18]

Evidence for the growth-promoting effects of AII in nonrenal tissue is also abundant and largely, but not entirely, derived from cell culture systems in vitro. Angiotensin II is a mitogen for cultured endothelial and adrenocortical cells.[19,20] Hypertrophic and/or hyperplastic growth of cultured rat and human vascular smooth muscle cells can be induced by AII.[21,22] This response in vascular smooth muscle is independent of intracellular alkalinization or activation of Na^+/H^+ exchange, but is dependent on mobilization of intracellular Ca^+ and protein kinase C activation.[23,24] In vivo blockade of AII formation by an ACE inhibitor reduces the vascular smooth muscle hypertrophy that occurs in SHR rats and blunts the myointimal proliferative response following vascular injury, effects independent of the antihypertensive action of these drugs as similar reductions in BP by other agents have minimal effect.[25,26] In addition, independent of BP reduction, ACE inhibition decreases the cardiac hypertrophy of chronic hypertension and aortic banding.[27] In cultured cardiac myocytes, AII increases total protein and protein synthesis, an effect blocked by AII antagonism.[28]

In contrast to the in vitro studies, the renal growth effects of AII in vivo have yielded inconsistent results. Enalapril failed to prevent whole-kidney and glomerular growth of the mature adult rat ingesting standard diets, although an inhibitory effect on maturational glomerular growth in young, immature rats was demonstrated.[29] However, captopril failed to alter the increase in renal mass after simple contralateral nephrectomy in adult rats.[31] Furthermore, dietary protein-induced renal growth is blunted in weanling rats but somatic growth was also retarded.[30] Chronic subcutaneous AII infusion at pressor doses also did not induce whole-kidney or glomerular growth in the adult rat.[32] However, acute infusion of AII into the renal artery stimulates the expression of the protooncogenes c-*fos* and Egr-1, cellular events known to precede a variety of growth states.[33] Angiotensin-converting enzyme inhibition imposed on the remnant kidney model of chronic renal disease and streptozotocin-induced diabetes has been reported to limit glomerular growth[34] and whole-kidney growth, respectively.[35] However, subsequent studies of diabetic rats receiving either captopril or another effective antihypertensive regimen (''triple therapy'': hydralazine, hydrochlorothiazide, reserpine) yielded similar inhibition of diabetic glomerular enlargement in both groups.[36] A recent report of RAS blockade in the remnant kidney model failed to demonstrate an effect on glomerular size, but did note a small inhibition of whole-kidney enlargement compared with triple therapy.[37] Activation and blockade of the RAS respectfully enhance and suppress growth of experimental, chemically induced renal cysts.[38] Thus, attenuation of renal growth in vivo by AII blockade seems to occur in some states but not others and may even be nonspecifically related to antihypertensive actions. Indeed, observation of an effect may depend in part on hemodynamic actions of such blockade as conditions in which growth inhibition has been reported (remnant kidney and diabetes) are associated, in the absence of AII blockade, with greater elevations in glomerular pressure than either high-protein feeding in normal rats or simple unilateral nephrectomy, reported circumstances in which AII blockade failed to alter renal growth.[34,35,39,40] Furthermore, not only the degree of hemodynamic perturbation but the severity of other intrarenal adaptations and pathology (transport and metabolic changes, ontogeny, scarring, cystogenesis, cellular invasion, etc) may condition the susceptibility of renal growth and remodeling to AII blockade.

Ineffectiveness of blockade seems an unlikely explanation of our results for several reasons. First, the doses used for both drugs were similar to or even greater than those used by other investigators to effect changes in functional and structural parameters, including growth, in other conditions in vivo.[29,30,34,35,37,41] Second, the basal levels of arterial pressure were depressed by both the ACE inhibitor and the AII receptor antagonist, indicating a hemodynamic effect of the drugs. Finally, we confirmed in preliminary studies that the pressor action of pharmacologic amounts of exogenous AII was markedly blunted by losartan.

When interpreting our results in light of the discordant literature, several other potential confounding factors also can be considered. The hemodynamic actions of AII blockade may have activated vascular responses and these, by their own growth-promoting effects, may have offset any action of AII blockade. For example, levels of vasopressin and endothelin,[42,43] both known to possess vasoconstrictive and renal growth-promoting properties, may increase in response to relative hypotension, perhaps negating any growth-inhibitory effect of AII blockade. On the other hand, endothelium-derived relaxing factor and atrial natriuretic factor[44,45] may have been inhibited in response to the vasodilation of AII blockade with consequent deletion of their growth inhibitory action, contributing to net growth in the AII-blocked state. While conceivable, we view these potential confounding scenarios as not only speculative but unlikely explanations of our results. However, we do acknowledge that if the RAS participates in protein-induced growth, it likely does so in conjunction with other factors. That is, dietary protein-induced renal growth probably represents a complex growth state under the influence of several redundant growth regulators. Thus, the ablation of one system alone may fail to alter net growth. In addition, other states of renal growth or pathology may depend more on the RAS. In any case, AII is not a necessary factor in dietary protein-induced renal growth in normal adult rats.

ADDENDUM

Despite normal to suppressed levels of renin activity in chronic renal disease, multiple lines of evidence suggest a role for the RAS, especially its intrarenal expression, in several critical aspects of this condition.[46] Alterations in the distribution and control of components of the renal RAS could account for localized areas of activation of this system. Renal scarring may be particularly important as a major stimulus to renin synthesis in the diseased kidney. Whereas both intrarenal and systemic hypertension may depend in part on actions of the RAS, other nonhemodynamic actions of the RAS may also contribute to the adaptation of residual nephrons as well as their progressive injury.

ACKNOWLEDGMENT

The authors thank R. D. Smith, PhD (DuPont, Wilmington, DE) for providing losartan and J. Burkhart for typing the manuscript.

REFERENCES

1. Paller MS, Hostetter TH: Dietary protein increases plasma renin and reduces pressor reactivity to angiotensin II. Am J Physiol 251:F34-F39, 1986

2. Fernández-Repollet E, Tapia E, Martínez-Maldonado M: Effects of angiotensin-converting enzyme inhibition on altered renal hemodynamics induced by low protein diet in the rat. J Clin Invest 80:1045-1049, 1987

3. Kapoor SC, Krishna GG: Protein-induced modulation of renin secretion is mediated by prostaglandins. Am J Physiol 260:F688-F694, 1991

4. Rosenberg ME, Chmielewski D, Hostetter TH: Effect of dietary protein on rat renin and angiotensinogen gene expression. J Clin Invest 85:144-1149, 1990

5. Halliburton IW: The effect of unilateral nephrectomy and of diet on the composition of the kidney, in Nowinski WW, Gross RJ (eds): Compensatory Renal Hypertrophy. New York, NY, Academic, 1969, pp 102-130

6. Brenner BM, Meyer TW, Hostetter TH: Dietary protein intake and the progressive nature of kidney disease: The role of hemodynamically mediated glomerular sclerosis in the pathogenesis of progressive glomerular sclerosis in aging, renal ablation, and intrinsic renal disease. N Engl J Med 307:652-659, 1982

7. Hostetter TH: Human response to a meat meal. Am J Physiol 250:F613-F618, 1986

8. Ray PE, Aguilera G, Kopp JB, Horikoshi S, Klotman PE: Angiotensin II receptor-mediated proliferation of cultured human fetal mesangial cells. Kidney Int 40:764-771, 1991

9. Wolf G, Neilson EG: Angiotensin II induces cellular hypertrophy in cultured murine proximal tubular cells. Am J Physiol 259:F768-F777, 1990

10. Smith LJ, Rosenberg ME, Correa-Rotter R, Hostetter TH: The renin-angiotensin system in chronic renal disease, in Mitch WE (ed): The Progressive Nature of Renal Disease. New York, NY, Churchill Livingstone, 1992, pp 55-76

11. Hirose K, Osterby R, Nozawa M, Gundersen HJG: Development of glomerular lesions in experimental long-term diabetes in the rat. Kidney Int 21:689-695, 1982

12. Nath KA, Salahudeen AK: Induction of renal growth and injury in the intact rat kidney by dietary deficiency of antioxidants. J Clin Invest 86:1179-1192, 1990

13. Fleck A, Munro HN: The precision of ultraviolet absorption measurements in the Schmidt-Thannhauser procedure for nucleic acid estimation. Biochem Biophys Acta 55:571-583, 1962

14. Giles K, Meyers A: An improved diphenylamine method for the estimation of deoxyribonucleic acid. Nature 206:93-96, 1965

15. Fujiwara Y, Takawa T, Shin S, Ochi S, Fukunaga M, Orita Y, Kamada T: Angiotensin II stimulates mesangial cell growth through phosphoinositide cascade. Kidney Int 35:172, 1989 (abstr)

16. Homma T, Hoover RL, Ichikawa I, Harris RC: Angiotensin II induces hypertrophy and stimulates collagen production in cultured rat glomerular mesangial cells. Clin Res 38:358, 1990 (abstr)

17. Norman J, Badie-Dezfooly B, Nord ET, Kurtz I, Schlosser J, Ghaudhari A, Fine LG: EGF-induced mitogenesis in proximal tubular cells: Potentiation by angiotensin II. Am J Physiol 253:299-309, 1987

18. Wolf G, Neilson EG, Goldfarb S, Ziyadeh FN: The influence of glucose concentration of angiotensin-II induced hypertrophy of proximal tubular cells in culture. Biochem Biophys Res Commun 176:902-909, 1991

19. Simonian MH, Gill GN: Regulation of deoxyribonucleic acid synthesis in bovine adrenocortical cells in culture. Endocrinology 104:588-595, 1979

20. Bagby SP, Holden W: Angiotensin II stimulates proliferation of aortic endothelial cells. Clin Res 36:259A, 1988 (abstr)

21. Campbell-Boswell M, Robertson AL, Jr: Effects of angiotensin II and vasopressin on human smooth muscle cells in vitro. Exp Mol Path 35:265-276, 1981

22. Geisterfer AAT, Peach MJ, Owens GK: Angiotensin II induces hypertrophy, not hyperplasia, of cultured rat aortic smooth muscle cells. Circ Res 62:749-756, 1988

23. Kawahara Y, Sunako M, Tsuda T, Fukuzaki H, Fukumoto Y, Takai Y: Angiotensin II induces expression of the *c-fos* gene through protein kinase C activation and calcium ion mobilization in cultured vascular smooth muscle cells. Biochem Biophys Res Commun 150:52-59, 1988

24. Taubman MB, Berk BC, Izumo S, Tsuda T, Alexander RW, Nadaz-Ginard B: Angiotensin II induces *c-fos* mRNA in aortic smooth muscle. Role of calcium mobilization and protein kinase C activation. J Biol Chem 264:526-530, 1988

25. Owens GK: Influence of blood pressure on development of aortic medial smooth muscle hypertrophy in spontaneously hypertensive rats. Hypertension 9:178-187, 1987

26. Powell JS, Clozel J-P, Muller RKM, Kuhn H, Hefti F, Hosang M, Baumgartner HR: Inhibitors of angiotensin-converting enzyme prevent myointimal proliferation after vascular injury. Science 245:186-188, 1989

27. Morgan HE, Baker KM: Cardiac hypertrophy. Mechanical, neural, and endocrine dependence. Circulation 83:13-25, 1991

28. Aceto JF, Baker KM: [Sar^1]angiotensin II receptor-mediated stimulation of protein synthesis in chick heart cells. Am J Physiol 258:H806-H813, 1990

29. Fogo A, Yoshida Y, Yared A, Ichikawa I: Importance of angiogenic action of angiotensin II in the glomerular growth of maturing kidneys. Kidney Int 38:1068-1074, 1990

30. Tufro-McReddie A, Arrizurieta EE, Brocca S, Gomez RA: Dietary protein modulates intrarenal distribution of renin and its mRNA during development. Am J Physiol 32:F427-F435, 1992

31. Valentin J-P, Ribstein J, Mimran A: Influence of angiotensin converting-enzyme inhibition on the renal compensatory hypertrophy following uninephrectomy in the rat. Med Sci Res 20:207-208, 1992

32. Miller PL, Rennke HG, Meyer TW: Glomerular hypertrophy accelerates hypertensive glomerular injury in rats. Am J Physiol 261:459-465, 1991

33. Rosenberg ME, Hostetter TH: Effect of angiotensin II on early growth genes in the kidney. J Am Soc Nephrol 1:426, 1990 (abstr)

34. Anderson S, Meyer TW, Rennke HG, Brenner BM: Control of glomerular hypertension limits glomerular injury in rats with reduced renal mass. J Clin Invest 76:612-619, 1985

35. Zatz R, Dunn BR, Meyer TW, Anderson S, Rennke HG, Brenner BM: Prevention of diabetic glomerulopathy by pharmacological amelioration of glomerular capillary hypertension. J Clin Invest 77:1925-1930, 1986

36. Anderson S, Rennke HG, Garcia DL, Brenner BM: Short and long-term effects of antihypertensive therapy in the diabetic rat. Kidney Int 36:526-536, 1989

37. Lafayette RA, Mayer G, Meyer TW: Angiotensin II receptor blockade limits glomerular injury in rats with reduced renal mass. J Clin Invest 90:766-771, 1992

38. Torres VE, Berndt TJ, Okamura M, et al: Mechanisms affecting the development of renal cystic disease induced by diphenylthiazole. Kidney Int 33:1130-1139, 1988

39. Ichikawa I, Purkerson ML, Klahr S, et al: Mechanism of reduced glomerular filtration rate in chronic malnutrition. J Clin Invest 65:982-988, 1980

40. Deen WM, Maddox DA, Robertson CR, et al: Dynamics of glomerular filtration in the rat. VII. Response to reduced renal mass. Am J Physiol 227:556-562, 1974

41. Hutchison FN, Webster SK: Effect of ANG II receptor antagonism on albuminuria and renal function in passive Heymann nephritis. Am J Physiol 263:F311-F318, 1992

42. Ganz MB, Pekar SK, Perfetto ME, et al: Arginine vasopressin promotes growth of rat glomerular mesangial cells in culture. Am J Physiol 255:898-906, 1988

43. Simonson MS, Wann S, Mené P, et al: Endothelin stimulates phospholipase C, Na^+/H^+ exchange, c-*fos* expression and mitogenesis in rat mesangial cells. J Clin Invest 83:708-712, 1989

44. Garg UC, Hassid A: Inhibition of rat mesangial cell mitogenesis by nitric-oxide generating vasodilators. Am J Physiol 257:60-66, 1989

45. Johnson A, Lermioglu F, Garg UC, et al: A novel biological effect of atrial natriuretic hormone: Inhibition of mesangial cell mitogenesis. Biochem Biophys Res Commun 152:893-897, 1988

46. Rosenberg ME, Smith LJ, Correa-Rotter R, Hostetter TH: The paradox of the renin-angiotensin system in chronic renal disease. Kidney Int 45:403-410, 1994

Effective Antihypertensive Treatment Postpones Renal Insufficiency in Diabetic Nephropathy

Hans-Henrik Parving, MD, Ulla M. Smidt, Eva Hommel, MD, Elisabeth R. Mathiesen, MD, Peter Rossing, MD, Flemming Nielsen, MD, and Mari-Anne Gall, MD

● The effect of long-term, aggressive, antihypertensive treatment on kidney function in diabetic nephropathy was studied prospectively in 11 insulin-dependent diabetic patients (mean age, 30 years). Renal function was assessed every 4 months by measurement of glomerular filtration rate (GFR) (single-bolus ^{51}Cr-EDTA technique) and by albuminuria (radial immunodiffusion). During the median pretreatment period of 2.4 years (range, 1.9 to 5.5 years), the GFR decreased significantly and albuminuria and the arterial blood pressure increased significantly. During the 9.7-year (range, 2.8 to 10.4 year) period of antihypertensive treatment with metoprolol, hydralazine, and furosemide, the arterial blood pressure decreased from 143/96 mm Hg to 130/84 mm Hg and albuminuria decreased from 1,038 μg/min to 547 μg/min. The rate of decline in GFR decreased from 10.7 mL/min/yr (range, 5.3 to 17.5 mL/min/yr) before treatment to 2.5 mL/min/yr (range, 0.5 to 4.8 mL/min/yr) during treatment. The rate of decline in GFR is significantly smaller during the last 6 years compared with the first 3 years in patients who received long-term antihypertensive treatment (≥9 years). One patient died from acute myocardial infarction (GFR, 46 mL/min/1.73 m^2). Effective antihypertensive treatment postpones renal insufficiency in diabetic nephropathy.

INDEX WORDS: Blood pressure; antihypertensive therapy; kidney function; diabetic nephropathy.

DIABETIC nephropathy is the single most important cause of end-stage renal disease in the Western world, accounting for more than 25% of all end-stage renal disease in adults.[1] The cost of care for renal failure in the United States currently exceeds $1.8 billion a year for diabetic nephropathy alone, and the amount is rapidly rising. Diabetic nephropathy is the main cause of the increased morbidity and mortality in insulin-dependent diabetes mellitus (IDDM) patients.[2-6] The excess mortality of the IDDM patients with clinical nephropathy is 70 to 100 times that of the age- and sex-matched backgroundpopulation and is due to an enormous excess of cardiovascular mortality (40 times the age-matched population) and end-stage renal disease (hundreds of times the age-matched population).[5,7]

The aims of our prospective study, which began in 1976, were to determine the initial clinical course of diabetic nephropathy[8] and to evaluate the long-term effect of antihypertensive treatment on the glomerular filtration rate (GFR) and albuminuria in hypertensive IDDM patients with diabetic nephropathy. Interim reports of this "self-controlled" study were published in 1983 and 1987.[9,10] The final analysis after 10 years' experience with antihypertensive treatment in diabetic nephropathy is presented.

RESEARCH DESIGN AND METHODS

We examined the records of all IDDM patients with proteinuria (positive "Albustix") visiting the outpatient clinic at Steno Memorial Hospital between June 1976 and January 1978. All patients (n = 18) aged less than 41 years with persistent proteinuria, onset of diabetes before age 31 years, serum creatinine less than 150 μmol/L, no antihypertensive treatment including diuretics, and no blindness were invited to join the study. Two women and one man declined to participate and one woman emigrated after the first investigation. The remaining 14 IDDM patients with persistent proteinuria were initially enrolled in our prospective study of the clinical course of diabetic nephropathy, as described previously.[8] One man left the study when he was admitted to a nursing home after a stroke, and another man was excluded because diabetic nephropathy was likely not to have been the cause of this renal disease.[9]

The remaining 12 patients were investigated (Table 1) after they had given their fully informed consent. The experimental design was approved by the local ethical committee. None of the patients received other drugs except case no. 11; she was using phenytoin (300 to 400 mg/d) for epilepsy. They had a normal diabetic diet containing 45% to 55% carbohydrate, 30% to 35% fat, and 15% to 20% protein throughout the study, and none of the patients had their intake of salt or protein restricted.

Metoprolol, furosemide, and hydralazine were used as antihypertensive drugs (Table 1). One patient (case no. 5) did not receive metoprolol because of a complete lack of hypoglycemic warning signs, and treatment with metoprolol was stopped after 2 years in case no. 3 because the patient suffered from two hypoglycemic attacks that required treatment with intravenous glucose. According to the protocol of our prospective study, antihypertensive treatment was initiated after a control period of at least 23 months if repeated recordings showed a diastolic blood pressure ≥100 mm Hg (eight patients) or if the patient had a sustained diastolic blood pressure of ≥90 mm Hg preceded by an increase in mean arterial blood pressure of ≥10 mm Hg during the past 2 years (four patients). The goal for the antihypertensive treatment was a stable reduction in mean arterial blood pressure (diastolic plus a third of the pulse amplitude) of at least 10 mm Hg.

All investigations were carried out on 1 day between 9 AM

Table 1. Clinical Data at Baseline From 12 Patients Who Had Insulin-Dependent Diabetes and Diabetic Nephropathy

Case No.	Sex	Age (yr)	Duration of Diabetes (yr)	Retinopathy	Antihypertensive Treatment (Dose in mg)
1	M	26	15	Proliferative	Metoprolol (200), hydralazine (100), furosemide (120)
2	M	35	6	None	Metoprolol (300), hydralazine (125), furosemide (200)
3	M	40	18	Background	Metoprolol (750), hydralazine (100), furosemide (120)
4	M	34	22	Proliferative	Metoprolol (400), hydralazine (200), furosemide (500)
5	F	20	16	Proliferative	Prazosin (4), spironolactone (50), furosemide (500)
6	M	24	12	Proliferative	Metoprolol (150), hydralazine (75), furosemide (360)
7	F	19	6	None	Metoprolol (400), hydralazine (150), furosemide (500)
8	F	31	21	Proliferative	Metoprolol (100), hydralazine (100), furosemide (80)
9	M	34	12	Background	Metoprolol (100), hydralazine (75), furosemide (120)
10	M	28	27	Proliferative	Metoprolol (300), hydralazine (200), furosemide (240)
11	F	39	25	Proliferative	Metoprolol (100), hydralazine (75), furosemide (1,000), spironolactone (100)
12	M	36	13	Background	Metoprolol (200), hydralazine (100), furosemide (500)

and 1 PM. Patients had their normal breakfast and morning insulin dose before the studies, during which they were resting in a supine position. The investigations were carried out four to 13 times (mean, five times) over 1.9 to 5.5 years before antihypertensive treatment and nine to 35 times (mean, 27 times) during the subsequent 2.8 to 10.4 years of treatment.

To measure GFR we gave the patients a single intravenous injection of 100 μCi sodium chromate-51 edetic acid at 9 AM and determined the plasma radioactivity in venous blood samples taken from the other arm 180, 200, 220, and 240 minutes after the injection.[11,12] The small underestimation (10%) of ^{51}Cr-edetic acid clearance versus clearance of inulin was corrected for by multiplying the cromate clearance by 1·10.[12] The results were standardized for 1.73 m^2 body surface area using the patients' surface area at the start of the study throughout. The mean coefficient of variation in the glomerular filtration rate of each patient from day to day was 4% (precision).

Urinary albumin excretion was measured by radial immunodiffusion during the 4-hour clearance period.[13] The blood pressure was taken with a standard clinical sphygmomanometer (cuff 25 cm × 12 cm) on the right arm, the patient having been in the supine position for at least 10 minutes. The blood pressure was measured twice during each investigation and visit to the outpatient clinic. The diastolic blood pressure was taken to be the point at which the Korotkoff sounds disappeared (phase V).

The patient visited the clinic every 2 to 4 months during the investigation. At each visit the postprandial blood glucose concentration was measured (with a glucose oxidase method), along with glucosuria, albuminuria, blood pressure, and body weight, and the insulin dose and antihypertensive treatment were adjusted. Ophthalmoscopy was carried out on dilated pupils at least every 6 to 12 months.

Wilcoxon's nonparametric test for paired comparisons (two-tailed) was used. All the results, including the rate of decline in GFR before antihypertensive treatment, were compared with all those during effective treatment. The main results are given with 95% confidence intervals. The rate of decline in GFR (mL/min/yr) was calculated by linear regression analysis (least squares method). The stochastic variation in GFR during the individual observation periods was calculated as the residual standard deviation and expressed as a percentage of the corresponding GFR value. The values given are means ± SEM.

RESULTS

Arterial blood pressure and albuminuria showed progressive increases during the control period ($P < 0.01$), whereas significant and stable reductions occurred during the antihypertensive treatment period ($P < 0.01$; Table 2, Fig 1). The average blood pressure just before the start of antihypertensive treatment was 154/100 ± 4/2. Case no. 11 is discussed separately, as arterial blood pressure increased during treatment. In one patient (case no. 4) who died from acute myocardial infarction after 35 months of antihypertensive treatment, the kidney function was well preserved, GFR being 46 mL/min/1.73 m^2.

The rate of decline in GFR diminished in all 11 effectively treated patients (mean, 10.7 mL/min/yr [95% confidence interval, 8.1 to 13.3 mL/min/yr] to mean, 2.5 [95% confidence interval, 1.2 to 3.4 mL/min/yr]); the rate of decline in case no. 11 remained about the same owing to insufficient treatment. Figure 1 shows the mean course of blood pressure and kidney function in the nine patients who received long-term (≥9 years) antihypertensive treatment. The rate of decline in GFR was significantly smaller during the last 6 years compared with the first 3 years of

Table 2. Course of Arterial Blood Pressure, Glomerular Filtration Rate, and Albuminuria Before and During Antihypertensive Treatment for Diabetic Nephropathy

	Investigation Period (yr)		Blood Pressure (mm Hg)*		Decrease in GFR (mL/min/yr)		Albuminuria (μg/min)*	
Case No.	Before Treatment	During Treatment	Before Treatment	During Treatment	Before Treatment	During Treatment	Before Treatment	During Treatment
1	2.3	10.2	141/88 ± 3/3	132/75 ± 1/1	9.2	1.8	803 ± 248	762 ± 120
2	2.1	10.3	148/108 ± 3/3	127/88 ± 1/1	10.8	3.0	1,131 ± 90	711 ± 105
3	2.0	10.3	149/96 ± 5/3	134/84 ± 1/1	8.4	1.7	633 ± 60	213 ± 24
4†	2.4	2.8	149/108 ± 5/2	132/98 ± 2/1	17.0	4.8	1,466 ± 430	328 ± 40
5	1.9	10.4	143/101 ± 1/1	118/82 ± 2/1	17.5	1.9	285 ± 107	69 ± 10
6	3.2	9.0	140/91 ± 4/2	131/85 ± 2/2	13.0	3.2	1,094 ± 254	1,201 ± 139
7	3.0	9.7	126/90 ± 2/4	129/81 ± 2/1	10.3	1.0	1,021 ± 166	393 ± 52
8	2.4	10.0	142/90 ± 2/3	134/78 ± 2/1	9.8	3.2	546 ± 98	281 ± 22
9	2.7	9.7	151/98 ± 5/3	132/82 ± 2/1	5.3	2.4	782 ± 196	429 ± 115
10	1.9	9.0	153/98 ± 3/1	134/80 ± 2/2	7.3	3.7	2,007 ± 493	678 ± 80
11‡	3.4	8.7	151/85 ± 2/1	162/84 ± 2/1	7.7	6.7	1,791 ± 190	3,559 ± 150
12	5.5	6.1	133/90 ± 2/1	132/86 ± 2/1	8.9	0.5	1,649 ± 401	947 ± 132
Mean ± SEM	2.6 ± 0.3	8.9 ± 0.7	143/96 ± 3/2	130/84 ± 1/2	10.7 ± 1.2	2.5 ± 0.4	1,038 ± 155	547 ± 99
			$P < 0.01$		$P < 0.01$		$P < 0.01$	

Note. Values are presented as means ± SEM.

* Average of all determinations before and during treatment.

† Died from acute myocardial infarction after 35 months of antihypertensive treatment.

‡ Insufficiently treated and excluded from mean values and from analyses of effect of antihypertensive treatment on kidney function.

treatment ($P < 0.02$; Fig 1, Table 3). The residual standard deviation of GFR (%) before and during antihypertensive treatment was a median of 5.1 (range, 3.2 to 8.4) and a median of 8.6 (range, 5.0 to 12.4), respectively ($P = 0.05$). The mean blood pressure, albuminuria, and postprandial blood glucose remained rather stable during the treatment period.

Figure 2 shows the individual time courses of GFR in all 12 patients. There was a close linear correlation between GFR and time before treatment (mean, $r = 0.92$; range, 0.82 to 0.97), but this correlation was weaker and completely lacking in four patients (cases no. 1, 5, 7, and 12) during treatment (mean $r = 0.66$; range, 0.01 to 0.92). These four patients had the smallest rate of decline in GFR (<2 mL/min/yr). A pronounced reduction in GFR was observed shortly after starting antihypertensive therapy in cases no. 4, 6, 7, 10, and 12. The rate of decline in GFR remained practically identical before and during treatment in case no. 11. We did not find any significant correlation between the rate of decline in GFR and albuminuria, systolic, diastolic, or mean blood pressures either before or during antihypertensive therapy.

Table 4 compares the measured GFR values at the end of the antihypertensive treatment period with those predicted from the individual rates of decline in GFR before treatment.

Four patients were initially treated with bendrofluazide (2.5 to 10 mg/24 hr), but this was stopped when treatment with furosemide became necessary to control fluid retention and arterial blood pressure. Several patients suffered from intermittent peripheral edema, but only one (case

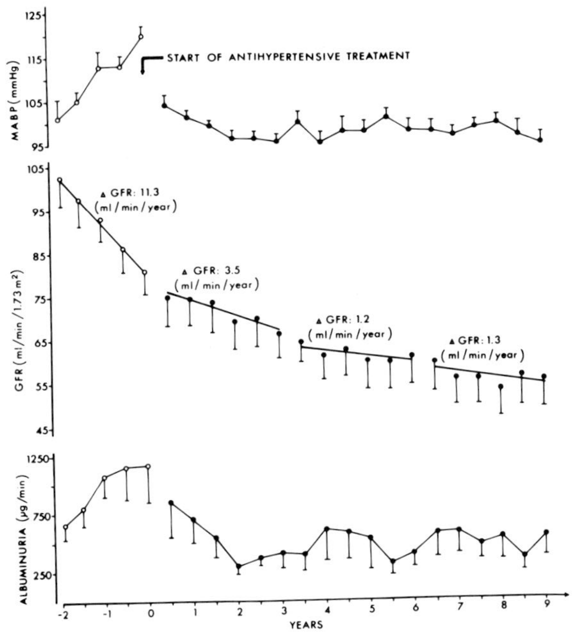

Fig 1. Average course of mean arterial blood pressure, GFR, and albumin before (○) and during (●) long-term effective antihypertensive treatment on nine IDDM patients suffering from diabetic nephropathy.

no. 11) had persistent edema during the whole treatment period. While frequent adjustment in diuretic therapy took place during the trial the dosage of the other antihypertensive drugs remained rather stable. The diet and body weight of the patients (65 ± 2 kg before treatment *v* 65.5 ± 2 kg during treatment) were unchanged. There were no alterations in average postprandial blood concentration (11.0 ± 1.0 mmol/L before *v* 10.3 ± 0.7 mmol/L during treatment) or daily insulin dose (36 ± 4 before treatment *v* 37 ± 2 IU during treatment) during the study. Retinopathy progressed in all 12 patients and 10 patients required laser treatment because of proliferative retinopathy (nine patients) and maculopathy (one patient).

DISCUSSION

Our long-term prospective trial has demonstrated that effective pharmacologic blood pressure lowering induces a reduction in albuminuria and in the rate of decline in GFR, thus postponing end-stage renal disease in IDDM patients suffering from diabetic nephropathy. This finding confirms and extends those of Mogensen[14] and Björck et al[15] and our own preliminary observations.[9,10,16] More important, the cumulative death rate was 9% (95% confidence interval, 0.2% to 41%) 13 years after onset of nephropathy in our patients, in contrast to previous reports of 50% to 77% 10 years after onset of nephropathy.[3,4,6] These three observational studies reflect the natural course of diabetic nephropathy in IDDM patients. Recently, two studies have demonstrated that the prognosis of diabetic nephropathy has improved during the past decade, largely because of effective antihypertensive treatment.[17,18]

We applied a self-controlled design because it was considered to be unethical to use a parallel, untreated hypertensive group of patients suffering from diabetic nephropathy and because prognostic evaluations can be made from the slope of decrease in GFR, as discussed in detail previously.[10] The validity of such a prediction depends on the precision of the method used for determining GFR and the stochastic variation in GFR. The mean coefficient of variation in GFR of each patient from day to day was 4% in our study applying plasma clearance of ^{51}Cr-edetic acid without urine collection. The mean coeffi-

Table 3. Course of Glomerular Filtration Rate, Mean Arterial Blood Pressure, Albuminuria, and Blood Gluclose Concentration During Long-term Antihypertensive Treatment for Diabetic Nephropathy in Nine Insulin-Dependent Diabetic Patients

Treatment Period (yr)	Decrease in GFR (mL/min/yr)	Mean Arterial Blood Pressure (mm Hg)	Albuminuria (μg/min)	Blood Glucose Concentration (mg/dL)
0-3	3.5 ± 0.8	98.5 ± 2	531 ± 107	182 ± 13
3-6	1.2 ± 0.5*	98.3 ± 1	472 ± 59	180 ± 11
6-9	1.3 ± 0.3*	97.7 ± 1	521 ± 33	172 ± 9

Note. Values are presented as means ± SE.
* $P < 0.02$ compared with treatment period 0 to 3 years.

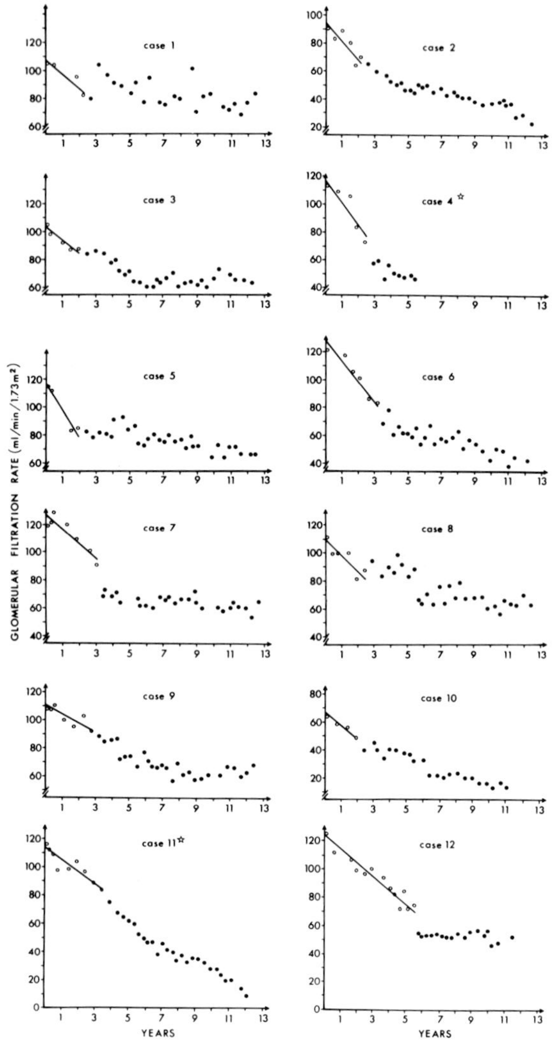

Fig 2. Individual courses of GFR before (○) and during (●) antihypertensive treatment in IDDM patients with diabetic nephropathy. Patient no. 4 died from acute myocardial infarction, and patient no. 11 was insufficiently treated.

cient of variation in GFR of each patient during the observation periods before and during antihypertensive treatment was 5.1% and 8.6%, respectively.

The coefficient of variation for renal clearance (n = 177) of ^{51}Cr-edetic acid, calculated from four urine collection periods of 40 minutes each, was as high as 20% in IDDM patients with diabetic nephropathy.[19] This is mainly due to residual urine, which is frequently (>30%) found in longstranding IDDM patients due to diabetic cystopathy.[20] We have demonstrated that correction for residual urine reduces the coefficient of variation in renal clearance from 23% to 6%.[21] The present GFR values are corrected for extrarenal loss of tracer (3.7 mL/min) and for the small underestimation (10%) versus clearance of inulin as described previously.[12] The present applied plasma clearance method overestimate GFR in case of severe edema; however, none of our patients had severe edema.

Approximately 40% (cases no. 4, 7, 10, and 12) of our patients showed a stepwise reduction in glomerular filtration rate ≥10% of GFR before treatment, at the start of aggressive antihypertensive treatment. We have demonstrated that the mechanism underlying the normal autoregulation of GFR (that is, the fairly constant GFR that occurs despite quite wide variations in perfusion

Table 4. Comparison of Glomerular Filtration Rate at End of Observation Period After Antihypertensive Treatment and Predicted Value After No Treatment in Insulin-Dependent Diabetic Patients With Diabetic Nephropathy

	GFR (mL/min/1.73 m²)	
Case No.	Predicted*	Actual
1	0	84
2	0	23
3	2	63
4	30	46
5	0	66
6	0	41
7	0	65
8	0	63
9	42	69
10	0	13
11†	24	9
12	24	52
Median	0	63
Range	0-42	13-84

$P < 0.01$

* Predicted from the rate of decline in GFR before treat ment, assuring unchanged slope during the whole observation period (median, 12.3 years).

† Patient in case no. 11 (insufficiently treated) is excluded
from the median value and from the analyses of effect of antihypertensive treatment on GFR.

pressure) is defective in IDDM patients suffering from diabetic nephropathy.[22] These observations might indicate that aggressive antihypertensive treatment would be ill advised and harmful to these patients. Fortunately, long-term observations clearly indicate that this is not the case, as discussed above.

We prescribed a normal diabetic diet to all our patients throughout the study. The diet was composed of 45% to 55% carbohydrate, 15% to 20% protein, and 30% to 35% fat. We did not apply dietary salt, phosphorous, or protein restriction unless GFR was below 20 mL/min (cases no. 10 and 11). We previously found a protein intake of 1.1 g/kg/d in our IDDM patients with nephropathy,[16] which is comparable to other studies in diabetic nephropathy.[23] Body weight and daily insulin dose remained unchanged during the study.

Improved metabolic control cannot explain the present results, as postprandial blood glucose concentrations remained unchanged during the study. Furthermore, long-term, near-normal blood glucose control achieved by continuous subcutaneous infusion of insulin does not reduce albuminuria or the rate of decline in GFR in diabetic nephropathy.[24]

In addition to the above-mentioned progression promoters in renal disease,[25] systemic and glomerular hypertension is suggested to play a major role in the initiation and progression of diabetic glomerulopathy.[26] Originally, Berkman and Rifkin[27] described the damaging effect of systemic hypertension on glomerular structure in a non–insulin-dependent diabetes mellitus patient suffering from unilateral renal artery stenosis. The unprotected kidney showed nodular diabetic glomerulosclerosis, while the stenotic kidney was protected and showed only ischemic lesions. Several studies have demonstrated a significant correlation between the rate of decline in GFR and diastolic blood pressure in IDDM patients suffering from diabetic nephropathy.[28,29] The same relationship also has been demonstrated in nondiabetic glomerulopathies.[30,31] The time interval between onset of persistent proteinuria and elevated serum creatinine above upper normal level is considerably shorter in hypertensive compared with normotensive IDDM patients with nephropathy.[32]

Hypertension may damage the kidney by vasoconstriction and by increasing arteriolar wall thickness, which leads to ischemia and subsequent glomerulopathy, or it may damage the glomeruli directly through increased glomerular capillary pressure. Raised systemic blood pressure is accompanied by raised pressure in the glomerular capillaries in numerous experimental models of hypertensive renal disease, including spontaneously hypertensive streptozotocin diabetic rats.[33,34] Elevated pressure has even been shown in normotensive insulin-treated streptozotocin diabetic rats.[35-37] Conversely, antihypertensive treatment or dietary protein restriction reduces glomerular hypertension and albuminuria, and mitigates the hemodynamically induced glomerular lesions.[38,39] More important, antihypertensive treatment reduces albuminuria, protects kidney function, and improves survival in IDDM patients with diabetic nephropathy, as in the present study.[9,10,14-18]

Experimental studies have suggested that all antihypertensive drugs are not equally effective in controlling progressive renal disease in rats with reduced renal mass or in insulin-treated streptozotocin diabetic rats.[33,39] Angiotensin-converting enzyme (ACE) inhibitors were more effective than triple therapy with reserpine, hydralazine, and hydrochlorothiazide, despite an equal reduction in systemic blood pressure. A recent meta-analysis of studies of long-term antihypertensive treatment in IDDM patients with diabetic nephropathy has revealed that the rate of decline in GFR was identical (4.4 mL/min/1.73 m^2) in patients given ACE inhibitors or cardioselective beta-blockers with or without diuretics, respectively.[40] However, mean systemic blood pressure was significantly lower 138/85 mm Hg in the group receiving beta-blockers as compared with the other group (146/90 mm Hg). This suggests that long-term ACE inhibitor treatment might protect kidney function (structure) in diabetic nephropathy to a greater extent than would be expected from the blood pressure-lowering effect alone (ie, renoprotection). Recently, Björck et al[41] reported that long-term treatment with ACE inhibition can protect kidney function in IDDM patients with diabetic nephropathy more than treatment with selective beta-blockers. These findings were obtained in a prospective randomized trial run for 3 years.

Sodium and water retention play a major role

in initiating and maintaining hypertension in diabetic nephropathy, while the contribution from the renin-angiotensin-altosterone system is smaller.[42-44] Therefore, it is rational to combine other antihypertensive drugs with diuretics (thiazide or furosemide), as done in all the abovementioned studies reporting a beneficial effect on rate of decline in GFR and survival of the patients.[9,10,14,16-18] By contrast, Warram et al[45] concluded that intervention with diuretics to reduce hypertension is associated with excess mortality in diabetics with and without proteinuria. This conclusion was based on a retrospective analysis of diabetics (mainly insulin users) participating in a multicenter clinical trial of laser therapy conducted between 1972 and 1979. The investigators claim that diuretics were used only as an antihypertensive drug and consequently classified all users of diuretics as hypertensive. This crucial suggestion is not supported by Klein et al[46] in the Wisconsin Epidemiologic Study of Diabetic Retinopathy, originally demonstrating that diuretic use is a significant predictor of diminished survival in IDDM and non–insulin-dependent diabetes mellitus patients. The association of decreased survival in diabetic patients taking diuretics may be due to a high proportion of such individuals being hypertensive (83%), having a history of heart disease (32%), or both, as suggested by Klein et al.[46]

In conclusion, antihypertensive treatment with selective beta-blockers or ACE inhibitors frequently combined with diuretics protects kidney function and enhance survival in IDDM patients with diabetic nephropathy.

REFERENCES

1. Eggers PW: Effect of transplantation on the medicare end-stage renal disease program. N Engl J Med 381:223-229, 1988

2. Deckert T, Poulsen JE, Larsen M: Prognosis of diabetics with diabetes onset before the age of thirthy-one. Survival, causes of death and complications. Diabetologia 14:363-370, 1978

3. Andersen AR, Christiansen JS, Andersen JK, Kreiner S, Deckert T: Diabetic nephropathy in type 1 (insulin-dependent) diabetes: An epidemiological study. Diabetologia 25:496-501, 1983

4. Krolewski AS, Warram JH, Christlieb AR, Busick EJ, Kahn CR: The changing natural history of nephropathy in type 1 diabetes. Am J Med 78:785-794, 1985

5. Borch-Johnsen K, Andersen PK, Deckert T: The effect of proteinuria on relative mortality in type 1 (insulin-dependent) diabetes mellitus. Diabetologia 28:590-596, 1985

6. Knowles HC, Jr: Long term juvenile diabetes treated with a measured diet. Trans Assoc Am Physicians 84:95-101, 1971

7. Borch-Johnsen K, Kreiner S: Proteinuria—Value as predictor of cardiovascular mortality in insulin dependent diabetes mellitus. Br Med J 294:1651-1654, 1987

8. Parving H-H, Smidt UM, Friisberg B, Bonnevie-Nielsen V, Andersen AR: A prospective study of glomerular filtration rate and arterial blood pressure in insulin-dependent diabetics with diabetic nephropathy. Diabetologia 20:457-461, 1981

9. Parving H-H, Andersen AR, Smidt UM, Svendsen PA: Early aggressive anti-hypertensive treatment reduces rate of decline in kidney function in diabetic nephropathy. Lancet 1:1175-1179, 1983

10. Parving H-H, Andersen AR, Smidt UM, Hommel E, Mathiesen ER, Svendsen PA: Effect of antihypertensive treatment on kidney function in diabetic nephropathy. Br Med J 294:1143-1147, 1987

11. Brøchner-Mortensen J: A simple method for determination of glomerular filtration rate. Scand J Clin Lab Invest 30:271-274, 1972

12. Brøchner-Mortensen J: Current status on assessment and measurement of glomerular filtration rate. Clin Physiol 5:1-17, 1985

13. Mancini G, Carbonara AO, Heremans JF: Immunochemical quantitation of antigens by single radial immunodiffusion. Immunochemistry 2:235-254, 1965

14. Mogensen CE: Long-term antihypertensive treatment inhibiting progression of diabetic nephropathy. Br Med J 285:685-688, 1982

15. Björck S, Nyberg G, Mulec H, Granerus G, Herlitz H, Aurell M: Beneficial effects of angiotensin converting enzyme inhibition on renal function in patients with diabetic nephropathy. Br Med J 293:471-474, 1986

16. Parving H-H, Hommel E, Smidt UM: Protection of kidney function and decrease in albuminuria by captopril in insulin dependent diabetics with nephropathy. Br Med J 297:1086-1091, 1988

17. Parving H-H, Hommel E: Prognosis in diabetic nephropathy. Br Med J 299:230-233, 1989

18. Mathiesen ER, Borch-Johnsen K, Jensen DV, Deckert T: Improved survival in patients with diabetic nephropathy. Diabetologia 32:884-886, 1989

19. Nordén G, Björck S, Granerus G, Nyberg G: Estimation of renal function in diabetic nephropathy. Nephron 47:36-42, 1987

20. Frimodt-Møller C: Diabetic cystopathy: epidemiology and related disorders. Ann Intern Med 92:318-321, 1980

21. Skøtt P, Vaag A, Bruun NE, Hother-Nielsen O, Gall M-A, Beck-Nielsen H, Parving H-H: Effect of insulin on renal sodium handling in hyperinsulinaemic type 2 (non–insulin-dependent) diabetic patients with peripheral insulin resistance. Diabetologia 34:275-281, 1991

22. Parving H-H, Kastrup J, Smidt UM, Andersen AR, Feldt-Rasmussen B, Christiansen JS: Impaired autoregulation of glomerular filtration rate in type 1 (insulin-dependent) diabetic patients with nephropathy. Diabetologia 27:547-552, 1984

23. Cohen D, Dodds R, Viberti GC: Effect of protein restriction in insulin dependent diabetics at risk of nephropathy. Br Med J 294:795-798, 1987

24. Viberti GC, Bilous RW, Mackintosh D, Bending JJ, Keen H: Long term correction of hyperglycaemia and progression of renal failure in insulin dependent diabetes. Br Med J 286:598-602, 1983

25. Jacobson HR: Chronic renal failure: Pathophysiology. Lancet 2:419-423, 1991

26. Hostetter TH, Rennke HG, Brenner BM: The case for intrarenal hypertension in the initiation and progression of diabetic and other glomerulopathies. Am J Med 72:375-380, 1982

27. Berkman J, Rifkin H: Unilateral nodular diabetic glomerulosclerosis (Kimmelstiel-Wilson). Report of a case. Metabolism 22:715-722, 1973

28. Mogensen CE: Progression of nephropathy in long-term diabetics with proteinuria and effects of initial antihypertensive treatment. Scand J Clin Lab Invest 36:383-388, 1976

29. Berglund J, Lins L-E, Lins P-E: Metabolic and blood pressure monitoring in diabetic renal failure. Acta Med Scand 218:401-408, 1985

30. Brazy PC, Slead WW, Fitzwilliam JF: Progression of renal insufficiency: Role of blood pressure. Kidney Int 35:670-674, 1989

31. Klahr S: The modification of diet in renal disease study. N Engl J Med 320:864-866, 1989

32. Hasslacher CH, Stech W, Wahl P, Ritz E: Blood pressure and metabolic control as risk factors for nephropathy in type 1 (insulin-dependent) diabetes. Diabetologia 28:6-11, 1985

33. Anderson S, Rennke HG, Brenner BM: Therapeutic advantage of converting enzyme inhibitors in arresting progressive renal disease associated with systemic hypertension in the rat. J Clin Invest 77:1993-2000, 1986

34. Bank N, Klose R, Aynedjian HS, Nguyen D, Sabtay LB: Evidence against increased glomerular pressure initiating diabetic nephropathy. Kidney Int 31:898-905, 1987

35. Hostetter TH, Troy JL, Brenner BM: Glomerular hemodynamics in experimental diabetes. Kidney Int 19:410-415, 1981

36. Jensen PK, Christiansen JS, Steven K, Parving H-H: Renal function in streptozotocin diabetic rats. Diabetologia 21:409-414, 1981

37. Jensen PK, Steven K, Blaehr H, Christiansen JS, Parving H-H: Effects of indomethacin on glomerular hemodynamics in experimental diabetes. Kidney Int 29:490-495, 1986

38. Zatz R, Dunn BR, Meyer TW, Anderson S, Rennke HG, Brenner BM: Prevention of diabetic glomerulopathy by pharmacological amelioration of glomerular capillary hypertension. J Clin Invest 77:1925-1930, 1986

39. Anderson S, Rennke HG, Garcia DL, Brenner BM: Short and long term effects of antihypertensive therapy in the diabetic rat. Kidney Int 36:526-536, 1989

40. Sawicki PT, Heinemann L, Mühlhauser J: Enalapril and metoprolol in diabetic nephropathy. Br Med J 300:1466, 1990 (abstr)

41. Björck S, Mulec H, Johnsen SA, Nordén G, Aurell M: Renal protective effect of enalapril in diabetic nephropathy. Br Med J 304:339-343, 1992

42. O'Hare JA, Ferriss JB, Brady D, Tworney B, O'Sullivan DJ: Exchangeable sodium and renin in hypertensive diabetic patients with and without nephropathy. Hypertension 7:43-48, 1985 (suppl 2)

43. Feldt-Rasmussen B, Mathiesen ER, Deckert T, Giese J, Christensen NJ, Bent-Hansen L, Nielsen MD: Central role for sodium in the pathogenesis of blood pressure changes independent of angiotensin, aldosterone and catecholamines in type 1 (insulin-dependent) diabetes mellitus. Diabetologia 30:610-617, 1987

44. Hommel E, Mathiesen ER, Giese J, Nielsen MD, Schütten HJ, Parving H-H: On the pathogenesis of arterial blood pressure elevation early in the course of diabetic nephropathy. Scand J Clin Lab Invest 49:537-544, 1989

45. Warram JH, Laffel LMB, Valsania P, Christlieb AR, Krolewski AS: Excess mortality associated with diuretic therapy in diabetes mellitus. Arch Intern Med 151:1350-1356, 1991

46. Klein R, Moss SE, Klein BEK, DeMets DL: Relation of ocular and systemic factors to survival in diabetes. Arch Intern Med 149:268-272, 1989

Angiotensin-Converting Enzyme Inhibition in Diabetic Nephropathy: Ten Years' Experience

Hans-Henrik Parving, MD, DMSc, Peter Rossing, MD, Eva Hommel, MD, and Ulla M. Smidt

● The aim of our prospective study was to evaluate putative progression promoters, kidney function, and prognosis during long-term treatment with angiotensin-converting enzyme inhibition in insulin-dependent diabetes mellitus patients suffering from diabetic nephropathy. Eighteen consecutive hypertensive insulin-dependent diabetes patients with nephropathy (mean age, 33 years) who had not been treated previously were all treated with captopril in combination with frusemide or bendrofluazide. The four patients who were refractory to this regimen also received nifedipine. Treatment was continued for a median of 8.9 years (range, 6.3 to 9.8, years). Renal function was assessed every 6 months by measurement of glomerular filtration rate (GFR) (single-bolus ^{51}Cr-EDTA technique) and albuminuria by radioimmunoassay. Baseline values (±SE) were mean arterial blood pressure 146/93 ± 3/1 mm Hg, albuminuria (geometric mean ± antilog SE) 982 ± 1.2 μg/min, and GFR 98 ± 5 mL/min/1.73 m^2. Angiotensin-converting enzyme inhibition induced a significant reduction during the whole treatment period of blood pressure (137/85 ± 3/1 mm Hg; $P < 0.01$) and albuminuria (392 ± 1.4 μ/min; $P < 0.01$), and the rate of decline in GFR was 4.4 ± 0.7 mL/min/yr, in contrast to previous reports of 10 to 14 mL/min/yr (natural history). Univariate analysis revealed a significant correlation between the rate of decline in GFR and mean arterial blood pressure ($r = 0.58$, $P = 0.01$), albuminuria ($r = 0.67$, $P < 0.01$), hemoglobin A_{1c} ($r = 0.69$, $P < 0.01$), and serum total cholesterol concentration ($r = 0.51$, $P < 0.05$). A multiple linear regression analysis including the four above-mentioned progression promoters showed that only albuminuria ($P < 0.05$) and hemoglobin A_{1c} ($P < 0.01$) correlated significantly with the rate of decline in GFR, explaining two thirds of the progression. The cumulative death rate was 11% (95% confidence interval, 0 to 25) 10 years after onset of nephropathy in patients receiving angiotensin-converting enzyme inhibition and diuretics, in contrast to previous reports of 50% to 77% 10 years after onset of nephropathy (natural history). In conclusion, long-term antihypertensive treatment with antiotensin-converting enzyme inhibition frequently combined with diuretics protects kidney function and enhances survival in hypertensive insulin-dependent diabetes patients with diabetic nephropathy.

INDEX WORDS: Insulin-dependent diabetes mellitus; diabetic nephropathy; hypertension; angiotensin-converting enzyme inhibition; antihypertensive treatment; glomerular filtration rate; renoprotection.

DIABETIC nephropathy is a clinical syndrome characterized by persistent albuminuria, increased arterial blood pressure, and a relentless decline in glomerular filtration rate (GFR). Blood pressure elevation is an early and frequent phenomenon, since approximately 50% of insulin-dependent diabetes mellitus (IDDM) patients with nephropathy and normal kidney function have a diastolic blood pressure ≥95 mm Hg.[1] Raised systemic blood pressure accelerates the progression of diabetic nephropathy,[2,3] probably due to downstream transmission resulting in glomerular capillary hypertension.[4,5] A link between glomerular hypertension and albuminuria and the development and progression of diabetic glomerulopathy has been suggested.[6] In accordance with that linkage, antihypertensive treatment mitigates albuminuria and diabetic glomerulopathy in streptozotocin diabetic rats[7,8] and reduces albuminuria and the rate of decline in kidney function in IDDM patients with diabetic nephropathy.[9-14] The beneficial effect of antihypertensive treatment on kidney function in diabetic nephropathy is highly variable and the factors responsible for this variability are not known. Several putative progression promoters, such as systemic blood pressure elevation,[2,3,9,10] albuminuria,[3,15-18] glycemic control,[11,14,19-22] and hyperlipidemia,[23-26] have been suggested in addition to the type of antihypertensive drugs.[13,27] However, these studies have yielded conflicting results.

The aim of our 10-year prospective study was to evaluate putative progression promoters, kidney function, and prognosis during treatment with ACEI in hypertensive IDDM patients suffering from diabetic nephropathy.

MATERIALS AND METHODS

We examined the records of all IDDM patients with proteinuria (positive on dipstick testing) who had visited the outpatient clinic at Hvidöre Hospital, Copenhagen, Denmark, during 1984.[28] We invited all hypertensive patients to join the study if they were younger than 50 years, had persistent albuminuria (>300 mg/d) and serum creatinine concentration less than 120 μmol/L and no edema, and had developed diabetes before the age of 31 years but were not receiving antihypertensive treatment (including diuretics). Twenty patients fulfilled these criteria and all gave fully informed consent.[12] At the beginning of the study one patient was excluded because therapy with thiazides had been started for edema.

Table 1. Clinical Data on Hypertensive Insulin-Dependent Diabetic Patients With Nephropathy Receiving Antihypertensive Treatment With Angiotensin-Converting Enzyme Inhibition

Case No.	Sex	Age (yr)	Duration of Diabetes (yr)	Retinopathy	Mean Dose of Insulin (U/kg/d)	Mean Body Mass Index (kg/m²)	Mean Energy Intake (MJ/d)	Antihypertensive Treatment (mg/d)
1	F	40	28	Proliferative	0.54	20.5	6.0	Captopril 50, furosemide 80
2	M	37	16	Proliferative	0.52	21.9	10.0	Captopril 100, furosemide 40, nifedipine 20
3	F	29	13	Simplex	0.64	24.3	8.0	Captopril 100, furosemide 160
4	M	43	20	Proliferative	0.49	24.6	8.8	Captopril 100, bendrofluazide 5
5	M	34	18	Proliferative	0.55	23.9	9.2	Captopril 100, furosemide 40
6	M	46	20	Proliferative	0.63	23.9	8.0	Captopril 75, furosemide 80, hydralazine 50
7	M	30	20	Proliferative	0.41	23.1	10.0	Captopril 100, furosemide 80
8	M	24	15	Simplex	0.80	20.7	10.0	Captopril 100, bendrofluazide 2.5
9	M	29	15	Proliferative	0.49	25.2	9.0	Captopril 100, bendrofluazide 10
10	M	31	27	Proliferative	0.80	24.6	8.0	Captopril 100, furosemide 240, nifedipine 40
11	M	19	13	Simplex	0.96	22.7	13.3	Captopril 100, bendrofluazide 2.5
12	M	34	28	Proliferative	0.62	24.0	9.0	Captopril 75, furosemide 320, nifedipine 40
13	M	26	19	Proliferative	0.75	21.5	10.0	Captopril 75, furosemide 160
14	F	25	18	Simplex	0.42	21.9	6.3	Captopril 100, furosemide 160, nifedipine 30
15	M	43	20	Proliferative	0.67	23.3	11.0	Captopril 100, bendrofluazide 5
16	F	23	22	Simplex	0.53	21.9	5.0	Captopril 100, furosemide 40
17	M	30	17	Simplex	0.50	26.6	10.4	Captopril 100, bendrofluazide 10
18	M	46	42	Simplex	0.56	25.8	9.0	Captopril 75
Mean ± SEM		33 ± 2	21 ± 2		0.60 ± 0.03	23.4 ± 0.4	9.0 ± 0.4	

After nearly 1 year of investigation, one man was excluded because renal biopsy showed measangioproliferative glomerulonephritis superimposed on a diffuse diabetic glomerulosclerosis.

After baseline investigation between December 1984 and April 1985, treatment with captopril (maximum dose, 50 mg twice a day) and frusemide or a thiazide was started in all 18 patients (Table 1). During the initial 12-week treatment period monotherapy with captopril was evaluated, which explains some of the above-mentioned inclusion/exclusion criteria.[29] The interim results after 3 years of treatment have been reported previously.[12]

All patients were dependent on insulin from the time of diagnosis, and all received at least two daily injections of highly purified porcine insulin (standard treatment in Denmark). They had a normal diabetic diet containing 45% to 55% carbohydrate, 30% to 35% fat, and 15% to 20% protein throughout the study. None of the patients had their intake of salt or protein restricted. Hypertension was diagnosed if the mean values of the last three recordings performed in the outpatient clinic before the start of the study were ≥160/90 mm Hg. With the antihypertensive treatment we aimed at achieving a stable reduction in diastolic blood pressure to below 90 mm Hg and at least 10 mm Hg in mean arterial blood pressure (diastolic pressure plus one third of the pulse amplitude), or both. Nearly all patients required diuretics to control blood pressure sufficiently and/or to treat edemata. If the antihypertensive treatment goals were still not achieved, nifedipine was added (maximum dose, 30 mg twice a day). Nephropathy was diagnosed clinically according to previously described criteria. The onset of nephropathy was taken as the date of the first persistent abnormal urine samples (albuminuria >300 mg/d).

All investigations were performed on one day between 8:00 AM and 2:00 PM. The patients had their normal breakfast and morning dose of insulin before the investigations, during which they rested supine and stood up only to pass urine. They drank 150 to 200 mL tap water/hr during the study. The investigations were carried out 14 to 18 times (median, 17 times).

To measure GFR we gave the patients a single intravenous injection of 3.7 MBq sodium chromate-51 edetic acid at 9:00 AM and determined the plasma radioactivity in venous blood samples taken from the other arm 180, 200, 220, and 240 minutes after the injection.[30] In case of GFR less than 25 mL/min, additional blood samples were taken after 270, 300, 330, and 360 minutes after the injection, in order to obtain the final slope. The small underestimation (10%) of ^{51}Cr-edetic acid clearance versus clearance of inulin was corrected for by multiplying the chromate clearance by 1.10. The results were standardized for 1.73 m^2 body surface area using the patient's surface area at the start of the study throughout. The mean coefficient of variation in the GFR of each patient from day to day was 4% (precision). Albuminuria was measured during the 4-hour clearance period by radioimmunoassay.[31]

Blood pressure was measured with a Hawksley random zero device (cuff size, 25 × 12 cm) on the right arm. Two readings were taken during each investigation between 9:00 and 10:00 AM, between 12:00 and 3:00 PM, and at each visit to the outpatient clinic (between 2:00 and 4:00 PM) after the patient had been supine for 10 minutes or more. Diastolic blood pressure was recorded at the disappearance of the Korotkoff sounds (phase V). Blood glucose concentration was measured hourly during the 4-hour clearance period and at each visit to the clinic by a glucose oxidase method.

The patients visited the clinic every 2 to 4 months (including the above-mentioned GFR investigations) during the study. The number of visits averaged 35 (range, 24 to 44). At each visit the stable hemoglobin A_{1c} concentration was measured (normal range, 4.1% to 6.1% of total hemoglobin along with postprandial glucose concentration, glucosuria, serum total cholesterol, albuminuria, blood pressure, and body weight, and the insulin dose and antihypertensive treatment were adjusted. Ophthalmoscopy and fundus photos were carried out on dilated pupils at least every 6 to 12 months.

Statistical Analysis

Results are expressed as mean values ± SEM. Values for urinary albumin excretion rate were logarithmically transformed before analysis because of their positively skewed distribution; the geometric mean and antilog SEM are given. All measurements made in each patient (including the two patients who died) during the entire treatment period were used to calculate the mean values during treatment. Linear regression analysis (least-squares method) was used to determine the rate of decline in GFR for each patient. The rate of decline was calculated from all values of GFR, including baseline values. Linear regression analysis and forward stepwise multiple regression were used to analyze data for correlations. The 95% confidence interval for the mortality was calculated by the exact binomial method. All calculations were made using Statgraphics (STSC, Rockville, MD). $P < 0.05$ was considered significant (two-tailed).

RESULTS

The pertinent clinical data are presented in Table 1. The individual and mean course of arterial blood pressure, albuminuria, and rate of decline in GFR are shown in Table 2 and Fig 1. All 18 patients experienced a decrease in blood pressure and in albuminuria, and four patients had albuminuria below 100 μg/min. The rate of decline in GFR varied between −1.6 and 9.1 mL/min/yr (mean, 4.4 mL/min/yr). A more pronounced

Table 2. Course of Arterial Blood Pressure, Albuminuria, and Glomerular Filtration Rate in Hypertensive Insulin-Dependent Diabetic Patients With Nephropathy Receiving Antihypertensive Treatment With Angiotensin-Converting Enzyme Inhibition

		Mean Baseline Values				Mean Values During the Investigation		
Case No.	Duration of Nephropathy (yr)*	Length of Investigation (yr)	Arterial Blood Pressure (mm Hg)	Albuminuria (μg/min)	Glomerular Filtration Rate (mL/min/1.73 m²)	Arterial Blood Pressure (mm Hg)	Albuminuria (μg/min)	Decrease in Glomerular Filtration Rate (mL/min/yr)
1	9.8	9.8	151/89	556	76	120/70	18	0.1
2	11.8	9.8	135/95	816	81	138/88	383	3.8
3	9.8	9.8	146/92	455	133	133/89	57	5.0
4	15.7	9.7	147/88	1,101	85	141/78	275	1.6
5	12.7	6.3	129/86	1,549	70	124/85	1,693	6.1
6	9.8†‡	7.8	158/92	2,238	82	163/83	2,041	8.2
7	9.6†	6.6	164/94	1,677	93	148/89	1,503	9.1
8	13.6	9.6	134/96	745	104	127/85	46	2.6
9	12.6	9.6	155/94	352	115	141/91	579	1.1
10	19.5	9.5	151/104	1,864	104	136/91	528	3.7
11	11.5	9.5	141/92	1,489	134	136/92	1,575	6.5
12	13.4	9.4	133/90	1,628	79	133/86	549	3.3
13	10.4	9.4	129/93	275	124	131/83	228	5.1
14	12.3	7.7	152/98	626	135	150/94	703	8.5
15	12.3	9.3	161/102	2,097	91	131/83	772	4.3
16	10.8‡	7.8	154/100	2,588	77	127/86	1,191	6.2
17	10.3	9.3	141/88	168	96	137/83	84	−1.6
18	13.2	9.2	156/85	2,946	89	148/80	1,873	4.8
Mean ± SEM	12.2 ± 0.6	8.9 ± 0.3	146/93 ± 3/1	982 ± 1.2	98 ± 5	137/85 ± 3/1	392 ± 1.4§	4.4 ± 0.7

* From onset of nephropathy to end of follow-up, death,† or renal death.‡
§ Geometric mean (antilog SEM).

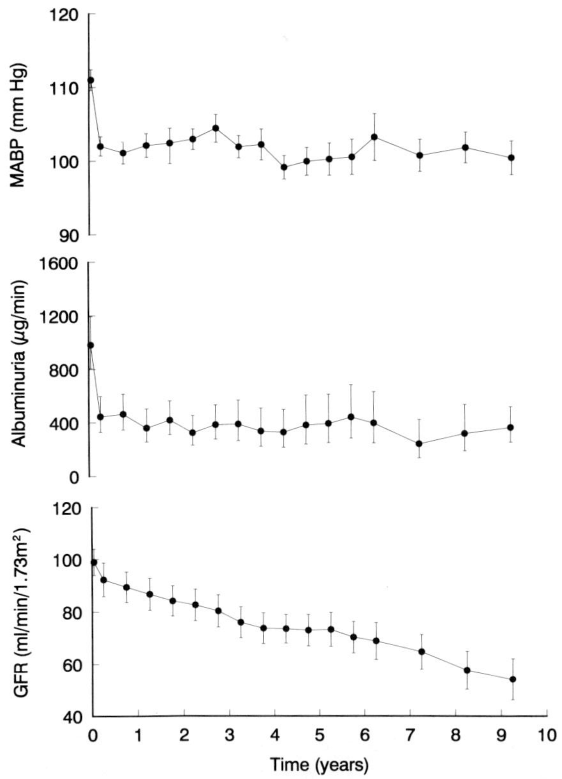

Fig 1. Mean course of mean arterial blood pressure, albuminuria, and GFR during long-term ACEI treatment in hypertensive IDDM patients with diabetic nephropathy. Bars represent the SEM.

reduction in GFR (6.1 mL/min) during the initial treatment period lasting 3.2 months was observed. This is equal to a monthly rate of decline in GFR of 1.9 mL/min as compared with 0.36 mL/min/mo during the following sustained treatment period.

We tried to determine whether the variables measured at baseline (diastolic, systolic, and mean blood pressures; albuminuria; hemoglobin A_{1c} [HbA_{1c}]; hemoglobin; serum total cholesterol; and serum albumin) predict the patient's rate of decline in GFR during the following antihypertensive treatment period. None of these variables had any predictive power, with the exception of albuminuria ($r = 0.53$, $P < 0.05$) and plasma albumin concentration ($r = -0.54$, $P < 0.05$).

Univariate analysis revealed a significant correlation between the rate of decline of GFR on the one hand and mean arterial blood pressure ($r = 0.58$, $P < 0.01$; Fig 2), albuminuria ($r = 0.67$, $P < 0.005$; Fig 3), HbA_{1c} ($r = 0.69$, $P < 0.005$; Fig 4), and serum total cholesterol ($r = 0.51$, $P < 0.05$; Fig 5) on the other. Forward stepwise multiple linear regression analysis, which included the four above-mentioned putative progression promoters, showed that only albuminuria ($P < 0.05$) and HbA_{1c} ($P < 0.01$) correlated significantly with the rate of decline in GFR, explaining two thirds of the progression in kidney function during antihypertensive treatment ($r^2 = 0.66$, $P < 0.001$).

The average courses of HbA_{1c}, serum cholesterol, serum potassium, and sodium are depicted in Fig 6. No significant changes occurred during the 10 years of study, and none of the patients developed hyperkalemia.

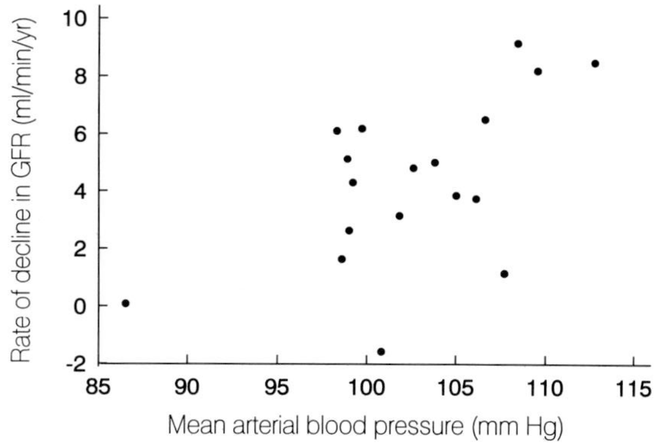

Fig 2. Mean arterial blood pressure and rate of decline in GFR during long-term ACEI treatment in hypertensive IDDM patients with diabetic nephropathy (n = 18; *r* = 0.58, *P* = 0.01).

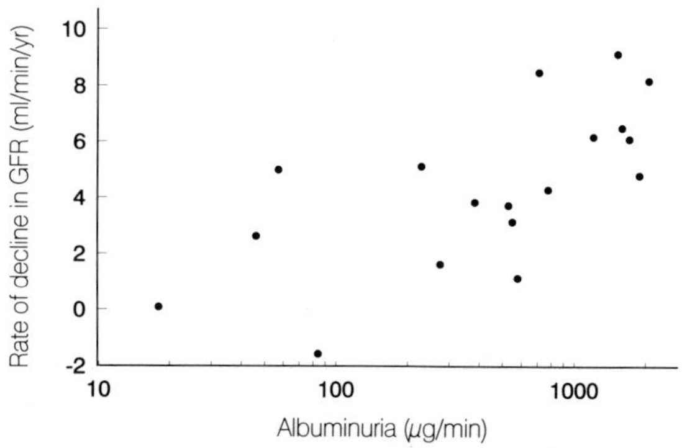

Fig 3. Albuminuria (log-scale) and rate of decline in GFR during long-term ACEI treatment in hypertensive IDDM patients with diabetic nephropathy (n = 18; *r* = 0.67, *P* < 0.01).

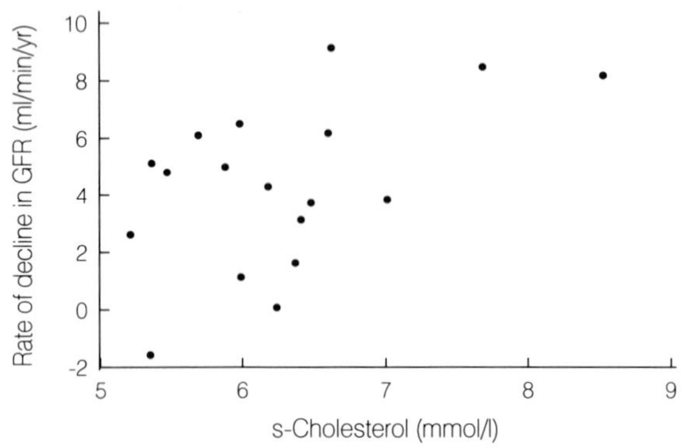

Fig 4. Serum cholesterol and rate of deline in GFR during long-term ACEI treatment in hypertensive IDDM patients with diabetic nephropathy (n = 18; *r* = 0.51, *P* < 0.05).

All patients were followed for at least 10 years or until death. The median length of follow-up from onset of persistent albuminuria was 12 years (range, 9.6 to 19.5 years) and the total mortality, including the "renal death" patient (no. 16), was 16.7% (95% confidence interval, 4% to 41%). The cumulative death rate (including "renal death") 10 years after onset of nephropathy was 11.1% (95% confidence interval, 0% to 25% (Fig 7, Table 3). One patient (no. 6) treated for end-stage renal disease died from cardiovascular cause, while another patient (no. 7) was found dead in bed, the cause of death unknown. His latest GFR was 34 mL/min/1.73 m^2. One patient (no. 16) had a kidney transplant due to end-stage renal disease after having diabetic nephropathy for 12 years. Finally, two patients (nos. 5 and 14) dropped out, but both are still alive without end-stage renal disease.

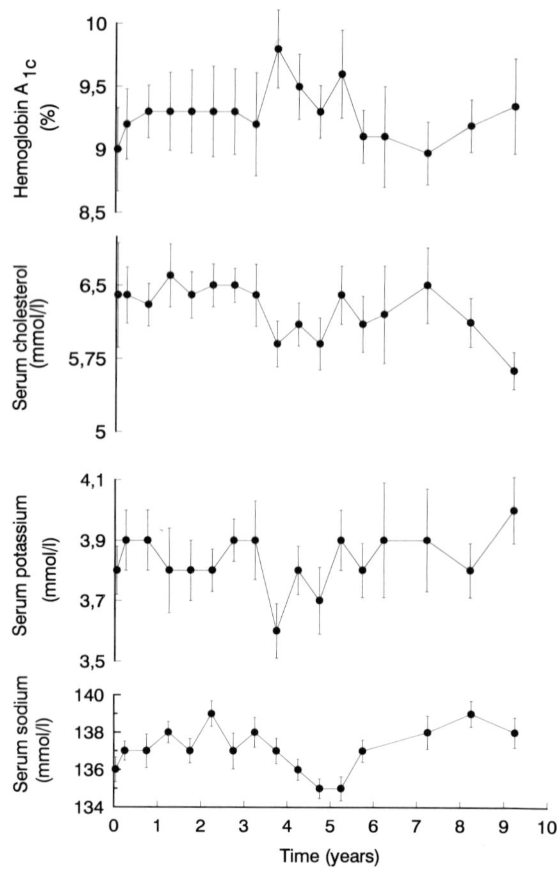

Fig 6. Mean course of hemoglobin A_{1c}, serum cholesterol, serum sodium, and serum potassium during long-term ACEI treatment in hypertensive IDDM patients with diabetic nephropathy. Bars represent the SEM.

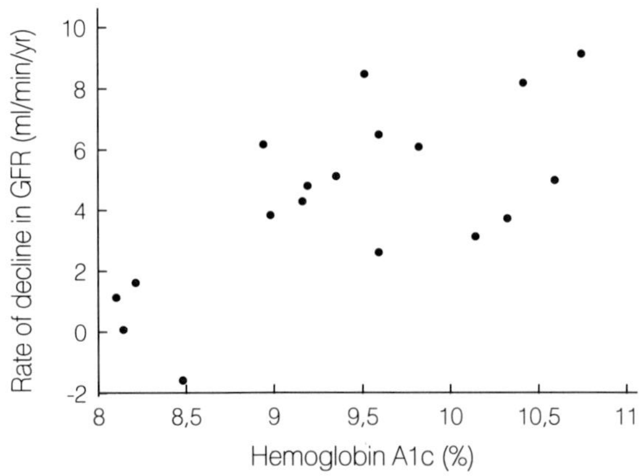

Fig 5. Hemoglobin A_{1c} and rate of deline in GFR during long-term ACEI treatment in hypertensive IDDM patients with diabetic nephropathy (n = 18; *r* = 0.69, *P* < 0.01).

Diet and body weight remained unchanged during the study and no severe side effects requiring withdrawal of angiotensin-converting enzyme inhibition (ACEI) took place.

DISCUSSION

Our 10-year prospective study in hypertensive IDDM patients with diabetic nephropathy revealed that ACEI in combination with diuretics induced a sustained reduction in systemic blood pressure, albuminuria, and a low but variable rate of decline in GFR. Part of this variability could be explained by the following progression pro-

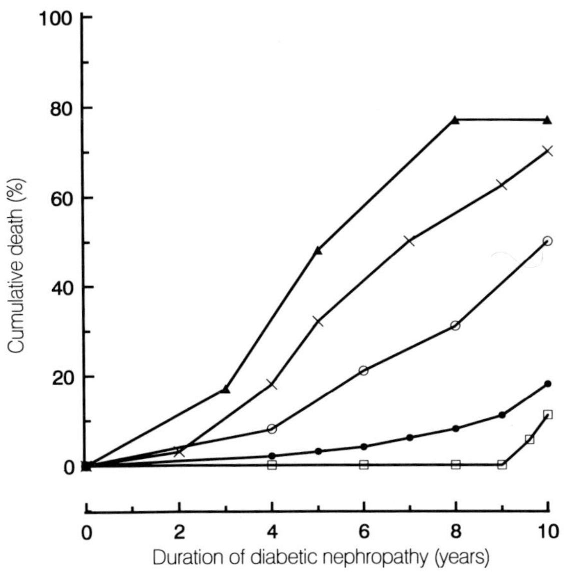

Fig 7. Deaths from diabetic nephropathy (natural history) in IDDM patients (▲ [n = 45], Knowles[39]; × [n = 360], Andersen et al[40]; o [n = 67], Krolewski et al[19]) compared with those who had effective antihypertensive treatment without ACEI (● [n = 45]; Parving and Hommel[41]) and with ACEI (□ [n = 18]).

moters: blood pressure, albuminuria, glycemic control, and serum cholesterol. Approximately two thirds of the variation in the progression rate of GFR could be explained by albuminuria and glycemic control. Finally, the ACEI treatment enhanced patient survival a considerable extent.

To obtain valid determination of the rate of decline in GFR in individual patients with chronic progressive kidney disease, the following requirements should be fulfilled[32]: the applied GFR method should be accurate and precise, repeated GFR measurements (approximately every 6 months) should be performed, and the observation period should be at least 2 years. The present GFR values are corrected for extrarenal loss of tracer (3.7 mL/min) and for the small underestimation (10%) versus renal clearance of inulin as described previously.[30] The present applied plasma clearance method overestimates GFR in case of severe edema. However, none of our patients had severe edema. The mean coefficient of variation in GFR of each patient from day to day (precision) was 4% in our study applying plasma clearance of ^{51}Cr-edetic acid without urine collection. Substitutes for GFR measurements, such as serum creatinine, are not good enough for scientific purposes and alone is not reliable for clinical use.[33]

Most studies dealing with the natural history of diabetic nephropathy have demonstrated a relentless linear and highly variable rate of decline in GFR ranging from 2 to 20 mL/min/yr, with a mean of 12 mL/min/yr as reviewed by Parving et al.[2,34] Systemic and glomerular hypertension enhance albuminuria and the development of diabetic glomerulopathy and accelerate the decrease in GFR both during the natural course of the disease[2-5] and during antihypertensive treatment,[2,7,8,34] as also demonstrated in our study. Conversely antihypertensive treatment reduces albuminuria, diminishes the loss of kidney func-

Table 3. Prognosis in Insulin-Dependent Diabetic Patients With Diabetic Nephropathy

	No. of Patients	Percentage of Female Patients	Percentage of Patients With Onset of Diabetes Before Age 21 yr	Age (yr) at Onset of Diabetes (Range)	Median Year of Onset of Diabetes (Range)	Antihypertensive Treatment	Cumulative Mortality (%) After 10 yr With Proteinuria (95% Confidence Interval)
Knowles (1971)[39]	45	48	100	9 (0-16)	1952 (1930–1962)	No	77
Andersen et al (1983)[40]	360	37	70	14 (0-30)	(1923–1952)	No	70
Krolewski et al (1985)[19]	67	46	100	12 (0-20)	1959	No	50*
Parving and Hommel (1989)[41]	45	44	82	12 (1-32)	1959 (1937–1971)	Years, without ACEI	18 (8-32)
Present study	18	22	78	11 (1-26)	1966 (1943–1971)	Years, with ACEI	11 (0-25)

* Deaths due to non-renal disease in patients who did not have serum creatinine concentrations > 2.5 mg/dL were not taken into account; deaths from end-stage renal failure only.

tion, and postpones renal insufficiency in diabetic nephropathy[2,9-12,14,34] as also documented in our long-term trial of ACEI. Renal protection, a beneficial effect on kidney function (and structure) above and beyond that expected from the blood pressure-lowering effect alone was originally suggested in diabetic nephropathy by Björck et al.[13] This suggestion has been confirmed in a recent randomized double-blind study comparing the effects of captopril (25 mg three times daily) versus placebo in normotensive and hypertensive (receiving conventional antihypertensive treatment) IDDM patients with diabetic nephropathy, whose baseline serum creatinine concentration was above 133 μmol/L.[27]

Our study revealed a significantly positive correlation between the decline in GFR and albuminuria measured at baseline and/or during the whole study period. Previous studies by Watkins et al[15] and Rossing et al[3] have demonstrated that the diabetic patients with the most marked proteinuria have the worse prognosis. It has been suggested recently that proteinuria is not simply a marker of the extent of glomerular damage, but that proteinuria per se may contribute to glomerular damage.[16] Furthermore, a decrease in albuminuria shortly after the onset of antihypertensive treatment predicts an attenuated rate of decrease in GFR in diabetic nephropathy.[17,18]

The degree of glycemic control is believed to have lost its significance as a risk factor for progression of kidney function when clinical overt diabetic nephropathy has developed.[11,19-22] This suggestion is based on studies frequently applying inappropriate methods for monitoring kidney function (eg, serum creatinine) and long-term integrated glycemic control (blood glucose concentration), in addition to small number of patients. Originally, Nyberg et al[14] found a significant positive correlation between the rate of decline in GFR and HbA_{1c} in 18 IDDM patients receiving antihypertensive treatment for diabetic nephropathy. Our long-term prospective study has confirmed and extended this observation by demonstrating that two thirds of the progression in GFR can be explained by glycemic control and albuminuria. While strict metabolic control can reduce the risk of progression from normoalbuminuria to microalbuminuria and macroalbuminuria,[35] we still lack information on the potential beneficial effect of improved glycemic control on kidney function in patients with overt diabetic nephropathy.

In addition to the above-mentioned progression promoters in chronic renal disease, hyperlipidemia is suggested to play a role.[23,24]. Mulec et al[25] found that raised serum concentrations of cholesterol were associated with a more rapid decline in GFR in diabetic nephropathy. We could not confirm that result in our 3-year prospective study of ACEI in diabetic nephropathy.[17] However, by extending that study, as done presently, we found a significant positive correlation between the level of serum cholesterol and the rate of decline in GFR. Finally, Krolewski et al[26] reported a greater loss of kidney function (serum creatinine) in hypercholesterolemic IDDM patients with intermittent or persistent proteinuria.

All our patients received a normal diabetic diet containing 15% to 20% protein. Protein intake was not restricted, and we have demonstrated previously that the average protein intake in the present patients was 1.1 g protein/kg/d during the initial 3 years of our study.

The decline in GFR early after start of antihypertensive treatment was four to five times higher than during the sustained treatment period lasting 7 to 9 years. The same phenomenon has been reported in other hypertensive IDDM and NIDDM patients with incipient and overt diabetic nephropathy[11,13,36] and in the Modification of Diet in Renal Disease study dealing with nondiabetic nephropathies.[37] The phenomenon is not dependent on the type of antihypertensive drug applied. The initial rapid loss of GFR may represent either a destruction of nephrons (progression in renal disease), or it may reflect a functional hemodynamic effect of low blood pressure and/or low protein diet intervention without a loss of nephrons. In case, the first mentioned event takes place then the initial decrease in GFR should be accounted for, when evaluating the long-term effect of intervention on progression of kidney disease. However, if the initial sleeper decrease in GFR is hemodynamically induced (reversible) then only the sustained effect on GFR reflecting progression of the renal disease should be analyzed in long-term intervention trials. Recently, we have presented data to support the hypothesis that the faster initial decline in GFR is due to a functional (hemodynamic) effect of antihypertensive treatment, which does not attenuate over time, while the subsequent slower decline reflects the beneficial effect on progression of diabetic nephropathy.[38]

The cumulative death rate was 11% (95% confidence interval, 0% to 25%) 10 years after onset of nephropathy in patients receiving ACEI and diuretics, in contrast to previous reports of 50% to 77% 10 years after onset of nephropathy (natural history).[19,39-41] Parving and Hommel[41] and Mathiesen et al[42] have shown that the survival of IDDM patients with nephropathy has improved substantially since the early use of effective antihypertensive treatment with conventional drugs. Recently, Lewis et al[27] demonstrated a significant risk reduction in patients with serum creatinine levels greater than 133 μmol/L for the occurrence of death or progression to dialysis or transplantation in IDDM patients with nephropathy treated with captopril versus placebo. The risk reduction was insignificant in the patients with serum creatinine less than 133 μmol/L, probably due to the relative short duration of the study (mean, 2.7 years).[27]

An ideal antihypertensive drug regimen is characterized by effectiveness, safety, and maintenance of the quality of life. The present treatment was effective, and as the adverse effects were only minimal, all patients continued to receive it.

In conclusion, long-term antihypertensive treatment with ACEI frequently combined with diuretics protects kidney function and enhances survival in hypertensive IDDM patients with diabetic nephropathy.

REFERENCES

1. Parving H-H, Andersen AR, Smidt UM, Oxenbøll B, Edsberg B, Christiansen JS: Diabetic nephropathy and arterial hypertension. Diabetologia 24:10-12, 1983

2. Parving H-H: Impact of blood pressure and antihypertensive treatment on incipient and overt nephropathy, retinopathy, and endothelial permeability in diabetes mellitus. Diabetes Care 14:260-269, 1991

3. Rossing P, Hommel E, Smidt UM, Parving H-H: Impact of arterial blood pressure and albuminuria on the progression of diabetic nephropathy in IDDM patients. Diabetes 42:715-719, 1993

4. Hostetter TH, Troy JL, Brenner BM: Glomerular hemodynamics in experimental diabetes mellitus. Kidney Int 19:410-415, 1981

5. Jensen PK, Steven K, Blæhr H, Christiansen JS, Parving H-H: The effects of indomethacin on glomerular hemodynamics in experimental diabetes. Kidney Int 29:490-495, 1986

6. Hostetter TH, Rennke HG, Brenner BM: The case for intrarenal hypertension in the initiation and progression of diabetic and other glomerulopathies. Am J Med 72:375-380, 1982

7. Zatz R, Dunn BR, Meyer TW, Anderson S, Rennke HG, Brenner BM: Prevention of diabetic glomerulopathy by pharmacological amelioration of glomerular capillary hypertension. J Clin Invest 77:1925-1930, 1986

8. Anderson S, Rennke HG, Garcia DL, Brenner BM: Short and long term effects of antihypertensive therapy in the diabetic rat. Kidney Int 36:526-536, 1989

9. Mogensen CE: Long-term antihypertensive treatment inhibiting progression of diabetic nephropathy. BMJ 285: 685-688, 1982

10. Parving H-H, Andersen AR, Smidt UM, Svendsen PA: Early aggressive antihypertensive treatment reduces rate of decline in kidney function in diabetic nephropathy. Lancet i:1175-1179, 1983

11. Parving H-H, Andersen AR, Smidt UM, Hommel E, Mathiesen ER, Svendsen PA: Effect of antihypertensive treatment on kidney function in diabetic nephropathy. BMJ 294:1443-1447, 1987

12. Parving H-H, Hommel E, Smidt UM: Protection of kidney function and decrease in albuminuria by captopril in insulin dependent diabetics with nephropathy. BMJ 297: 1086-1091, 1988

13. Björck S, Mulec H, Johnsen SA, Nordén G, Aurell M: Renal protective effect of enalapril in diabetic nephropathy. BMJ 304:339-343, 1992

14. Nyberg G, Blohmé G, Nordén G: Impact of metabolic control in progression of clinical diabetic nephropathy. Diabetologia 30:82-86, 1987

15. Watkins PJ, Blainey JD, Brewer DB, Fitzgerald MG, Malins JM, O'Sullivan DJ, Pinto J: The natural history of diabetic renal disease. A follow-up study of series of renal biopsies. Q J Med 41:437-456, 1972

16. Remuzzi G, Bertani T: Is glomerulosclerosis a consequence of altered glomerular permeability to macromolecules?. Kidney Int 38:384-394, 1990

17. Rossing P, Hommel E, Smidt UM, Parving H-H: Reduction in albuminuria predicts a beneficial effect on diminishing the progression of human diabetic nephropathy during antihypertensive treatment. Diabetologia 37:511-516, 1994

18. Rossing P, Hommel E, Smidt UM, Parving H-H: Reduction in albuminuria predicts diminished progression in diabetic nephropathy. Kidney Int 45:S145-S149, 1994 (suppl 45)

19. Krolewski AS, Warram JH, Christlieb AR, Busick EJ, Kahn CR: The changing natural history of nephropathy in type 1 diabetes. Am J Med 78:785-794, 1985

20. Parving H-H, Smidt UM, Friisberg B, Bonnevie-Nielsen V, Andersen AR: A prospective study of glomerular filtration rate and arterial blood pressure in insulin-dependent diabetics with diabetic nephropathy. Diabetologia 20:457-461, 1981

21. Viberti GC, Bilous RW, Mackintosh D, Keen H: Monitoring glomerular function in diabetic nephropathy. Am J Med 74:256-264, 1983

22. Hasslacher C, Stech W, Wahl P, Ritz E: Blood pres-

sure and metabolic control as risk factors for nephropathy in type 1 (insulin-dependent) diabetes. Diabetologia 28:6-11, 1985

23. Jacobson HR: Chronic renal failure: Pathophysiology. Lancet 338:419-423, 1991

24. Kasiske BL, O'Donnell MP, Cleary MP, Keane WF: Treatment of hyperlipidemia reduces glomerular injury in obese Zucker rats. Kidney Int 33:667-672, 1988

25. Mulec H, Johnsen SA, Wiklund D, Björck S: Cholesterol: A renal risk factor in diabetic nephropathy? Am J Kidney Dis 22:196-201, 1993

26. Krolewski AS, Warram JH, Christlieb AR: Hypercholesterolemia—A determinant of renal function loss and deaths in IDDM patients with nephropathy. Kidney Int 45:S125-S131, 1994 (suppl 45)

27. Lewis E, Hunsicker L, Bain R, Rhode R: The effect of angiotensin-converting-enzyme inhibition on diabetic nephropathy. N Engl J Med 329:1456-1462, 1993

28. Parving H-H, Hommel E, Mathiesen ER, Skøtt P, Edsberg B, Bahnsen M, Lauritzen M, Hougaard P, Lauritzen E: Prevalence of microalbuminuria, arterial hypertension, retinopathy and neuropathy in patients with insulin-dependent diabetes. Br Med J 296:156-160, 1988

29. Hommel E, Parving H-H, Mathiesen ER, Edsberg B, Nielsen MD, Giese J: Effect of captopril on kidney function in insulin-dependent diabetic patients with nephropathy. BMJ 293:466-470, 1986

30. Bröchner-Mortensen J: A simple method for the determination of glomerular filtration rate. Scand J Clin Lab Invest 30:271-274, 1972

31. Miles DW, Mogensen CE, Gundersen HJG: Radioimmunoassay for urinary albumin using a single antibody. Scand J Clin Lab Invest 26:5-11, 1970

32. Modification of Diet in Renal Disease Study Group, Levey AS, Gassman J, Hall PM, Walker WG: Assessing the progression of renal disease in clinical studies: Effects of duration of follow-up and regression to the mean. J Am Soc Nephrol 1:1087-1094, 1991

33. Shemesh O, Golbetz HV, Kriss JP, Myers BD: Limitations of creatinine as a filtration marker in glomerulopathic patients. Kidney Int 28:830-838, 1985

34. Parving H-H, Rossing P: The use of antihypertensive agents in prevention and treatment af diabetic nephropathy. Curr Opin Nephrol Hypertens 3:292-300, 1994

35. The Diabetes Control and Complications Trial Research Group: The effect of intensive treatment of diabetes on the development and progression of long-term complications in insulin-dependent diabetes mellitus. N Engl J Med 329:977-986, 1993

36. Lebovitz HE, Wiegmann TB, Cnaan A, Shahinfar S, Sica D, Broadstone V, Schwartz SL, Mengel MC, Segal R, Versaggi JA, Bolten WK: Renal protective effects of enalapril in hypertensive NIDDM: Role of baseline albuminuria. Kidney Int 45:S150-S155, 1994 (suppl 45)

37. Klahr S, Levey AS, Beck GJ, Caggiula AW, Hunsicker L, Kusek JW, Striker G, for the Modification of Diet in Renal Disease Study Group: The effects of dietary protein restriction and blood-pressure control on the progression of chronic renal disease. N Engl J Med 330:877-884, 1994

38. Hansen HP, Rossing P, Tarnow L, Nielsen FS, Jensen B, Parving H-H: Elevated GFR after withdrawal of chronic antihypertensive treatment in diabetic nephropathy. J Am Soc Nephrol 5:378, 1994 (abstr)

39. Knowles HCJ: Long term juvenile diabetes treated with unmeasured diet. Trans Assoc Am Phys 84:95-101, 1971

40. Andersen AR, Christiansen JS, Andersen JK, Kreiner S, Deckert T: Diabetic nephropathy in type 1 (insulin-dependent) diabetes: An epidemiological study. Diabetologia 25:496-501, 1983

41. Parving H-H, Hommel E: Prognosis in diabetic nephropathy. BMJ 299:230-233, 1989

42. Mathiesen ER, Borch-Johnsen K, Jensen DV, Deckert T: Improved survival in patients with diabetic nephropathy. Diabetologia 32:884-886, 1989

Monitoring Diabetic Nephropathy: Glomerular Filtration Rate and Abnormal Albuminuria in Diabetic Renal Disease—Reproducibility, Progression, and Efficacy of Antihypertensive Intervention

C.E. Mogensen, MD, K.W. Hansen, MD, S. Nielsen, MD, M. Mau Pedersen, MD, M. Rehling, MD, and A. Schmitz, MD

● The principal end point in the evaluation of treatment in incipient and overt diabetic nephropathy is rate of decline in glomerular filtration rate (GFR). Therefore, information on reproducibility of GFR measurements is essential in the planning and evaluation of clinical trials. We studied reproducibility of GFR measurements in insulin-dependent and non–insulin-dependent diabetes mellitus patients using, respectively, a constant-infusion technique with urine collection and labeled iothalamate as a tracer marker and a single-shot procedure using Cr-EDTA, measuring the GFR from the decline in plasma level after bolus injection. The coefficient of variance in the insulin-dependent patients was from 7.5% to 8.8% with repeated measurements. In longitudinal studies with several measurements the mean coefficient of variances varied between 7.4% and 3.4%. In the non–insulin-dependent patients the coefficient of variances between two tests were 7.0% and 5.3% for normoalbuminuric and microalbuminuric patients, respectively. In cross-sectional studies as well as in longitudinal studies, it has been consistently shown that GFR is well preserved and at a supranormal level in patients with normoalbuminuria and microalbuminuria. A decline in GFR appears to start around the transition from microalbuminuria to overt diabetic renal disease, although more detailed studies are needed to support this finding. With regard to intervention trials, several studies document that microalbuminuria can be reduced by effective antihypertensive treatment, particularly with angiotensin-converting enzyme inhibitors, also in patients with normal or close to normal blood pressure. Preliminary results from long-term studies suggest that reduction in microalbuminuria in these patients is associated with preservation of GFR and, thus, apparently renoprotection. In patients with overt renal disease, it has been consistently shown that antihypertensive treatment reduces albuminuria as well as the rate of decline in GFR. This is also observed with combined treatment regimens, for instance beta blockers or angiotensin-converting enzyme inhibitors combined with diuretics, or the three types of drugs in combination.

INDEX WORDS: Glomerular filtration rate; renal plasma flow; diabetic nephropathy; microalbuminuria; blood pressure; proteinuria; angiotensin-converting enzyme inhibitors; antihypertensive treatment.

MANY STUDIES have emphasized the role of abnormal albuminuria in the prediction and possibly also the genesis of diabetic renal disease.[1] Thus, it is clear that the earliest phase of abnormal albuminuria, so-called microalbuminuria,[2] predicts overt renal disease with clinical proteinuria, also termed macroalbuminuria, the well-known clinical entity characterized by blood pressure elevation and the approximate linear decline in glomerular filtration rate (GFR). On the other hand, patients with normoalbuminuria usually have a good long-term prognosis.[3,4] However, measurement of albuminuria should always be linked to the determination of GFR, since the rate of decline of GFR probably more directly relates to future reduction in renal function and, thus, end-stage renal failure.[5] Importantly, reducing the rate of decline of GFR and albuminuria by antihypertensive intervention suggests a more beneficial course of renal disease.[5]

Therefore, the exact measurement of GFR, along with the measurement of blood pressure and the degree of abnormal albuminuria are key features in studies of the natural history of diabetic renal disease, as well as in trials attempting to ameliorate its malignant course. The purpose of this article is to report on new reproducibility studies in the various phases of renal disease in both types of diabetes. Additionally, this report will review previous studies on the natural course of diabetic renal disease as related to abnormal albuminuria. Finally, a brief review will be given regarding antihypertensive treatment as a key measure to ameliorate the progression of renal disease, with emphasis on insulin-dependent diabetes mellitus (IDDM) patients with microalbuminuria. In addition, appropriate end points used in the documentation of a beneficial effect on the course of renal disease will be discussed briefly.

REPRODUCIBILITY STUDIES OF GLOMERULAR FILTRATION RATE MEASUREMENTS

Although there is some documentation about reproducibility of GFR measurements in healthy individuals,[6] there is in fact only very limited data available on reproducibility of this parameter in diabetic patients.[7] We studied the reproducibility of GFR measurements in a series of diabetic patients followed in the placebo arms of intervention studies. These studies refer to patients with normal albumin excretion rates and to patients with microalbuminuria. The results of studies of IDDM patients with longitudinal follow-up with multiple measurements of GFR will also be shown in microalbuminuria as well as overt diabetic nephropathy, and the clinical data from these patient studies are shown in subsequent tables. Eighty-nine diabetic individuals were studied with two or several measurements of GFR. One problem, of course, is that patients with overt diabetic nephropathy may show a time-dependent decline in GFR unless treatment is very effective in stabilizing the course of renal disease.

Glomerular Filtration Rate and Renal Plasma Flow Determinations

In IDDM patients the constant-infusion technique was used with ^{125}I-iothalamate as the filtration marker and ^{131}I-hippuran as a measurement of effective renal plasma flow (RPF).[8] In non–insulin-dependent diabetes mellitus (NIDDM) patients a single-shot procedure was used with calculation of the GFR from the plasma clearance of ^{51}Cr-EDTA, a standard procedure in many European laboratories.[6] The technicians and doctors calculating the values were all unaware that the data being obtained was part of a reproducibility study. All GFR and RPF values are corrected to 1.73 m^2 body surface.

Definition of Abnormal Albuminuria

Microalbuminuria is usually defined as the excretion rate of albumin in an overnight or 24-hour urine collection of 20 to 200 μg/min.[2] Three collections are usually necessary, and at least two should be in the 20 to 200 μ/min range. In defining the degree of renal involvement, a level above 200 μg/min is designated as proteinuria or macroalbuminuria and a level below 20 μg/minis designated as normoalbuminuria. These levels are relevant in patients without antihypertensive treatment. With antihypertensive treatment urinary albumin excretion (UAE) is usually reduced. Proteinuric patients may show decreases to the microalbuminuric, or even in some cases,

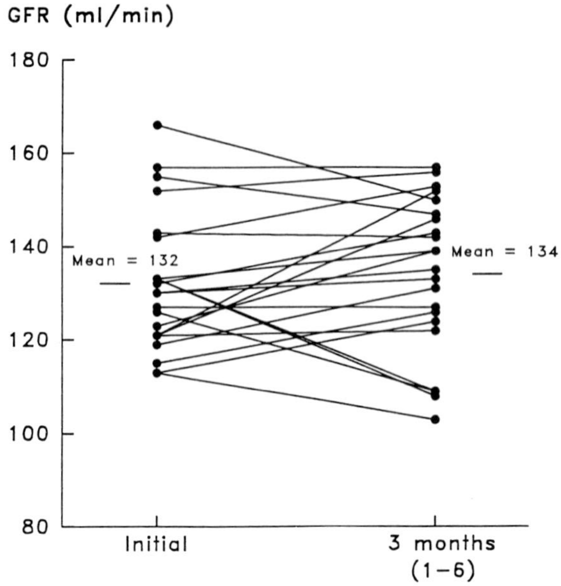

Fig 1. Normoalbuminuria in IDDM patients. The results are from repeated measurements (Table 1).

to the normoalbuminuric level. It is now well established that glomerular structural damage is present in microalbuminuric patients.[1]

Insulin-Dependent Diabetes Mellitus Patients

Twenty-two normoalbuminuric IDDM patients were studied twice; the relevant data are shown in Fig 1 and Table 1 with respect to GFR, RPF, mean arterial pressure (MAP), and rate of UAE. Prior to the calculations a plot of the day-to-day differences versus the average of the values obtained on 2 separate days indicated that the percentage differences were independent of the actual level of the parameter measured in the range of GFR observed. The mean interval between the measurements is 3 months. The mean GFR value was approximately the same on the 2 study days. The mean coefficient of variance is 7.5% between the two measurements of GFR. Slightly higher values are found for RPF, whereas the measurement of mean arterial blood pressure is somewhat less variable. In individual patients the maximal difference in GFR between two tests were 31 mL/min (HbA_{1c}-increase from 8.8% to 9.7% in this patient). A greater coefficient of variance is found with respect to the measurement of UAE rate, which is shown as log values.

Table 4. Insulin-Dependent Diabetes Mellitus Patients With Early Nephropathy: Longitudinal Study (During Long-Term Triple Treatment)

		Baseline	Follow-up	CV%
No. of patients (male/female)	8 (7/1)			
Age (yr)	39 ± 6 (29-51)			
Duration of diabetes (yr)	26 ± 5 (17-37)			
HbA_{1c} (%)	8.7 ± 1.1 (7.9-9.8)			
Follow-up period (mo)*	18			
No. of measurements*	4 (in one, only 3)			
GFR (mL/min), constant infusion (five periods)		108 ± 20 (74-133)	107 ± 17 (78-133)	3.4 ± 1.7 (1.6-5.5)
RPF (mL/min), constant infusion (five periods)		476 ± 81 (369-590)	452 ± 66 (395-556)	4.8 ± 2.6 (2.2-9.7)
MAP (mm Hg), renal clearance, sphygmomanometry (five measurements)		96 ± 11 (79-111)	98 ± 8 (87-110)	3.3 ± 1.3 (1.5-5.5)
UAE† (μg/min), renal clearance (five periods)		90 ×/÷ 2.9 (18-283)	81 ×/÷ 1.4 (14-290)	7.9 ± 4.2 (4.7-16.7)

Note. Data are presented as means ± SD. Ranges are presented in parentheses. Follow-up values were not significantly different from baseline values.

Abbreviation: MAP, mean arterial pressure.

* Median ×/÷ tolerance factor.

† Geometric mean ×/÷ tolerance factor.

urine collection, in contrast to the constant-infusion technique. Therefore, it may be the method of choice in elderly people, in whom complete voiding cannot always be expected (for example, due to prostatic hypertrophy). In our experience the same may be the case in some patients with proteinuria and long-term diabetes who have associated autonomic neuropathy. Such patients may have difficulties in voiding, so it cannot be taken for granted that the bladder is emptied after each voiding during a clearance procedure.

Table 5 shows that the coefficient of variance in 15 normoalbuminuric patients is 7.0% in studies in which the interval between the two measurements is a mean of 15 months (Fig 4). In 10 microalbuminuric NIDDM patients studied with an interval of 18 weeks the coefficient of variance is 5.3% (Table 5 and Fig 5). No data are available in the NIDDM patients with overt proteinuria.

Conclusion Concerning Reproducibility Studies

These reproducibility studies, which were mainly documented from the placebo arms of intervention studies, clearly suggest good reproducibility in both types of diabetes, with a coefficient of variance between two tests of 5.3% to 8.8%. In the constant-infusion technique studies the mean coefficient of variance between the individual periods (most often three or four periods) of the separate GFR determination are from 5.9% to 8.6%. Some of the variability is caused by physiologic variation and some by the nature of the measurement.[9]

NATURAL COURSE OF GLOMERULAR FILTRATION RATE CHANGES IN DIABETES

Cross-sectional Studies in Insulin-Dependent Diabetes Mellitus Patients

Data on cross-sectional material recently have been documented,[8] as shown in Table 6 which compares diabetic patients with healthy individuals. It is clear that both normoalbuminuric and microalbuminuric patients show evidence of hyperfiltration. There is a tendency to higher GFR values in the microalbuminuric patients, but no correlation between GFR and the degree of albuminuria is found within the microalbuminuric range. Thus, this material shows that GFR is still well preserved in microalbuminuric patients, and may first start to decline with the transition from microalbuminuria to macroalbuminuria; however, further studies are needed to support this theory.

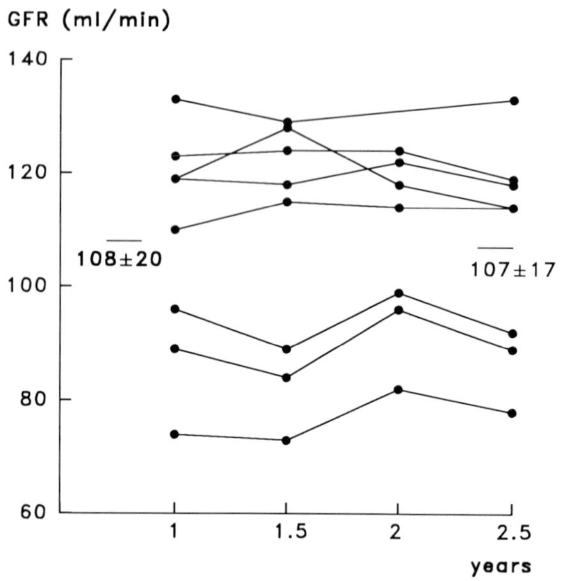

Fig 3. Longitudinal study of early proteinuria in IDDM patients. All patients were receiving triple treatment (β_1-blockers, diuretics, ACE inhibitors) (Table 3). The mean doses were metoprolol 140 mg/24 hr, bendroflumethiazide (with KCl) 3.8 mg/24 hr, and ramipril 5 mg/24 hr.

Longitudinal Studies in Insulin-Dependent Diabetes Mellitus Patients

Table 7 summarizes the data from several studies[10-15] in which the relationship between albuminuria and the rate of change in GFR was examined in 70 patients followed for a mean of 3.3 years. Data are shown graphically in Fig 6 in which the letters indicate the material described in Table 7. It is clear that patients with a normal albumin excretion rate preserve intact renal function even in long-term studies (approximately 12 years),[16] although with extremely long follow-up (approximately 20 years) there may be a small and probably age-related reduction in GFR.[4] In addition, patients with persistent microalbuminuria usually maintain intact renal function (usually hyperfiltration) (Table 7), but a subsequent decrease in GFR can be predicted. Thus, with the development of proteinuria there is a significant decline in GFR.[14] Feldt-Rasmussen et al[13] also observed a significant decrease in GFR with the development ofclinical nephropathy (UAE > 300 mg/24 hr), but most of their patients received antihypertensive treatment, which may modify the level of UAE. In 1976, patients with more advanced renal disease were documented to have a very significant decrease in the mean GFR, around 1 mL/min/mo (Table 7).[15] This study also suggested the presence of glomer-ular hyperfiltration in microalbuminuric patients but not a time-dependent decline in GFR.[15]

Cross-sectional Studies in Non–Insulin-Dependent Diabetes Mellitus

Data from a recently published study of NIDDM patients using single-shot ^{51}Cr-EDTA clearance clearly document that microalbuminuric patients still have well-preserved GFR and that renal size is increased in such patients.[17] The mean GFR in these normoalbuminuric NIDDM patients was 94 ± 13 mL/min (SD)[17]; in the microalbuminuric patients mean GFR was 91 ± 20 mL/min.[17]

Longitudinal Studies in Non–Insulin-Dependent Diabetes Mellitus Patients

Recent studies have documented that normoalbuminuric NIDDM patients preserve intact renal function (no decline in GFR) even after 4 years of follow-up.[18] There is a tendency for a decline in GFR in patients with microalbuminuria, but the difference from normoalbuminuric patients is not significant. However, with overt diabetic nephropathy there is a clear reduction in GFR.[18] The rate of decline in GFR is related to systolic blood pressure, as also observed in IDDM patients.[15]

Insulin-Dependent Versus Non–Insulin-Dependent Diabetes Mellitus Patients

The same pattern in longitudinal GFR studies is found when comparing IDDM with NIDDM patients. The GFR seems to be well preserved, even with the occurrence of microalbuminuria. In our experience there is a difference between the two types of diabetes since we did not find clear hyperfiltration in NIDDM patients; hyperfiltration was also not found in microalbuminuric patients.[17] In the Pima Indians, hyperfiltration was only found to a limited extent when correcting for (obese) body size (namely, 7%; when uncorrected for body size, the increase in GFR may be considerable[19] (that is, when obesity is not taken into consideration). The exact point at which GFR starts to decline during the transition

Table 5. Normoalbuminuric and Microalbuminuric Non–Insulin-Dependent Diabetes Mellitus Patients Studied Twice

	NIDDM Normoalbuminuria	NIDDM Microalbuminuria
No. of patients (male/female)	15 (9/6)	10 (6/4)
Age (yr)	65 ± 5 (57-72)	65 ± 4 (60-70)
Known duration of diabetes (yr)	6.5 ± 4.4 (1-18)	11 ± 6 (1-26)
HbA_{1c} (%)	8.4 ± 1.4 (5.7-11.7)	7.1 ± 0.9 (4.9-8.6)
Interval between investigations (mo)*	15 (13-22)	4

	NIDDM Normoalbuminuria				NIDDM Microalbuminuria			
	Day 1	Day 2	(Day 2 − Day 1)	CV %	Day 1	Day 2	(Day 2 − Day 1)	CV %
GFR (mL/min), single shot	88 ± 21 (41-118)	87 ± 24 (43-133)	−1 ± 9 (−19-17)	7.0	97 ± 21 (63-138)	96 ± 21 (64-129)	−1 ± 7 (−12-12)	5.3
MAP (mm Hg), sphygmomanometry (I measurement)	103 ± 15 (73-127)	103 ± 11 (75-117)	−1 ± 9‡ (−11-19)	5.9	110 ± 10 (95-127)	105 ± 12 (83-125)	−5 ± 9‡ (−5-10)	6.1
UAE† (μg/min)	6.9 ×/÷ 1.76 (3.1-19.6)	6.7 ×/÷ 1.93 (2.3-23.7)	0.98 ×/÷ 1.38 (0.50-1.59)	11.4	33 ×/÷ 2.35 (8-131)	30 ×/÷ 2.74 (9-122)	0.91 ×/÷ 1.63 (0.40-2.24)	9.7

Note. Data are presented as means ± SD. No difference was found between day 1 and day 2 values. The UAE was assessed from one 24-hour collection at each visit in normoalbuminuric patients and from three overnight collections at each visit in microalbuminuric patients.

Abbreviation: MAP, mean arterial pressure.

* Median.

† Geometric mean ×/÷ tolerance factor.

‡ Geometric mean and tolerance factor for log (day 2/day 1).

between microalbuminuria and macroalbuminuria is not clearly defined. This cut-off point may be highly variable in individual patients and may require a multitude of studies in individual patient follow-up, eg, measurements every 6 months. However, in the studies of IDDM patients by Mathiesen et al and Feldt-Rasmussen et al, it was documented that GFR declines with the transition from microalbuminuria to macroalbuminuria.[13,14]

CHANGING THE COURSE OF DIABETIC RENAL DISEASE WITH ANTIHYPERTENSIVE TREATMENT IN INSULIN-DEPENDENT DIABETES MELLITUS PATIENTS

Evaluation of treatment effect has to be differentiated according to degree of abnormal albuminuria. Due to elevated blood pressure, IDDM patients with normoalbuminuria rarely need antihypertensive treatment, but prophylaxis (with, for example, ACE inhibitors) could be considered (according to well-defined criteria) to prevent the transition from normoalbuminuria to microalbuminuria and patients should in such a trial be treated irrespective of actual blood pressure. Long-term follow-up will be needed since only 2% to 4% of such patients progress from normoalbuminuria to microalbuminuria yearly.

With microalbuminuria there is well-preserved renal function; thus, the effect parameter is reduction of albuminuria or prevention of increase; however, with very long-term follow-up the effect parameter is the prevention of fall in GFR.[5] In patients with overt nephropathy the main effect parameter is the rate of decline of GFR, with albuminuria and blood pressure reduction as secondary parameters.

Normoalbuminuria

In a double-blind, placebo-controlled, 3-month intervention study of 10 patients we have shown that filtration fraction as well as albumin excretion even in the normal range can be reduced with enalapril.[20] In these normotensive individuals blood pressure and hyperfiltration were not reduced. A potential study to document prevention of transition to microalbuminuria should last several years and probably comprise several hundred patients to have enough power to document an effect. Since approximately 25% of the IDDM

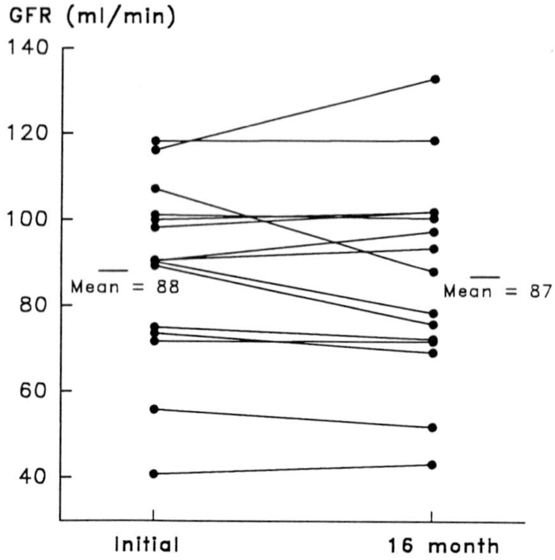

Fig 4. Normoalbuminuria in NIDDM patients. The results are from repeated measurements (Table 5).

patients progress to renal disease (or used to progress) this may be a high-priority study.

Incipient Diabetic Nephropathy

Several intervention studies have been published, some with a self-controlled design and some randomized, but not masked, as outlined in Table 8.[12-14,21-31] Table 8 provides information on the data from 12 trials, including a recent randomized, double-blind, large-scale, placebo-controlled, 2-year study published in abstract form.[31] Blood pressure was reduced in practically all studies or an increase in blood pressure was prevented. In the large multicenter study,[31] the effect of captopril was investigated with respect to progression to clinical nephropathy in normotensive IDDM patients with microalbuminuria. The study end points were the progression to persistent proteinuria (UAE >200 μg/min) and an increase in UAE of 30% or more. Twelve of 44 patients in the placebo group and four of 44 patients in the captopril group progressed to clinical proteinuria (Fisher's exact test, $P = 0.05$). Thus, treatment with captopril delayed the progression to overt renal disease in normotensive IDDM patients with microalbuminuria,[31] as was also seen in another long-term study.[14] The mean rate of progression of albuminuria was also significantly reduced by ACE inhibition.

Interestingly, in all the studies from 1985 to 1992 included in Table 8, the patients were included purely on the basis of microalbuminuria and, indeed, patients could not be overtly hypertensive (an exclusion criterion for participation). In most of these studies blood pressure was close to normal, meaning that the blood pressure was in the middle of the range seen in healthy young individuals around the age of 30 years (mean arterial pressure, approximately 90 mm Hg).[32] There seems to be a tendency to correlation between reduction in blood pressure and reduction in albuminuria,[33] and a recent analysis concluded that approximately 50% of the anti-albuminuric effect in one study[14] could be caused by the blood pressure reduction.[1] Importantly, early treatment may also prevent the increase in blood pressure seen in the spontaneous course of microalbuminuria.[11]

The clinical consequence is that the indication for antihypertensive treatment should be microalbuminuria (as in the clinical trials) rather than some elevation of blood pressure, an elevation that may be difficult to define considering the overlap in blood pressure between normoalbuminuric and microalbuminuric patients.[1] Obviously, clear elevation of blood pressure would further strengthen the indication, because there is a correlation between rate of progression of microal-

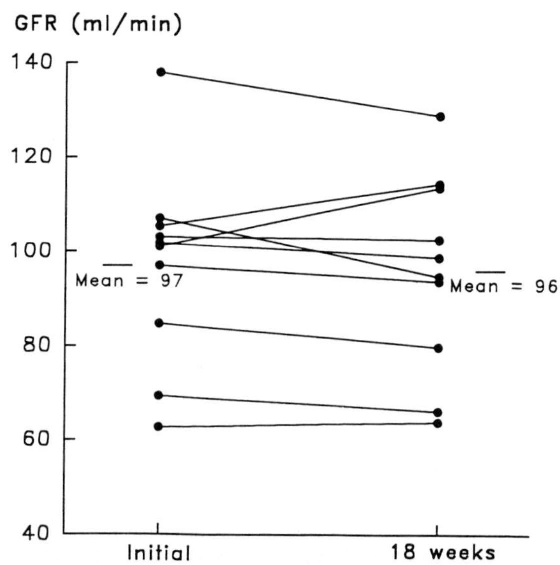

Fig 5. Microalbuminuria in NIDDM patients. The results are from repeated measurements (Table 5).

Table 6. Clinical Data and Results From Renal Clearance Investigations in Insulin-Dependent Diabetes Mellitus Patients

	Microalbuminuric Patients		Normoalbuminuric Patients		Healthy Subjects
No. of patients	50		134		27
Sex (male/female)	34/16	NS*	95/39	NS‡	19/8
Age (yr)	31 ± 10 (19-56)	NS†	33 ± 8 (18-55)	NS†	30 ± 5 (23-42)
Duration of diabetes (yr)	18 ± 6 (8-31)	NS*	19 ± 9 (1-40)		
UAE (μg/min)	53.1 ×/÷ 1.86 (20.8-147.5)		4.5 ×/÷ 1.65 (1.0-19.3)	NS‡	4.0 ×/÷ 1.7 (2.1-17.9)
GFR (mL/min)	142 ± 21 (100-186)	$P < 0.05$	135 ± 16 (97-198)	$P < 1 \cdot 10^{-6}$	118 ± 13 (94-139)
RPF (mL/min)	576 ± 88 (338-700)	NS†	542 ± 82 (325-764)	NS†	536 ± 75 (385-729)
Systolic BP (mm Hg)	129 ± 15 (107-177)	$P < 1 \cdot 10^{-8}$	118 ± 9 (100-148)	$P < 0.05$	114 ± 8 (97-128)
Diastolic BP (mm Hg)	83 ± 10 (60-108)	$P < 0.0001$	77 ± 7 (62-95)	NS‡	77 ± 6 (62-90)
Blood glucose (mmol/L)	13.1 ± 5.3 (2.8-20.8)	NS*	11.7 ± 5.0 (2.3-22.0)		

Note. Data are presented as means ± SD or geometric mean ×/÷ tolerance factor. Ranges are presented in parentheses. The GFR and RPF are corrected to a standard body surface of 1.73 m^2. Healthy subjects are nondiabetic persons without hypertension.[8]

Abbreviation: BP, blood pressure; NS, not significant.

* Comparison between microalbuminuric and normoalbuminuric patients.

† Analysis of variance.

‡ Comparison between normoalbuminuric patients and healthy subjects.

buminuria and blood pressure.[11] A more cautious view would be to start antihypertensive treatment if microalbuminuria is clearly increasing. As seen in Table 8 all studies document a reduction in microalbuminuria, irrespective of the type of treatment used. However, most studies were conducted with ACE inhibitors as a principal agent, sometimes with the addition of diuretics.[14] There were few or no side effects. Thus, the scenario for antihypertensive treatment, particularly ACE inhibitors, is changing from the indication of elevated blood pressure[34,35] to the indication of increased or increasing UAE.[36]

As discussed elsewhere,[1,37] abnormal albuminuria correlates stronger to organ damage (in the kidney and elsewhere) than to blood pressure elevation in not overtly hypertensive diabetic individuals.[1] This concept further strengthens the view that microalbuminuria could be an independent indicator for the start of antihypertensive treatment, particularly ACE inhibitors, often combined with a small dose of diuretics. This idea was proposed in 1985, using a β_1-blocker as the principal agent.[21] New studies show that the addition of ACE inhibitors to β_1-blockers combined with diuretics may be beneficial.[28,29] The risk with this approach, which is not very costly, is limited or nonexistent, and the potential benefit is enormous (increased life expectancy by postponing end-stage renal failure) provided the sustained long-term effect persists, as suggested in a cohort of patients with overt nephropathy.[38]

The long-term, antialbuminuric effect of ACE inhibitors cannot be ascribed to an acute hemodynamic response, since albumin excretion is only slightly decreased acutely by thcse agents.[28] In addition, after discontinuation of ACE inhibitors the reduced albumin excretion persists, at least for the 1 month after stopping therapy.[26]

Overt Diabetic Nephropathy

In the untreated situation there is a correlation between the rate of decline of GFR and blood

Table 7. Stability or Change in Glomerular Filtration Rate and Albuminuria in Insulin-Dependent Diabetes Mellitus Patients (Without Antihypertensive Treatment)

Reference (Designation in Fig 6)	No. of Patients	Mean Duration of Diabetes (yr)	Follow-up Period (mo)	Mean Albumin Excretion of Period (μg/min) (Geometric Mean ×/÷ Confidence Factor)	GFR (mL/min) (Initial → Follow-up)	Mean Blood Pressure of Period
Christensen et al.[10,11] (A)	12	8	24	4.8 ×/÷ 1.3	138 → 139*	113/77
Mau Pedersen (unpublished data) (B_1)	14	20 ± 6	20	29.9 ×/÷ 2.0	147 → 146*	121/80
Christensen and Mogensen[11,12] (B_2)	6	20	78	84.5 ×/÷ 1.5	142 → 141*	134/87
Feldt-Rasmussen et al[13] (C_1)	15	15	≈78	≈36	116 → 116†	128/82
Mathiesen et al[14] (C_2)	16	17	48	55.6 ×/÷ 1.2	117 → 114†	125/76
Mathiesen et al[14] (C_3)	7	17	48	268.7 ×/÷ 1.1	Fall in GFR,† 0.33 mL/min/mo	127/80
Mogensen[15] (D)	7	18 ± 2	28	2689.7 ×/÷ 1.3	Fall in GFR,* 0.96 mL/min/mo	161/101

* Constant-infusion technique for GFR determination.
† Single shot technique for GFR determination.
Note. The letters in column 1 (A, B_1, B_2, C_1, C_2, C_3, and D) refer to Fig 6.

pressure,[15] but, interestingly, the correlation between the rate of decline of GFR and the degree of albuminuria is equally strong.[15] Recently, it has been documented that a pronounced decrease in proteinuria after the start of antihypertensive treatment predicts a more benign course of renal disease in IDDM patients, also suggesting an important role of the level of albuminuria for rate of progression in renal disease,[33] at least in the prediction process. Several studies have documented that antihypertensive treatment clearly reduces the rate of decline of GFR, and this effect is always accompanied by the reduction of albuminuria.[5,39,40] Antihypertensive treatment is the major therapeutic option for these patients. The use of ACE inhibitors (with diuretics) is clearly popular, but antihypertensive programs with β_1-blockers also seem to be equally effective, possi-

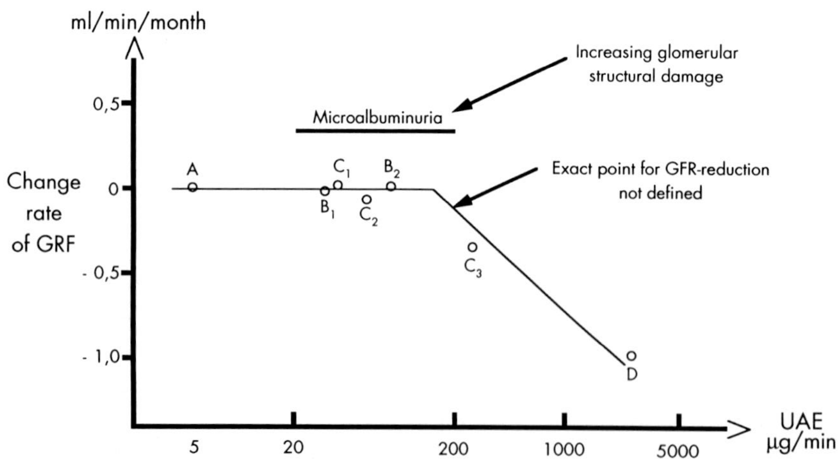

Fig 6. Decline in GFR (mean) as related to different levels of UAE (geometric mean and confidence intervals) in IDDM patients without antihypertensive treatment (n = 70). The letters (A, B_1, B_2, C_1, C_2, C_3, and D) refer to data in Table 7.

Table 8. Trial in Young Nonhypertensive Microalbuminuric or Early Nephropathy Insulin-Dependent Diabetes Mellitus Patients (Resulting in Slightly Reduced Blood Pressure)

	Nature of Trial	Intervention	Pretreatment BP	No. of Patients and Duration of Treatment	Microalbuminuria	Remarks
Christensen and Mogensen[12,21]	Self-controlled, open	β_1-blocker + diuretics	135/93	6, 5 yr	Reduced	Gradual reversal by antihypertensive treatment
Marre et al[22]	Double-blinded, randomized with parallel controls	ACE inhibition	≈100 (MAP)	20, 1 yr	Reduced by ACE inhibition	Untreated patients showed rapid increase in UAE
Brichard et al[23]	Open	ACE inhibition	169/101	7, 1 yr	Reduced by ACE inhibition	Open study
Rudberg et al[24]	Open	ACE inhibition	135/85 and 113/72	12, 6 mo	Reduced by ACE inhibition	Young patients
Cook et al[25]	Cross-over, double-blinded	ACE inhibition	108/64	12, 3 mo	Reduced by ACE inhibition	Children
Melbourne Diabetic Nephropathy Study Group[26]	Open, randomized with parallel controls	ACE inhibition *v* calcium blocker	102 (MAP)	43, 1 yr	Reduced by ACE inhibition and by calcium blocker	Effect mostly seen with elevated blood pressure
Mathiesen et al[14]	Open, randomized with parallel controls	ACE inhibition	125/77	44, 4 yr	Reduced by ACE inhibition	First study to indicate preservation of GFR; proteinuria prevented
Marre et al[27]	Double-blinded, randomized with parallel controls	ACE inhibition	132/79	16, 6 wk	Reduced	Effect not dose dependent
Mau Pedersen et al[28]	Open, cross-over	β_1-blocker thiazide + ACE inhibition	129/84	8, 3 mo	Albuminuria reduced	Triple treatment may be useful (early nephropathy)
Mau Pedersen et al[29]	Cross-over, double-blinded	β_1-blocker thiazide + ACE inhibition	133/85	10, 4 mo	Albuminuria reduced	Triple treatment may be useful (early nephropathy) (results similar to open study[28])
Hallab et al[30]	Randomized with parallel controls	ACE inhibition *v* thiazide	134/78	21, 1 yr	Reduced by ACE inhibition	ACE inhibition more efficient than thiazide
Mogensen[31] (European Microalbuminuria Study Group)	Multicenter, double-blinded, randomized with parallel controls	ACE inhibition	124/77	92, 2 yr	Reduced by ACE inhibition	First large-scale, double-blind study; increase in albuminuria and development of proteinuria prevented

Abbreviations: BP, blood pressure; MAP, mean arterial pressure.

bly with more side effects, especially hypo-glycemic unawareness.[34-39] A low-protein diet may also reduce the rate of decline of GFR in these patients,[41,42] but in most of the trials with antihypertensive treatment, which had an excellent effect on the rate of decline of GFR, dietary protein restriction was not used.[39,40] Thus, the results presented by Zeller et al[42] have been debated by Parving[43] simply because Parving et al and Björck et al found a low decline in the rate of GFR without dietary protein restriction but with efficient antihypertensive therapy.[39,40]

Triple Treatment Using Diuretics, Beta Blockers, and Angiotensin-Converting Enzyme Inhibitors in Early Diabetic Nephropathy

This treatment modality seems to have a clear pathophysiologic rationale.[29] Angiotensin-converting enzyme inhibition has shown promising results in diabetic nephropathy, but the long-term results concerning survival are not available, in contrast to data concerning β_1-blockers.[38] In a cohort of patients receiving antihypertensive treatment predominantly consisting of beta blockers in combination with diuretics, support for an improved survival has been presented.[38] The addition of angiotensin-converting enzyme inhibition to such a combination treatment may be favorable both due to the suggested renoprotective effects of ACE inhibitors and because diuretics activate the renin angiotensin system. Diabetic patients often show sodium retention.[44,45] The IDDM patients with early diabetic nephropathy (UAE $< 1{,}000$ μg/min) who were receiving continuous therapy with metoprolol and bendroflumethiazide were included in a double-blind cross-over study with 4 months' addition of ramipril 5 mg (Ramace) and placebo.[29] Urinary albumin excretion and fractional albumin excretion were significantly reduced after the 4 months of ramipril administration. The GFR (^{125}I-iothalamate clearance) remained unchanged (121 ± 8 v 120 ± 9 mL/min/1.73 m^2), and the mean arterial pressure during clearance studies decreased moderately (95 ± 3 v 101 ± 1 mm Hg, $P < 0.05$), correlated to changes in UAE. Angiotensin-converting enzyme activity was suppressed in all patients. It can be concluded that the addition of an ACE inhibitor reduces UAE in patients receiving ongoing antihypertensive therapy. Qualitatively, the renal response to ACE inhibition in the present patients receiving beta blocker and thiazide treatment corresponds to the hemodynamic effects observed in previously untreated diabetic patients.[28]

The GFR continues to be stable on a long-term basis (3 years) using this therapy, as seen in Fig 3. It is important to exclude initial GFR values during treatment because of a potential short-term hemodynamic effect, and Fig 3 only shows data after 1 year of treatment, as seen in Table 4. No significant change in any of the parameters is seen (blood pressure, UAE, GFR, and RPF). Before adding the ACE inhibitor, the mean GFR was 114 mL/min; after 3.3 years the final data concerning combination therapy show the mean GFR to be 107 mL/min. The results from this small study suggest stable renal function and GFR with triple treatment in early diabetic nephropathy, but further long-term studies are needed.

CONCLUSION

This study documents a good reproducibility in repeated measurements of GFR in diabetic patients with coefficients of variance of approximately 7% to 8%. However, in few individual patients difference in GFR in two tests may be approximately 25% (associated with marked change in HbA_{1c}). This is observed in IDDM patients using the constant-infusion technique using labeled iothalamate clearance with urine collection procedures. A similar mean low degree of variability is also observed by the single-shot procedure in NIDDM patients. Generally, the coefficient of variance between two measurements is from 5% to 8%. This is also seen with high GFR values in patients with normoalbuminuria and microalbuminuria as well as in patients with early overt proteinuria. In cross-sectional studies of IDDM patients published to date, it is well documented that normoalbuminuric and microalbuminuric IDDM patients still have a well-preserved GFR, most often with GFR values higher than in healthy controls. This concept has been confirmed, in longitudinal studies, and the studies also suggest that GFR starts to decline with the transition from microalbuminuria to macroalbuminuria, although the exact cut-off point for GFR loss is not yet clearly defined and may not be the same in all patients. In addition, in NIDDM patients the GFR starts to decline with the transition from microalbuminuria to macroalbuminuria.

Multiple intervention studies with antihypertensive treatment suggest the beneficial effect by reducing abnormal albuminuria. Most studies are short term, but one long-term study documents that the GFR is preserved by ACE inhibition in microalbuminuric patients. This is consistent with the observation that the rate of decline of GFR is reduced by antihypertensive treatment in overt renal disease. Differences between various antihypertensive regimens (eg, ACE inhibitors v β_1-blockers) may be documented in favor of ACE inhibitors,[40,46] but this is not the case in all studies.[5,47] However, there are fewer side effects from ACE inhibitors. When evaluating the general effect of antihypertensive treatment it is important to view abnormal albuminuria as a continuous documentation of increasing severity of renal disease. Therefore, if reduction of abnormal albuminuria means a decreased decline of GFR in overt proteinuria, it is also likely that reduction of abnormal albuminuria in the microalbuminuric range means preservation of GFR, which is also suggested in one long-term study. Effective antihypertensive treatment, mainly with ACE inhibitors and diuretics, possibly combined with other agents (β_1-blockers) is at present the main method of ameliorating the malignant course of renal disease in IDDM patients. However, intervention over a decade may be needed to adequately document a beneficial effect in microalbuminuric patients. Monitoring of structural damage under therapy may present an opportunity to obtain results over a shorter period of time.

ADDENDUM

Recent literature has explored the role of hyperfiltration,[48] exercise,[49] and hypertension[50] in diabetic nephropathy. The management of the condition,[51-53] the history of hypertension in diabetes,[54] and microalbuminuria[55-57] have also been discussed.

REFERENCES

1. Mogensen CE, Østerby R, Hansen KW, Damsgaard EM: Blood pressure elevation versus abnormal albuminuria in the genesis and prediction of renal disease in diabetes. Diabetes Care 15:1192-1204, 1992

2. Mogensen CE, Hansen KW, Klebe J, Christensen CK, Schmitz A, Mau Pedersen M, Pedersen EB, Jespersen B, Petersen RS, Christiansen JS, Schmitz O, Damsgaard EM, Frøland A: Microalbuminuria: Studies in diabetes, essential hypertension, and renal diseases as compared with the background population, in Grünfeld JP (ed): Advances in Nephrology, vol 20. Chicago, IL, Mosby Year Book, 1991, pp 191-228

3. Messent JWC, Elliott TG, Hill RD, Jarrett RJ, Keen H, Viberti GC: Prognostic significance of microalbuminuria in insulin-dependent diabetes mellitus: A twenty-three year follow-up study. Kidney Int 41:836-839, 1992

4. Mau Pedersen M, Christensen CK, Mogensen CE: Long-term (18 year) prognosis for normo- and microalbuminuric type 1 (insulin-dependent) diabetic patients. Diabetologia 35:A60, 1992 (abstr)

5. Mogensen CE: Angiotensin converting enzyme inhibitors and diabetic nephropathy. Br Med J 304:227-228, 1992 (editorial)

6. Brøchner-Mortensen J: Routine methods and their reliability for assessment of glomerular filtration rate in adults. With special reference to total (^{51}Cr)EDTA plasma clearance. Dan Med Bull 25:181-202, 1978

7. Hommel E, Parving H-H, Mathiesen E, Edsberg B, Nielsen MD, Giese J: Effect of captopril on kidney function in insulin-dependent diabetic patients with nephropathy. Br Med J 293:479-480, 1986

8. Hansen KW, Mau Pedersen M, Christensen CK, Schmitz A, Christiansen JS, Mogensen CE: Normoalbuminuria ensures no reduction of renal function in type 1 (insulin-dependent) diabetic patients. J Intern Med 232:161-167, 1992

9. Mau Pedersen M, Christiansen JS, Pedersen EB, Mogensen CE: Determinants of intra-individual variation in kidney function in normoalbuminuric insulin-dependent diabetic patients: Importance of atrial natriuretic peptide and glycaemic control. Clin Sci 83:445-451, 1992

10. Christensen CK, Christiansen JS, Schmitz A, Christensen T, Hermansen K, Mogensen CE: Effect of continuous subcutaneous insulin infusion on kidney function and size in IDDM-patients: A 2 year controlled study. J Diabet Complications 1:91-95, 1987

11. Christensen CK: The pre-proteinuric phase of diabetic nephropathy. Dan Med Bull 38:145-159, 1991

12. Christensen CK, Mogensen CE: Antihypertensive treatment: Long-term reversal of progression of albuminuria in incipient diabetic nephropathy. A longitudinal study of renal function. J Diabet Complications 1:45-52, 1987

13. Feldt-Rasmussen B, Mathiesen ER, Jensen T, Lauritzen T, Deckert T: Effect of improved metabolic control on loss of kidney function in type 1 (insulin-dependent) diabetic patients: An update of the Steno studies. Diabetologia 34:164-170, 1991

14. Mathiesen ER, Hommel E, Giese J, Parving H-H: Efficacy of captopril in postponing nephropathy in normotensive insulin-dependent diabetic patients with microalbuminuria. Br Med J 303:81-87, 1991

15. Mogensen CE: Progression of nephropathy in long-term diabetics with proteinuria and effect of initial anti-hypertensive treatment. Scand J Clin Lab Invest 36:383-388, 1976

16. Mogensen CE, Christensen CK: Blood pressure changes and renal function in incipient and overt diabetic nephropathy. Hypertension 7:II-64-II-73, 1985

17. Schmitz A, Christensen T, Møller A, Mogensen CE:

Kidney function and cardiovascular risk factors in non–insulin-dependent diabetics (NIDDM) with microalbuminuria. J Intern Med 228:347-352, 1990

18. Nielsen S, Schmitz A, Rehling M, Mogensen CE: Systolic blood pressure determines the rate of decline of glomerular filtration rate in Type 2 (non-insulin-dependent) diabetes mellitus. Diabetes Care 16:1427-1432, 1993

19. Myers BD, Nelson RG, Williams GW, Bennett PH, Hardy SA, Berg RL, Loon N, Knowler WC, Mitch WE: Glomerular function in Pima Indians with noninsulin-dependent diabetes mellitus of recent onset. J Clin Invest 88:524-530, 1991

20. Mau Pedersen M, Schmitz A, Pedersen EB, Danielsen H, Christiansen JS: Acute and long-term renal effects of angiotensin converting enzyme inhibition in normotensive, normoalbuminuric insulin-dependent diabetic patients. Diabetic Med 5:562-569, 1988

21. Christensen CK, Mogensen CE: Effect of antihypertensive treatment on progression of incipient diabetic nephropathy. Hypertension 7:II-109-II-113, 1985 (suppl II)

22. Marre M, Chatellier G, Leblanc H, Guyenne T-T, Ménard J, Passa Ph: Prevention of diabetic nephropathy with enalapril in normotensive diabetics with microalbuminuria. Br Med J 297:1092-1095, 1988

23. Brichard SM, Santoni JPh, Thomas JR, van de Voorde K, Ketelslegers JM, Lambert AE: Long term reduction of microalbuminuria after 1 year of angiotensin converting enzyme inhibition by perindropil in hypertensive insulin-treated diabetic patients. Diabete Metab 16:30-36, 1989

24. Rudberg S, Aperia A, Freyschuss U, Persson B: Enalapril reduces microalbuminuria in young normotensive type 1 (insulin-dependent) diabetic patients irrespective of its hypotensive effect. Diabetologia 33:470-476, 1990

25. Cook JJ, Daneman D, Spino M, Sochett E, Perlman K, Balfe JW: Angiotensin converting enzyme inhibitor therapy to decrease microalbuminuria in normotensive children with insulin-dependent diabetes mellitus. J Pediatr 117:39-45, 1990

26. Melbourne Diabetic Nephropathy Study Group: Comparison between perindopril and nifedipine in hypertensive and normotensive diabetic patients with microalbuminuria. Br Med J 302:210-216, 1991

27. Marre M, Hallab M, Billiard A, Le Jeune JJ, Bled F, Girault A, Fressinaud Ph: Small doses of ramipril to reduce microalbuminuria in diabetic patients with incipient nephropathy independently of blood pressure changes. J Cardiovasc Pharmacol 18:S165-S168, 1991 (suppl 2)

28. Mau Pedersen M, Christensen CK, Hansen KW, Christiansen JS, Mogensen: ACE-inhibition and renoprotection in early diabetic nephropathy. Response to enalapril acutely and in long-term combination with conventional antihypertensive treatment. Clin Invest Med 14:642-651, 1991

29. Mau Pedersen M, Hansen KW, Schmitz A, Sørensen K, Christensen CK, Mogensen CE: Effect of ACE-inhibition supplementary to beta-blockers and diuretics in early diabetic nephropathy. Kidney Int 41:883-890, 1992

30. Hallab M, Gallois Y, Chatellier G, Rohmer V, Fressinaud P, Marre M: Comparison of reduction in microalbuminuria by enalapril and hydrochlorothiazide in normotensive patients with insulin dependent diabetes. Br Med J 306:175-182, 1993

31. Viberti GC, Mogensen CE, Groop L, Pauls JF for the European Microalbuminuria Captopril Study Group: Effect of captopril on progression to clinical proteinuria in patients with insulin-dependent diabetes mellitus and microalbuminuria. JAMA 271:275-279, 1994

32. Mogensen CE, Hansen KW, Mau Pedersen M, Christensen CK: Renal factors influencing blood pressure threshold and choice of treatment for hypertension in IDDM. Diabetes Care 14:13-26, 1991 (suppl 4)

33. Rossing P, Hommel E, Smidt UM, Parving H-H: Reduction in albuminuria predicts diminished progression in diabetic nephropathy. Kidney Int 45:S145-S149, 1994 (suppl 45)

34. Mogensen CE: Long-term antihypertensive treatment inhibiting progression of diabetic nephropathy. Br Med J 285:685-688, 1982

35. Mogensen CE: Management of diabetic renal involvement and disease. Lancet 1:867-870, 1988

36. Mogensen CE, Poulsen PL, Heinsvig EM: Abnormal albuminuria in the monitoring of early renal changes in diabetes, in Mogensen CE, Standl E (eds): Concepts for the Ideal Diabetes Clinic. Diabetes Forum Series, vol 4. Berlin, Germany, Walter de Gruyter, 1993, pp 289-313

37. Mogensen CE, Mau Pedersen M, Hansen KW, Christensen CK: Micro-albuminuria and the organ-damage concept in antihypertensive therapy for patients with insulin-dependent diabetes mellitus. J Hypertens 10:S43-S51, 1992 (suppl 1)

38. Mathiesen ER, Borch-Johnsen K, Jensen DV, Deckert T: Improved survival in patients with diabetic nephropathy. Diabetologia 32:884-886, 1989

39. Parving H-H, Andersen AR, Smidt UM, Hommel E, Mathiesen ER, Svendsen PA: Effect of antihypertensive treatment on kidney function in diabetic nephropathy. Br Med J 294:1443-1447, 1987

40. Björck S, Mulec H, Johnsen SA, Nordén G, Aurell M: Renal protective effect of enalapril in diabetic nephropathy. Br Med J 304:339-343, 1992

41. Walker JD, Dodds RA, Murrells TJ, Bending JJ, Mattock MB, Keen H, Viberti GC: Restriction of dietary protein and progression of renal failure in diabetic nephropathy. Lancet 2:1411-1415, 1989

42. Zeller KR, Whittaker E, Sullivan L, Raskin P, Jacobson HR: Effect of dietary protein on the progression of renal failure in patients with insulin-dependent diabetes mellitus. N Engl J Med 324:78-84, 1991

43. Parving H-H: Protein restriction and renal failure in diabetes mellitus. N Engl J Med 324:1743-1744, 1991

44. Feldt-Rasmussen B, Mathiesen ER, Deckert T, Giese J, Christensen NJ, Bent-Hansen L, Nielsen MD: Central role for sodium in the pathogenesis of blood pressure changes independent of angiotensin, aldosterone and catecholamines in type 1 (insulin-dependent) diabetes mellitus. Diabetologia 30:610-617, 1987

45. Weidmann P, Ferrari P: Central role of sodium in hypertension in diabetic subjects. Diabetes Care 14:220-232, 1991

46. Kasiske BL, Kalil RSN, Ma JZ, Liao M, Keane WF: Effect of antihypertensive therapy on the kidney in patients with diabetes: A meta-regression analysis. Ann Intern Med 118:129-138, 1993

47. Parving H-H, Rossing P, Hommel E, Smidt UM: Renal protective effects of captopril and metoprolol in diabetic nephropathy. J Am Soc Nephrol 3:337, 1992 (abstr)

48. Mogensen CE: Glomerular hyperfiltration in human diabetes. Diabetes Care 17:770-775, 1994

49. Mogensen CE: Nephropathy: Early, in The Handbook of Diabetes and Exercise. American Diabetes Association (in press)

50. Mogensen CE: Systemic blood pressure and glomerular leakage with particular reference to diabetes and hypertension. J Intern Med 235:297-316, 1994

51. Mogensen CE: Management of the diabetic patient with elevated blood pressure or renal disease. Early screening and treatment programs: Albuminuria and blood pressure, in Laragh JH, Brenner BM (eds): Hypertension: Pathology, Diagnosis and Management (ed 2). New York, NY, Raven, 1995, pp 2335-2365

52. Mogensen CE: Management of early nephropathy in diabetic patients. Annu Rev Med 46:79-94, 1995

53. Bennett PH, Haffner S, Kasiske BL, Keane WF, Mogensen CE, Parving H-H, Steffes MW, Striker GE: Screening and management of microalbuminuria in patients with diabetes mellitus—Recommendations to the scientific advisory board of the National Kidney Foundation from an ad hoc committee of the Council on Diabetes Mellitus of the National Kidney Foundation. Am J Kidney Dis 25:107-112, 1995

54. Mogensen CE: Diabetic renal disease: The quest for normotension—and beyond. Including some personal experiences and observations. Diabet Med (in press)

55. Mogensen CE, Vestbo E, Poulsen PL, Christiansen C, Damsgaard E, Eiskjaer H, Frøland A, Hansen KW, Nielsen S, Mau Pedersen M: Microalbuminuria and potential confounders. A review and some observations on variability of urinary albumin excretion. Diabetes Care 18:572-581, 1995

56. Mogensen CE, Christensen CK, Christensen PD, Hansen KW, Molgaard H, Mau Pedersen M, Poulsen PL, Schmitz A, Thuesen L, Østerby R: The abnormal albuminuria syndrome in diabetes. Microalbuminuria: Key to the complications, in Belfiore F, Bergman RN, Molinatti GM (eds): Current Topics in Diabetes Research. Front Diabetes. Basel, Karger, 1993, pp 86-121

57. Poulsen PL, Mogensen CE: Evaluation of a new semiquantitative stix for microalbuminuria. Diabetes Care 18:732-733, 1995

Studies of the Renal Effects of Angiotensin II Receptor Blockade: The Confounding Factor of Acute Water Loading on the Action of Vasoactive Systems

M. Burnier, MD, A. Pechère-Bertschi, MD, J. Nussberger, MD, B. Waeber, MD, and H.R. Brunner, MD

● The acute renal tubular effects of two pharmacologically distinct angiotensin II receptor antagonists have been evaluated in normotensive volunteers on various salt diets. In the first study, the renal response to a single oral dose of losartan (100 mg) was assessed in subjects on a low (50 mmol Na/d) and on a high (200 mmol Na/d) salt intake. In a second protocol, the renal effects of 50 mg irbesartan were investigated in subjects receiving a 100 mmol Na/d diet. Both angiotensin II antagonists induced a significant increase in urinary sodium excretion. With losartan, a modest, transient increase in urinary potassium and a significant increase in uric acid excretion were found. In contrast, no change in potassium and uric acid excretions were observed with irbesartan, suggesting that the effects of losartan on potassium and uric acid are due to the intrinsic pharmacologic properties of losartan rather than to the specific blockade of renal angiotensin II receptors. Assessment of segmental sodium reabsorption using lithium as a marker of proximal tubular reabsorption demonstrated a decreased distal reabsorption of sodium with both antagonists. A direct proximal tubular natriuretic effect of the angiotensin II antagonist could be demonstrated only with irbesartan. This apparent discrepancy allowed us to reveal the importance of acute water loading as a possible confounding factor in renal studies. The results of the present analysis show that acute water loading per se may enhance renal sodium excretion and hence modify the level of activity of the renin-angiotensin system expected from a given sodium diet. Since acute water loading is a common practice in clinical renal studies, this confounding factor should be taken into account when investigating the renal effects of vasoactive systems.

INDEX WORDS: Angiotensin II; receptor antagonists, human; renal sodium; uric acid.

BESIDES its ability to control vascular tone and hence the renal and glomerular hemodynamics, to stimulate aldosterone secretion, and to modulate neural catecholamine release, angiotensin II is a potent regulator of transepithelial sodium transport in renal tubular cells. Thus, in microperfused, subcortical rabbit proximal convoluted tubules, angiotensin II has been shown to increase sodium and water absorption at physiologic low concentrations (10^{-11} and 10^{-10} mol/L), whereas sodium transport is reduced by higher concentrations of the peptide (10^{-8} and 10^{-6} mol/L).[1] In vitro, angiotensin II modulates sodium and water reabsorption both in the S_1 and S_2 segments of the proximal tubule, but its effect is quantitatively larger in the former segment than in the latter.[2] These effects of angiotensin II occur independently of changes in renal or systemic hemodynamics.

Angiotensin II can regulate the epithelial cell function either directly by occupancy of both luminal and basolateral membrane receptors, or indirectly by activation of presynaptic receptors controlling catecholamine release from nerves having terminals on the tubular cells.[3] In the proximal tubule, sodium is reabsorbed together with either chloride or bicarbonate. Angiotensin II appears to affect predominantly the sodium bicarbonate transport via epithelial receptors, whereas changes in sodium chloride reabsorption are predominantly mediated via presynaptic angiotensin II receptors on nerve terminals.[3] Angiotensin II increases transport primarily by a Gi protein-mediated decrease in intracellular cyclic adenosine monophosphate, which enhances the affinity of the Na^+-H^+ antiporter.[4]

Sodium excretion in postproximal segments also is modulated by angiotensin II, mainly through its effect on aldosterone secretion. However, autoradiographic studies have demonstrated the presence of angiotensin II receptors in the outer medulla, which contains medullary and cortical thick ascending limbs as well as thin limbs of Henle's loops.[5,6] In addition, the medullary vasa recta flow is under the control of angiotensin II.[7] A decrease in sodium reabsorption in the loop of Henle may thus occur in response to a vasodilation of the medullary circulation.

Clinically, the ability of angiotensin II to affect sodium excretion has been demonstrated with the use of angiotensin-converting enzyme (ACE) inhibitors, which reduce the generation of angiotensin II. Thus, ACE inhibitors have been shown

Supported by a grant from the Fonds National de la Recherche Scientifique, Bern, Switzerland.

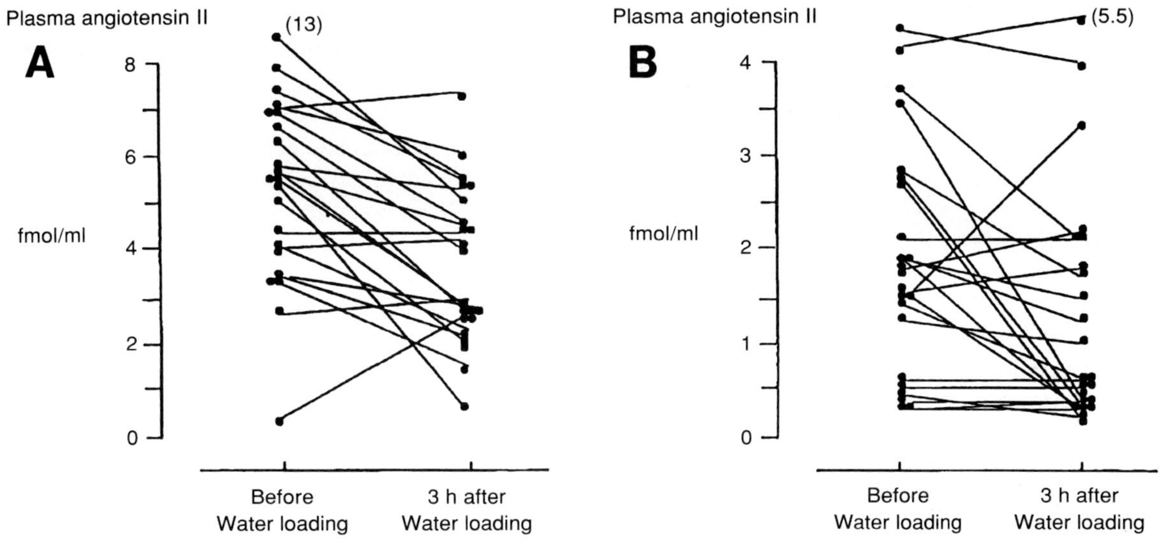

Fig 4. Individual changes in plasma angiotensin II levels observed before and after acute water loading in salt-depleted (50 mmol Na/d; n = 23) (A) and salt-loaded (200 mmol Na/d; n = 23) (B) normotensive subjects.

panel). Plasma angiotensin II correlates with the sodium excretion rate, thereby confirming the known relationship between urinary sodium excretion and plasma renin activity.[23] However, because massive water loading increased sodium excretion in salt-depleted subjects, moderately water-loaded volunteers on the 100 mmol salt diet (closed triangles) end up with higher plasma angiotensin II levels than those on the low salt intake (open circles). The lower panel of Fig 3 illustrates that urine flow rate can markedly influence the baseline activity of the renin-angiotensin system. Indeed, plasma angiotensin II levels are lower in subjects on a low salt diet who have a urine flow rate above 10 mL/min than in subjects on a higher salt-intake but a reduced urine output. Figure 4 depicts the individual changes in plasma angiotensin II levels before and 3 hours after maintenance of a high urine flow rate by water loading. A clear decrease in plasma angiotensin II levels is observed in both salt-depleted and, to a certain degree, salt-repleted subjects. Together, these observations indicate that acute water loading enhances renal sodium excretion. Although not investigated in the present studies, this effect of water might be linked to the stimulation of atrial natriuretic peptide secretion. Other substances may contribute to these effects, including prostaglandins and vasopressin. Yet, in our experience, vasopressin levels are hardly measurable after acute water loading. Thus, when performing renal studies in humans, water loading should be kept as low as possible to obtain accurate urine collections. If necessary, the duration of the urine collection should be prolonged rather than the volume of the water load augmented.

Uric acid excretion is sometimes used as a marker of proximal tubular reabsorption. Thus, the 10% to 30% increase in uric acid excretion observed under ACE inhibition has been attributed to a reduced activity of angiotensin II on proximal uric acid reabsorption. In the present studies, losartan induced a very marked increase in uric acid excretion (+300%), which is out of proportion with the previous observations using ACE inhibitors or calcium channel blockers.[24,25] In fact, the uricosuric effect of losartan is closer to that of probenecid than that of ACE inhibitors.[26] In our studies, the increase in uric acid excretion induced by losartan was independent of salt intake and hence of the degree of stimulation of the renin angiotensin system. Moreover, no increased uricosuria was found with irbesartan. These data suggest that the effect of losartan on uric acid excretion is the result of a pharmacologic interaction between the losartan molecule and uric acid transport in the proximal tubule and is not linked to the blockade of angiotensin II receptors on the proximal tubule. The recent demonstration that E-3174, the active metabolite of losartan, has no effect on uric acid excretion goes along with a specific effect of the losartan molecule.[27] In addition, urinary pH and urine flow rate, two important determinants of uric acid excretion, were not different in the placebo and losartan groups. It may seem surprising that the fractional excretion of lithium increased with irbesartan whereas uric acid excretion did not change, since both parameters are supposed to be markers of proximal tubular reabsorption. In our opinion, this apparent discrepancy is due to the fact that lithium is a much more sensitive index of proximal reabsorption than uric acid, as we demonstrated recently in the context of the diagnosis of acute renal failure.[28]

Urinary potassium excretion is known to decrease during long-term inhibition of the renin-angiotensin system. Surprisingly, an increase rather than a decrease in urinary potassium excretion has been reported to occur on the acute administration of losartan in rats and dogs.[17,18] In normotensive subjects, an increase in urinary potassium excretion also was found with losartan.[12] With irbesartan a slight increase in potassium excretion was noted, but the change did not reach statistical significance. The acute kaliuretic response to angiotensin II receptor blockade may be the consequence of the increased natriuresis, since an increased sodium delivery to distal tubules may lead to a reduced reabsorption of potassium. This mechanism likely contributes to the slight kaliuresis observed with irbesartan. However, during salt depletion, losartan produced an increase in sodium excretion comparable to that of irbesartan, as shown in Fig 1. Yet, the kaliuretic effect of losartan was more pronounced. This suggests that another parameter contributes to the effect of losartan on potassium excretion. An alternative explanation is that the high uric acid concentration in the distal tubule enhances potassium excretion by increasing the number of negative charges in the lumen. To support this hypothesis, a positive relationship recently was found between the changes in urinary potassium excretion and urinary uric acid excretion.[26] An increased distal delivery could theoretically also play a role because angiotensin II receptor blockade is known to inhibit sodium bicarbonate reabsorption in the proximal tubule.[21] However, under normal conditions, a decreased reabsorption of bicarbonate in the S1 segment of the proximal tubule is generally fully compensated by an increased reabsorption in the S2 segment. At last, differences in urine flow rate could modulate potassium secretion in the distal tubule. The results obtained in the two placebo groups (Fig 2) do not favor this hypothesis since potassium excretion was lower in subjects receiving the placebo of losartan, which had a high urine flow rate, than in those given the placebo of irbesartan.

In conclusion, we recently investigated the acute renal tubular effects of two pharmacologically different longacting angiotensin II receptor antagonists in normotensive volunteers. After a single administration of both compounds, a significant increase in urinary sodium excretion occurred. Concomitantly, a transient increase in urinary uric acid and potassium excretion was found with losartan, but not with irbesartan, thereby suggesting that these effects are due to the intrinsic properties of the losartan molecule and not to the specific blockade of angiotensin II receptors. Whether the tubular responses of these agents persist during long-term administration, particularly in patients, and are clinically relevant to their antihypertensive efficacy will be the topic of further studies. In addition, this new analysis of our results demonstrates that acute water loading is an important methodologic aspect to consider when assessing the renal effects of vasoactive drugs in humans, as it may increase sodium excretion if too abundant.

REFERENCES

1. Schuster VL, Kokko JP, Jacobson HR: Angiotensin II directly stimulates sodium transport in rabbit proximal convoluted tubules. J Clin Invest 73:507-515, 1984

2. Liu F-Y, Cogan MG: Angiotensin II: A potent regulator of acidification in the rat early proximal convoluted tubule. J Clin Invest 80:272-275, 1987

3. Liu F-Y, Cogan MG: Angiotensin II stimulation of hydrogen ion secretion in the rat early proximal tubule. Modes of action, mechanisms, and kinetics. J Clin Invest 82:601-607, 1988

4. Liu F-Y, Cogan MG: Angiotensin II stimulates early proximal bicarbonate absorption in the rat by decreasing cyclic adenosine monophosphate. J Clin Invest 84:83-91, 1989

5. Mendelsohn FAO: Localization and properties of angiotensin receptors. J Hypertens 3:307-316, 1985

6. Douglas JG: Angiotensin receptor subtypes of the kidney cortex. Am J Physiol 253:F1-F7, 1987

7. Faubert PF, Chou SY, Porush JG: Regulation of papillary plasma flow by angiotensin II. Kidney Int 32:472-478, 1987

8. McNabb WR, Noormohamed FH, Brooks BA, Till AE, Lant AF: Effects of repeated doses of enalapril and renal function in man. Br J Clin Pharmacol 19:353-361, 1985

9. Strocchi E, Malini PL, Ambrosioni E: Lisinopril and

renal tubular function. J Hypertension 5:S401-S402, 1987 (suppl 5)

10. MacGregor GA, Markandu ND, Roulston JF, Jones JC, Morton JJ: The renin-angiotensin-aldosterone system in the maintenance of blood pressure, aldosterone secretion and sodium clearance in normotensive subjects. Clin Sci 59:95s-99s, 1980

11. McNabb WR, Noormohamed FH, Lant AF: The effects of enalapril on blood pressure and the kidney in normotensive subjects under altered sodium balance. J Hypertens 4:39-47, 1986

12. Burnier M, Rutschmann B, Nussberger J, Versaggi J, Shahinfar S, Waeber B, Brunner HR: Salt-dependent renal effects of an angiotensin II antagonist in healthy subjects. Hypertension 22:339-347, 1993

13. Burnier M, Hagman M, Nussberger J, Armagnac C, Brouard R, Waeber B, Brunner HR: Short-term and sustained renal effects of angiotensin II receptor blockade in healthy subjects. Hypertension 25:602-609, 1995

14. Ribstein J, Sissmann J, Picard A, Bouroudian M, Mimran A: Effect of the angiotensin II antagonist SR 47436 (BMS 186295) on the pressor response to exogenous angiotensin II and the renin-angiotensin system in sodium replete normal subjects. J Hypertens 12:131, 1994 (suppl 3) (abstr)

15. Magnin JL, Munafo A, Steinhauslin F, Burnier M, Diezi J, Biollaz J: Endogenous lithium: A new tool in nephrology. Experientia 47:A30, 1991 (abstr)

16. Nussberger J, Keller I, Waeber B, Brunner HR: Angiotensin II measurement with high affinity monoclonal antibodies. J Hypertens 6:S424-S425, 1988 (suppl 4)

17. Fenoy FJ, Milicic I, Smith RD, Wong PC, Timmermans PBMWM, Roman R: Effects of Dup 753 on renal function of normotensive and spontaneously hypertensive rats. Am J Hypertens 4:321S-326S, 1991

18. Bovee KC, Wong PC, Timmermans PBMWM, Thoolen MJMC: Effects of nonpeptide angiotensin II receptors antagonist DuP 753 on blood pressure and renal functions in spontaneously hypertensive PH dogs. Am J Hypertens 4:327S-333S, 1991

19. Chan DP, Sandok EK, Aarhus LL, Heublein DM, Burnett JC Jr: Renal-specific actions of angiotensin II receptor antagonism in the anesthetized dog. Am J Hypertens 5:354-360, 1992

20. Zhuo J, Thomas D, Harris PJ, Skinner SL: The role of endogenous angiotensin II in the regulation of renal haemodynamics and proximal fluid reabsorption in the rat. J Physiol 453:1-13, 1992

21. Xie MH, Liu FY, Wong PC, Timmermans PBMWM, Cogan MG: Proximal nephron and renal effects of Dup 753, a nonpeptide angiotensin II receptor antagonist. Kidney Int 38:473-479, 1990

22. Munafo H, Christen Y, Nussberger J, Shum LY, Borland RM, Lee RJ, Waeber B, Biollaz J, Brunner HR: Drug concentration response relationships in normal volunteers after oral administration of losartan, an angiotensin II receptor antagonist. Clin Pharmacol Ther 51:513-521, 1992

23. Brunner HR, Laragh JH, Baer L, Newton MA, Goodwin FT, Krakoff LR, Bard RH, Buehler FR: Essential hypertension: Renin and aldosterone, heart attack and stroke. N Engl J Med 286:441-449, 1972

24. Vos PF, Boer P, Koomans HA: Effects of enalapril on renal sodium handling in healthy subjects on low, intermediate, and high sodium intake. J Cardiovasc Pharmacol 22:27-32, 1993

25. Krusell LR, Jespersen LT, Schmitz A, Thomsen K, Pedersen OL: Repetitive natriuresis and blood pressure. Long-term calcium entry blockade with isradipine. Hypertension 10:577-581, 1987

26. Burnier M, Waeber B, Brunner HR: Clinical pharmacology of the angiotensin II receptor antagonist losartan-potassium in healthy subjects. J Hypertens 1995 (in press)

27. Sweet CS, Bradstreet DC, Berman RS, Jallard N, Saenz A, Weidler DJ: Pharmacodynamic activity of intravenous E-3174, an angiotensin II antagonist, in patients with essential hypertension. Am J Hypertens 7:1035-1040, 1994

28. Steinhauslin F, Burnier M, Magnin JL, Munafo A, Buclin T, Diezi J, Biollaz J: Fractional excretion of trace lithium and uric acid in acute renal failure. J Am Soc Nephrol 4:1429-1437, 1994

Long-Term Benefits of the Antiproteinuric Effect of Angiotensin-Converting Enzyme Inhibition in Nondiabetic Renal Disease

Ron T. Gansevoort, MD, Dick de Zeeuw, MD, and Paul E. de Jong, MD

● The long-term (1.5 years) effects of angiotensin-converting enzyme inhibition were evaluated in 22 mostly normotensive patients with nondiabetic renal disease and moderate to severe proteinuria. The nephrotic-range proteinuria of 7.5 g/24 hr fell to 2.9 g/24 hr (−62%) after 2 months' treatment with an angiotensin-converting enzyme inhibitor and remained relatively stable at this level during continued treatment. The antiproteinuric response varied between study days and between individuals. Of note was the fact that the best antiproteinuric response was observed on those study days when no more than the instituted daily sodium intake (50 to 100 mEq/24 hr) was excreted. The sustained reduction in urinary protein excretion was accompanied by an increase in serum albumin and a slight but significant decrease in serum cholesterol. Those patients with the most pronounced initial antiproteinuric response showed less deterioration of renal function, estimated from the slope of the inverse serum creatinine value in time. These data suggest that long-term angiotensin-converting enzyme inhibitor treatment may be beneficial in normotensive patients with nephrotic-range proteinuria, not only to reduce the symptoms of a nephrotic syndrome, but also to prevent further renal damage.

INDEX WORDS: Proteinuria; renal disease; angiotensin-converting enzyme inhibition; progression renal disease.

MANY renal diseases are accompanied by overt proteinuria, which may have certain pathologic consequences. First, in case of marked proteinuria, serum albumin levels may decrease, cholesterol levels may increase, and edema may develop. This nephrotic condition is associated with increased morbidity and mortality rates.[1-3] Second, although the evidence is still debated, proteinuria itself may be related to or induce renal damage, resulting in a progressive decline of renal function.[4-6] Curative treatment of the underlying disease entities is seldom available. Thus, symptomatic treatment of the nephrotic condition is often indicated in these patients with non–steroid-sensitive proteinuria. The reduction of urinary protein excretion can be achieved by only a limited number of therapeutic options, among which angiotensin-converting enzyme (ACE) inhibitors appear to be effective and promising tools. Indeed, many investigators have demonstrated that various ACE inhibitors are effective antiproteinuric agents in renal disease.[7] Most of these studies, however, focussed either on the short-term effects of such a treatment or the long-term effects were monitored in hypertensive patients with mild proteinuria. The question remains whether continued long-term reduction of moderate to severe proteinuria indeed relieves the typical symptoms associated with continued loss of protein in the urine.

Supported by Grants No. C87-691 and C90-963 from the Dutch Kidney Foundation.

We therefore evaluated the rationale of long-term symptomatic antiproteinuric treatment with ACE inhibition, studying 22 nephrotic-range proteinuric patients with nondiabetic renal disease of different etiology. The patients were all followed for 1.5 years after the start of ACE inhibitor treatment, and the effects on relevant systemic and renal parameters were monitored.

PATIENTS AND METHODS

Patients

Twenty-two patients were enrolled in this long-term treatment protocol; five were women and 17 were men with a mean age of 38.8 years (range, 20 to 66 years) at the start of the study. Mean blood pressure was systolic 139 mm Hg (range, 107 to 177 mm Hg) and diastolic 85 mm Hg (range, 61 to 119 mm Hg). Only four patients were considered to be hypertensive (diastolic blood pressure >95 mm Hg). Mean glomerular filtration rate was 77 mL/min (range, 17 to 134 mL/min) and mean proteinuria was 7.5 g/24 hr (range, 3.4 to 18.4 g/24 hr). Histologically proven diagnoses were membranous glomerulopathy (n = 8), glomerulosclerosis (n = 8), and IgA nephropathy (n = 6).

Protocol

In case patients were on antihypertensive medication, this therapy was withdrawn at least 6 weeks before start of the study, except for three patients needing continued diuretic therapy. A dietary intake of 50 to 100 mEq sodium/d and 1 to 1.5 g protein/kg body weight/d were prescribed. This diet remained unaltered during the entire follow-up period. None of the patients used cholesterol-lowering drugs. After establishing the baseline data, the ACE inhibitor lisinopril was given at a dose of 10 mg/24 hr. During follow-up the dose was titrated down to 5 mg/24 hr in two patients because of hypotensive complaints. In four patients, 20 mg/24 hr was prescribed to achieve adequate blood pressure control. One of these four patients needed the addition of another antihypertensive (atenolol). All patients visited the outpatient clinic every 2 to 4 weeks during the first months of treatment, and subsequently once every 3 months. During each visit blood pressure was measured and blood was drawn for determination of creatinine, cholesterol, and albumin. Urinary protein, sodium, creatinine, and urea were measured in 24-hour urine collected on the day prior to the outpatient clinic visit.

Methods

Blood pressure was measured after at least 5 minutes of supine rest with either a standard sphygmomanometer or an automated device (Dinamap, Critikon GmbH, Norderstedt, Germany). Albumin, sodium, cholesterol, urea, and creatinine were measured with a standard auto-analyzer (SMAC, Technicon Instruments, Tarrytown, NY). Urinary protein was determined by the pyrogallol-red-molybdate method. Progression of renal disease was estimated for each individual by calculating the slope of the linear regression derived from the 3-month inverse serum creatinine data (L/serum creatinine) plotted against time.[8] Data collected at baseline and at 2, 6, 12, and 18 months after the start of ACE inhibitor treatment are given. Results are expressed as mean ± standard error (SEM). Statistical analysis was performed by analysis of variance for repeated measurements followed by Student's paired *t*-test, and by Pearson's correlation coefficient for correlation between variables. Significant differences were tested at a 5% level.

RESULTS

Angiotensin-converting enzyme inhibition resulted in a sustained decrease in systemic mean arterial pressure from baseline 103.0 ± 3.5 mm Hg to 86.0 ± 2.1 mm Hg, 89.9 ± 1.8 mm Hg, 94.5 ± 2.2 mm Hg, and 93.9 ± 2.2 mm Hg, at 2, 6, 12, and 18 months, respectively. This decrease in blood pressure was accompanied by a decrease in urinary protein excretion, a slow progressive increase in serum albumin to normal levels, and a slight but significant decrease in serum cholesterol, as shown in Fig 1. Figure 1 also shows that renal function progressively declines during follow-up, as estimated from the mean inverse serum creatinine values. Serum potassium levels increased slightly, from 4.5 ± 0.1 mEq/L at baseline to 4.8 ± 0.1 mEq/L after 2 months of ACE inhibitor treatment, remaining stable at this level: 5.0 ± 0.1 mEq/L, 4.9 ± 0.1 mEq/L, and 4.9 ± 0.1 mEq/L at 6, 12, and 18 months, respectively.

In general, patients complied with the instituted dietary restrictions as reflected by a stable urinary sodium excretion: 86 ± 10 mEq/24 hr at baseline, 77 ± 6 mEq/24 hr at 2 months, 111 ± 10 mEq/24 hr at 6 months, 111 ± 9 mEq/24 hr at 12 months, and 114 ± 11 mEq/24 hr at 18 months. Similarly, urinary urea excretion remained stable (18.9 ± 1.5 g/24 hr, 22.0 ± 1.8 g/24 hr, 23.1 ± 2.0 g/24 hr, 22.5 ± 1.9 g/24 hr, and 21.7 ± 1.7 g/24 hr at baseline and at 2, 6, 12, and 18 months, respectively), indicating an adequate compliance to the dietary protein restriction.

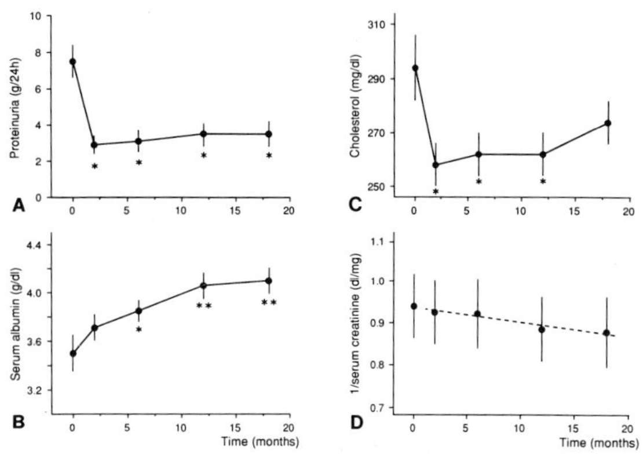

Fig 1. The effect of long-term ACE inhibitor treatment on (A) proteinuria, (B) serum albumin, (C) cholesterol, and (D) the course of the inverse serum creatinine. All data are expressed as mean ± SEM. Pretreatment values are given at time 0. Asterisks denote a significant ($P < 0.05$) change compared with baseline (j) or compared with values obtained at baseline and at 2 months (jj).

Although the antiproteinuric response appears to be quite stable in time (−62% ± 3%, −59% ± 5%, −53% ± 6%, and −53% ± 6% at 2, 6, 12, 18 months, respectively) and quite uniform throughout the studied population, variation was observed both between individuals and within one individual in time. Interestingly, the variation in antiproteinuric response could be partly explained by the compliance to the dietary sodium restriction. When correlating the individual antiproteinuric response (percentage decrease in protein excretion compared with baseline) with the urinary sodium excretion at that study day for all study periods, a significant relationship was found, indicating that at times of higher sodium excretion a less antiproteinuric response was present ($r = 0.54$; $P < 0.001$; Fig 2). Such a correlation was also found for most single follow-up periods: 2 months ($r = 0.42$; $P = 0.05$), 6 months ($r = 0.41$; $P =$ NS), 12 months ($r = 0.60$; $P < 0.01$), and 18 months ($r = 0.62$; $P < 0.01$). A possible bias in the observed relation-

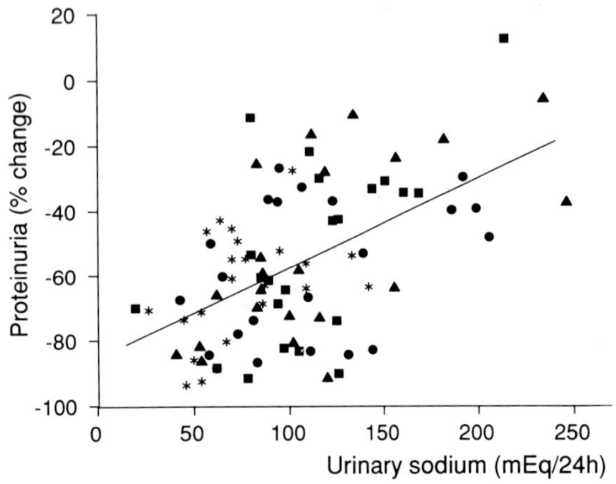

Fig 2. Correlation between the antiproteinuric response (percentage of change compared with baseline) and the urinary sodium excretion (r = 0.54; P < 0.001). Each data point represents the antiproteinuric and sodium excretion value of one individual at the time point of 2 months (j), 6 months (●), 12 months (■), or 18 months (▲) after the start of treatment.

ship could be the fact that low urinary protein values are accompanied by low sodium values due to inadequate urine collection. Although this bias may be present it does not appear to explain the observation, since correction for urine collection using urinary creatinine levels did not markedly attenuate the correlation (r = 0.53; P < 0.001).

The overall antiproteinuric response was found to correlate (r = 0.47; P < 0.05) with the increase in serum albumin (baseline *v* 18 months). The antiproteinuric response did not correlate with baseline renal function (r = 0.26; P = NS) or the decrease in serum cholesterol (r = 0.20; P = NS). The observed change in systemic blood pressure did not appear to explain the decrease in proteinuria, since the decrease in mean arterial pressure did not correlate with the change in protein excretion (r = 0.14; P = NS).

The mean progressive decline in renal function with a slope of −0.027 ± 0.009 dL/mg/yr varied considerably between the individual patients, ranging from −0.113 dL/mg/yr to +0.044 dL/mg/yr. Unfortunately, no sufficient pretreatment creatinine data are available to evaluate whether a change in slope was induced by the ACE inhibitor treatment. However, an intriguing observation was made in the fact that the individual initial antiproteinuric response (measured at 2 months compared with baseline) correlated with the individual inverse creatinine slope calculated over the total follow-up period (r = 0.68; P < 0.001; Fig 3). A similar correlation was found between the remaining proteinuria after 2 months' treatment and the inverse creatinine slope (r = 0.60; P < 0.01). These correlations suggest that the alleged renoprotective effect of ACE inhibition can be at least partly explained by the successful reduction of urinary protein excretion. No such correlation was found plotting the rate of progression against baseline renal function, mean individual sodium excretion, the changes in serum cholesterol, or the changes in mean arterial pressure.

Evaluating the different parameters discussed above for each group of patients with the same histologic diagnosis revealed no significant differences between these groups.

DISCUSSION

The present study shows that prolonged treatment with an ACE inhibitor in proteinuric, predominantly normotensive patients with renal disease has beneficial effects on those parameters typically associated with excess urinary protein: the sustained decrease in urinary protein excretion is accompanied by an increase in serum albu-

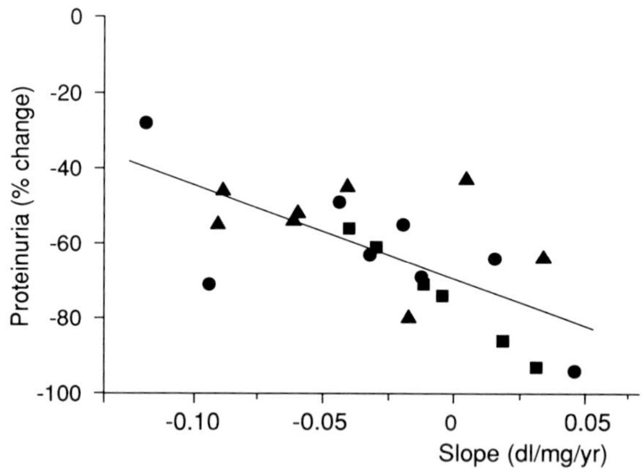

Fig 3. Correlation between the initial antiproteinuric response (percentage of change of proteinuria comparing the 2-month value with baseline) and the progression of renal function deterioration (r = 0.68; P < 0.001). The latter is expressed as the slope of the regression line plotted using the individual inverse serum creatinine levels at multiple study time points. Patients with membranous glomerulopathy (●), IgA nephropathy (■), and glomerulosclerosis (▲) are separately identified.

min and a decrease, albeit limited, in serum cholesterol levels. No serious side effects of the treatment were observed.

Although many previous studies have documented the efficacy of short-term treatment with ACE inhibitors to reduce urinary protein excretion, the merit of this treatment still has to be proven. Hypothetically, at least two beneficial effects can be linked to the sustained reduction in protein excretion. First, the improvement of all those parameters associated with the nephrotic state may reduce morbidity and mortality in these patients. Indeed, we found that serum albumin increases and cholesterol slightly decreases. Data on such long-term ACE inhibitor effects in patients with nephrotic-range proteinuria are scarce. In a small subgroup of hypertensive patients with renal disease and proteinuria of more than 3 g/d, Rodicio et al found that captopril treatment induced both a small increase in serum albumin and a small decrease in serum cholesterol.[9] It is clear that these data together do not allow a firm conclusion on morbidity or mortality, and that larger placebo-controlled studies are needed to prove this hypothesis.

Second, the reduction of protein loss may improve the progressive character of renal function loss so often encountered in patients with renal disease. Indeed, Williams et al and Hunt et al have shown that the degree of progression appears to be related to the degree of proteinuria.[4,5] These studies do not reveal whether proteinuria is the result of progressive renal disease or that proteinuria causes the progression. However, Remuzzi and Bertani recently reviewed the experimental evidence for protein excretion to play a major role in the progressive nature of different experimental renal disease models.[6] If true, a sustained reduction of protein excretion as induced by the ACE inhibitor in the present study would benefit the individual patient by reducing the rate of decline of progressive renal function. We have no direct evidence to substantiate this hypothesis with the present data, since the present study did not include a parallel control group or a pretreatment control period. Moreover, the rate of renal function decline measured by inverse serum creatinine should be treated with caution, as this is not always a reliable marker of renal function. However, despite these drawbacks, the observation that the patients with the most marked antiproteinuric response and the patients with the lowest proteinuria during treatment show the least progression of renal function deterioration may suggest that lowering of proteinuria is indeed beneficial for renal function survival. This is supported by data that Praga et al, who found that renal function remained stable in a subgroup of patients with a more than 45% reduction of proteinuria during 2 years of treatment with captopril, whereas a similarly treated subgroup with less antiproteinuric response showed a progressive decrease in creatinine clearance.[10]

Other factors that may determine the progression of renal disease also have to be taken into account, such as the decrease in systemic blood pressure. It has been documented that lowering of blood pressure per se, not only in diabetic[11-13] but also in nondiabetic renal disease, reduces the decline in renal function.[14] Whether ACE inhibitors have additional benefits in this respect remains to be proven, and large prospective trials are still ongoing. The fact that we observed beneficial effects of ACE inhibitor treatment in a group of patients largely consisting of normotensive patients prompted us to question whether ACE inhibitor therapy should be restricted only to treatment of high blood pressure per se, with the renal benefits as a positive "side effect." It seems appropriate to consider whether ACE inhibitor treatment should be given in proteinuric patients merely with the intention to lower proteinuria.

Besides the decreases in proteinuria and blood pressure, the reduction in serum cholesterol also may be of importance in reducing the progressive decrease in renal function. In several animal models, such a relationship has been demonstrated.[15] Given the fact that the decrease in serum cholesterol in the present study was relatively small, it seems unlikely that this had a major impact on renal function in the long term. However, more specific studies on the effect of ACE inhibitor treatment on specific lipid profiles and specific lipid risk factors have to be carried out.

The present data again demonstrate the importance of an adequate restriction of dietary sodium intake during ACE inhibitor treatment to achieve an optimal and sustained antiproteinuric response. We have previously demonstrated that the antiproteinuric effect of lisinopril is nearly completely abolished after switching from a low (50 mEq/24 hr) to a high (200 mEq/24 hr) sodium intake.[16] In the present study we even found that during prolonged ACE inhibitor treatment a single high urinary sodium measurement is often accompanied by a reduced antiproteinuric response at that moment in that patient.

In conclusion, the data of the present study suggest that long-term ACE inhibitor treatment may be beneficial in normotensive patients with nephrotic-range proteinuria, not only to reduce the symptoms of a nephrotic syndrome, but also to prevent further renal damage. Prospective controlled trials using more reliable means of measuring renal function will have to be carried out to give more support to this latter hypothesis.

REFERENCES

1. Wass V, Cameron JS: Cardiovascular disease and the nephrotic syndrome: The other side of the coin. Nephron 27:54-57, 1981
2. Llach F: Hypercoagulability, renal vein thrombosis and other thrombotic complications of nephrotic syndrome. Kidney Int 28:429-439, 1985
3. Bernard DB: Extrarenal complications of the nephrotic syndrome. Kidney Int 33:1184-1202, 1988
4. Hunt LP, Short CD, Mallick NP: Prognostic indicators in patients presenting with the nephrotic syndrome. Kidney Int 34:382-388, 1988
5. Williams PS, Fass G, Bone JM: Renal pathology and proteinuria determine progression in untreated mild/moderate chronic renal failure. Q J Med 67:343-354, 1988
6. Remuzzi G, Bertani T: Is glomerulosclerosis a consequence of altered glomerular permeability to macromolecules? Kidney Int 38:384-394, 1990
7. de Zeeuw D, Heeg JE, de Jong PE: The antiproteinuric effect of angiotensin-converting-enzyme inhibitors in human renal disease, in Andreucci VE, Fine LG (eds): International Yearbook of Nephrology. London, UK, Springer Verlag, 1991, pp 95-113
8. Mitch WE, Walser M, Buffington GA, Lemann J: A simple method for estimating progression of chronic renal failure. Lancet 298:122-126, 1976
9. Rodicio JL, Alcazar JM, Ruilope LM: Influence of converting enzyme inhibition on glomerular filtration rate and proteinuria. Kidney Int 38:590-594, 1990
10. Praga M, Hernandez E, Monyoyo C, Andres A, Ruilope LM, Rodicio JL: Long-term beneficial effects of ACE-inhibition in patients with nephrotic proteinuria. Am J Kidney Dis 20:240-248, 1992
11. Parving HH, Andersen AR, Smidt UM, Svendsen PA: Early aggressive antihypertensive treatment reduces rate of decline in kidney function in diabetic nephropathy. Lancet 1:1175-1179, 1983
12. Mogensen CE: Long-term antihypertensive treatment inhibiting progression of diabetic nephropathy. B Med J 285:658-688, 1982
13. Parving HH, Andersen AR, Smidt UM, Hommel E, Mathiesen ER, Svendsen PA: Effect of antihypertensive treatment on kidney function in diabetic nephropathy. B Med J 294:1443-1447, 1987
14. Brazy PC, Stead WW, Fitzwilliam FJ: Progression of renal insufficiency: Role of blood pressure. Kidney Int 35:670-674, 1989
15. Keane WF, Kasiske BL, O'Donnell MP, Kim Y: The role of altered lipid metabolism in the progression of renal disease: Experimental evidence. Am J Kidney Dis 17:38-42, 1991 (suppl 1)
16. Heeg JE, de Jong PE, van der Hem GK, de Zeeuw D: Efficacy and variability of the antiproteinuric effect of ACE-inhibition by lisinopril. Kidney Int 36:272-279, 1989

Erythropoietin in Diabetic Macular Edema and Renal Insufficiency

Eli A. Friedman, MD, Clinton D. Brown, MD, and David H. Berman, MD

● Erythropoietin was administered to five anemic azotemic diabetic subjects for 1 year to assess the effect of increasing red cell mass on clinical well-being and the course of renal functional decline. None of the subjects manifested worsened hypertension or cerebrovascular or cardiovascular complications despite an increase in mean hematocrit from a baseline mean of 29.6% to a mean of 39.5%. The serum creatinine concentration after 1 year of treatment with erythropoietin was 3.7 mg/dL, which was unchanged from the baseline value of 3.5 mg/dL. Plasma viscosity remained constant as red cell mass increased. Although the viscosity of whole blood rose as the hematocrit increased, it was within the range of normal blood viscosity for an equivalent hematocrit. The favorable impact of erythropoietin treatment on three diabetic subjects who had macular edema and anemia is described. One hypothesis to explain the benefit of a raised hematocrit on both diabetic nephropathy and retinopathy is that the metabolic, hormonal, and hemodynamic components of the diabetic syndrome, in concert, produce tissue and cellular hypoxia that is ameliorated in part by the greater oxygen-transporting capacity of a raised red cell mass. The pseudohypoxia of diabetes may be implicated in the pathogenesis of diabetic neuropathy, retinopathy, muscular dysfunction, and nephropathy.

INDEX WORDS: Diabetes; nephropathy; erythropoietin; hypoxia; pseudohypoxia; retinopathy; macular edema.

THE PATHOGENESIS of diabetic complications is debated; hyperglycemia,[1] growth factors,[2] vascular defects,[3] and hemodynamic perturbations[4] are proposed as primary factors leading to microvasculopathy. Over the past 5 years, growing evidence supports the hypothesis that hypoxia, at the organ, tissue, or cellular level, contributes to progression of tissue injury in diabetic individuals.[5] If this thinking is correct, raising tissue oxygen tension might slow the course of microvasculopathic complications. Increasing the blood hemoglobin level by administration of recombinant erythropoietin is one means of improving oxygen carriage to peripheral tissues. In this report, we describe preliminary trials of the effect of erythropoietin in diabetic subjects with eye and kidney complications attributable to diabetes.

PATIENTS AND METHODS

Volunteers for the predialysis study were solicited from the renal clinic of University Hospital of Brooklyn. The study was approved by the Institutional Review Board. All subjects gave informed consent. Adult diabetic subjects who had anemia attributed to renal insufficiency, after confirmation of normal iron stores, were treated with erythropoietin. Inclusion criteria included anemia not caused by extrarenal disease; absence of gastrointestinal and urinary blood loss; a serum creatinine concentration of between 2.0 and 5.0 mg/dL; and absence of concurrent disorders likely to progress to a life-threatening degree. The effect of erythropoietin on anemia in the five diabetic subjects cited herein has previously been presented, in part, without peer review.[6] Three patients with macular edema whose course is detailed later were previously reported.[7]

On initiation of study, each subject had a physical examination, measurement of seated blood pressure, ophthalmologic evaluation including retinal photography, and, where indicated, fluorescein angiography of the retina, and an electrocardiogram. Patients were followed on an ambulatory basis, at weekly to monthly intervals determined by their course and complications. At each visit, a physical examination including seated blood pressure measurement was performed, and a hemogram and chemical screen were obtained.

End points for the trial were either death or progression to end-stage renal disease (ESRD). Erythropoietin prepared by the Amgen Corp. (Thousand Oaks, CA) and provided by Ortho Pharmaceutical Corp. (Raritan, NJ) was administered intravenously in doses of 50 to 150 U/kg three times weekly until the mean hematocrit increased to 40%. Maintenance doses of erythropoietin were given to sustain the hematocrit above 32%. Dietary protein was restricted to 60 g/day. Antihypertensive and diuretic medications were continued, as needed, in the judgment of the primary nephrologist. Metabolic control of hyperglycemia was optimized using multiple daily fingerstick glucose measurements in conjunction with fractional doses of insulin or oral hypoglycemic agents.

The viscosity of an aliquot of heparinized venous whole blood or plasma was determined with an LTV-CP II Wells-Brookfield cone plate viscometer (Brookfield Engineering Laboratories, Stoughton, MA) at 37°C as detailed by Wells et al.[8] Viscosity is expressed in units of milli-pascal · second (mPas). Blood viscosity was measured at high and low rates of shear (4.35 ± 0.53 and 6.83 ± 0.79 mPas), respectively, and plasma viscosity ($230\ s^{-1}$) of 1.57 ± 0.11 mPas for high and low rates of shear, respectively. All measurements were made in duplicate. Instrument accuracy and precision was checked daily by repeated measures of viscosity of distilled water and standard fluids (with viscosities in the range of human blood) supplied by Brookfield Engineering Laboratories. All measurements were made within 2 hours of venepuncture. For comparison with a control population of anemic but not azotemic subjects, normal blood was diluted to lower hematocrits by adding autologous plasma to attain a hematocrit of 30%.

The cohort of three women with macular edema were col-

Table 1. Response of Azotemic Diabetic Patients to 1 Year of Erythropoietin Treatment (n = 5)

	Hematocrit (%)	Serum Creatinine (mg/dL)	Blood Viscosity (230/s)	Blood Viscosity (23/s)	Plasma Viscosity (230/s)	Blood Pressure (mm Hg)
Pre-erythropoietin	29.6 ± 2.0	3.5 ± 0.4	3.62 ± 0.32	4.96 ± 0.98	1.55 ± 0.16	149.0/87.8
Post-erythropoietin	39.5 ± 2.4	3.7 ± 0.4	4.27 ± 0.28	6.99 ± 0.88	1.60 ± 0.07	149.0/76.0
P	$<$0.005	NS	$<$0.001	$<$0.001	NS	NS

NOTE. Results expressed as mean ± standard deviation.
Abbreviation: NS, not significant.

lected from a referral base of approximately 40 diabetic patients sent for eye evaluation to a single ophthalmologist (D.H.B.). Their evaluation reflects the retrospective collection of a clinical experience rather than a prospective study. Lacking concurrent control groups, and with groups of only five azotemic diabetics and three individuals with macular edema, statistical analysis of treatment groups is inappropriate for comparison with a control population. A comparison of pre-erythropoietin and post-erythropoietin values in the five predialysis azotemic diabetic subjects is provided in Table 1.

RESULTS

A total of five azotemic diabetic subjects were treated with erythropoietin. All five subjects reported improved well-being and greater tolerance for effort. Urine protein excretion was not altered over the course of study. One patient was hospitalized during the year because of transient hyperkalemia attributed to treatment with enalapril. There were no cardiovascular or cerebrovascular events. Mean systolic and diastolic blood pressures were unchanged. None of the patients were catabolic though azotemic; mean body weight at the start (76.9 ± 19.7 kg) was unchanged after 1 year (76.3 ± 19.7 kg). Mean serum creatinine concentration was unchanged after 1 year.

Viscosity of whole blood and plasma at baseline level and after treatment with erythropoietin, for 1 year, are shown in Table 1. Whole blood viscosity for diluted ''normal'' blood with hematocrit reduced to 30% was 3.49 ± 0.27 and 5.05 ± 0.63 mPa for high and low rates of shear, respectively. Plasma viscosity was unchanged throughout the course of observation. Whole blood viscosity increased with the rise in hematocrit as measured at both shear rates. There were no changes in plasma lipids or serum protein concentration throughout the study.

Summative data on three patients who evinced improvement in macular edema after treatment with erythropoietin are given.

CASE REPORTS

Case 1

A 63-year-old hypertensive diabetic (non–insulin-dependent diabetes mellitus [NIDDM]) woman with azotemia (serum creatinine of 3.7 mg/dL) and anemia (hematocrit of 22%) attributed to her kidney disease was seen for deteriorating visual acuity. At initial examination, the blood pressure was 150/90 mm Hg, and the visual acuity was 20/200 in the right eye and 20/20 in the left eye. Funduscopic examination showed a dense lipid exudate at the foveal center in the right eye, assigned a grade of 5 (Fig 1A) according to the Early Treatment Diabetic Retinopathy Study (ETDRS).[9] Treatment with erythropoietin, at a dose of 4,000 IU injected subcutaneously twice weekly, was begun. The patient was also treated with tolazamide, metolazone, furosemide, and lisinopril. After 8 months of treatment with erythropoietin, the hematocrit increased to 33%, the visual acuity in the right eye improved to 20/60, and funduscopic examination showed complete resolution of the foveal hard exudates with an ETDRS grade of 3 (Fig 1B). Repeat fluorescein angiography confirmed the absence of new leakage and a stable pattern of nonperfusion found on the first study. During the interval between Figs 1A and 1B, the blood pressure and serum lipid profile were stable, and no laser treatments were given.

Case 2

A 60-year-old formerly hypertensive diabetic (IDDM) woman on maintenance hemodialysis because of diabetic nephropathy had severe visual loss with diminished visual acuity of 20/400 due to diabetic retinopathy. The right eye had extensive vitreous hemorrhage, and the left eye had parafoveal hard exudates and macular edema designated ETDRS fundus photo grade 5 (Fig 2A). Fluorescein angiography was not attempted because of the patient's prior anaphylactic reaction to fluorescein dye 1 year earlier when panretinal photocoagulation had been performed for proliferative retinopathy. The blood pressure was 110/70 mm Hg and the hematocrit was 21%. Treatment with erythropoietin was initiated at a dose of 4,000 IU injected subcutaneously twice weekly. The patient was also treated with insulin and calcium carbonate.

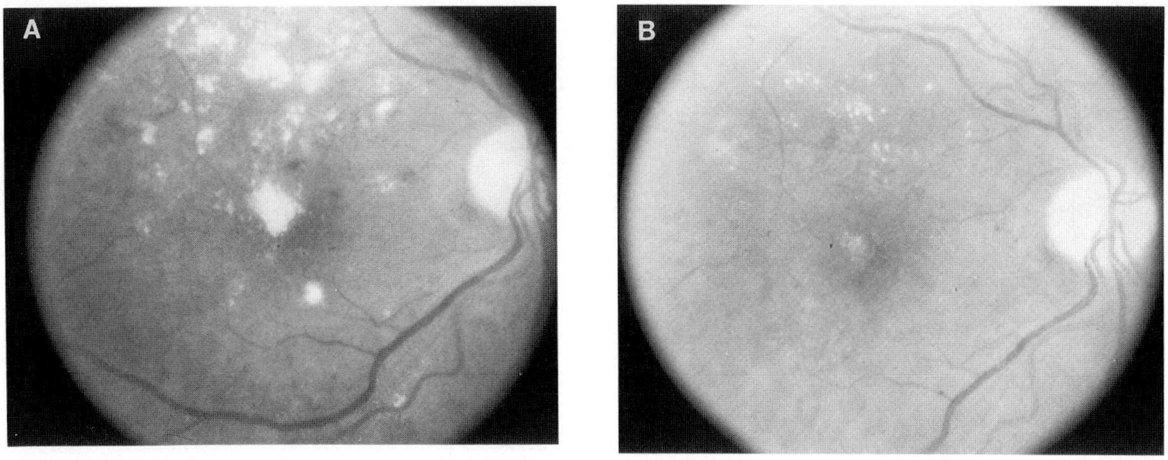

Fig 1. (A) Patient 1. Right eye before treatment with erythropoietin, showing central hard exudates. (B) Right eye during treatment with erythropoietin, demonstrating significant clearing of central exudates.

After 6 months of erythropoietin injections, the hematocrit increased to 31%, the blood pressure remained normal, and the visual acuity had improved to 20/200 while funduscopy indicated an ETDRS photo grade 4 (Fig 2B). No laser treatment was administered.

Case 3

A 55-year-old hypertensive diabetic (IDDM) woman undergoing maintenance hemodialysis because of diabetic nephropathy had visual acuity of 20/50 in the right eye and 20/40 in the left eye. Funduscopic examination showed photocoagulation scars in the right eye and parafoveal hard exudates and an old laser scar in the left eye designated as ETDRS fundus photo grade 5 (Fig 3A). Fluorescein angiography showed focal nonperfusion and mild leakage. The blood pressure was 149/92 mm Hg, and the hematocrit was 24%. A regimen of insulin, furosemide, and metolazone was established and maintained over the course of study. Erythropoietin treatment was started at a dose of 4,000 IU injected subcutaneously twice weekly. Eleven months later, the hematocrit increased to 32%, and the patient's visual acuity improved to 20/40 in the left eye, with substantial resorption of the macular edema and hard exudates equivalent to ETDRS fundus photo grade 3 (Fig 3B). During the interval between Figs 3A and 3B, the blood pressure was unchanged, and no laser therapy was administered. Repeat fluorescein angiography demonstrated no change in the leak-

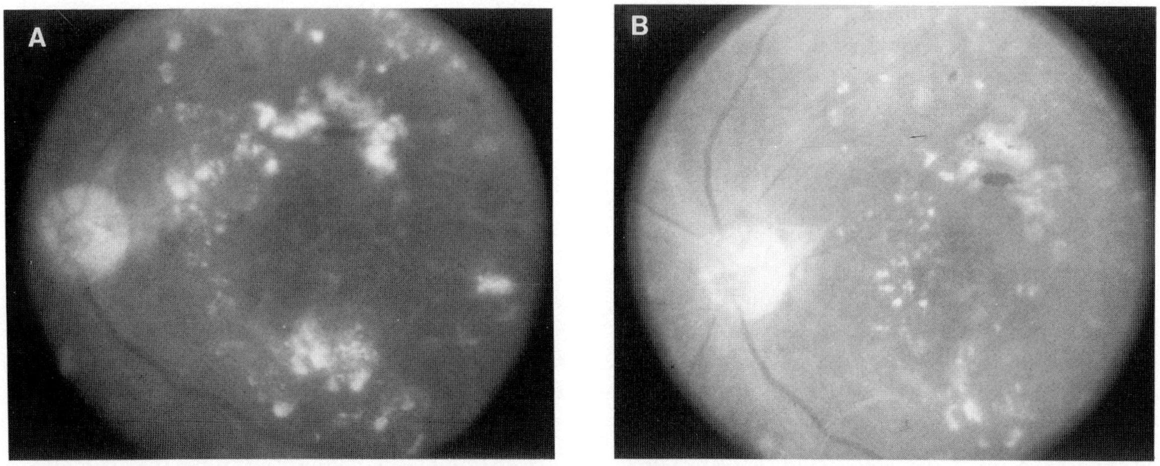

Fig 2. (A) Patient 2. Left eye showing diffused macular exudates before erythropoietin treatment. (B) Same eye during treatment with erythropoietin, indicating significant resorbtion of exudates.

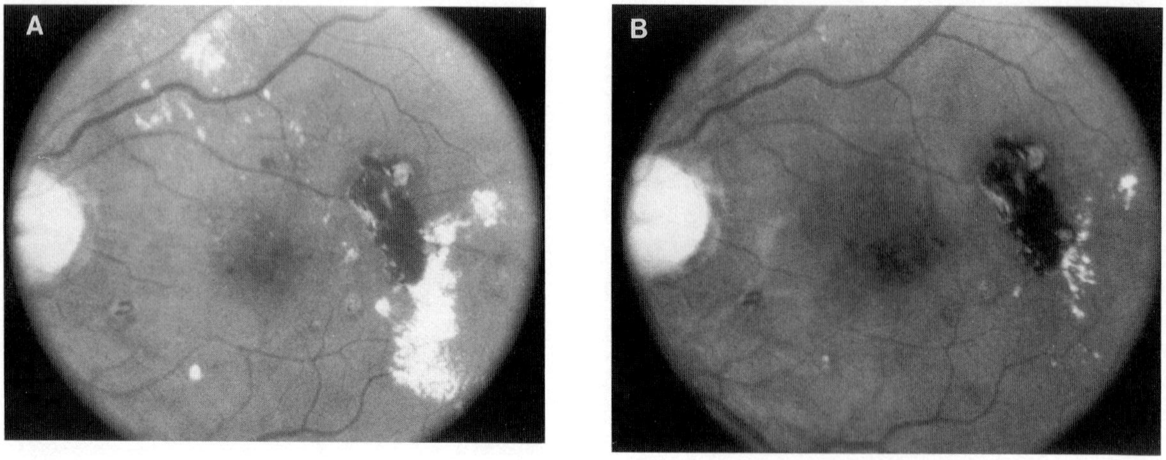

Fig 3. (A) Patient 3. Left eye before treatment with erythropoietin showing peripheral macular exudates. (B) Same eye in which nearly complete clearing of exudates is evident during treatment with erythropoietin.

age pattern and no further decrease in microcirculatory perfusion.

DISCUSSION

Erythropoietin is remarkable safe and effective when administered to patients undergoing maintenance hemodialysis.[10] Extension of the application of erythropoietin to azotemic patients who do not require dialytic therapy expanded the indication for this hormone replacement.[11] Fear that a higher hematocrit and associated raised blood viscosity might accelerate the rate of decline of renal function in azotemic patients has been assuaged.[12] Our report is consistent with prior reports in documenting the absence of cerebrovascular or cardiovascular complications precipitated by erythropoietin-induced increased blood mass. Indeed, we note the stability in renal function over 1 year of a small group of diabetic patients who might have been expected to lapse into ESRD. Whether the steadiness of serum creatinine levels reflects a statistical quirk or a generalized response that can be anticipated in larger groups of azotemic diabetic patients followed prospectively is the subject of a controlled trial in progress.

Macular edema, the most common finding in diabetic people losing visual acuity is usually the consequence of focal, and rarely diffuse, capillary leakage.[13] Retinal thickening, the main associated finding in macular edema, correlates with hard exudates[14] and focal leakage. Consisting mainly of polyunsaturated fats deposited in the outer plexiform layer of the retina, hard exudates are derived from hyperpermeable microaneurysms.[15] Hard exudates may resorb spontaneously or after treatment of hypertension and uremia. Focal laser treatment by sealing incompetent microaneurysms may reduce focal leakage, promoting resorption of hard exudates, thereby stabilizing visual acuity. Bresnick[16] believes that the frequency of diabetic macular edema is reduced when hypertension is treated, but the relationship between blood lipids[17] and macular edema and hard exudate production is unclear.[18] Of a total of eight historical control diabetic azotemic patients with macular edema, none evinced resolution or improvement over 1 year of observation. So-called residual hard exudates, as found in cases 1, 2, and 3, may persist without evidence of vascular incompetence after maximal laser photocoagulation of the retina. In our three cases, blood pressure, serum lipid levels, and degree of retinal angiopathy as judged by fluorescein angiography were unchanged when the hematocrit increased during erythropoietin treatment.

Retinal neovascularization is thought to follow the release of angiogenic factors (vasoformative factor) by an ischemic and hypoxic retina[19] (Fig 4). Although the pathophysiologic events leading to angiogenesis is obscure,[20] antiangiogenic agents are under evaluation as a means of ar-

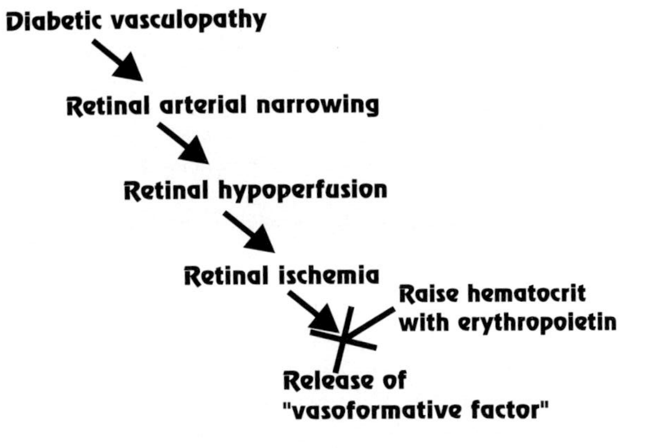

Fig 4. Raising red cell mass by treating with erythropoietin should increase retinal oxygenation, thereby reducing the stimulus for release of factors (kinines, autocrines?, hormones?) that induce retinal neovascularization. Variously termed vasoformative factor, angiogenesis factor, or neovascular factor by different investigators, the underlying hypothesis that retinal hypoxia is the main stimulus for release is the consensus view.

resting retinal neovascularization.[21] Decreased transcutaneous oxygen tension was measured in 119 diabetic subjects by an Oxymonitor at 45°C at the dorsum of the foot.[22] In this study, tissue hypoxia was found to precede clinical signs of angiopathy while correlating with abnormal microrheological parameters including plasma viscosity, red cell aggregation times, disaggregation threshold, and red cell aggregate structure index. Tissue hypoxia, specifically arterial wall hypoxia—independent of insulin treatment—is proposed by Santilli, Fiegel, and Knighton[23] as an initiator and continuing stimulus for atherosclerotic vascular occlusive disease in diabetes. Williamson et al[5] use the term *pseudohypoxia* to characterize the vasodilation and increased blood flow characteristic of the early vascular response to acute hyperglycemia that in hypoxic tissues are linked with impaired oxidation of the reduced form of nicotinamide-adenine dinucleotide phosphate (NADH) to the oxidized form of nicotinamide-adenine dinucleotide (NAD+), resulting in an increased ratio of NADH/NAD+ (Fig 5). An increased cytosolic ratio of free NADH/NAD+ caused by hyperglycemia is typical of poorly controlled diabetes and mimics effects of true hypoxia on vascular and neural function, promoting diabetic complications. These effects are postulated to stimulate production of superoxide anion and increased nitric oxide formation.

From an obverse perspective of the pathogenesis of diabetic complications, it is pertinent that based on the electrophysiologic measurement of ischemic conduction failure in the median nerve of diabetic subjects, Hampton et al[24] suggest that hypoxia contributes to resistance to ischemic conduction failure, a characteristic feature of diabetic neuropathy. Consistent with this observation is the report of Low et al[25] that in induced-diabetic rats, hyperbaric oxygenation partially reversed the neuropathy of chronic diabetes. Supportive of the case for hypoxia as a pathogenetic mechanism in diabetes is the finding that hyperbaric oxygen heals otherwise hopeless foot ulcers in diabetic individuals by enhancing oxygenation of affected tissues while accelerating collagen production, thereby enhancing tissue repair.[26] However, cautious interpretation of this study is appropriate because there are no reported controlled prospective trials of the utility of hyperbaric oxygen therapy in the treatment of ulcers of the feet in diabetes. Additionally, ventricular muscle from diabetic rats of longer than 30 weeks' duration is more susceptible to hypoxic injury than is normal rat heart muscle.[27]

A rationale for administration of erythropoietin to anemic diabetic subjects cannot be based on an absolute deficiency of this hormone. Indeed, erythropoietin activity in plasma, as assessed in

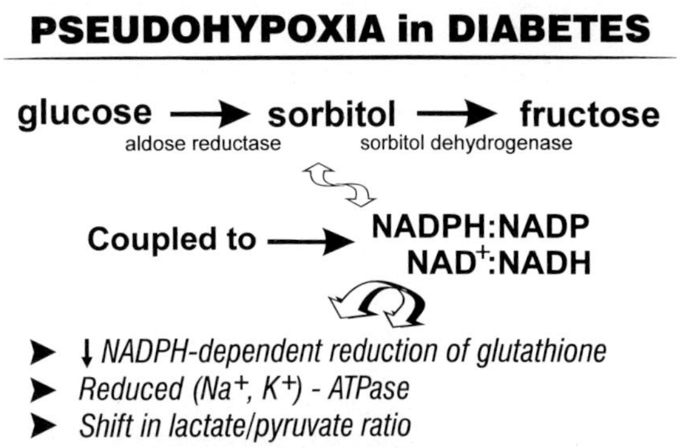

Fig 5. Hypoxia (actual or relative) is thought to be present in the diabetic eye, heart, nervous system, and possibly kidney. As theorized by Stevens et al[30], hyperglycemia can be linked to biochemical events that reduce tissue oxygenation, a sequence that may be ameliorated by increasing red cell mass with erythropoietin treatment.

posthypoxic polycythemic mice, is higher in diabetic individuals than in clinically healthy subjects.[28] Individuals with IDDM are not deficient in erythropoietin synthesis.[29] As is true for the apparently "normal" insulin level typically found in NIDDM even in the presence of hyperglycemia, a "normal" erythropoietin level in an anemic diabetic subject may be disproportionately low for the actual red cell mass. Just as the blood sugar decreases with exogenous insulin treatment in the hyperglycemia of NIDDM, so does the hematocrit increase in azotemic diabetic subjects with purportedly "normal" endogenous erythropoietin secretion.

Our preliminary trial of erythropoietin in azotemic diabetic patients supports three main inferences: (1) Erythropoietin is well tolerated without major complication. (2) Anemic azotemic diabetic patients respond promptly with a vigorous increase in red cell mass to doses of erythropoietin that are effective in the nondiabetic azotemic patients. (3) An increased hematocrit may slow the progression of diabetic nephropathy and improve visual acuity because of resolution of macular edema in diabetic retinopathy. It must be appreciated that no reference population documenting the natural history of macular edema in azotemic diabetic patients has been studied, limiting the extent of generalization permitted by our small experience.

REFERENCES

1. Brownlee M: Glycation and diabetic complications. Diabetes 43:836-841, 1994

2. Woolf AS, Bosch RJ, Fine LG: TI growth factors in the pathogenesis of renovascular complications of diabetes mellitus. J Hypertens Suppl 10:S11-6, 1992

3. Cameron NE, Cotter MA, Robertson S: Angiotensin converting enzyme inhibition prevents development of muscle and nerve dysfunction and stimulated angiogenesis in streptozotocin-diabetic rats. Diabetologia 35:12-18, 1992

4. Earle K, Viberti GC: Familial, hemodynamic and metabolic factors in the predisposition to diabetic kidney disease. Kidney Int 452:434-437, 1994

5. Williamson JR, Chang K, Frangos M, Hasan KS, Ido Y, Kawamura T, Nyengaard JR, van den Enden M, Kilo C, Tilton RG: Hyperglycemic pseudohypoxia and diabetic complications. Diabetes 42:801-813, 1993

6. Brown CD, Friedman EA: Stable renal function and benign course in azotemic diabetics treated with erythropoietin for one year. Contrib Nephrol 88:182-191, 1991

7. Berman D, Friedman EA: Absorption of hard exudates after treatment with erythropoietin. Retina 14.1-5, 1994

8. Wells RF Jr, Denten R, Merrill EW: Measurement of viscosity of biologic fluids by cone plate viscometer. J Lab Clin Med 57:646-656, 1961

9. Early Treatment Diabetic Retinopathy Study: Manual of Operations. Springfield, VA, United States Department of Commerce, National Technical Information Service, 1979; chap 18

10. Eschbach JW, Egrie JC, Downing MR, Browne JK, Adamson JW: Correction of the anemic of end-stage renal disease with recombinant human erythropoietin: Results of a phase I and II clinical trial. N Engl J Med 316:73-78, 1987

11. Kulzer P, Schaefer RM, Krahn R, Schaefer L, Heidland A: Effectiveness and safety of recombinant human erythropoietin (r-HuEPO) in the treatment of anemia of chronic renal failure in non dialysis patients. European Multicentre Study Group. Int J Artif Organs 17:195-202, 1994

12. Koene RA, Frenken LA: Does treatment of predialysis patients with recombinant human erythropoietin compromise renal function? Contrib Nephrol 87:105-112, 1990

13. Bresnick G: Background diabetic retinopathy, in Ryan SJ, Schachat AP, Murphy RP, Patz A (eds): Retina. St. Louis, MO, CV Mosby, 1989, pp 327-366

14. Bresnick GH: Diabetic maculopathy: A critical review highlighting diffuse macular edema. Ophthalmology 90:1301-1317, 1983

15. Green WR: Retina, in Specer WH (ed): Ophthalmic Pathology. Philadelphia, PA, Saunders, 1985, pp 589-1291

16. Bresnick GH: Diabetic maculopathy: A review. Ophthalmology 93:989-997, 1986

17. Duncan LJP, Cullen JF, Ireland JT, Nmolan J, Clarke BF, Oliver MF: A three year trial of atromid therapy in exudative diabetic retinopathy. Diabetes 17:458-459, 1968

18. Gordon B, Chang S, Kavangh M, Berrocal M, Yannuzzi L, Robertoson C, Drexler A: The effects of lipid lowering on diabetic retinopathy. Am J Ophthalmol 112:385-391, 1992

19. Frank RN: On the pathogenesis of diabetic retinopathy: A 19900 update. Ophthalmology 98:586-593, 1991

20. D'Amico DJ: Diseases of the retina. N Engl J Med 331:95-106, 1994

21. Ingber D, Fujita T, Kishimoto S, Sudo K, Kanamaru T, Brem H, Folkman J: Synthetic analogues of fumagillin that inhibit angiogenesis and suppress tumour growth. Nature 348:555-557, 1990

22. Le Devchat C, Khodabandehlou T: Transcutaneous oxygen pressure and hemorheology in diabetes mellitus. Int Angiol 9:259-262, 1990

23. Santilli SM, Fiegel VD, Knighton DR: Alloxan diabetes alters the rabbit transarterial wall oxygen gradient. J Vasc Surg 18:227-233, 1993

24. Hampton KK, Alani SM, Wilson JI, Price DE: Resistance to ischaemic conduction failure in chronic hypoxaemia and diabetes. J Neurol Neurosurg Psychiatry 52:1303-1305, 1989

25. Low PA, Schmelzer JD, Ward KK, Curran GL, Podusol JF: Effect of hyperbaric oxygenation on normal and chronic strptozotocin diabetic peripheral nerves. Exp Neurol 99:201-212, 1988

26. Weisz G, Ramon Y, Melamed Y: Treatment of the

diabetic foot by hyperbaric oxygen. Harefuah 124:678-681, 1993

27. Aomine M, Nobe S, Srita M: Increased susceptibility to hypoxia of prolonged action potential duration in ventricular papillary muscles from diabetic rats. Diabetes 39:1485-1489, 1990

28. Nikolov V, Kalaydjieva V, Logofetov A: Plasma erythropoietin activity in diabetes patients, studied by determining the 59Fe incorporation in posthypoxic polycythemic mice. Acta Physiol Pharmacol Bulg 15:37-40, 1989

29. Nielsen OJ, Mandrup-Poulsen T, Nerup J: Deficiency of erythropoietin is not responsible for the anaemia associated with cyclosporin treatment of insulin-dependent diabetes mellitus. Canadian-European Randomized Control Trial Group. J Intern Med 233:471-476, 1993

30. Stevens MJ, Danabery J, Feldman EL, Lattimer SA, Kamijo M, Thomas TP, Shindo H, Sima AAF, Greene DA: The linked roles of nitric oxide, aldose reductase, and (Na, K)-ATPase in the slowing of nerve conduction in the streptozotocin diabetic rat. J Clin Invest 94:853-859, 1994

CYTOKINES AND VASOACTIVE AGENTS IN RENAL DISEASE

Introduction

Our increasing understanding of the differences between healing with preservation of normal structure and function, on the one hand, and healing with scarring on the other, has focused on the local balance between endocrine, paracrine, and autocrine factors (including cytokines and vasoactive agents) that regulate proliferation and function of fibroblasts. Particular attention has been focused on growth factors such as transforming growth factor-β (TGF-β) and vasoactive compounds, such as endothelin, prostaglandins, nitric oxide, and angiotensin II, in the progression of renal disease. Also, the role of invading macrophages in the production of some of the factors that may affect progression of renal disease has come into more clear focus.

Border and Noble present a compelling discussion of the cytokine TGF-β. Cytokines regulate the basic processes of cell homeostasis and tissue repair in all organs. In a model of glomerulonephritis, the authors present evidence that TGF-β mediates the accumulation of extracellular matrix by inducing matrix synthesis, inhibiting matrix degradation, and modulating matrix receptors. Transforming growth factor-β may also cause matrix accumulation in diabetic nephropathy. The authors also report new evidence that human decorin can block scar formation in a glomerulonephritis model and thus offer hope that this drug can be used in the future for treatment of fibrotic disease caused by the overexpression of TGF-β.

Chou and Porush demonstrate that the endothelins ET-1 and ET-3 activate the endothelium-derived relaxation factor (EDRF)/nitric oxide (NO) system, producing early renal vasodilatation and direct effects on vascular smooth muscle, leading to prolonged vasoconstriction. This late effect was modulated by inhibition of cyclooxygenase but in divergent ways (ie, increased vasoconstriction with ET-1, whereas ET-3-evoked vasoconstriction was abolished). ET-3 causes natriuresis and diuresis, which was inhibited by NO synthase inhibition.

Neugarten and Silbiger note that there are well-described gender differences in renal disease progression, explaining that sex hormones can directly influence many of the mechanisms implicated in progressive renal disease, including mesangial cell proliferation and matrix accumulation as well as the synthesis and release of cytokines, vasoactive agents, and growth factors. In addition, estrogens may exert potent antioxidant actions in the mesangium, which may contribute to the protective effect on the female gender.

D'Amico et al review the evidence that tubulointerstitial inflammation and fibrosis occur in glomerular diseases, nonimmunologically as well as immunologically mediated, and stress the importance of tubulointerstitial damage as a marker of progression and unfavorable prognosis. In addition to interstitial recruitment of leukocytes and fibroblast proliferation, the role of persistent heavy proteinuria and exposure to proinflammatory cytokines in inducing damage of tubular epithelial cells, and the ultimate activation of T-lymphocytes, is suggested. The authors propose that measures to reduce urinary protein excretion and decrease oxygen consumption by tubular cells, such as dietary restriction of protein, phosphorus, and lipids, as well as the use of angiotensin-converting enzyme inhibitor (ACEI), should be effective therapeutic interventions.

Diamond, using a rat model of unilateral ureteral obstruction, demonstrates the role of the infiltrating renal macrophage as a mediator of interstitial fibrosis. He proposes that increased expression of macrophage-derived fibrogenic cytokines, especially TGF-β, is pathogenetically important.

Klahr et al present work illustrating the importance of angiotensin II in the development of tubulointerstitial fibrosis following unilateral ureteral obstruction. The use of an ACEI, enalapril, or an angiotensin II receptor antagonist reduced extracellular matrix protein in the tubulointerstitium, lessened the levels of mRNA for TGF-β and collagen IV, and almost completely abolished the mononuclear cell infiltration seen in this model.

Cytokines in Kidney Disease: The Role of Transforming Growth Factor-β

Wayne A. Border, MD, and Nancy A. Noble, PhD

● Cytokines such as transforming growth factor-β (TGF-β) are peptide factors that regulate embryogenesis, development, inflammation, tissue repair, and carcinogenesis. Growing evidence indicates that dysregulation of cytokine actions may underlie the pathogenesis of serious autoimmune, degenerative, and fibrotic diseases. Studies in a model of acute mesangial proliferative glomerulonephritis show that overproduction of TGF-β is the cause of pathologic accumulation of extracellular matrix in the nephritic glomeruli. Transforming growth factor-β acts to increase matrix production, inhibit matrix degradation, and modulate matrix receptors in the glomerulonephritic rats. It may also play a role in the glomerular matrix build-up that is a central feature of diabetic nephropathy. Elevated expression of TGF-β mRNA and TGF-β protein were found in the glomeruli of diabetic rats along with increased levels of proteoglycans and other matrix components that are known to be induced by TGF-β. The study of human diabetic glomeruli has also shown markedly elevated levels of TGF-β protein. Glomeruli from normal kidneys and nonprogressive kidney disorders were negative. The striking ability of TGF-β to cause exuberant matrix formation may be due to the fact that TGF-β can induce its own production by resident cells at a site of injury. Thus, the potential for TGF-β to do harm may be due to this autoinduction mechanism whereby TGF-β expression can become chronic, creating a vicious circle. As the role that TGF-β plays in chronic fibrotic diseases becomes better understood, it is likely that TGF-β inhibitors will become important future drugs for treating these conditions. To date, TGF-β activity has been successfully blocked in the kidney, in the skin, and in the central nervous system by neutralizing antibodies. In each case, inhibiting TGF-β significantly decreased the accumulation of excessive extracellular matrix but did not interfere with normal tissue repair. Recently, it has been discovered that the proteoglycan decorin may be a natural regulator of TGF-β. Injection of recombinant human decorin into glomerulonephritic rats significantly blocked extracellular matrix build-up in the nephritic glomeruli and suppressed the development of proteinuria. Since decorin is a natural human compound that can be produced as a recombinant molecule, it is likely not to be immunogenic compared with antibodies. Decorin offers hope as a treatment for chronic diseases associated with the overproduction of TGF-β.

INDEX WORDS: Cytokines; tumor necrosis factor-β; extracellular matrix; glomerulonephritis; diabetic nephropathy.

A GROWING BODY of evidence, recently reviewed by Sporn and Roberts, indicates that cytokines regulate essential biologic events, such as embryogenesis, development, inflammation and tissue repair, and carcinogenesis.[1,2] Cytokines act to maintain tissue homeostasis, but dysregulation of cytokine action results in autoimmune, degenerative, and fibrotic diseases. Thus, the improved understanding of cytokine function promises to lead to a unified pathogenesis of disease. An example of this common basis for health and disease is the profound proposal that "a wound is a tumor that heals itself" and the corollary that "tumors are wounds that do not heal."[3,4] Advances in cytokine research are likely to lead to a new molecular medicine in which cytokines and their antagonists, produced by biotechnology, will provide innovative therapies for the prevention and treatment of serious disorders, such as progressive kidney disease.[5]

Cytokines are peptide regulatory factors, also known as growth factors, that are produced by cells for the purpose of communication.[1] Transforming growth factor-β (TGF-β) is a prototypical cytokine. Other cytokines include platelet-derived growth factor (PDGF), fibroblast growth factor (FGF), tumor necrosis factor (TNF), epidermal growth factor (EGF), insulin-like growth factor (IGF), and the interleukins (IL) and colony-stimulating factors (CSF). Cytokines are the alphabet of the language that cells use to talk to each other (paracrine) or to themselves (autocrine). The purpose of cell communication is to regulate functions in order to maintain internal and tissue homeostasis. Cytokines are multifunctional and contextual, unique properties that provide the cell with a range of responses to a stimulus.[6,7] That is, cytokines do not have intrinsic positive or negative actions. They can stimulate or inhibit the same action (multifunctional) depending on the cell's memory of past experience and the present environment (contextual).[8]

Pathologic accumulation of extracellular matrix is the central biologic feature of glomerulo-

Supported by Grant No. DK 43609 from the National Institute of Diabetes and Digestive and Kidney Diseases-Department of Health and Human Services and a grant from Telios Pharmaceuticals, Inc.

sclerosis and interstitial fibrosis that leads to end-stage renal disease.[9] This is true whether the initial stimulus to injury is immunologic, hemodynamic, or metabolic. Production and deposition of extracellular matrix is a key part of tissue repair and remodeling that occurs following a stimulus such as a dermal wound. Transforming growth factor-β plays a central role in regulating wound repair by acting as a molecular switch that turns the repair process on and off. In this process, TGF-β has widespread effects on extracellular matrix; it is unique among cytokines in stimulating matrix production, inhibiting matrix degradation, and modulating matrix receptors to increase cell adhesion to matrix. All these effects lead to deposition and accumulation of matrix in the wound. Platelet-derived growth factor and FGF are also expressed in wounds and seem to be mitogenic and angiogenic, respectively. Neither directly stimulate matrix production and both seem to be regulated in complex ways by TGF-β. The molecular events that occur in response to kidney injury and that lead to matrix deposition have been unknown. Consequently, limited understanding of the molecular pathogenesis of renal fibrosis has hindered the development of new and more effective therapies. Despite current treatment, many patients have progressive loss of renal function and ultimately require dialysis or transplantation at a huge cost to the federal government.

There is now convincing evidence that the process of matrix deposition in the diseased kidney is regulated by TGF-β and involves other cytokines, in a manner identical to tissue repair in the skin and other organs.[5] There is also evidence that overproduction or persistent production of TGF-β (and possibly other cytokines) can lead to scarring and tissue damage. The pathologic consequences of the excessive action of TGF-β has been termed the "dark side" of tissue repair.[10] As shown in Fig 1, TGF-β is released from platelets following tissue damage. Transforming growth factor-β induces the local cells to produce extracellular matrix and more TGF-β, while PDGF seems to stimulate cell proliferation and possibly augment TGF-β production. Unknown mechanisms shut down the production of matrix and TGF-β when the repair is completed. A failure to shut down TGF-β, caused by continuous injury or a defect in TGF-β regulation, may lead to a vicious circle in which there is accelerated production of TGF-β and persistent production and deposition of extracellular matrix. Evidence that TGF-β plays a central role in experimental glomerulonephritis by (1) inducing matrix production, (2) inhibiting matrix degradation, and (3) modulating matrix receptors is presented below.

GLOMERULONEPHRITIS

Our work began with the observation that in human and experimental glomerular disease there was often continued accumulation of extracellular matrix despite cessation of injury. This suggested the presence of an intervening process, a missing link between the injury and the progressive build-up of glomerular matrix. We hypothesized that the missing link was the activation of TGF-β. Nearly all cells and tissues are capable of producing TGF-β and other cytokines, meaning that cytokine production does not equal cytokine action. Thus, we planned our studies to show that if TGF-β was present in the disease, it was biologically active in stimulating matrix production.

We started by testing the effects of TGF-β and, as control cytokines, PDGF, IL-1, and TNF on cultured rat mesangial and glomerular epithelial cells. (For a review of experimental techniques see ref 11.) The third resident cell in the glomerulus, the endothelial cell, cannot easily be cultured and is not thought to contribute to matrix production in the mature glomerulus. The addition of TGF-β, but not other cytokines, dramatically increased the production of proteoglycans by both cell types. Production of fibronectin, type IV collagen, and, to a lesser extent, laminin was stimulated in the epithelial cells.[12,13] Two of the increased proteoglycans are decorin and biglycan. We and others have shown that the ability to stimulate the production of these proteoglycans is a relatively specific property of TGF-β.[12,13] Decorin is also known to bind TGF-β and neutralize its biologic actions.[14]

To determine the relevance of the glomerular cell culture results to disease, we studied a rat model of acute mesangial proliferative glomerulonephritis induced by the injection of antithymocyte serum, which selectively injures mesangial cells. Initially there is a decrease in glomerular matrix due to lysis of a portion of the mesangial

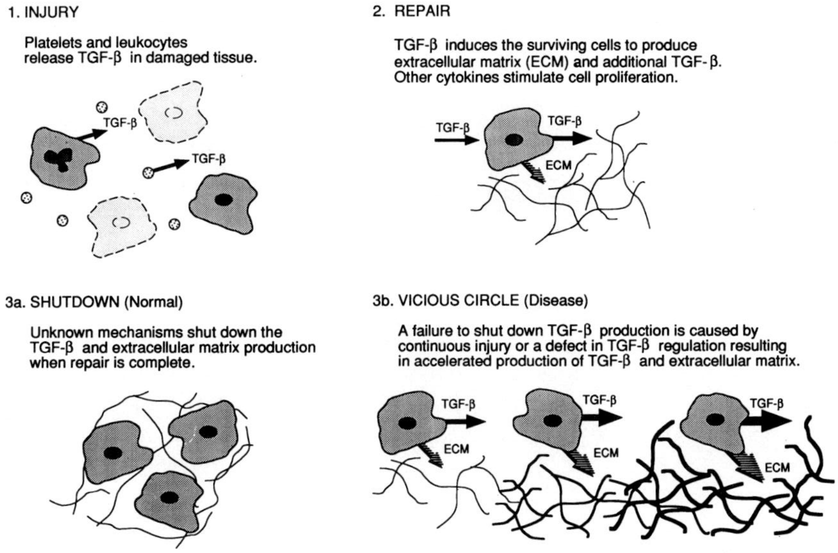

Fig 1. A schematic depiction of the role that TGF-β is believed to play in the repair of tissue injury throughout the body, including the kidney. The ability of TGF-β to induce the production of TGF-β by target cells may underly the conversion of the repair process into a chronic fibrotic disease. (Reproduced from *The Journal of Clinical Investigation*, 1992, vol 90, p 5 by copyright permission of the American Society for Clinical Investigation.[10])

cells; however, by days 7 and 14 of disease there is a striking increase in matrix accumulation, which then begins to decrease and within several weeks returns to normal. A powerful tool in studying this model is the ability to isolate and culture glomeruli as though they were cells. Nephritic glomeruli on days 1, 4, 7, 14, and 28 of disease were isolated. We examined the production of the most abundant component of matrix, fibronectin, production of proteoglycans, and expression of TGF-β mRNA and TGF-β protein.[15]

On day 1 of disease proteoglycan and fibronectin synthesis were the same as in the control glomeruli. By day 4 there was a steady increase in proteoglycan synthesis, reaching a nearly 50-fold increase by day 7, along with an elevation in fibronectin production (Fig 2). The nephritic glomeruli also showed a significant increase in the expression of TGF-β mRNA and TGF-β protein that temporally correlated with the induction of glomerular matrix production and deposition (Fig 3). Additional experiments confirmed that the nephritic glomeruli were releasing large amounts of active TGF-β. This TGF-β could stimulate normal mesangial cells to produce proteoglycans; anti–TGF-β blocked this stimulation. To further show that TGF-β was the cause of increased matrix production in the nephritic glomeruli, we added anti–TGF-β to cultured nephritic glomeruli isolated on day 7 of disease. Anti–TGF-β effectively suppressed nearly 80% of the elevated matrix production.

Since anti–TGF-β suppressed matrix production in vitro, we next tested its potential by injecting it or a control serum into glomerulonephritic rats beginning on day 1 of disease.[16] The effects of anti–TGF-β were assessed by using histologic evaluation of glomerular matrix accumulation as a measure of disease activity. Glomeruli from the anti–TGF-β–treated group contained much less matrix than glomeruli from animals treated with control serum (Fig 4). To determine the mechanism of the protective effect of anti–TGF-β, we measured proteoglycan production in the glomeruli from the experimental groups. In the animals treated with anti–TGF-β, proteoglycan production by the nephritic glomeruli was suppressed by 60% to 80% compared with controls (Fig 5). Thus, the therapeutic effect of anti–TGF-β in blocking matrix deposition in this model is directly linked to suppression of matrix production.

Transforming growth factor-β also inhibits matrix degradation, an effect that is potentially important in the accumulation of pathologic matrix in glomerular disease. The plasminogen/plasmin system is thought to play a key role in the normal degradation and turnover of extracellular matrix.[17] This system is regulated by the balance between plasminogen activators (PA), which convert plasminogen to the potent protease plasmin, and plasminogen activator inhibitors (PAI). In many other cell lines TGF-β decreases the secretion of PA and stimulates the production of

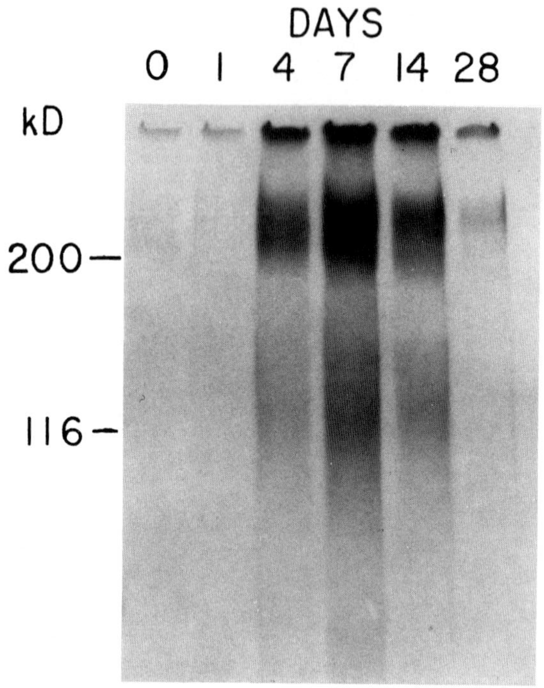

Fig 2. Proteoglycan production by cultured glomeruli isolated from glomerulonephritic rats on days 0 (control), 1, 4, 7, 14, and 28 after induction of disease. Compared with the controls, there is a striking increase in proteoglycan production on days 4, 7, and 14. (Reproduced from *The Journal of Clinical Investigation*, 1990, vol 86, p 457 by copyright permission of the American Society for Clinical Investigation.[15])

PAI.[18] We found that the same is true when TGF-β is added to cultured normal glomeruli.[19] As little as 1 ng/mL of TGF-β caused the disappearance of secreted PA activity, which correlated with the strong stimulation of PAI production. We then examined glomerulonephritic rats to determine whether the same changes occurred in disease. On day 3 of disease PA activity was nearly undetectable in the nephritic glomeruli compared with controls and PAI production was greatly elevated, the same sequence of events that was observed with addition of TGF-β in vitro.[19] On days 7 and 14 of disease, PAI-1 was progressively deposited into the glomerular matrix. It is thought that when PAI-1 is bound to the matrix it is active in inhibiting the formation of plasmin. We studied the kidneys from the glomerulonephritic rats that were treated with anti–TGF-β. Compared with the untreated rats, the kidneys from the anti–TGF-β–treated rats showed significantly ($P < 0.005$) less PAI-1 in the glomerular matrix, again demonstrating a causal role for TGF-β in matrix build-up.

The third action of TGF-β on extracellular matrix in tissue repair is to modulate matrix receptors termed "integrins."[20,21] These transmembrane receptors are expressed on the cell surface, where they interact with specific matrix components, while a cytoplasmic portion is connected to the internal cytoskeleton and ultimately the cell nucleus.[22] Thus, these receptors "integrate" extracellular stimuli from the matrix with the interior of the cell. Integrins are composed of different α and β subunits, the specific combination determining ligand specificity. Since fibronectin is a major matrix component whose production and deposition is increased in nephritic glomeruli, we examined $\alpha5\ \beta1$, an important fibronectin receptor. The addition of TGF-β to cultured normal glomeruli stimulated an increase in production of both $\alpha5$ and $\beta1$, which were shown by immunoprecipitation of the fibronectin receptor, $\alpha5\ \beta1$, at the cell surface. In glomeruli of ne-

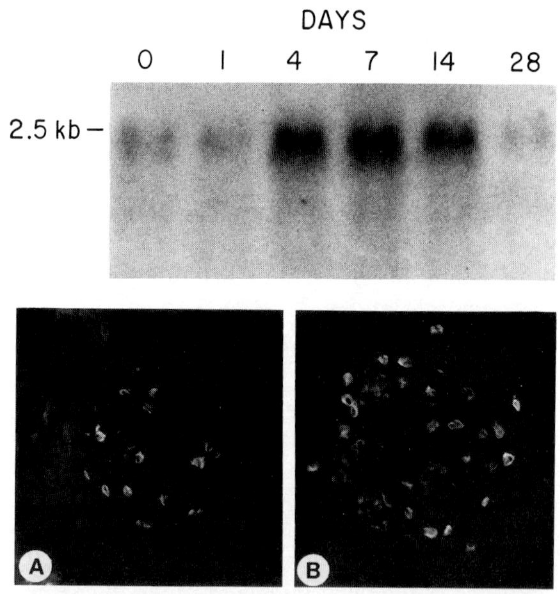

Fig 3. (Top) Northern blotting of TGF-β mRNA in kidneys isolated from glomerulonephritic rats at the same time points as described in Fig 2. (Bottom) Immunofluorescence micrographs of glomeruli stained with anti–TGF-β antibody: (A) normal glomerulus and (B) nephritic glomerulus on day 7 of disease. (Reproduced from *The Journal of Clinical Investigation*, 1990, vol 86, p 459 by copyright permission of the American Society for Clinical Investigation.[15])

phritic rats isolated on day 7 of disease there was a striking increase in the $\alpha5\ \beta1$ receptor demonstrated by immunofluores-cence microscopy and by immunoprecipitation studies using specific antibodies (Kagami et al, unpublished observations). In cultured cells, overexpression of this receptor is associated with increased incorporation of fibronectin into the matrix. It is reasonable to believe, but difficult to prove, that increased expression of the receptor would have the same effect in nephritic glomeruli.

DIABETIC NEPHROPATHY

The three actions of TGF-β that are central to normal tissue repair, stimulation of matrix synthesis, inhibition of matrix degradation, and modulation of matrix receptors have now been demonstrated to underlie matrix accumulation in experimental glomerulonephritis. Although fundamentally different in pathogenesis from glomerulonephritis, diabetic nephropathy does share the common feature of mesangial matrix expansion. This fact caused us to question whether TGF-β expression might be involved in diabetic kidney disease. We studied rats made diabetic by the administration of streptozotocin, a chemical that produces insulin deficiency. The rats then develop kidney disease that closely resembles human diabetic nephropathy. After the onset of diabetes, we found progressively elevated levels of TGF-β mRNA and TGF-β protein in the glomeruli of the diabetic rats.[23] The expression of TGF-β was somewhat reduced, but still abnormal, in diabetic rats treated with insulin compared with age-matched normal rats with or without identical insulin treatment. We also found elevated levels of proteoglycans and other matrix components known to be induced by TGF-β, indicating increased TGF-β biologic activity in the diabetic glomeruli. The relevance of these findings in the experimental model of the human disease was confirmed by the demonstration of similarly elevated levels of TGF-β protein and matrix in the glomeruli of patients with diabetic nephropathy (Fig 6). Glomeruli from normal kidneys or from patients with nonprogressive glomerular diseases (minimal change disease and thin basement mem-

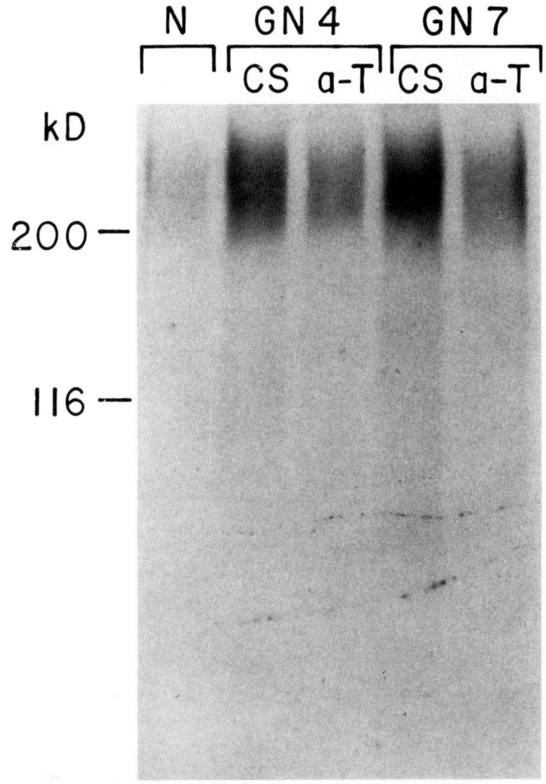

Fig 5. Proteoglycan synthesis by glomeruli from glomerulonephritic rats treated with anti–TGF-β (a-T) or control serum (CS) on days 4 (GN 4) and 7 (GN 7) of disease. There is a marked reduction in proteoglycan production in the anti–TGF-β–treated rats. (Reprinted with permission from *Nature*, Copyright 1990 Macmillan Magazines Limited.[16])

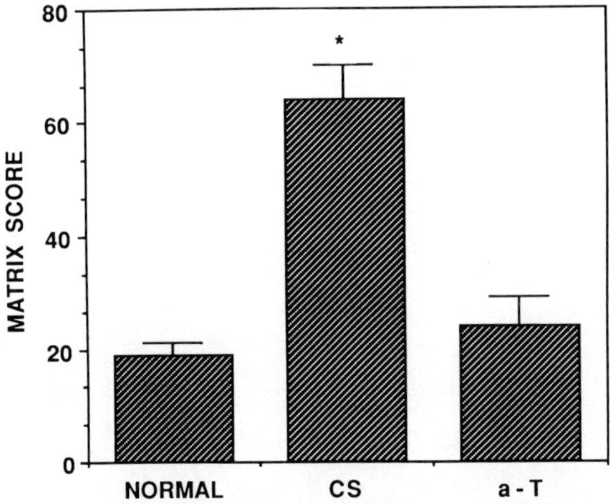

Fig 4. Quantitation of extracellular matrix in nephritic glomeruli. *$P < 0.001$ for glomerulonephritic rats treated with control serum (CS) compared with anti–TGF-β (a-T) on day 7 of glomerulonephritis. (Reprinted with permission from *Nature*, Copyright 1990 Macmillan Magazines Limited.[16])

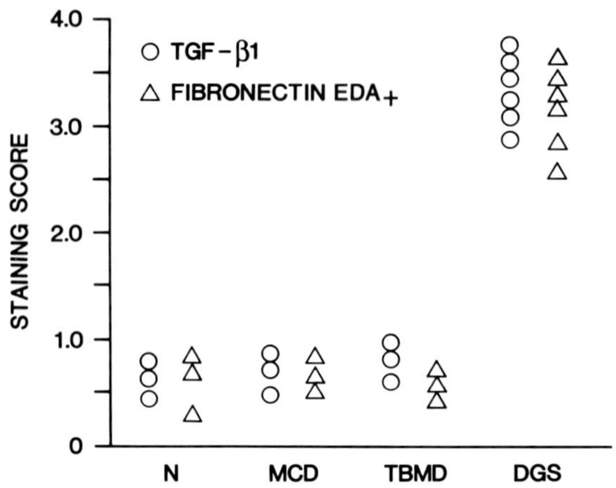

Fig 6. Staining of TGF-β protein and fibronectin EDA+ in human glomeruli. Kidney tissues from normals (N), minimal change disease (MCD), thin basement membrane disease (TBMD), and diabetic glomerulosclerosis (DGS) cases were studied. (Reprinted with permission.[23])

brane disease) were negative for TGF-β. Thus, TGF-β may play a key role in the development of glomerular matrix accumulation in both glomerulonephritis and diabetic nephropathy.

TUBULOINTERSTITIAL FIBROSIS

Several studies have shown that in many forms of glomerular disease the development of tubulointerstitial fibrosis is closely correlated with progressive kidney failure. We have found that in animals who receive a second injection of antithymocyte serum, unlike the single injection model, there is sustained expression of TGF-β (Yamamoto et al, unpublished observation). The elevated expression of TGF-β is accompanied by the development of glomerulosclerosis, tubulointerstitial fibrosis, persistent proteinuria, and decreased kidney function. In glomerular injury induced by repeated injections of aminonucleoside of puromycin, increased TGF-β expression was also detected in association with the development of tubulointerstitial fibrosis.[24] It has been suggested that TGF-β plays a role in cortical collagen deposition in experimental anti-glomerular basement membrane glomerulonephritis.[25]

TRANSFORMING GROWTH FACTOR-β AND DIET

Transforming growth factor-β may also play a role in the protective effect of a low-protein diet in progressive kidney disease. Dietary protein restriction has been shown to slow the rate of loss of kidney function in humans with glomerulonephritis and diabetic nephropathy. We administered a low-protein diet to rats with experimental glomerulonephritis.[26] Compared with a normal-protein diet, glomerulonephritic rats receiving the low-protein diet did not develop an increase in glomerular extracellular matrix (Fig 7). Glomeruli from the nephritic rats fed the normal protein diet showed a striking increase in extracellular matrix production and were shown to be producing large amounts of TGF-β. In contrast, glomeruli isolated from rats on a low-protein diet at the same point of disease showed no increase in matrix production of TGF-β secretion (Fig 8). Thus, a mechanism of the therapeutic effect of dietary protein restriction may be the suppression of TGF-β expression and the prevention of increased extracellular matrix production in the diseased glomeruli.

TRANSFORMING GROWTH FACTOR-β ANTAGONISTS AS FUTURE DRUGS

As the critical role that TGF-β and possibly other cytokines play in chronic diseases becomes better understood, it is likely that cytokine inhibitors will become important future drugs in con-

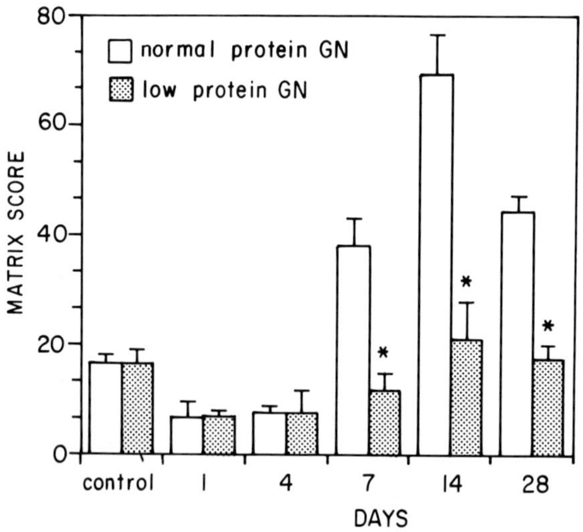

Fig 7. Quantitation of the effect of dietary protein on glomerular extracellular matrix in experimental glomerulonephritis (GN) at several time points following induction of disease. The low-protein diet prevented matrix build-up. (Reprinted with permission.[26])

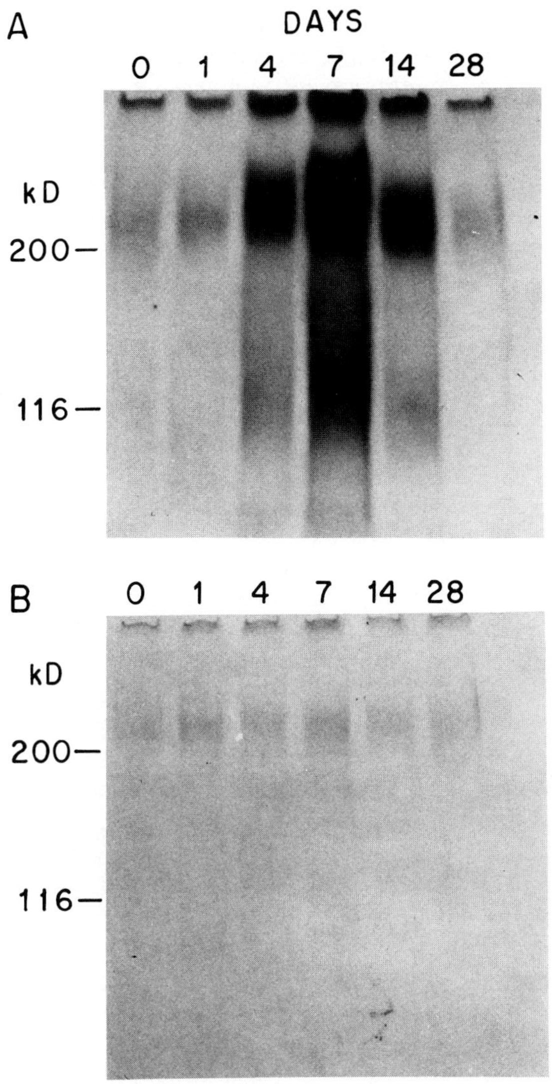

Fig 8. **Proteoglycan production by cultured nephritic glomeruli from rats fed a normal-protein diet (A) or a low-protein diet (B) at the same time points as described in Fig 6. Induction of proteoglycan synthesis was suppressed by a low-protein diet. (Reprinted with permission.[26])**

trolling these conditions. The complex manner in which TGF-β production and activity is regulated offers several targets for TGF-β suppression. Transforming growth factor-β is produced as a latent precursor protein that requires proteolytic processing for activation.[27] A large peptide derived from TGF-β activation can bind mature, active TGF-β and inhibit it, possibly by blocking interaction with TGF-β receptors. Soluble forms of the receptors also may be effective in blocking TGF-β by the same mechanism. Several members of the steroid receptor super-family can regulate transcription of the TGF-β gene and thus might be used to suppress TGF-β.[28] To date, TGF-β activity has been successfully blocked by neutralizing antibodies in the kidney[16] and the skin.[29] The anti–TGF-β antibodies appear to work by preventing TGF-β binding to receptors. In each example, inhibiting TGF-β significantly decreased the accumulation of excessive extracellular matrix, but did not interfere with normal healing of the tissue. In the case of dermal wounds treated with anti–TGF-β, there was dramatically less collagen and no scar formation, but the healed wound possessed the same tensile strength as the control wounds.[29]

The action of TGF-β in causing scar formation is particularly interesting. It is known that fetal skin heals normally without a scar, whereas in the adult scarring occurs. An explanation for this observation recently was found. The lack of scarring in fetal wounds correlates with negligible expression of TGF-β in the wound. Transforming growth factor-β was found only in platelets that had aggregated at the wound site.[30] In contrast, adult wounds contained large amounts of TGF-β. Thus, the ability to heal a wound rapidly with exuberant matrix formation is a feature in the adult that may not be a necessity. In addition, the ability of TGF-β to mount such an effective healing response may account for the unusual feature of TGF-β regulation that TGF-β can induce its own production by local cells. As suggested earlier this may be the mechanism by which TGF-β expression can become chronic, creating a vicious circle.

It recently has been found that the proteoglycans decorin and biglycan can bind TGF-β and neutralize its biologic activity.[14] Since the production of decorin and biglycan is induced by TGF-β, it was suggested that these proteoglycans may be natural regulators of the action of TGF-β.[31] We hypothesized that if decorin is a natural regulator of TGF-β, it would be an ideal molecule to use therapeutically to antagonize the action of TGF-β in the glomerulonephritis model. We intravenously administered recombinant human decorin or tissue-derived decorin for 2, 4, or 6 days to test for the ability to block matrix accumulation in the nephritic kidneys.[32] As control injections we used another proteoglycan that does not bind TGF-β, a protein that resembles the core protein of decorin, an unrelated protein, and buffer alone.

To assess the efficacy of decorin, we stained the nephritic glomeruli with antibodies that detect an isoform of fibronectin and tenascin, because these matrix components are relatively specifically induced by TGF-β and are barely detectable in normal glomeruli. We found that both these matrix components were greatly increased in nephritic glomeruli in rats treated with no or two injections of decorin. However, four or six injections of decorin greatly reduced the deposition of these two markers of TGF-β activity, as well as that of whole fibronectin. Histologic analysis showed a comparable effect of decorin in preventing the increase in extracellular matrix that occurs in this disease. Decorin also suppressed the development of proteinuria. None of the control molecules had an effect on any of the manifestations of disease.

These results show a dramatic effect of decorin in preventing the deposition of extracellular matrix in injured glomeruli from the nephritic animals. That matrix accumulation in this model was prevented by injecting decorin demonstrates an in vivo activity of decorin in suppressing TGF-β and supports the idea that decorin is a natural regulator of TGF-β. Decorin may be particularly suitable for the treatment of kidney disease because it accumulates in the kidney after intravenous administration. Furthermore, decorin is a natural human compound that can be produced as a recombinant molecule and is not likely to be immunogenic compared with antibodies. Thus, decorin offers hope as a novel treatment for glomerulonephritis and diabetic nephropathy as well as other diseases associated with the overproduction of TGF-β.[10]

ADDENDUM

New studies[33] involving the addition of angiotensin to rat mesangial cells in culture demonstrated increased TGF-β and matrix components biglycan, fibronectin, and collagen type I at both mRNA and protein levels. A competitive inhibitor of angiotensin II, saralasin, abrogated the stimulation. Angiotensin II also promoted the conversion of latent TGF-β to the biologically active form. Coincubation of mesangial cells with angiotensin II and neutralizing antibody to TGF-β blocked the angiotensin II-induced increases in matrix protein expression. Continuous in vivo administration of angiotensin II to normal rats for 7 days resulted in 70% increases in glomerular mRNA for both TGF-β and collagen type I. The effects of angiotensin II on matrix formation seem to be mediated through TGF-β expression. This mechanism may contribute to glomerulosclerosis in vivo.

Transforming growth factor-β expression and increased matrix production is transient and self-limited in nephritic glomeruli from rats with acute, reversible glomerulonephritis induced by a single injection of an antibody reactive with glomerular mesangial cells.[34] In contrast, in rats given a second antibody injection, 1 week later, the glomerular expression of TGF-$\beta 1$ mRNA and TGF-$\beta 1$ protein remained elevated through 18 weeks and was associated with a large infiltration of mononuclear cells, with staining features of fibroblastic/myofibroblastic cells, strongly expressing TGF-$\beta 1$ in the tubulointerstitium of the kidney. By 18 weeks, kidneys from animals receiving two antibody injections showed glomerulosclerosis and tubulointerstitial fibrosis with striking deposition of collagens type I and III, whereas kidney tissue from animals given one antibody injection was indistinguishable from the normal control. The histological changes were accompanied by persistent proteinuria and elevated levels of blood urea nitrogen. Extracellular matrix markers of TGF-$\beta 1$ activity, a special isoform of fibronectin, tenascin, biglycan, and PAI-1, were significantly elevated in kidneys undergoing fibrosis. These data suggest that sustained TGF-$\beta 1$ expression contributes to the development of progressive kidney fibrosis.

REFERENCES

1. Sporn MB, Roberts AB: Autocrine secretion—10 years later. Ann Intern Med 117:408-414, 1992

2. Sporn MB, Roberts AB: Peptide growth factors and inflammation, tissue repair, and cancer. J Clin Invest 78:329-332, 1986

3. Haddow A: Molecular repair, wound healing, and carcinogenesis: Tumor production a possible overhealing? Adv Cancer Res 16:181-234, 1972

4. Dvorak HF: Tumors: Wounds that do not heal. N Engl J Med 313:1650-1659, 1986

5. Border WA, Noble NA, Yamamoto T, Tomooka S, Kagami S: Antagonists of transforming growth factor-β: A novel approach to treatment of glomerulonephritis and prevention of glomerulosclerosis. Kidney Int 41:566-570, 1992

6. Sporn MB, Roberts AB: Peptide growth factors are multifunctional. Nature 332:217-219, 1988

7. Nathan C, Sporn M: Cytokines in context. J Cell Biol 113:981-986, 1991

8. Moses HL, Yang EY, Pietenpol JA: TGF-β stimulation and inhibition of cell proliferation: New mechanistic insights. Cell 63:245-247, 1990

9. Border WA, Okuda S, Nakamura T: Extracellular matrix and glomerular disease. Semin Nephrol 9:307-317, 1989

10. Border WA, Ruoslahti E: Transforming growth factor-β in disease: The dark side of tissue repair. J Clin Invest 90:1-7, 1992

11. Miller DE, Noble NA, Yu X, Border WA: Molecular and cellular biological techniques in the study of glomerular diseases. Semin Nephrol 12:506-515, 1992

12. Border WA, Okuda S, Languino LR, Ruoslahti E: Transforming growth factor-β regulates production of proteoglycans by mesangial cells. Kidney Int 37:689-695, 1990

13. Nakamura T, Miller D, Ruoslahti E, Border WA: Production of extracellular matrix by glomerular epithelial cells is regulated by transforming growth factor-$\beta 1$. Kidney Int 41:1213-1221, 1992

14. Yamaguchi Y, Mann DM, Ruoslahti E: Negative regulation of transforming growth factor-β by the proteoglycan decorin. Nature 346:281-284, 1990

15. Okuda S, Languino LR, Ruoslahti E, Border WA: Elevated expression of transforming growth factor-β and proteoglycan production in experimental glomerulonephritis. Possible role in expansion of the mesangial extracellular matrix. J Clin Invest 86:453-462, 1990

16. Border WA, Okuda S, Languino L, Sporn MB, Ruoslahti E: Suppression of experimental glomerulonephritis by antiserum against transforming growth factor $\beta 1$. Nature 346:371-374, 1990

17. Vassalli J-D, Sappino A-P, Belin D: The plasminogen activator/plasmin system. J Clin Invest 88:1067-1072, 1991

18. Laiho M, Saksela O, Andreasen PA, Keski-Oja J: Enhanced production and extracellular deposition of the endothelial-type plasminogen activator inhibitor in cultured human lung fibroblasts by transforming growth factor-β. J Cell Biol 103:2403-2410, 1986

19. Tomooka S, Border WA, Marshall BC, Noble NA: Glomerular matrix accumulation is linked to inhibition of the plasmin protease system. Kidney Int 42:1462-1469, 1992

20. Ignotz RA, Massague J: Cell adhesion protein receptors as targets for transforming growth factor-β action. Cell 51:189-197, 1987

21. Heino J, Ignotz RA, Hemler ME, Crouse C, Massague J: Regulation of cell adhesion receptors by transforming growth factor-β. Concomitant regulation of integrins that share a common $\beta 1$ subunit. J Biol Chem 264:380-388, 1989

22. Ruoslahti E: Integrins. J Clin Invest 87:1-5, 1991

23. Yamamoto T, Nakamura T, Noble NA, Ruoslahti E, Border WA: Diabetic kidney disease is linked to elevated expression of transforming growth factor-β. Proc Natl Acad Sci U S A 90:1814-1818, 1993

24. Jones CL, Buch S, Post M, McCulloch L, Liu E, Eddy AA: Pathogenesis of interstitial fibrosis in chronic purine aminonucleoside nephrosis. Kidney Int 40:1020-1031, 1991

25. Coimbra T, Wiggins R, Noh JW, Merritt S, Phan SH: Transforming growth factor-β production in anti-glomerular basement membrane disease in the rabbit. Am J Pathol 138:223-234, 1991

26. Okuda S, Nakamura T, Yamamoto T, Ruoslahti E, Border WA: Dietary protein restriction rapidly reduces transforming growth factor β-1 expression in experimental glomerulonephritis. Proc Natl Acad Sci U S A 88:9765-9769, 1991

27. Roberts AB, Sporn MB: The transforming growth factor-βs, in Sporn MB, Roberts AB (eds): Peptide Growth Factors and Their Receptors I. Basal, Switzerland, Springer-Verlag, 1990, pp 419-472

28. Roberts AB, Sporn MB: Mechanistic interrelationships between two superfamilies: The steroid/retinoid receptors and transforming growth factor-β. Cancer Surv 14:205-220, 1992

29. Shah M, Foreman DM, Ferguson WJ: Control of scarring in adult wounds by neutralizing antibody to transforming growth factor β. Lancet 339:213-214, 1992

30. Whitby DJ, Ferguson MWJ: Immunohistochemical localization of growth factors in fetal wound healing. Dev Biol 147:207-215, 1991

31. Ruoslahti E, Yamaguchi Y: Proteoglycans as modulators of growth factor activities. Cell 64:867-869, 1991

32. Border WA, Noble NA, Yamamoto T, Harper J, Yamamguchi Y, Pierschbacher MD, Ruoslahti E: Natural inhibitor of transforming growth factor-β protects against scarring in experimental kidney disease. Nature 360:361-364, 1992

33. Kagami S, Border WA, Miller DE, Noble NA: Angiotensin II stimulates extracellular matrix protein synthesis through induction of transforming growth factor-beta expression in rat glomerular mesangial cells. J Clin Invest 93:2431-2437, 1994

34. Yamamoto T, Noble NA, Miller DE, Border WA: Sustained expression of TGF-beta 1 underlies development of progressive kidney fibrosis. Kidney Int 45:916-927, 1994

Renal Actions of Endothelin-1 and Endothelin-3: Interactions With the Prostaglandin System and Nitric Oxide

Shyan-Yih Chou, MD, and Jerome G. Porush, MD

● Endothelins (ET) possess both vasodilatory and vasoconstrictive properties. The renal actions of ET-1 and ET-3, as well as in vivo interactions of these two isopeptides with the prostaglandin and endothelium-derived relaxation factor/nitric oxide systems were studied in anesthetized dogs. The ETs were infused intrarenally at doses not affecting systemic hemodynamics. Both ET-1 and ET-3 induced an early transient renal vasodilation, followed by a prolonged vasoconstriction. Inhibition of nitric oxide synthase with N^G-monomethyl-L-arginine completely abolished the renal vasodilation induced by either ET-1 or ET-3 and enhanced the vasoconstriction. Endothelin-1 was associated with an increase in the renal release of prostacyclin, while urinary thromboxane A_2 was increased after ET-3 administration. Inhibition of cyclooxygenase (with indomethacin) augmented the renal vasoconstriction induced by ET-1, but inhibition of cyclooxygenase (with meclofenamate) abolished the ET-3–evoked vasoconstriction. Endothelin-1 showed little effects on urinary water and sodium excretion; however, ET-3 displayed significant diuretic and natriuretic effects, which were inhibited by nitric oxide synthase inhibition. These findings suggest that these two isopeptides activate the endothelial endothelium-derived relaxation factor/nitric oxide system, which elicits early renal vasodilation, whereas direct effects on the vascular smooth muscle leads to vasoconstriction. Endothelin-3 causes diuresis and natriuresis, possibly by inducing release of nitric oxide in medullary collecting duct cells.

INDEX WORDS: Endothelin-1; endothelin-3; prostacyclin; nitric oxide; thromboxane.

IN 1985, Hickey et al[1] observed that the media derived from cultured endothelial cells elicited a slowly developing, longlasting vasoconstrictive response in the coronary artery. In 1988, Yanagisawa et al[2] isolated and purified a potent polypeptide vasoconstrictor, termed endothelin (ET), from the cultured porcine endothelial cells. This 21-amino acid peptide, now designated as ET-1, produces a marked and prolonged pressor response when administered intravenously.[2] In a short period of time following this discovery, cloning and sequencing of preproendothelin complementary DNA and the proteolytic process necessary to generate this peptide have been elucidated in a number of species.[2,3] In addition, three structurally distinct isopeptides (ET-1, ET-2, and ET-3) have been identified.[3] These isopeptides share a common structure consisting of a hairpin loop, two disulfide bonds, an amino terminus, and a hydrophobic C-terminal end. Endothelin-1 differs from ET-2 and ET-3 by two and six amino acids, respectively.[3] The three ETs are encoded by separate genes at different chromosomal loci. The human ET-1, ET-2, and ET-3 genes are localized to chromosomes 6p23-24, 1p34, and 20q31.2-13.3, respectively.[4] Human ET-1 mRNA encodes 212 amino acid prepropeptide, which is cleaved by endopeptidases to yield a 38 amino acid big ET-1.[2,5] Endothelin-converting enzyme, a membrane-bound phosphoramidon-inhibitable metalloprotease, converts big ET-1 to the mature 21 amino acid ET-1.[6] The released ET-1 either binds to specific receptors or is quickly degraded.

Two ET receptors have been identified and cloned: ET-A and ET-B.[7-9] Human ET-A receptor contains 427 amino acids and binds ETs in the following order: ET-1 > ET-2 >> ET-3.[7,8] The human ET-B receptor contains 422 amino acids and binds the three ETs with equal affinity.[9] The location and function of these two receptors have not been well defined. In the kidney, radioligand-binding studies and measurement of ET receptor mRNA in microdissected nephron segments show that ET-A receptors are located mainly on vascular smooth muscle cells and ET-B receptors are present on the vascular endothelial and tubular epithelial cells.[10,11] Several antagonists specific to ET-A or to both ET-A and ET-B receptors have been developed recently[12-16] and are beginning to provide insight into the role of ETs in pathophysiologic events, such as ischemic acute renal failure.[17]

Endothelin-1 binding to ET-A receptors in mesangial and vascular smooth muscle cells stimulates phosphatidylcholine hydrolysis and ultimately mediates contraction.[18-20] After activating phospholipase C through inhibitory G protein, ET-1 induces hydrolysis of phosphoinosi-

Supported by a research grant from Nephrology Foundation of Brooklyn.

tate-bisphosphate in the plasma membrane to form inositol 1,4,5-trisphosphate and diacylglycerol. After diffusing into the endoplasmic reticulum through the cytosol, inositol 1,4,5-trisphosphate opens calcium channels and activates transient calcium release from its stores. This is followed by calcium influx through receptor-operated and voltage-dependent calcium channels in the cell membrane. The calcium influx then leads to a sustained increase in cytosolic calcium after ET stimulation, thereby mediating vasoconstriction.

Studies undertaken to identify the sites of ET synthesis in the kidney have been limited mainly to those performed in the rat. In the glomerulus, ET-1 and ET-3 are produced by endothelial, epithelial, and mesangial cells.[21-23] In the tubules, the collecting ducts (particularly the inner medullary collecting duct) are the major nephron segments producing ET-1 and ET-3.[24,25] Factors stimulating the production of ET-1 have been primarily studied in vitro and include shear stress, hypoxia, vasoactive agents (angiotensin II, vasopressin, bradykinin, and epinephrine), inflammatory agents (tumor necrosis factor, interleukin-1, and transforming growth factor-β), and thrombin.[26-28]

Both the kidney and lung participate in the clearance of ET-1 from the blood. Little circulating ET-1 is found in the urine, but inhibition of neutral endopeptidase markedly increases urinary excretion of both endogenous and exogenous ET-1.[29] Since ET-1 is a relatively small peptide (molecular weight, 2,490 d), it is readily filtered into the proximal tubules. The brush border of the proximal tubules is richly endowed with neutral endopeptidases, which degrade filtered peptides, including atrial natriuretic peptide, angiotensin II, and bradykinin, as well as ET-1.[29,30] Since circulating ET-1 is extensively degraded in the proximal tubules, it is likely that most of the measurable urinary ET-1 derives from the nephron segments beyond this site.

There have been an abundance of in vitro studies addressing synthesis of ETs in various nephron components, characterization of ET receptors, transmembrane signaling pathways of ETs, and transcriptional control of the ET genes.[26-28] In contrast, there are relatively few in vivo studies and they have been performed mostly in the rat; in addition, studies to clarify renal physiologic actions of ETs in other species are scarce. Furthermore, most of the studies examine the properties of ET-1 and little is known about the renal actions of ET-3. This report describes and compares the vascular and tubular actions of ET-1 and ET-3 in the canine kidney as well as in vivo interactions of these two peptides with the prostaglandin and endothelium-derived relaxation factor (EDRF)/nitric oxide (NO) systems.

RENAL ACTIONS OF ENDOTHELIN-1

Intravenous infusion of ET-1 increases arterial blood pressure, decreases cardiac output, and affects several hormonal systems, including the renin-angiotensin system and release of aldosterone and atrial natriuretic peptide.[31,32] When ET-1 disturbs other hormonal systems, the renal effects of this peptide differ markedly from those observed when other systems are kept intact. These confounding effects due to altering systemic hemodynamics can be avoided by intrarenal infusion of ET-1.[33]

We have infused ET-1 intrarenally in dogs at the rate of 4 ng/kg/min and noted an early transient increase in renal blood flow (RBF) by 13%, lasting approximately 12 minutes, followed by a progressive decline in RBF by 26% (Fig 1) and a decrease in glomerular filtration rate (GFR) by 23%.[33] The intrarenal infusion of this dose of ET-1 avoided the systemic effects of ET-1 on renal function since arterial pressure, cardiac output, and total peripheral resistance did not change. In addition, the renal vasoconstrictive response to ET-1 did not result from stimulation of the renin-angiotensin or renal adrenergic systems.

In contrast to ET-1, intrarenal infusion of other vasoconstrictors, including angiotensin II, vasopressin, and norepinephrine leads to an immediate renal vasoconstriction without early transient vasodilation.[34] This initial decrease in renal vascular resistance induced by ET-1 suggests that some potent renal vasodilator is released in response to ET-1. After ET-1 infusion, renal output of 6-keto-$PGF_{1\alpha}$, a prostacyclin metabolite, increased by 184%, suggesting that ET-1 stimulated renal prostacyclin production (Fig 2), a finding also noted by Miura et al.[35] Inhibition of prostacyclin synthesis with indomethacin allowed the ET-1–induced vasoconstriction to be fully expressed, resulting in a more pronounced

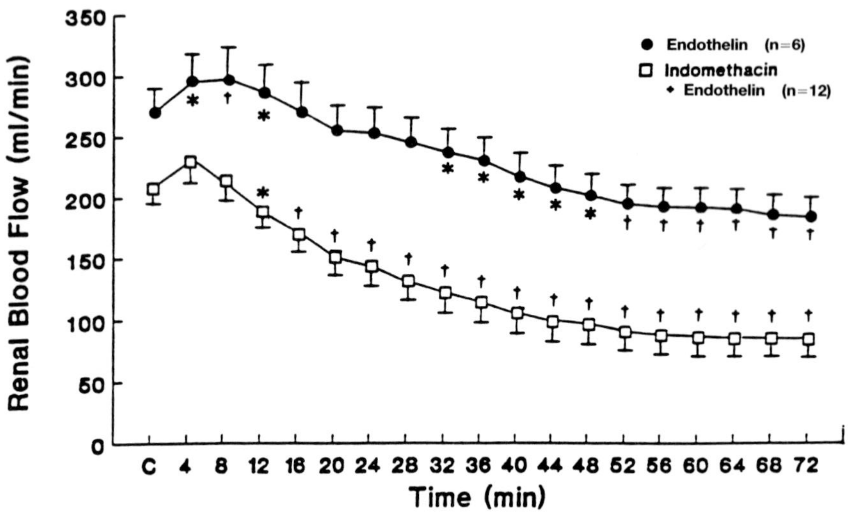

Fig 1. Renal blood flow during the control period (C) and after intrarenal infusion of ET-1. $^*P < 0.05$ and $^+P < 0.01$ compared with the control value. Solid circles, dogs receiving ET-1 alone (n = 6); open squares, dogs pretreated with indomethacin followed by intrarenal ET-1 infusion (n = 12). (Reprinted with permission.[33])

decline in RBF and GFR (by 65% and 54%, respectively) than noted without indomethacin pretreatment, and somewhat attenuated the early vasodilation, but failed to completely abolish it. This observation strongly suggests that a potent vasodilator other than prostacyclin is released in response to ET-1 administration and, in conjunction with prostacyclin, modifies the vascular effects of ET-1.

In addition to the production of ET and prostacyclin, the endothelium also produces EDRF.[36] It has been established that several chemically diverse endogenous substances (such as acetylcholine, bradykinin, and interleukin-1) interact with specific receptors on endothelial cells to induce the formation and release of EDRF.[37,38] The principal EDRF is identified as NO, which causes smooth muscle relaxation that is closely associated with activation of soluble guanylate cyclase and intracellular cyclic guanosine monophosphate accumulation.[39,40]

Recent evidence indicates that NO is produced enzymatically from the guanidino nitrogen of L-arginine.[41,42] The production of NO in endothelial cells as well as the endothelium-dependent vasodilatation is inhibited by L-NMMA, an L-arginine analogue with a methylated guanidino nitrogen.[43] Inhibition effect is achieved by L-NMMA com-

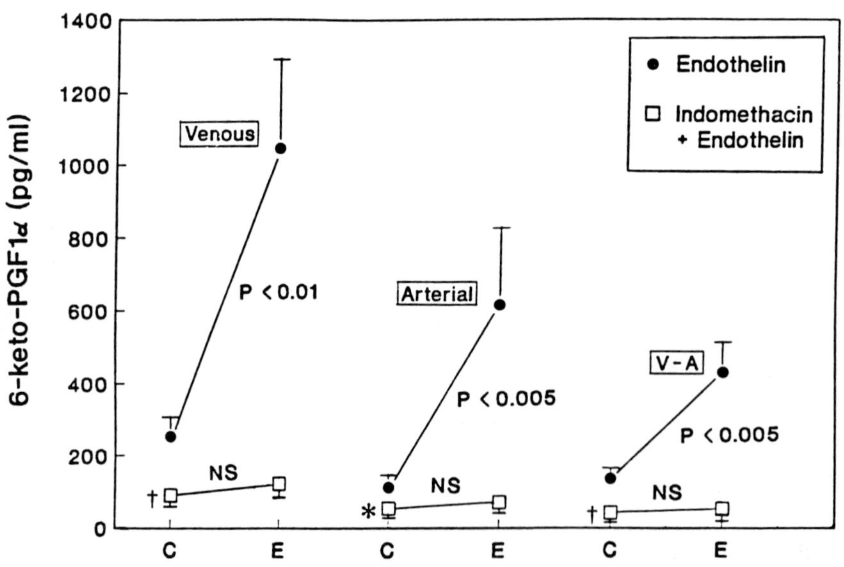

Fig 2. Effects of indomethacin on the levels of 6-keto-$PGF_{1\alpha}$ in renal venous and arterial plasma during the control period (C) and after intrarenal ET-1 infusion. V-A indicates the difference between the renal venous and arterial plasma levels. Solid circles, dogs receiving ET-1 alone; squares, dogs pretreated with indomethacin followed by intrarenal ET-1 infusion (E). $^*P < 0.05$ and $^+P < 0.01$ compared between the two groups. NS, statistically not significant between C and E. (Reprinted with permission.[33])

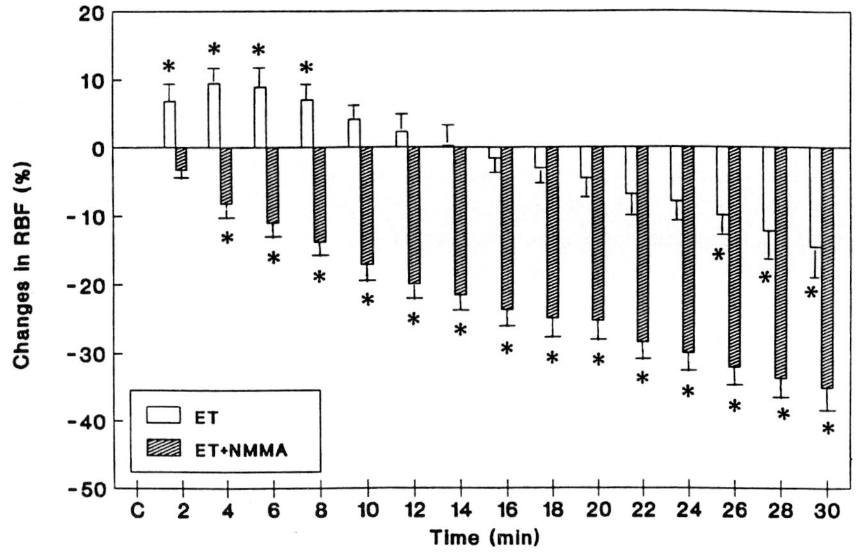

Fig 3. Percent change in RBF in dogs after intrarenal infusion of ET-1 (open bars) and after receiving an intrarenal infusion of N^G-monomethyl-L-arginine (NMMA) and ET-1 (shaded bars). $^*P < 0.05$ **compared with the control value (C).**

peting with L-arginine for binding to NO synthase. The effect of L-NMMA is specific in that it is reversed by an excess of L-arginine but not by D-arginine.[44,45]

We have examined the possibility that EDRF/NO participated in the early vasodilatory event elicited by ET-1 and attenuated the ET-1 vasoconstriction.[46] To be certain about avoiding alterations in systemic hemodynamics, ET-1 was infused into the renal artery of dogs at 2 ng/kg/min. Intrarenal infusion of ET-1 at this dose again elicited a transient renal vasodilation, followed by a progressive decrease in RBF. In a separate group of dogs, the specific inhibitor of EDRF/NO formation, L-NMMA (50 μg/kg/min), was infused intrarenally prior to intrarenal infusion of ET-1. In each dog the initial renal dilatory response induced by ET-1 was completely abolished (Fig 3). In addition, a greater decrease in RBF and GFR was observed when compared with that obtained with ET-1 infusion alone (Fig 4). These findings demonstrate that ET-1 stimulates the production of both prostacyclin and NO, which are responsible for the transient vasodilation and attenuate the renal vasoconstriction induced by ET-1.

Despite the modulating effects of prostacyclin and NO in the kidney, renal vessels are more sensitive to the vasoconstrictive action of ET-1 than other vascular beds. For instance, in a study using anesthetized dogs, coronary blood flow did not decrease after injection of ET-1 at doses between 0.1 and 0.3 μg directly into the coronary artery, and declined only at doses greater than 1 μg.[47] In another study, intravenous infusion of ET-1 (50 ng/kg/min) did not significantly alter coronary blood flow in anesthetized dogs, but produced reductions in RBF by 49% to 76%.[32] In addition, coronary vasoconstriction elicited by intracoronary injection of ET-1 was immediate and was neither augmented by prostaglandin synthesis inhibition nor preceded by a vasodilatory response.[47] These findings are distinct from the renal vascular responses, suggesting variable counterregulatory mechanisms for ET-1 in different regions of the circulation.

Intrarenal infusion of ET-1 without affecting

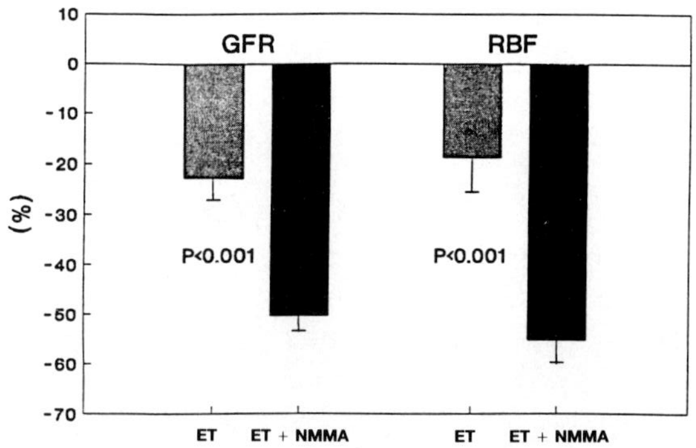

Fig 4. Percent change in GFR and RBF in ET-1 alone (shaded bars) and in dogs receiving an intrarenal infusion of N^G-monomethyl-l-arginine (NMMA) and ET-1 (solid bars).

systemic hemodynamics did not change urinary water and sodium excretion. In contrast, intravenous infusion of ET-1 in the rat at doses not severely compromising renal hemodynamics led to significant diuresis and natriuresis.[48,49] This has been attributed to pressure natriuresis, since intravenous ET-1 infusion increases arterial pressure.[50] The natriuresis after intravenous ET-1 administration also has been attributed to the renal effects of atrial natriuretic peptide, which is released into the systemic circulation following ET-1 administration.[51] In healthy humans, intravenous infusion of ET-1 sufficient to increase the diastolic blood pressure by 7.8% leads to a marked decrease in urine volume and sodium excretion.[52] The dose used in this study did not alter plasma concentrations of angiotensin II, aldosterone, vasopressin, and atrial natriuretic peptide. Thus, whether ET-1 participates in the water and sodium homeostasis remains unknown.

RENAL ACTION OF ENDOTHELIN-3

Being an isopeptide of ET-1, ET-3 is thought to have a pharmacologic profile qualitatively similar to ET-1 but differing in vasoactive potency. In vitro studies in the rat suggest that ET-3 possesses a greater vasodilatory property and a weaker vasoconstrictor effect than ET-1.[53] Recently, Yamashita et al[54] showed that a brief intrarenal injection of ET-3 led to renal vasodilation with no vasoconstriction noted. This latter observation may have resulted from the rapid degradation and renal excretion of the infused ET-3, since ETs have a short plasma half-life of 1 to 2 minutes in vivo.[52] Since the renal effects of ET-3 in vivo have not been well studied, we examined the renal effects of ET-3 by continuous intrarenal infusion of the peptide for 70 minutes in anesthetized dogs with a dose (0.8 pmol/kg/min) that does not affect systemic hemodynamics, as described with ET-1.[55] As observed with ET-1, ET-3 caused an early transient but significant increase in RBF, lasting approximately 10 minutes, followed by a significant decrease in 60 minutes by 24%, associated with a decrease in GRF by 35%. Urinary thromboxane B_2 excretion increased significantly (42%) following ET-3 infusion. In addition, a significant correlation was observed between increments in urinary thromboxane B_2 excretion and decrements in RBF.

In another group of dogs, prostaglandin synthesis was inhibited with meclofenamate (5 mg/kg intravenously). After intrarenal infusion of ET-3, a similar transient but significant increase in RBF occurred; however, the renal vasoconstriction seen with ET-3 infusion alone was completely abolished as RBF and GFR were unchanged.

Renal hemodynamic responses to ET-1 and ET-3 are similar in that early transient renal vasodilatation is followed by profound vasoconstriction. Furthermore, the magnitude of the vasodilation and vasoconstriction also is similar for these two isopeptides. However, the use of prostaglandin synthesis inhibitors underscores the distinct roles of prostaglandins in influencing renal hemodynamic responses to ET-1 and ET-3. While ET-1 stimulated renal prostacyclin formation, ET-3 activated thromboxane production. As a result, cyclooxygenase inhibition augmented ET-1–induced renal vasoconstriction by suppressing prostacyclin synthesis. In contrast, suppression of thromboxane formation by inhibiting cyclooxygenase activity abolished the renal vasoconstriction caused by ET-3.

Since intrarenal ET-3 infusion led to an initial transient renal vasodilatory response similar to ET-1, it is likely that ET-3 stimulates the EDRF/NO system, thereby mediating this vasodilatory response. In another group of dogs, NO formation was inhibited by intrarenal infusion of L-NMMA, followed by intrarenal infusion of ET-3 at 0.8 pmol/kg/min. In each dog the early renal vasodilatory response was completely abolished. In addition, the pretreatment with L-NMMA caused a more profound decrease in RBF and GFR than when ET-3 was infused alone. Thus, the stimulation of NO by ET-3 is responsible for the transient vasodilatory phase as well as attenuating the renal vasoconstriction caused by ET-3. In this regard, the interactions between ET-3 and the EDRF/NO system are similar to those noted for ET-1.

In a previous study in the dog, Yamashita et al[56] infused ET-3 at 5 ng/kg/min into the renal artery for 25 minutes and observed that RBF increased in the first 10 minutes and returned to baseline within 20 minutes. Pretreatment with a NO synthase inhibitor abolished the renal vasodilatory response and unmasked the renal vasoconstrictor action of ET-3 within 20 minutes. Inhibition of prostaglandin synthesis with ibuprofen did not eliminate the initial vasodilatory effect of ET-3, but did lead to vasoconstriction within 20 minutes. In this study, NO mediates the vasodilating action of ET-3, similar to our findings; however, the vasoconstricting effect of ET-3 is independent of prostanoids. The reason for this discrepancy is not clear, but may be related to the differences in the doses of ET-3 used as well as the relatively short duration of infusion.

In a final group of dogs, simultaneous intrarenal infusion of L-arginine (a NO synthase substrate; 2 mg/kg/min) along with ET-3 did not potentiate or prolong the early renal vasodilation, nor did it attenuate the ET-3-induced decrease in RBF or GFR. Thus, the addition of the substrate for NO fails to alter the vasodilatory response of ET-3, although an intact EDRF/NO system is required for ET-3 to express its vasodilatory action. These findings suggest that ET-3 enhances NO synthase activity but to a limited extent.

In contrast to ET-1, ET-3 infusion caused a marked diuresis and natriuresis that was not affected by cyclooxygenase inhibition or the addition of L-arginine to ET-3 infusion. On the other hand, when the EDRF/NO system was inhibited by L-NMMA, the diuresis and natriuresis induced by ET-3 was completely abolished. Although it is not clear whether ET-3 is produced in the dog kidney, significant ET-3 production has been found in the rabbit inner medullary collecting duct cells.[57] In addition, high levels of ET-3 mRNA has been identified in the rat kidney, including glomeruli, proximal tubules, the cortical collecting tubule, and the medullary collecting duct; ET-3 protein also has been detected in tubule suspensions from the outer and inner medulla.[58,59] Binding to ET-B receptors has been associated with activation of NO formation.[28,60,61] Thus, it is conceivable that ET-3 stimulates NO production and increases cytosolic cyclic guanosine monophosphate, which serves as a second messenger and ultimately blocks the sodium channel on the luminal side of the inner medullary collecting duct, a sequence of events analogous to those for atrial natriuretic peptide.[62] Since inhibition of NO synthase in our study led to a profound decrease in GFR, which in itself may have reduced natriuresis, the proposed mechanism of cyclic guanosine monophosphate as a second messenger for natriuresis induced by ET-3 remains speculative.

In summary, the two isopeptides, ET-1 and ET-3, share certain vascular properties; both elicit early renal vasodilatation, followed by prolonged vasoconstriction. The vasodilatation induced by both peptides is abolished by inhibition of NO synthase. It is likely that both ET-1 and ET-3 bind to the ET-B receptors on the endothelial cell and stimulate EDRF/NO release, which in turn mediates vasodilatation. In contrast, the interactions between the two ET isopeptides with the prostaglandin system differ strikingly. While inhibition of cyclooxygenase intensifies renal vasoconstriction caused by ET-1, it abolishes vasoconstriction induced by ET-3. Endothelin-1 stimulates renal prostacyclin production, whereas ET-3 increases thromboxane release. With respect to the effects of ETs on tubular function, the two isopeptides also differ markedly. Endothelin-1 shows little effects on urinary water and sodium excretion; however, ET-3 possesses significant diuretic and natriuretic properties, possibly by binding to ET-B receptors in the inner medullary collecting duct. It is important to emphasize that our findings pertain to the dog kidney and may not be entirely applicable to other species. The differences in the renal actions of ETs may be related to the distribution of and affinity to ET-A and ET-B receptors in the kidney in a given species as well as among different species. Antagonists to ET-A and ET-B receptors are being rapidly developed and are very promising in delineating the physiologic and pathophysiologic roles of each ET isopeptide.

REFERENCES

1. Hickey KA, Rubanyi G, Paul RJ, Highsmith RF: Characterization of a coronary vasoconstrictor produced by cultured endothelial cells. Am J Physiol 248:C550-C556, 1985

2. Yanagisawa M, Kunhara H, Kimura S, Tomobe Y, Kobayashi M, Mitsui Y, Yazaki Y, Goto K, Masaki T: A novel potent vasoconstrictor peptide produced by vascular endothelial cells. Nature 332:411-415, 1988

3. Inoue A, Yanagisawa M, Kimura S, Kasuya Y, Miyauchi T, Goto K, Masaki T: The human endothelin family: Three structurally and pharmacologically distinct isopeptides predicted by three separate genes. Proc Natl Acad Sci U S A 86:2863-2867, 1989

4. Arinami T, Ishikawa M, Inoue A, Yanagisawa M, Masaki T, Yoshida MC, Hamaguchi H: Chromosomal assignments of the human endothelin family genes: The endothelin-1 gene (EDN1) to 6p23-p24, the endothelin-2 gene (EDN2) to 1p34, and the endothelin-3 gene (EDN3) to 20q13.2-q13.3. Am J Hum Genet 48:990-996, 1991

5. Masaki T, Kimura S, Yanagisawa M, Goto K: Molecu-

lar and cellular mechanism of endothelin regulation: Implications for vascular function. Circulation 84:1457-1468, 1991

6. McMahon EG, Palomo MA, Moore WM, McDonald JF, Stern MK: Phosphoramidon blocks the pressor activity of porcine big endothelin-1 (1-39) in vivo and conversion of big endothelin-1-(1-39) to endothelin 1-(1-21) in vitro. Proc Natl Acad Sci U S A 88:703-707, 1991

7. Arai H, Hon S, Aramori I, Ohkubo H, Nakanishi S: Cloning and expression of a cDNA encoding an endothelin receptor. Nature 348:730-732, 1990

8. Hosoda K, Nakao K, Tamura N, Arai H, Ogawa Y, Suga S, Nakanishi S, Imura H: Organization, structure, chromosomal assignment and expression of the gene encoding the human endothelin-A receptor. J Biol Chem 267:18797-18804, 1992

9. Sakamoto A, Yanagisawa M, Sakurai T, Takuwa Y, Yanagisawa H, Masaki T: Cloning and functional expression of human cDNA for the ET_B endothelin receptor. Biochem Biophys Res Commun 178:656-663, 1991

10. Wilkes BM, Ruston AS, Mento P, Girardi E, Hart D, Vander M, Barnett R, Nord EP: Characterization of the endothelin-1 receptor and signal transduction mechanisms in rat renal medullary interstitial cells. Am J Physiol 260:F579-F589, 1991

11. Terada Y, Tomita K, Nonoguchi H, Marumo F: Different localization of two types of endothelin receptor mRNA in microdissected rat nephron segments using reverse transcription and polymerase chain reaction assay. J Clin Invest 90:107-112, 1992

12. Ihara M, Nonoguchi K, Sacki T, Fukuroda T, Tsuchida S, Kimura S, Fukami T, Ishikawa K, Nishikibe M, Yano M: Biological profiles of highly potent novel endothelin antagonists selective for the ET_A receptor. Life Sci 50:247-255, 1992

13. Sogabe K, Nirei H, Shoubo M, Nomoto A, Ao S, Notsu Y, Ono T: Pharmacological profile of ER139317, a novel, potent endothelin ET_A receptor antagonist. J Pharmacol Exp Ther 264:1040-1046, 1993

14. Urade Y, Fujitani Y, Oda K, Watakabe T, Umemura I, Takai M, Okada T, Sakata K, Karaki H: An endothelin B receptor-selective antagonist: IRL 1038, [Cys^{11}-Cys^{15}]-endothelin-1(11-21). FEBS Lett 311:12-16, 1992

15. Ikeda S, Awane Y, Kusumoto K, Wakimasu M, Watanabe T, Fujino M: A new endothelin receptor antagonist, TAK-044, shows long-lasting inhibition of both ET_A- and ET_B-mediated blood pressure responses in rats. J Pharmacol Exp Ther 270:728-733, 1994

16. Brook DP, DePalma PD, Pullen M, Nambi P: Characterization of canine renal endothelin receptor subtypes and their function. J Pharmacol Exp Ther 268:1091-1097, 1994

17. Gellai M, Jugus M, Fletcher T, DeWolf R, Nambi P: Reversal of postischemic acute renal failure with a selective $endothelin_A$ receptor antagonist in the rat. J Clin Invest 93:900-906, 1994

18. Simonson MS, Wann S, Mene P, Dubyak GR, Kester M, Nakazato Y, Sedor JR, Dunn MJ: Endothelin stimulates phospholipase C, Na/H exchange, c-*fos* expression, and mitogenesis in rat mesangial cells. J Clin Invest 83:708-712, 1989

19. Baldi E, Musial A, Kester M: endothelin stimulates phosphatidylcholine hydrolysis through both PLC and PLD pathways in mesangial cells. Am J Physiol 266:F957-F965, 1994

20. Mitsuhashi T, Morris RC Jr, Ives HE: Endothelin-induced increases in vascular smooth muscle Ca++ do not depend on dihydropyridine-sensitive Ca++ channels. J Clin Invest 84:635-639, 1989

21. Kohan DE: Production of endothelin-1 by rat mesangial cells: Regulation by tumor necrosis factor. J Lab Clin Med 119:477-484, 1992

22. Sakamoto H, Sasaki S, Nakamura Y, Fushimi K, Marumo F: Regulation of endothelin-1 production in cultured rat mesangial cells. Kidney Int 41:350-355, 1992

23. Kasinath BS, Fried TA, Davalath S, Marsden PA: Glomerular epithelial cells synthesize endothelin peptides. Am J Pathol 141:279-283, 1992

24. Kohan DE, Fiedorek FTJ: Endothelin synthesis by rat inner medullary collecting duct cells. J Am Soc Nephrol 2:150-155, 1991

25. Ujiie K, Terada Y, Nonoguchi H, Shinohara M, Tomita K, Marumo F: Messenger RNA expression and synthesis of endothelin-1 along rat nephron segments. J Clin Invest 90:1043-1048, 1992

26. Simonson MS: Endothelins: Multifunctional renal peptides. Physiol Rev 73:375-411, 1993

27. Kohan DE: Endothelins in the kidney: Physiology and pathophysiology. Am J Kidney Dis 22:493-510, 1993

28. Marsen TA, Schramek H, Dunn MJ: Renal actions of endothelin: Linking cellular signaling pathways to kidney disease. Kidney Int 45:336-344, 1994

29. Abassi ZA, Tate JE, Golomb E, Keiser HR: Role of neutral endopeptidase in the metabolism of endothelin. Hypertension 20:89-95, 1992

30. Erdos EG, Skigel RA: Neutral endopeptidase 24.11 (enkephalinase) and related regulators of peptide hormones. FASEB J 3:145-151, 1989

31. Goetz KL, Wang BC, Madwed JB, Zhu JL, Leadley RJ Jr: Cardiovascular, renal and endocrine responses to intravenous endothelin in conscious dogs. Am J Physiol 255:R1064-R1068, 1988

32. Miller WL, Redfield MM, Burnett JC Jr: Integrated cardiac, renal, and endocrine actions of endothelin. J Clin Invest 83:317-320, 1989

33. Chou S-Y, Dahhan A, Porush IG: Renal actions of endothelin: Interaction with prostacyclin. Am J Physiol 259:F645-F652, 1990

34. Banks RO: Vasoconstrictor-induced changes in renal blood flow: Role of prostaglandins and histamine. Am J Physiol 254:F470-F476, 1988

35. Miura K, Yukimura T, Yamashita Y, Shimmen T, Okumura M, Yamanaka S, Imanishi M, Yamamoto K: Renal and femoral vascular responses to endothelin-1 in dogs: Role of prostaglandins. J Pharmacol Exp Ther 256:11-17, 1991

36. Furchgott RF, Zawadzki JV: The obligatory role of endothelial cells in the relaxation of arterial smooth muscle by acetylcholine. Nature 288:373-376, 1980

37. Furchgott RF, Vanhoutte PM: Endothelium-derived relaxing and contracting factors. FASEB J 3:2007-2018, 1989

38. Beasley D, Schwartz JH, Brenner BM: Interleukin 1 induces prolonged L-arginine–dependent cyclic guanosine monophosphate and nitrite production in rat vascular smooth muscle cells. J Clin Invest 87:602-608, 1991

39. Ignarro LJ: Biological actions and properties of endothelium-derived nitric oxide formed and released from artery and vein. Circ Res 65:1-21, 1989

40. Murad F: Cyclic guanosine monophosphate as a mediator of vasodilation. J Clin Invest 78:1-5, 1986

41. Palmer RMJ, Ferrige AG, Moncada S: Nitric oxide release accounts for the biological activity of endothelium-derived relaxing factor. Nature 327:524-526, 1987

42. Palmer RMJ, Ashton DS, Moncada S: Vascular endothelial cells synthesize nitric oxide from L-arginine. Nature 333:644-646, 1988

43. Sukuma I, Stuehr DJ, Gross SS, Nathan C, Levi R: Identification of arginine as a precursor of endothelium-derived relaxing factor. Proc Natl Acad Sci U S A 85:8664-8667, 1988

44. Marletta MA, Yoon PS, Iyengar R, Leaf CD, Wishnok JS: Macrophage oxidation of L-arginine to nitrite and nitrate: Nitric oxide is an intermediate. Biochem 27:8706-8711, 1988

45. Palmer RMJ, Rees DD, Ashton DS, Moncada S: L-Arginine is the physiological precursor for the formation of nitric oxide in endothelium-dependent relaxation. Biochem Biophys Res Commun 153:1251-1256, 1988

46. Chou S-Y, Ramamurthy G, Porush JG: Endothelin stimulates renal production of endothelium-derived relaxing factor. J Am Soc Nephrol 3:397A, 1992 (abstr)

47. Clozel JP, Clozel M: Effects of endothelin on the coronary vascular bed in open-chest dogs. Circ Res 65:1193-1200, 1989

48. Perico N, Cornejo RP, Benigni A, Malanchini B, Ladny JR, Remuzzi G: Endothelin induces diuresis and natriuresis in the rat by acting on proximal tubular cells through a mechanism mediated by lipoxygenase products. J Am Soc Nephrol 2:57-69, 1991

49. Takabatake T, Ise T, Ohta K, Kobayashi K-I: Endothelin effects on renal function and tubulo-glomerular feedback. Kidney Int 39:S122-S124, 1991 (suppl 32)

50. Uzunder K, Banks RO: Endothelin-induced natriuresis and diuresis are pressure-dependent events in the rat. Am J Physiol 265:R90-R96, 1993

51. Munger KA, Sugiura M, Takahashi K, Inagami T, Badr KF: A role for atrial natriuretic peptide in endothelin-induced natriuresis. J Am Soc Nephrol 1:1278-1283, 1991

52. Sorensen SS, Madsen JK, Pedersen EB: Systemic and renal effect of intravenous infusion of endothelin-1 in healthy human volunteers. Am J Physiol 266:F411-F418, 1994

53. Edwards RM, Trizna W, Ohlstein EH: Renal microvascular effects of endothelin. Am J Physiol 259:F217-F221, 1990

54. Yamashita Y, Yukimura T, Miura K, Okumura M, Yamanaka S, Yamamoto K: Effects of NG-nitro-L-arginine on renal hemodynamic responses to endothelin-3 in anesthetized dogs. J Cardiovasc Pharmacol 17:S332-S334, 1991 (suppl 7)

55. Greenberg S, Chou S-Y, Porush JG: Endothelin-3 causes renal vasoconstriction via a cyclooxygenase-dependent prostaglandin. J Am Soc Nephrol 4:551A, 1993 (abstr)

56. Yamashita Y, Yukimura T, Miura K, Okumura M, Yamamoto K: Effects of endothelin-3 on renal functions. J Pharmacol Exp Ther 259:1256-1260, 1991

57. Kohan DE: Endothelin synthesis by rabbit renal tubule cells. Am J Physiol 261:F221-F226, 1991

58. Firth JD, Ratcliffe PJ: Organ distribution of the three rat endothelin messenger RNAs and the effects of ischemia on renal gene expression. J Clin Invest 90:1023-1031, 1992

59. Terada Y, Tomita K, Nonoguchi H, Yang T, Marumo F: Expression of endothelin-3 mRNA along rat nephron segments using polymerase chain reaction. Kidney Int 44:1273-1280, 1993

60. Edwards RM, Pullen M, Nambi P: Activation of endothelin ET_B receptors increases glomerular cGMP via an L-arginine–dependent pathway. Am J Physiol 263:F1020-F1025, 1992

61. Owada A, Tomita K, Terada Y, Sakamoto H, Nonoguchi H, Marumo F: Endothelin (ET)-3 stimulates cyclic guanosine 3′, 5′-monophosphate production via ET_B receptor by producing nitric oxide in isolated rat glomerulus, and in cultured rat mesangial cells. J Clin Invest 93:556-563, 1994

62. Brenner BM, Ballermann BJ, Gunning ME, Zeidel ML: Diverse biological actions of atrial natriuretic peptide. Physiol Rev 70:665-699, 1990

Effects of Sex Hormones on Mesangial Cells

Joel Neugarten, MD, and Sharon R. Silbiger, MD

• Male gender is associated with a more rapid progression of chronic renal disease. In various experimental models of renal injury, manipulation of the hormonal milieu can replicate the effects of gender on the course of renal disease. These observations suggest that sex hormones per se may be important determinants of the greater susceptibility of the male kidney to progressive renal injury. Sex hormones may influence many of the processes implicated in the pathogenesis of renal disease progression, including cell proliferation and the synthesis and degradation of collagen and proteoglycans. In addition, sex hormones may indirectly influence these processes by modulating the synthesis and release of vasoactive agents, cytokines, and other growth factors, which in turn are capable of altering mesangial cell function. Finally, estrogens also exert potent antioxidant effects that may contribute to the protective effect of female gender on the course of renal disease.

INDEX WORDS: Estrogen; testosterone; mesangial cells; lipids.

MALE GENDER is associated with a more rapid progression of chronic renal disease.[1,2] In various experimental models of renal injury, modulation of the hormonal milieu can replicate the effects of gender on the course of renal disease. These observations suggest that sex hormones per se may be important determinants of the greater susceptibility of the male kidney to progressive renal injury. Thus, orchiectomy reverses the adverse effect of male gender on renal disease progression, while testosterone replacement exacerbates disease progression.[3-7] A recent study of glomerulosclerosis in aging rats suggested that it is the presence of androgens rather than the absence of estrogens that promotes glomerular injury.[8] In contrast, other studies of aging male rats have demonstrated that estrogen administration attenuates the progression of glomerular injury, suggesting a protective role for female sex hormones.[9,10]

Sex hormones may influence many of the cellular processes implicated in the pathogenesis of renal disease progression. Studies in a variety of tissues suggest that sex hormones directly influence cell proliferation and the synthesis and degradation of collagen and proteoglycans through receptor-mediated mechanisms.[1] In addition, sex hormones may indirectly influence these processes by modulating the synthesis and release of vasoactive agents, cytokines, and other growth factors, which in turn are capable of altering mesangial cell function.[1] Finally, estrogens also exert potent antioxidant effects that may contribute to the protective effect of female gender on the course of renal disease (Fig 1).[1]

Supported by a grant-in-aid from the American Heart Association NY-NJ Affiliate, New York, NY.

MESANGIAL CELL RECEPTORS FOR SEX HORMONES

If the influence of gender on the course of renal disease is mediated through direct cellular effects of sex hormones, then receptors for these hormones must exist in the kidney. Receptors for estradiol and testosterone have been demonstrated in the nuclear and cytosolic fractions of renal tissue homogenates.[1] In addition, autoradiographic studies have shown binding of estradiol and testosterone to glomeruli, arterioles, and tubular cells.[11] We were able to demonstrate nuclear receptors for estradiol and testosterone in cultured mesangial cells obtained from male rats.[12] Studies were performed in which mesangial cells were incubated with radiolabeled estradiol or testosterone. DNA isolated from these cells demonstrated specific binding of both hormones.[12]

COLLAGEN SYNTHESIS

It has been suggested that the accumulation of glomerular extracellular matrix may be a precursor to the development of glomerular sclerosis.[13] In the renal ablation model of glomerulosclerosis in the rat, mRNA for glomerular $\alpha 1$ (IV) procollagen is higher in males than in females, and this increase is correlated with mesangial expansion and the severity of glomerulosclerosis.[14] Moreover, castration ameliorates and exogenous androgens exacerbate the rate at which glomerular sclerosis develops in this model.[4,5,15] These data are consistent with the hypothesis that direct effects of sex hormones on mesangial cells may influence matrix accumulation and thereby contribute to the adverse effect of male gender on renal disease progression.

Sex hormones have been shown to influence the synthesis and degradation of collagen and

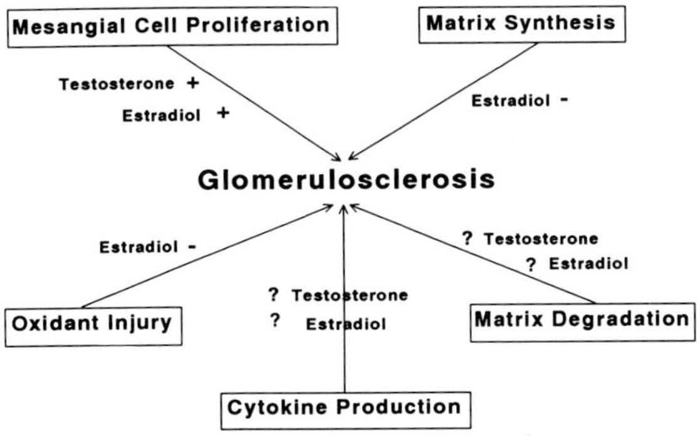

Fig 1. Potential mechanisms whereby sex hormones may influence the development of glomerulosclerosis.

proteoglycans in a variety of tissues.[1,16] Estradiol suppresses collagen synthesis in cultured vascular smooth muscle cells, a cell type similar in phylogeny, structure, and function to the glomerular mesangial cell.[17,18] In bovine aortic smooth muscle, estradiol decreases synthesis of procollagen type III and in high concentrations also decreases synthesis of procollagen type I.[17,18] The direct effects of testosterone on cellular collagen synthesis have not been extensively studied; however, most available data suggest a stimulatory effect.[19-25] For example, testosterone increases collagen synthesis by vascular smooth muscle cells in culture.[24]

We have studied the direct effects of sex hormones on collagen synthesis by cultured rat mesangial cells by measuring ^{3}H proline incorporation into collagenase sensitive protein and by performing immunoprecipitation studies. We found that estradiol in micromolar concentrations suppressed total collagen, type I collagen, and type IV collagen synthesis, and decreased steady state mRNA levels for type I collagen.[26] In contrast, testosterone had no effect on collagen synthesis by mesangial cells.

MATRIX DEGRADATION

Matrix accumulation in vivo depends on the balance between the rates of synthesis and degradation of matrix proteins, both of which are influenced by sex hormones. In a variety of tissues, sex hormones influence the level and activity of collagenase, a key enzyme that digests collagen.[20,27-30] Sex hormones also influence the activity of the enzymes responsible for collagen cross-linking, which enhances the resistance of collagen to degradation.[1,25] Although basic mechanisms have not yet been well defined, it has been observed that estrogen reduces the accumulation of collagen and elastin in the kidney of hypertensive rats, in the vascular wall of normal rats, in the aorta of rabbits fed an atherogenic diet, and in rat connective tissue.[1] In contrast, administration of testosterone increases the accumulation of collagen and elastin in the aorta of normal and cholesterol-fed animals.[1]

Collagen-degrading metalloproteases, synthesized and secreted by resident glomerular epithelial and mesangial cells, play an important role in limiting glomerular matrix accumulation.[31] Although glomerular metalloprotease activity was found to be similar in young male and young female rats, activity increased in aging female rats but not in aging male rats.[31] Glomerular metalloprotease activity was found to correlate inversely with glomerular sclerosis, suggesting that these enzymes may play an important role in protecting aging females from glomerulosclerosis.[31] However, other investigators have concluded the opposite, based on finding that urinary proteinase activity increased with age in male but not female rats.[32] These researchers suggested that glomerular proteinases may damage glomerular basement membrane proteins and contribute to glomerular injury in aging male rats.[32]

CELL PROLIFERATION

Conflicting effects of sex hormones on cell proliferation have been reported in various studies. These variable results may reflect differences in species, cell type, cell density, and the nature of the culture medium used. A mitogenic effect of estrogen has been demonstrated in estrogen-responsive breast cancers, bone, most cell lines derived from female reproductive organs, and in some proximal tubular epithelia.[1] However, estradiol has no effect on cell proliferation in several other non-renal cell types, including vascular smooth muscle cells, which are analogous in structure and function to renal mesangial cells.[1,16,17,33]

The mechanisms whereby estrogen exerts a mitogenic effect in responsive cell types is not well established. At the transcriptional level, estrogens induce the synthesis of proto-oncogenes, proliferation-related proteins, and enzymes involved in nucleic acid synthesis.[34-37] mRNAs for c-*fos* and c-*myc* are induced within 4 hours after exposure to estradiol, and c-*ras* mRNA increases at 12 hours.[35-37] Estradiol also modulates expression of cytokines, which may act in a paracrine or autocrine manner to influence cell proliferation. Sex hormones influence the synthesis of transforming growth factor-β, insulin-like growth factor-I, and epidermal growth factor and its receptor.[1] In this context, a variety of cell types are induced to synthesize growth-promoting factors after exposure to estrogen.[34,38,39] Estradiol exerts a mitogenic effect on rat ovary granulosa cells in association with enhanced synthesis of transforming growth factor-β, on osteoblast cells in association with enhanced synthesis of insulin-like growth factor-I, and on mouse uterine and vaginal cells in association with enhanced synthesis of epidermal growth factor.[1] In each case, neutralizing antibody to the specific cytokine reverses the mitogenic effect of estradiol.[1]

Androgens also have been reported to be either proproliferative or antiproliferative, depending on the cell type studied and the culture conditions.[20,21] Testosterone stimulates proliferation of cultured chondrocytes and normal human bone cells and has been reported both to increase and decrease proliferation in human osteosarcoma cells.[20,21]

It recently has been suggested that mesangial cell proliferation precedes glomerulosclerosis.[13] It is possible that gender differences in progression of renal disease reflect differences in the mitogenic effects of sex hormones on mesangial cells. We have studied the direct effects of estradiol, estriol, estrone, and testosterone on the proliferation of cultured mesangial cells obtained from male rats.[26] Estradiol in micromolar concentrations stimulated ^3H thymidine incorporation into DNA at 24, 48, and 72 hours and at 7 days. The mitogenic effects of estradiol were receptor mediated, as shown by their reversal with tamoxifen, a competitive receptor antagonist. Among the estrogens, estriol showed the greatest mitogenic activity. In contrast, the proliferative activity of estrone was minor and did not achieve statistical significance. Testosterone had a modest mitogenic effect on mesangial cells at 48 hours, which also did not achieve statistical significance. However, when mesangial cell proliferation was assessed after incubation with sex hormones for 7 days, the proliferative effects of estradiol and testosterone were similar. Although cell proliferation may contribute to progressive renal injury, it is unlikely that gender-related differences in renal disease progression can be explained on this basis, given the similar long-term effects of estrogens and testosterone on cell proliferation.

ANTIOXIDANT ACTIVITY OF SEX HORMONES

The development of atherosclerotic lesions has been linked to local accumulation of low-density lipoprotein (LDL) and its oxidation in the microenvironment of the vessel wall.[40] Similarly, oxidized LDL has been postulated to play a role in the evolution of glomerular sclerosis.[40] The influence of estrogens on lipid metabolism, serum lipoprotein levels, and tissue antioxidant activity may protect against the development of glomerulosclerosis analogous to the protective role they play in atherosclerosis. Estradiol contains a phenolic hydroxyl group that is responsible for its potent antioxidant properties.[41] Estradiol can insert into the lipid core of LDL and donate hydrogen atoms from its phenolic hydroxyl group to lipid radicals to inhibit lipid peroxidation.[41-49] In an in-vitro system using reactions with substituted phenoxyl radicals as a model for reactions with lipid peroxyl radicals, the antioxidant activities of various estrogen compounds were assessed.[41] The antioxidant activity of estradiol was found to be more than 1.5 times greater than that of butylated hydroxytoluene, a commonly used antioxidant in tissue culture studies. 2-Hydroxyestrone, a major hepatic metabolite of estradiol, had an antioxidant activity threefold greater than that of α-tocopherol, which is among the most potent of the lipid soluble natural antioxidants.[41] Moreover, estradiol is capable of regenerating α-tocopherol by donating an H^+ atom to the tocopheroxyl radical.[41,49]

The antioxidant properties of estrogens have been demonstrated by their ability to inhibit peroxidation of lipoproteins induced by UV irradiation or exposure to Fe^{3+}-adenosine 5′-diphosphate.[47-49] Estradiol also has been shown to inhibit cell-free, copper-mediated oxidation of LDL in a dose-dependent manner.[42-44,49] As predicted, estradiol is a potent inhibitor of LDL oxidation by cells in culture.[42-45,49] Estradiol inhibits oxidation of LDL by endothelial cells, mononuclear cells, lymphoblastoid cells, and macrophages.[42-44,49] In addition, we have recently shown that estrogen inhibits mesangial cell-mediated oxidation of LDL.[45] Estrogens in physiologic concentrations possess antioxidant activity in vivo.[46] The administration of estrogen replacement therapy to postmenopausal women increases the resistance of their circulating LDL to oxidation.[46] Estrogens also have been shown to modulate the levels of cellular LDL receptors and the activity of intracellular enzymes involved in lipoprotein metabolism.[1] In contrast, testosterone, which lacks a phenolic hydroxyl group, is devoid of antioxidant properties in all systems studied.[42-45]

In addition to inhibiting cell-mediated oxidation of LDL, estradiol protects cultured endothelial cells from cytotoxicity following exposure to preformed oxidized LDL.[49] The mechanism of this cytoprotective effect has not been elucidated. Pretreatment of mononuclear cells with estradiol inhibits subsequent cell-mediated LDL oxidation in estrogen-free media.[44] This observation led to the hypothesis that estrogens may directly inhibit cellular generation of reactive oxygen species.[44] However, the inhibitory effects of estrogen on macrophage-mediated oxidation of LDL were found to be independent of cellular generation of superoxide anion.[42]

CONCLUSION

Sex hormones directly influence many of the processes implicated in the pathogenesis of renal disease progression, including mesangial cell proliferation and matrix accumulation, as well as the synthesis and release of cytokines, vasoactive agents, and growth factors. In addition, estrogens may exert potent antioxidant actions in the mesangial microenvironment, which may contribute to the protective effect of female gender on renal disease progression. The role played by each of these potentially important mechanisms may vary in different types of renal disease and requires further investigation.

REFERENCES

1. Silbiger S, Neugarten J: The impact of gender on progressive renal functional impairment. Am J Kidney Dis 25:515-533, 1995

2. Glassock R, Ferris T, Hull A, Herrera-Acosta J, Grunfeld J, Salant D, Williams D: Modification of diet and renal disease: Progression. External advisory group: Recommendations, in Prevention of Progression in Chronic Renal Disease: Development of Management Recommendations Symposium. Bethesda, MD, National Institutes of Diabetes and Digestive and Kidney Diseases, 1994

3. Sakemi T, Toyoshima H, Morito F: Testosterone eliminates the attenuating effect of castration on the progressive glomerular injury in hypercholesterolemic male Imai rats. Nephron 67:469-476, 1994

4. Zeier M, Schonherr R, Geberth S, Ritz E: Effects of testosterone on glomerular growth, permeability and scarring after uninephrectomy. J Am Soc Nephrol 4:788, 1993 (abstr)

5. Zeier M, Schonherr S, Geberth S, Wagner J, Ritz E: Does testosterone enhance glomerular injury? J Am Soc Nephrol 3:754, 1992 (abstr)

6. Sakemi T, Baba N: Castration attenuates proteinuria and glomerular injury in hyperlipidemic male Imai rats. Nephron 64:429-435, 1993

7. Gilboa N, Magro AM, Han Y, Rudofsky UH: Contrasting effects of early and late orchiectomy on hypertension and renal disease in Fawn-hooded rats. Life Sci 41:1629-1634, 1987

8. Baylis C: Age-dependent glomerular damage in the rat. Dissociation between glomerular injury and both glomerular hypertension and hypertrophy. Male gender as a primary risk factor. J Clin Invest 94:1823-1829, 1994

9. Hajdu A, Rona G: The protective effect of estrogens against spontaneous pancreatic islet and renal changes in aging male rats. Experientia 27:956-957, 1971

10. Sakemi T, Toyoshima H, Shono Y, Ikeda Y: Protective effect of estrogen on the progressive glomerular injury in hypercholesterolemic male Imai rats. J Am Soc Nephrol 4:630, 1993 (abstr)

11. Davidoff M, Caffier H, Schiebler TH: Steroid hormone binding receptors in the rat kidney. Histochemistry 69:39-48, 1980

12. Neugarten J, Silbiger S: Nuclear receptors for estradiol and testosterone in mesangial cells. J Am Soc Nephrol 5:951, 1994 (abstr)

13. Eng E, Floege J, Young BA, Couser WG, Johnson RJ: Does extracellular matrix expansion in glomerular disease require mesangial cell proliferation? Kidney Int 45:S45-S47, 1994

14. Lombet JR, Adler SG, Anderson PS, Nast CC, Olsen DR, Glassock RJ: Sex vulnerability in the subtotal nephrectomy model of glomerulosclerosis in the rat. J Lab Clin Med 114:66-74, 1989

15. Gafter U, Ben-Bassat M, Levi J: Castration inhibits glomerular hypertrophy and proteinuria in uninephrectomized male rats. Eur J Clin Invest 20:360-365, 1990

16. Chander CL, Spector TD: Oestrogens, joint disease, and cartilage. Ann Rheum Dis 50:139-140, 1991

17. Beldekas JC, Smith B, Gerstenfeld LC, Sonenshein GE, Franzblau C: Effects of 17β-estradiol on the biosynthesis of collagen in cultured bovine aortic smooth muscle cells. Biochemistry 20:2162-2167, 1981

18. Beldekas JC, Gerstenfeld L, Sonensheim GE, Franzblau C: Cell density and estradiol modulation of procollagen type III in cultured calf smooth muscle cells. J Biol Chem 257:12252-12256, 1982

19. Fischer GM, Bashey RI, Rosenbaum H, Lyttle CR: A possible mechanism in arterial wall for mediation of sex difference in atherosclerosis. Exp Mol Pathol 43:288-296, 1985

20. Franchimont P, Bassleer C: Effects of hormones and local growth factors on articular chondrocyte metabolism. J Rheumatol 18:68-70, 1991 (suppl 27)

21. Benz DJ, Haussler MR, Thomas MA, Speelman B,

Komm BS: High-affinity androgen binding and androgenic regulation of $\alpha 1$(I)-procollagen and transforming growth factor-β steady state messenger ribonucleic acid levels in human osteoblast-like osteosarcoma cells. Endocrinology 128:2723-2730, 1991

22. Black MM, Shuster S, Bottoms E: Osteoporosis, skin collagen and androgen. BMJ 4:773-774, 1994

23. Mariotti A, Mawhinney M: The hormonal maintenance and restoration of guinea pig seminal vesicle fibromuscular stroma. J Urol 128:852-857, 1982

24. Leitman DC, Benson SC, Johnson LK: Glucocorticoids stimulate collagen and noncollagen protein synthesis in cultured vascular smooth muscle cells. J Cell Biol 98:541-549, 1994

25. Bronson RE, Calaman SD, Traish AM, Kagan HM: Stimulation of lysyl oxidase (EC 1.4.3.13) activity by testosterone and characterization of androgen receptors in cultured calf aorta smooth-muscle cells. Biochem J 244:317-323, 1987

26. Kwan G, Neugarten J, Sherman M, Silbiger S: The effects of sex hormones on mesangial cell proliferation and collagen synthesis. J Am Soc Nephrol 5:947, 1994 (abstr)

27. Sakyo K, Ito A, Mori Y: Dehydroepiandrosterone sulfate stimulates collagenase synthesis without affecting the rates of collagen and noncollagen protein synthesis by rabbit uterine cervical fibroblasts. Biol Reprod 36:277-281, 1987

28. Ryan JN, Woessner JF Jr: Oestradiol inhibition of collagenase: Role in uterine involution. Nature 218:526-528, 1974

29. Oursler MJ, Pederson L, Pyfferoen J, Osdoby P, Fitzpatrick L, Spelsberg TC: Estrogen modulation of avian osteoclast lysosomal gene expression. Endocrinology 132:1373-1380, 1993

30. Rajabi MR, Solomon S, Poole AR: Activation of protein kinase C stimulates collagenase production by cultured cells of the cervix of the pregnant guinea pig. Am J Obstet Gynecol 167:194-200, 1992

31. Reckelhoff JF, Baylis C: Glomerular metalloprotease activity in the aging rat kidney: Inverse correlation with injury. J Am Soc Nephrol 3:1835-1838, 1993

32. Battaglia C, Remuzzi G, Remuzzi A: Urinary proteinases activity (UPA) increases in male MWF/Ztm rats with age. J Am Soc Nephrol 4:764, 1993 (abstr)

33. Hosokawa M, Ishii M, Inoue K, Yao CS, Takeda T: Estrogen induces different responses in dermal and lung fibroblasts: Special reference to collagen. Connective Tissue Res 9:115-120, 1981

34. Dickson RB, Lippman ME: Estrogenic regulation of growth and polypeptide growth factor secretion in human breast carcinoma. Endocr Rev 8:29-43, 1987

35. Pollard JW: Regulation of polypeptide growth factor synthesis and growth factor-related gene expression in the rat and mouse uterus before and after implantation. J Reprod Fertil 88:721-731, 1990

36. Murphy LJ, Murphy LC, Friesen HG: Estrogen induction of N-*myc* and c-*myc* proto-oncogene expression in the rat uterus. Endocrinology 120:1882-1888, 1987

37. Huet-Hudson YM, Andrews GK, Dey SK: Cell-type specific localization of c-*myc* protein in the mouse uterus: Modulation by steroid hormones and analysis of the periimplantation period. Endocrinology 125:1683-1690, 1989

38. Ikeda T, Sirbasku DA: Purification and properties of a mammary-uterine-pituitary tumor cell growth factor from pregnant sheep uterus. J Biol Chem 259:4049-4064, 1984

39. Sirbasku DA: Estrogen induction of growth factors specific for hormone-responsive mammary, pituitary, and kidney tumor cells. Proc Natl Acad Sci U S A 75:3786-3790, 1978

40. Neugarten J, Schlondorff D: Lipoprotein interactions with glomerular cells and matrix, in Keane WE, Stein JH (eds): Lipids and Renal Disease. Contemporary Issues in Nephrology. New York, NY, Churchill Livingstone, 1991, pp 173-205

41. Mukai K, Daifuku K, Yokoyama S, Nakano M: Stopped-flow investigation of antioxidant activity of estrogens in solution. Biochim Biophys Acta 1035:348-355, 1990

42. Rifici VA, Khachadurian AK: The inhibition of low-density lipoprotein oxidation by 17-β estradiol. Metabolism 41:1110-1114, 1992

43. Huber LA, Scheffler E, Poll T, Ziegler R, Dresel HA: 17 beta-estradiol inhibits LDL oxidation and cholesteryl ester formation in cultured macrophages. Free Radic Res Commun 8:167-173, 1990

44. Maziere C, Auclair M, Ronveaux MF, Salmon S, Santus R, Maziere JC: Estrogens inhibit copper and cell-mediated modification of low density lipoprotein. Atherosclerosis 89:175-182, 1991

45. Ghossein C, Silbiger S, Neugarten J: Effect of estradiol on mesangial cell-mediated oxidation of low density lipoprotein. J Am Soc Nephrol 4:769, 1994 (abstr)

46. Sack MN, Rader DJ, Cannon RO III: Oestrogen and inhibition of oxidation of low-density lipoproteins in postmenopausal women. Lancet 343:269-270, 1994

47. Sugioka K, Shimosegawa Y, Nakano M: Estrogens as natural antioxidants of membrane phospholipid peroxidation. FEBS Lett 210:37-39, 1987

48. Yagi K, Komura S: Inhibitory effect of female hormones on lipid peroxidation. Biochem Int 13:1051-1055, 1986

49. Negre-Salvayre A, Pieraggi M-T, Mabile L, Salvayre R: Protective effect of 17β-estradiol against the cytotoxicity of minimally oxidized LDL to cultured bovine aortic endothelial cells. Atherosclerosis 99:207-217, 1993

Tubulointerstitial Damage in Glomerular Diseases: Its Role in the Progression of Renal Damage

Giuseppe D'Amico, MD, Franco Ferrario, MD, and Maria Pia Rastaldi, MD

● The evidence that tubular damage, interstitial infiltration, and interstitial fibrosis occur in all glomerular diseases, either immunologically or non-immunologically mediated, is reviewed on the basis of personal data and data from the literature. The proposed mechanisms linking glomerular and tubular damage to the interstitial recruitment of mononuclear leukocytes and fibroblast proliferation, with abnormal extracellular matrix production leading to interstitial fibrosis, also are analyzed. The role of persistent heavy proteinuria and exposure to proinflammatory cytokines in inducing the damage of the tubular epithelial cells, with consequent acquisition by these cells of the ability to interact as antigen-presenting cells with T lymphocytes, is especially emphasized. Finally, the importance of the tubulointerstitial damage as a marker of unfavorable prognosis in glomerular diseases is documented.

INDEX WORDS: Tubulointerstitial damage; interstitial infiltration; renal disease progression; glomerulonephritis.

UP TO THE END of the 1960s, the tubulointerstitial changes accompanying glomerular diseases were believed to be trivial.[1] Between 1968 and 1979 three groups of investigators in London, UK,[2] Seattle, WA,[3,4] and Tübingen, Germany[5,6] demonstrated for the first time that the impairment of glomerular filtration rate in glomerular diseases correlated better with the extent of tubulointerstitial damage than with the degree of the glomerular damage, and suggested that the major events that determine outcome in these diseases probably occur in the interstitium.

In the last decade, many groups of investigators have renewed interest in the role of the tubulointerstitial changes on the progression of renal damage in glomerular diseases because of two new factors: (1) the availability of monoclonal antibodies that recognize specific surface antigens on extrinsic cells infiltrating the interstitium and on tubular cells, with which investigators can characterize and quantitate these cells and their activity better, and (2) the data emerging from the study of the natural history of large populations of patients with various immunologically and non-immunologically mediated glomerular diseases.

IMMUNOPHENOTYPING OF INTERSTITIAL MONONUCLEAR LEUKOCYTES AND OF TUBULAR CELLS IN PRIMARY AND SECONDARY GLOMERULAR DISEASE

In 1986 and 1987, three groups of investigators[7-9] first reported data on the interstitial leukocyte subpopulations identified by monoclonal antibodies to cell surface antigens in renal biopsy specimens from small numbers of patients with different types of glomerulonephritis (GN), documenting that there is significant interstitial infiltration, predominantly of T lymphocytes, not only in proliferative immune-mediated glomerular disease (lupus nephritis, acute postinfectious GN, crescentic GN, immunoglobulin A [IgA] nephropathy, membranoproliferative GN) but also in membranous nephropathy, focal segmental glomerulosclerosis, and diabetic nephropathy. The entity of these infiltrates was strongly correlated with impairment of renal function.[9] Subsequent studies[10-20] of larger numbers of patients, the results of which are summarized in Table 1, confirmed these data. Both T lymphocytes and monocytes were increased, T lymphocytes being the prevalent infiltrating cells, with a trend toward an increased CD4+ to CD8+ cell ratio in all diseases, except systemic lupus erythematosus and cryoglobulinemic nephritis, in which CD8+ cells increased more than CD4+ cells. Some of the investigators of these studies[13-18,20] stained the interstitial cells with surface markers of activation to study the expression of HLA class II antigens, intercellular adhesion molecule-1 (ICAM-1), and cytokine receptor interleukin-2R (IL-2R), demonstrating that part of the leukocytes infiltrating the interstitium in many glomerular diseases expressed one or more of these antigens (Table 1). We have enlarged our previous study[12] of IgA nephropathy, looking also to the markers of activation, confirming that infiltrating leukocytes overexpress DR antigens and have an abnormal expression of ICAM-1, vascular cell adhesion molecule-1 (VCAM-1), and IL-2R antigens (Table 2). The correlation of the intensity of the interstitial infiltration with the impairment of renal function and with the subsequent rate of

Table 1. Immunophenotyping of Interstitial Infiltrating Mononuclear Leukocytes in Glomerular Diseases

Source	No. of Patients	All Leukocytes	T Lymphocyte	Monocytes	CD4 to CD8 Ratio	HLA-DR DR + Leukocytes	ICAM-1 + Leukocytes	IL-2R + Leukocytes
IgAN								
Alexopoulos et al[13]	34	↑	↑	↑	↑	↑	ND	ND
Sabadini et al[12]	21	↔	↑	↔	↔	ND	ND	ND
Li et al[16]	23	↑	↑	↑	↑	ND	ND	↑
Bohle et al[20]	10	↑	↑	↑	↑	↑	↑	ND
Personal data*	57	↑	↑	↑	↑	↑	↑	↑
MGN								
Alexopoulos et al[14]	36	↑	↑	↑	↑	↑	ND	ND
FSGS								
Markovic-Lipkovski et al[18]	15	↑	↑	↑	↑	↑	↑	ND
RPGN								
Markovic-Lipkovski et al[17]	9	↑↑	↑↑	↑	↑↑	↑	↑	ND
Sabadini et al[19]	11	↑↑	↑↑	↑	↔	ND	ND	ND
Personal data*	15	↑↑	↑↑	↑↑	↑↑	↑	↑	↑
SLE								
D'Agati et al[10]	26	↑	↑	↔	↓	ND	ND	ND
Castiglione et al[11]	18	↑	↑	↑	↓	ND	ND	ND
Alexopoulos et al[15]	35	↑	↑	↑	↔	↑	↔	↑
Cryo-GN								
Castiglione et al[11]	26	↑	↑	↑	↓	ND	ND	ND

Symbols: ↑, increased; ↔, unchanged; ↓, decreased.

Abbreviations: IgAN, immunoglobulin A nephritis; MGN, membranous glomerulonephitis; FSGS, focal segmental glomerulosclerosis; RPGN, rapidly progressive glomerulonephritis; SLE, systemic lupus erythematosus; Cryo-GN, cryoglobulinemic glomerulonephritis; ND, not done.

* Unpublished.

progression also was studied by our group and by Alexopoulos et al.[13] We found[12] that the mean numbers of infiltrating T lymphocytes and monocytes were greater in a subgroup of our patients with IgA nephropathy who, no matter what their serum creatinine levels were at the time of biopsy, showed deterioration of renal function at the end of a postbiopsy follow-up of more than 3 years (Fig 1). In the larger population of 57 patients with the same glomerular disease, reported in Table 2, we also demonstrated a significant correlation between the number of infil-

Table 2. Personal Data on Interstitial Leukocyte Infiltration for 57 Patients With Immunoglobulin A Nephropathy

Monoclonal Antibody	Specificity	Interstitial Cells (No. of Cells/mm² ± SD): Normals	Interstitial Cells (No. of Cells/mm² ± SD): IgA GN Patients	Probability Value
CD45	All leukocytes	72.1 ± 53.8	243.2 ± 185.9	0.006
CD68	Monocytes/macrophages	44.1 ± 32.8	86.4 ± 66.2	0.05
CD3	T lymphocytes	26.5 ± 23.3	167.7 ± 133.4	0.001
CD4	CD4+ lymphocytes	11.8 ± 11.7	103.8 ± 70.5	0.0001
CD8	CD8+ lymphocytes	10.6 ± 9.1	55.5 ± 45.5	0.003
	CD4+ to CD8+ ratio	1.1	1.8	
HLA-DR	HLA-DR+ leukocytes	4.2 ± 2.1	12.1 ± 5.9	0.005
CD25	Il-2R+ leukocytes	0.2 ± 0.4	5.5 ± 3.1	0.002
CD54	ICAM+ leukocytes	2.2 ± 1.5	6.8 ± 2.9	0.002
VCAM-1	VCAM+ leukocytes	2.8 ± 1.3	8.4 ± 3.1	0.001

trating total leukocytes and T lymphocytes, and the value of serum creatinine (Fig 2). The same significant correlation between number of infiltrated interstitial cells (both T lymphocytes and monocytes) and the glomerular filtration rate at the time of biopsy and at the end of a mean follow-up of 49 months also was found by Alexopoulos et al in their 28 patients with membranous nephropathy.[14]

An abnormal expression of molecules completely absent in the tubular cells of normal kidney, such as HLA-DQ and HLA-DP antigens and ICAM-1, also was found by the Tübingen group[21] in the proximal tubular cells of patients with various glomerular diseases. The two surface antigens were concomitantly detectable in six of 14 patients with IgA nephritis, in seven of 13 patients with membranoproliferative GN, in 13 of 15 patients with focal segmental glomerulosclerosis, and in 11 of 14 patients with rapidly progressive glomerulonephritis (RPGN). In IgA nephropathy, RPGN, lupus nephritis, and diabetic nephropathy, Seron et al[22] documented an increased expression of VCAM-1 on tubular epithelial cells. Several investigators[23,24] also demonstrated a different pattern of expression of these molecules at the tubular level, where ICAM-1 is only present on the luminal side, but VCAM-1 is positive also on the basolateral membrane. These results, which we confirmed in patients with IgA nephropathy and with renal vasculitis (unpublished data), are of particular importance, since they demonstrate that tubular

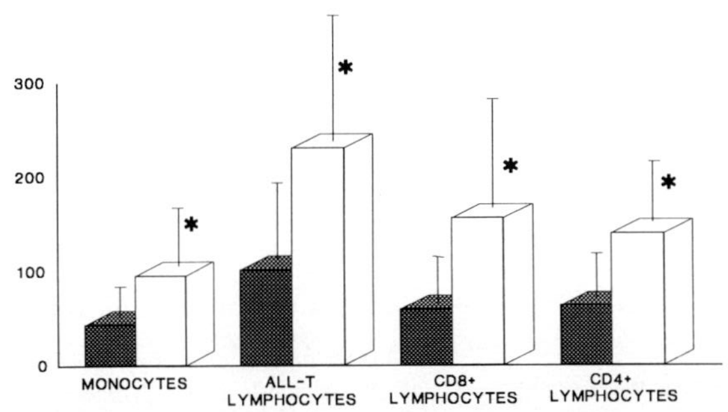

Fig 1. Immunoglobulin A nephropathy. Average numbers of interstitial leucocytes at the time of biopsy for 17 patients with stable renal function and 16 patients with further impairment of the glomerular filtration rate at the end of a mean follow-up period of 5.4 ± 2.3 years. (▩) Stable GRF (no. 17); (□) worsening GFR (no. 16); * $P < 0.001$.

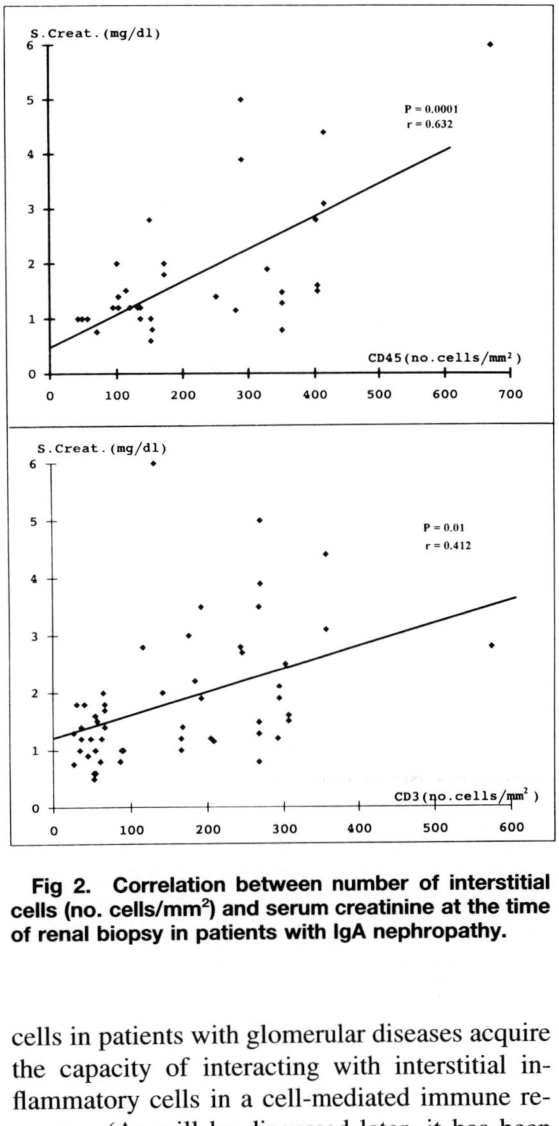

Fig 2. Correlation between number of interstitial cells (no. cells/mm^2) and serum creatinine at the time of renal biopsy in patients with IgA nephropathy.

cells in patients with glomerular diseases acquire the capacity of interacting with interstitial inflammatory cells in a cell-mediated immune response. (As will be discussed later, it has been demonstrated that this interaction requires the inducible surface co-expression of HLA class II molecules and adhesion molecules.)

STUDIES OF THE NATURAL HISTORY OF GLOMERULAR DISEASES: ROLE OF TUBULOINTERSTITIAL DAMAGE AS A PROGNOSTIC INDICATOR

We reviewed[25] the most recent studies, based on actuarial life-table analysis, of long-term renal outcome and factors that influence it in adult patients with one of the three most common types of chronic idiopathic GN: IgA nephropathy, membranous nephropathy, and type I membranoproliferative GN. According to Cox's model, the presenting histologic factor that most strongly predicted subsequent poor outcome in the multivariate analysis in all three types of GN was tubulointerstitial damage, while severe proteinuria, together with the impairment of renal function, was the most powerful clinical predictor of subsequent progression. The same statistical analysis of 250 patients with focal glomerulosclerosis and 488 patients with diabetic nephropathy, performed by the Tübingen investigators,[26,27] gave similar results.

We have just completed a comparative study of the histologic features of 22 patients with IgA nephropathy who we re-biopsied after a long follow-up period (average interval, 10.5 years) because they did not show any sign of progression of functional impairment. Interstitial infiltration and fibrosis were evaluated separately on a semiquantitative basis, grading the lesions from 0 to 2+. As shown in Table 3, both leukocytic infiltration and fibrosis had been absent or moderate in the first biopsy of the great majority of these patients with remarkably favorable courses and remained almost unchanged in the second biopsy. We counted the total number of interstitial leukocytes in the second biopsy of 17 of these 22 patients, and found that their average number was significantly ($P < 0.01$) less than in all the other IgA patients studied by us during the past years.

MECHANISMS OF THE TUBULOINTERSTITIAL DAMAGE IN GLOMERULAR DISEASES

A lot of effort is now being devoted to the study of the mechanisms through which tubulointerstitial lesions are induced and can progressively aggravate the overall renal damage in diseases initially involving the glomerular structures, without concomitant deposition of immunoreactants in the tubules. Many reviews have been published.[19-21,28-35] We will briefly summarize the existing experimental and clinical experience.

Table 3. Semiquantitative Evaluation of Interstitial Infiltrates and Fibrosis for 22 Immunoglobulin A Nephritis Patients Re-biopsied Because of a Nonprogressive Course After an Interval of 10.5 ± 5.0 Years

	0	+	++
Infiltrates			
First biopsy	12 (54.5%)	8 (36.4%)	2 (9.1%)
Second biopsy	9 (40.9%)	12 (54.5%)	1 (4.6%)
Fibrosis			
First biopsy	9 (40.9%)	10 (45.5%)	3 (13.6%)
Second biopsy	5 (22.7%)	15 (68.2%)	2 (9.1%)

NOTE. Mean proteinuria at first renal biopsy = 0.9 ± 0.2 g/d; mean proteinuria at second renal biopsy = 0.7 ± 0.1 g/d.

Mechanisms of Tubular Damage Related to Heavy Proteinuria

Tubular damage (increased mitotic activity of epithelial cells, transient expression of vimentin) has been documented during the acute phase of GN.[36,37] Even in chronic GN, with persistent severe urinary protein loss, the tubular cell damage induced by proteinuria probably is the most important phenomenon linking the glomerular inflammatory processes to the interstitial leukocytic infiltration and fibrosis,[38,39] as has been demonstrated in many experimental models of GN with nephrotic-range proteinuria, such as puromycin aminonucleoside (PAN) nephritis,[40-42] Heymann's nephritis,[43] and overload proteinuria.[44]

At least eight different mechanisms have been proposed to explain how an increased trafficking of proteins across the proximal tubular epithelial cells might induce tubular damage:

1. Increased urinary excretion of many normal proteins overloads the reabsorbing tubular epithelial cells, with consequent release of lysosomal degradative enzymes and complement proteins.[36,43-46]

2. Increased uptake of albumin by tubular cells induces release of an epithelium-derived chemotactic lipid generated in tubular metabolism of albumin-associated fatty acids.[47,48]

3. Increased urinary excretion of complement favors activation of the alternative complement cascade by the brush-border of the proximal tubule.[49]

4. Metabolic degradation of the increased filtered load of proteins by tubules leads to increased production of ammonia and consequent generation of amidated C3.[50]

5. Low molecular weight cytokines entering the urinary space from diseased glomeruli may induce widespread inflammatory damage and generation of nitric oxide by the tubular cells.[51]

6. Increased urinary excretion of transferrin

induces the release of iron, which damages tubular cells through the generation of hydroxyl ion.[52]

7. Heavy proteinuria obstructs single nephrons through interaction with Tamm-Horsfall glycoprotein elaborated by the distal tubular cells, with consequent tubular damage.[53]

8. Detachment of podocytes from the glomerular basement membrane favors direct passage of basement membrane components produced by these cells into the urinary space, with absorption in the proximal tubule.[20]

Several of the above-listed mechanisms may operate concomitantly to induce the tubular damage.

Mechanisms of Tubular Damage Independent of the Proteinuria

1. The results of in vitro studies[54] suggest that the direct activation of tubular cells by cytokines produced in the glomerulus by invading or resident cells may lead to the expression of HLA class II antigens and adhesion molecules. This mechanism also might trigger the tubulointerstitial damage through a direct action on the recruitment of leukocytes in the interstitium.

2. Antigenic molecules unmasked as a consequence of tubular damage or neoantigens, such as heat shock proteins,[55,56] can be expressed by tubules themselves in response to injury and contribute to interstitial monocyte recruitment via a T cell-dependent pathway.

3. Another mechanism is the tubular ischemia due to the reduced blood flow in the postglomerular capillary network, which can be a consequence of the same hemodynamic factors that cause microvascular injury in the diseased glomerulus,[33] but is probably accentuated when there is interstitial damage, with the consequent increase of the cortical interstitial volume and separation of the tubular epithelium from its feeding capillaries.[57]

4. There is progressively increasing tubular cell injury when the glomerular damage, reducing the surviving nephrons, increases the rates of oxygen consumption in each of them, with a consequent increase of ammonia production and generation of reactive oxygen species by the tubular cells (reviewed in ref 32).

Mechanisms Linking Tubular Cell Damage to Interstitial Infiltration

There is continuously increasing evidence in support of the assumption that "far from being an innocent bystander during immune injury, the cells of tubules (and of glomerulus) participate actively in inflammatory events."[31]

First, it is well known that co-expression of HLA class II antigens and adhesion molecules on renal tubular epithelial cells enables them to act as antigen-presenting cell with T lymphocytes (reviewed in ref 54). Since, as we reported above, there is increased expression of HLA-DR antigens and abnormal expression of HLA-DQ/DP molecules, frequently associated with an aberrant expression of ICAM-1, in proximal tubular epithelial cells after exposure to the proinflammatory cytokines that diffuse down from the glomerulus and the non-immune processes (such as chemical injury and renal ischemia) that accompany the glomerular diseases, it is highly probable that these cells acquire the ability to interact as antigen-presenting cells with T lymphocytes, which usually are sparsely distributed between tubular epithelial cells even in normal renal tissue. Recruitment and infiltration of mononuclear leukocytes in the interstitium may be a consequence of this T-lymphocyte activation and cell–cell interaction.[21,31,33,35,54]

Second, however, it is becoming clear that the stimulated or damaged tubular cells of patients with glomerular diseases can trigger recruitment and proliferation of interstitial leukocytes directly through the production of various growth factors and cytokines. Their increased expression may cause chemoattraction (granulocyte-macrophage colony-stimulating factor, monocyte chemoattractant protein-1, platelet-derived growth factor, transforming growth factor-β, IL-6, IL-8, osteopontin) and activation (tumor necrosis factor-α, IL-1, IL-6) of mononuclear inflammatory cells. For example, a correlation between IL-6 expression and extent of interstitial infiltrate has been documented.[35,58-61]

Finally, it has been suggested that tubular rupture associated with increased intratubular pressure or nonspecific tubular damage might permit access to the interstitium of Tamm-Horsfall protein, which activates and recruits inflammatory cells.[62]

Mechanisms Linking Tubular Damage and Interstitial Infiltration to Interstitial Fibrosis and Tubular Atrophy

The final step in the process of tubulointerstitial damage is the interstitial fibrosis induced by the growth, proliferation, increased motility, and secretion of various extracellular matrix components by interstitial fibroblasts. As Müller and Rodemann have recently shown,[63,64] fibroblasts in biopsy specimens taken from patients with interstitial fibrosis are more numerous than in biopsy specimens of healthy transplant donors. They are prevalently in the mitotic stage and produce more type III than type I collagen and a novel protein, yet to be fully characterized, which has been named "fibrosin."

Both activated tubular cells and recruited interstitial leukocytes might stimulate fibroblast proliferation through the secretion of cytokines and growth factors. There is some evidence, although not yet conclusive, that tubular epithelial cells might act mainly through the secretion of transforming growth factor-β and granulocyte-macrophage colony-stimulating factor,[21,35,61,65] and that interstitial inflammatory cells act mainly through the secretion of transforming growth factor-β and IL-4,[21,35,65-69] although other mediators, not yet studied, also could be involved.

Moreover, it has been suggested recently that damage or stimulation of the tubular epithelial cells might also modify the rate of secretion of the various type of collagen by those cells, resulting in an upregulation of the production of interstitial collagens favoring fibrosis and in a downregulation of type IV collagen, which is a normal constituent of tubular basement membrane, with consequent deformative remodeling of this basement membrane and consequent tubular atrophy (reviewed in ref 69).

There have been recent reports[70-72] that in normal kidney a population of interstitial cells with some muscle-like features (expression of α-smooth muscle actin) can be identified in the cortex. Immunoelectron microscopy has shown that these cells are fibroblasts and not endothelial cells or leukocytes. Their accumulation has been identified in human and experimental GN at sites of interstitial damage and may be induced by the nerve growth factor and platelet-derived growth factor, because these cells constitutively express their receptors at the surface.

It is important to realize that once all the mechanisms discussed above have led to the installation of an interstitial fibrosis, a vicious circle that progressively aggravates the overall renal damage is automatically triggered. Activated or damaged tubular cells, infiltrating interstitial leukocytes, and fibroblasts interact continuously between themselves and the resident glomerular cells through the action of cytokines, with consequent amplification of the immune injury, which obviously also is the primary triggering mechanism. It also has been postulated that activated fibroblasts may be involved in an autocrine production of a growth factor that then continues to modulate its own production by positive feedback.[73]

Two additional nonimmunologic mechanisms contribute to this progressive aggravation of the renal damage: first, interstitial fibrosis obliterates postglomerular capillaries, with consequent anoxia,[20] additional tubular damage, and tubular atrophy,[20,33,74] and second, tubular atrophy can produce atubular glomeruli, with a consequent decrease of functioning nephrons.[20,75]

It is worth stressing that the extent of the chronic fibrotic damage, more than the acute inflammatory response, is the predictor of the decline in renal function and of a worse long-term prognosis.

THERAPEUTIC IMPLICATIONS

The extent of interstitial leukocytic infiltration should, in our opinion, be one of the determinant morphologic parameters for the decision to administer steroids and/or cytotoxic drugs to patients with glomerular diseases.

A beneficial effect on the progression of the interstitial damage is suggested by the results of the study of Saito and Atkins.[76] In a rat model of progressive focal glomerular sclerosis, treatment with oral steroids reduced interstitial infiltration and improved renal function in spite of the lack of any beneficial effect on glomerular leukocyte accumulation and sclerosis. Alexopoulos et al[77] very recently demonstrated that responsiveness of proteinuria to steroids in human idiopathic membranous nephropathy was significantly correlated with the extent of interstitial infiltration at the start of treatment: the patients who had complete remission of proteinuria were those who before treatment had larger numbers of interstitial cells.

The mechanisms of the tubulointerstitial damage that we have illustrated strengthen the rationale for the use of such therapeutic tools as dietary manipulation and angiotensin-converting enzyme inhibitor administration. Dietary manipulation, especially reduced protein, phosphorus, and lipid intake, can reduce urinary protein loss as well as decrease metabolic work and oxygen consumption by the tubular cells. Angiotensin-converting enzyme inhibitors might be useful, since they reduce urinary protein loss and, probably, renal ammonia production (angiotensin II is a potent stimulus for its production); moreover, as suggested by Klahr et al in this symposium, they can reduce interstitial leukocyte infiltration.

ACKNOWLEDGMENT

The authors wish thank to Drs Stefania Tunesi and Lin Yang for their technical assistance and Carmen Racco for typing the manuscript.

REFERENCES

1. Allen AC: The Kidney. Grune and Stratton, New York, NY, 1951

2. Risdon RA, Sloper JAC, de Wardener HE: Relationship between renal function and histological changes found in renal biopsy specimens from patients with persistent glomerular nephritis. Lancet 2:363-366, 1968

3. Striker GE, Schainuck LI, Cutler RE, Benditt EP: Structural-functional correlations in renal disease. Part I: A method for assaying and classifying histopathologic changes in renal disease. Hum Pathol 1:615-630, 1970

4. Schainuck LI, Striker GE, Cutler RE, Benditt EP: Structural-functional correlations in renal disease. Part II: The correlations. Hum Pathol 1:631-641, 1970

5. Bohle A, Grund KE, Mackensen S, Tolon M: Correlations between renal interstitium and level of serum creatinine. Virchows Arch A Pathol Anat Histol 373:15-23, 1977

6. Mackensen S, Grund KE, Sindjie M, Bohle A: Influence of the renal cortical interstitium on the serum creatinine clearance in different chronic sclerosing interstitial nephritides. Nephron 24:30-34, 1979

7. Boucher A, Droz D, Adafer E, Nöel LH: Characterization of mononuclear cell subsets in renal cellular interstitial infiltrates. Kidney Int 29:1043-1049, 1986

8. Brunati C, Brando B, Confalonieri R, Belli SL, Lavagni MG, Minetti L: Immunophenotyping of mononuclear cell infiltrates associated with renal disease. Clin Nephrol 26:15-20, 1986

9. Hooke DH, Gee DC, Atkins RC: Leukocyte analysis using monoclonal antibodies in human glomerulonephritis. Kidney Int 31:964-972, 1987

10. D'Agati VD, Appel GB, Estes D, Knowles D, Pirani C: Monoclonal antibody (Mab) identification of infiltrating mononuclear leukocytes in lupus nephritis. Kidney Int 30:573-581, 1986

11. Castiglione A, Bucci A, Fellin G, D'Amico G, Atkins RC: The relationship of infiltrating renal leucocytes to disease activity in lupus and cryoglobulinemic glomerulonephritis. Nephron 50:14-23, 1988

12. Sabadini E, Castiglione A, Colasanti G, Ferrario F, Civardi R, Fellin G, D'Amico G: Characterization of interstitial infiltrating cells in Berger's disease. Am J Kidney Dis 12:307-315, 1988

13. Alexopoulos E, Seron D, Hartley RB, Nolasco F, Cameron JS: The role of interstitial infiltrates In IgA nephropathy: A study with monoclonal antibodies. Nephrol Dial Transplant 4:187-195, 1989

14. Alexopoulos E, Seron D, Hartley RB, Nolasco F, Cameron JS: Immune mechanisms in idiopathic membranous nephropathy. The role of interstitial infiltrates. Am J Kidney Dis 13:404-412, 1989

15. Alexopoulos E, Seron D, Hartley BR, Cameron JS: Lupus nephritis: Correlation of interstitial cells with glomerular function. Kidney Int 37:100-109, 1990

16. Li HL, Hancock WW, Hooke DH, Dowling JP, Atkins RC: Mononuclear cell activation and decreased renal function in IgA nephropathy with crescents. Kidney Int 37:1552-1556, 1990

17. Markovic-Lipkovski J, Müller CA, Risler T, Bohle A, Müller GA: Association of glomerular and interstitial mononuclear leukocytes with different forms of glomerulonephritis. Nephrol Dial Transplant 5:10-17, 1990

18. Markovic-Lipkovski J, Müller CA, Risler T, Bohle A, Müller GA: Mononuclear leukocytes, expression of HLA class II antigens and intercellular adhesion molecule 1 in focal segmental glomerulosclerosis. Nephron 59:286-293, 1991

19. Sabadini E, Gandini E, Castiglione A, Gaimarri M, Ferrario F, D'Amico G: Interstitial infiltrates in secondary glomerulonephritis, in D'Amico G. Colasanti G (eds): Dialysis Strategies—Interstitial Infiltrates in GN—Diabetic Nephropathy. Milano, Italy, Wichtig, 1991, pp 106-112

20. Bohle A, Strutz F, Müller GA: On the pathogenesis of chronic renal failure in primary glomerulopathies: A view from the interstitium. Exp Nephrol 2:205-210, 1994

21. Müller GA, Markovic-Lipkovski J, Rodemann HP: The progression of renal diseases: On the pathogenesis of renal interstitial fibrosis. Klin Wochenschr 69:576-586, 1991

22. Seron D, Cameron JS, Haskard DO: Expression of VCAM-1 in the normal and diseased kidney. Nephrol Dial Transplant 6:917-922, 1991

23. Wuthrich RP: Intercellular adhesion molecules and vascular cell adhesion molecule-1 and the kidney. J Am Soc Nephrol 3:1201-1211, 1992

24. Hill PA, Lan HY, Nikolic-Paterson DJ, Atkins RC: The ICAM-1/LFA-1 interaction in glomerular leukocytic accumulation in anti-GBM glomerulonephritis. Kidney Int 45:700-708, 1994

25. D'Amico G: Influence of clinical and histological features on actuarial renal survival in adult patients with idiopathic IgA nephropathy, membranous nephropathy and membranoproliferative glomerulonephritis: Survey of the recent literature. Am J Kidney Dis 20:315-323, 1992

26. Wehrmann M, Bohle A, Held H, Schumm G, Kendziorra H, Presslar H: Long-term prognosis of focal sclerosis glomerulonephritis. An analysis of 250 cases with particular regard to tubulointerstitial changes. Clin Nephrol 33:115-122, 1990

27. Bohle A, Wehrmann M, Bogenschütz O, Batz C, Müller CA, Müller GA: The pathogenesis of chronic renal failure in diabetic nephropathy: Investigation of 488 cases of diabetic glomerulosclerosis. Pathol Res Pract 187:251-259, 1991

28. Cameron JS: Interstitial changes in glomerulonephritis, in Buccianti G (ed): Prevention in Nephrology. Milan, Italy, Massons, 1987, pp 8-18

29. D'Amico G: Role of interstitial infiltration of leucocytes in glomerular diseases. Nephrol Dial Transplant 3:596-600, 1988

30. Yee J, Kuncio GS, Neilson EG: Tubulointerstitial injury following glomerulonephritis. Semin Nephrol 11:361-366, 1991

31. Cameron JS: Tubular and interstitial factors in the progression of glomerulonephritis. Pediatr Nephrol 6:292-303, 1992

32. Nath KA: Tubulointerstitial changes as a major determinant in the progression of renal damage. Am J Kidney Dis 20:1-17, 1992

33. Fine LG, Ong ACM, Norman JT: Mechanisms of tubulo-interstitial injury in progressive renal diseases. Eur J Clin Invest 23:259-265, 1993

34. Atkins RC, Lan HY, Paterson DJ: Pathogenic mechanisms of interstitial leucocyte infiltration in glomerulonephritis, in D'Amico G, Colasanti G (eds): Dialysis Strategies—Interstitial infiltrates in GN—Diabetic Nephropathy. Milano, Italy, Wichtig, 1991, pp 123-122

35. Strutz F, Müller GA: The role of tubulo-interstitial processes in progression of primary renal diseases. Nephrol Dial Transplant 9:S10-S22, 1994

36. Eddy AA: Interstitial nephritis induced by protein-overload proteinuria. Am J Pathol 135:719-733, 1989

37. Szabolcs MJ, Inghirami G, Liu J, Ward L, D'Agati V: Analysis of cellular proliferation in human glomerulopathies (G) using KI-67 and PCNA. J Am Soc Nephrol 4:690, 1993 (abstr)

38. Cameron JS: Proteinuria and progression in human glomerular diseases. Am J Nephrol 10:81-87, 1990 (suppl 1)

39. D'Amico G: The clinical role of proteinuria. Am J Kidney Dis 17:48-52, 1991

40. Eddy AA, Michael AF: Acute interstitial nephritis associated with aminonucleoside nephrosis. Kidney Int 33:719-733, 1988

41. Mampaso FM, Egido J, Martinez-Montero JC, Bricio T, Gonzales E, Cobo ME, Pirotzky E, Braquet P, Hernando L: Interstitial mononuclear cell infiltrates in experimental nephrosis: Effect of PAF antagonist. Nephrol Dial Transplant 4:1037-1044, 1989

42. Diamond JR, Anderson S: Irreversible tubulointerstitial damage associated with chronic aminonucleoside nephrosis. Am J Pathol 137:1323-1332, 1990

43. Hutchinson FN, Kaysen GA: Albuminuria causes lysozymuria in rats with Heymann nephritis. Kidney Int 33:787-791, 1988

44. Zamlauski-Tucker MJ, Van Liew JB, Goldinger J, Noble B: Persistent proximal tubule disfunction late in Heymann nephritis. Kidney Int 37:1536-1542, 1990

45. Olbricht CJ, Cannon JK, Garg LC, Tisher CC: Activities of cathepsin B and L in isolated nephron segments from proteinuric and non-proteinuric rats. Am J Physiol 250:F1055-F1062, 1986

46. Welch TR, Beischel LS, Witte DP: Differential expression of complement C3 and C4 in the human kidney. J Clin Invest 92:1451-1458, 1993

47. Thomas ME, Schreiner GF: Contribution of proteinuria to progressive renal injury: Consequences of tubular uptake of fatty acid bearing albumin. Am J Nephrol 13:385-398, 1993

48. Kees-Folts D, Lewis Sadow J, Schreiner GF: Tubular catabolism of albumin is associated with the release of an inflammatory lipid. Kidney Int 45:1697-1709, 1994

49. Camussi G, Tetta C, Mazzucco G, Vercellone A: The brush border of proximal tubules of normal human kidney activates the alternative pathway of the complement system in vitro. Ann N Y Acad Sci 420:321-324, 1983

50. Rustom R, Jackson MJ, Critchley M, Bone JM: Tubular metabolism of aprotinin ^{99m}Tc and urinary ammonia: Effects of proteinuria. Miner Electrolyte Metab 18:108-112, 1992

51. Markewitz BA, Michael JR, Kohan DE: Cytokine-induced expression of a nitric oxide synthase in rat renal tubule cells. J Clin Invest 91:2138-2143, 1993

52. Alfrey AC, Foment DH, Hammond WS: Role of iron in tubulo-interstitial injury in nephrotoxic serum nephritis. Kidney Int 36:753-759, 1989

53. Klahr S: Pathophysiology of obstructive nephropathy, in Hatano M (ed): Proceedings of the XIth International Congress of Nephrology, vol 1. New York, NY, Springer-Verlag, 1991, pp 77-93

54. Rubin-Kelley VE, Jevnikar AM: Antigen presentation by renal tubular epithelial cells. J Am Soc Nephrol 2:13-26, 1991

55. Komatsuda A, Wakui H, Imai H, Nakamoto Y, Miura AB, Itoh H, Tashima Y: Renal localization of the constitutive 73-kDa heat-shock protein in normal and PAN rats. Kidney Int 41:1204-1212, 1992

56. Weiss RA, Kelly CJ, Madaio MP: Heat shock protein (HSP)-reactive T-cells eluted from the kidneys of nephritic mice are nephritogenic and cytotoxic to stressed renal tubular cells. J Am Soc Nephrol 4:641, 1993 (abstr)

57. Bohle A, Gise HV, Mackensen-Haen S, Stark-Jakob B: The obliteration of the postglomerular capillaries and its influence upon the function of both glomeruli and tubuli. Klin Wochenschr 59:1043-1051, 1981

58. Eddy AA: Experimental insights into the tubulointerstitial disease accompanying primary glomerular lesions. J Am Soc Nephrol 5:1273-1287, 1994

59. Schmouder RL, Strieter RM, Wiggins RC, Chensue WS, Kunkel SL: In vitro and in vivo interleukin-8 production in human renal cortical epithelia. Kidney Int 41:191-198, 1992

60. Frank J, Engler-Blum G, Rodemann HP, Müller GA: Human renal tubular cells as a cytokine source: PDGF-B, GM-CSF and IL6 mRNA expression in vitro. Exp Nephrol 1:26-35, 1993

61. Jevnikar AM, Wuthrich RP, Brennan DC, Maslinski W, Glimcher LH, Rubin-Kelley VE: TNF-α is expressed on the surface of kidney proximal tubular cells. Transplant Proc 23:231-232, 1991

62. Thomas DBL, Davies M, Williams JD: Tamm-Horsfall protein: An aetiological agent in tubulointerstitial disease? Exp Nephrol 1:281-284, 1993

63. Müller GA, Rodemann HP: Characterization of human renal fibroblasts in health and disease: I. Immunophenotyping of cultured tubular epithelial cells and fibroblasts derived from kidneys with histologically proven interstitial fibrosis. Am J Kidney Dis 17:680-683, 1991

64. Rodemann HP, Müller GA: Characterization of human renal fibroblasts in health and disease: II. In vitro growth, differentiation, and collagen synthesis of fibroblasts from kidneys with interstitial fibrosis. Am J Kidney Dis 17:684-686, 1991

65. Alpers CE, Seifert RA, Hudkins KL, Johnson RJ, Bowen-Pope DF: PDGF-receptor localizes to mesangial, parietal epithelial, and interstitial cells in human and primate kidneys. Kidney Int 43:286-294, 1993

66. Monroe JG, Haldar S, Prystowsky MB, Lammie P: Lymphokine regulation of inflammatory processes: Interleukin-4 stimulates fibroblast proliferation. Clin Immunol Immunopathol 49:292-298, 1988

67. Holter W: Regulation of interleukin 4 production and of interleukin 4-producing cells. Int Arch Allergy Immunol 98:273-278, 1992

68. Kovacs EJ, Brock B, Varesio L, Young HA: IL-2 induction of IL-1 b mRNA expression in monocytes. Regulation by agents that block second messenger pathways. J Immunol 143:3532-3537, 1989

69. Strutz F, Neilson EG: The role of lymphocytes in the progression of interstitial disease. Kidney Int 45:S106-S110, 1994

70. Alpers CE, Hudkins KL, Gown AM, Johnson RJ: Enhanced expression of ''muscle-specific'' actin in glomerulonephritis. Kidney Int 41:1134-1142, 1992

71. MacPherson BR, Leslie KO, Lizaso KV, Schwarz JE: Contractile cells of the kidney in primary glomerular disorders: An immunohistochemical study using an anti–alpha-smooth muscle actin monoclonal antibody. Hum Pathol 24:710-716, 1993

72. Alpers CE, Kelly LH, Floege J, Johnson RJ: Human renal cortical interstitial cells with some features of smooth muscle cells participate in tubulointerstitial and crescentic glomerular injury. J Am Soc Nephrol 5:201-210, 1994

73. Ong ACM, Fine LG: Loss of glomerular function and tubulointerstitial fibrosis: Cause or effect? Kidney Int 45:345-351, 1994

74. Bohle A, Kressel G, Müller CA, Müller GA: The pathogenesis of chronic renal failure. Pathol Res Pract 185:421-440, 1989

75. Marcussen N: Biology of disease: Atubular glomeruli and the structural basis for chronic renal failure. Lab Invest 66:265-284, 1992

76. Saito T, Atkins RC: Contribution of mononuclear leucocytes to the progression of experimental focal glomerular sclerosis. Kidney Int 37:1076-1083, 1990

77. Alexopoulos E, Leontsini M, Papadimitriou M: Relationship between interstitial infiltrates and steroid responsiveness of proteinuria in membranous nephropathy. Nephrol Dial Transplant 9:623-629, 1994

Macrophages and Progressive Renal Disease in Experimental Hydronephrosis

Jonathan R. Diamond, MD

● Many recent clinical and experimental studies have clearly demonstrated that one of the initial events taking place in the process of progressive renal injury is monocytic infiltration of the glomerular and tubulointerstitial compartments. In this report, experimental data supporting the role of the infiltrating renal macrophage (Mø) as a mediator of interstitial fibrosis during the course of obstructive nephropathy will be reviewed as it pertains to the unilateral ureteral obstruction model in the rat. The central pathobiologic theme drawn on data from this model is that fibrogenic cytokines, especially transforming growth factor-β, are, in part, Mø-derived and represent pivotal links between the initial postobstructive renal inflammation and the late development of renal scarring. The tubular epithelium, as a consequence of the mechanical disturbance produced by ureteral obstruction, may elaborate a host of Mø chemoattractant moieties. Many substances can be released by these infiltrating Mø; however, our studies have focused on transforming growth factor-β1. Transforming growth factor-β is an important regulator of extracellular matrix, through its direct effects and modulation of other growth factors to maintain matrix homeostasis. We propose that the markedly increased expression of transforming growth factor-β1 following ureteral ligation, as detected by a number of laboratories, induces a profibrogenic state and initiates a cascade of dysregulatory events, including the upregulation of tissue inhibitors of metalloproteinase. Transforming growth factor-β1 also may serve as a potent stimulus for the modulation of quiescent interstitial fibroblasts into myofibroblasts. From a therapeutic standpoint, targeting these early cellular and molecular events may be extremely important in interrupting the interstitial fibrotic response to long-term obstructive uropathy.

INDEX WORDS: Obstructive nephropathy; macrophages; cytokines; interstitial fibrosis.

MANY RECENT clinical and experimental studies have clearly demonstrated that one of the initial events taking place in the process of progressive renal injury is monocytic infiltration of the glomerular and tubulointerstitial compartments (for review see ref 1). These bone marrow-derived macrophages (Møs) release a potent armamentarium of proinflammatory mediators, including cytokines, growth factors, oxygen-free radicals, proteases, and extracellular matrix products, and have been implicated in a diverse number of nonimmune models of progressive renal disease, such as the experimental nephrotic syndrome produced by either puromycin aminonucleoside or doxorubicin, renal ablation (''remnant kidney''), and protein overload proteinuria.[1]

In this report, experimental data supporting the role of the infiltrating renal Mø as a mediator of interstitial fibrosis during the course of obstructive nephropathy will be reviewed as it pertains to the unilateral ureteral obstruction (UUO) model in the rat. The central pathobiologic theme drawn on data from this model is that fibrogenic cytokines, especially transforming growth factor-β (TGF-β), are, in part, Mø-derived and represent pivotal links between the initial postobstructive renal inflammation and the late development of renal scarring.

We recently focused our attention on this model, in sharp contradistinction to the abovementioned models,[1] because ureteral obstruction is a nonproteinuric and nonhyperlipidemic disorder. Review of our experimental studies will demonstrate that there is yet another nonimmune stimulus (ie, the mechanical disturbance produced by urinary tract obstruction), which is capable of eliciting a florid Mø infiltration of the kidney and, if unrelieved, contributes to the cascade of events that ultimately leads to the development of interstitial fibrosis.

Obstructive uropathy refers to a group of parenchymal and extraparenchymal renal disorders that exhibit an impaired flow of urine or tubular fluid as a consequence of structural or functional abnormalities in the urinary tract. The functional and morphologic derangements that develop as sequelae to urinary tract obstruction constitutes obstructive nephropathy.

The seminal investigations into the pathobiology of obstructive nephropathy were pioneered

The experimental studies referred to in this article were funded by a Baxter Healthcare (McGaw Park, IL) Extramural Research Grant and an American Heart Association (Pennsylvania Affiliate; Camp Hill, PA) Research Grant-in-Aid. Dr Diamond is a recipient of an Established Investigator Award of the American Heart Association (Dallas, TX) and the Alyce G. Spector Research Award from the Central Pennsylvania Kidney Foundation (Harrisburg, PA).

by Klahr.[2] The acute hemodynamic abnormalities have been well described by his group[2]; however, the cellular and molecular aberrations,[3-5] which mediate the development of interstitial fibrosis[6] and, ultimately, renal failure, are only recently becoming evident. Recent evidence has demonstrated that the process of fibrosis represents an imbalance between extracellular matrix protein synthesis and degradation.[7] In this review, experimental evidence supporting an Mø–TGF-β–renal fibrosis axis will be presented.

CHEMOATTRACTANT SIGNALS AND MACROPHAGE INFILTRATION IN OBSTRUCTIVE NEPHROPATHY

There is an increase in the interstitial Mø content at 4 to 12 hours after obstruction, which continues to increase rapidly thereafter.[5,8,9] The signal responsible for the recruitment of leukocytes into the kidney after ureteral obstruction appears to be specific for Møs because polymorphonuclear leukocytes are not seen in the kidney after ureteral obstruction of less than 24 hours' duration.[8,9] Rovin et al[10] demonstrated that acute ureteral obstruction results in the release of a specific monocyte chemoattractant from the affected kidney. Initial analysis suggested that this released factor was a lipid in nature.[10]

We recently observed[5] that monocyte chemoattractant peptide-1 (MCP-1) mRNA was detected between 12 and 96 hours in the obstructed rat kidney, but was absent in the contralateral unobstructed kidney specimens at all time points. In addition, apical tubular MCP-1 expression in the renal cortex at the time of immunolabeling was present from 12 through 96 hours after UUO in the obstructed kidney but not the contralateral unobstructed kidney specimen. This is not the first demonstration of renal tubular epithelial MCP-1 expression in vivo. Safirstein et al[11] noted epithelial immunolocalization for MCP-1 in renal tubules in a rat model of ischemic acute renal failure, which was associated with an interstitial Mø infiltrate. In studying the proinflammatory conditions in cultured human renal cortical epithelial cells, Schmouder et al[12] noted fourfold to fivefold increments in steady-state mRNA levels of MCP-1 as well as antigenic peptide in the conditioned media of these cells after cytokine stimulation. Thus, the cortical tubular epithelium appears to be a ready source of MCP-1 during acute inflammatory states.

Other proteins with potential chemoattractant activity also may be involved in the Mø infiltration of the renal interstitium. In a model of focal tubulointerstitial injury associated with angiotensin II infusion, Giachelli et al[13] recently observed a dramatic increase in the focal expression of osteopontin mRNA and protein in renal distal cortical tubules and surrounding Bowman's capsules. Osteopontin is a highly acidic, secreted glycoprotein, also known as uropontin, eta-1, secreted phosphoprotein I, and bone sialoprotein I.[13] A number of inflammatory cytokines (eg, TGF-β, interleukin-1, tumor necrosis factor, etc) have been shown to stimulate osteopontin synthesis in various cell types.[13]

Giachelli et al[13] noted that the elevated expression of osteopontin occurred early and was followed by a monocyte/Mø influx. The Møs localized almost exclusively to sites of tubular osteopontin, suggesting that inappropriate expression of osteopontin by kidney tubules might be an important chemoattractant mechanism in directing an inflammatory response, which would be necessary for the subsequent development of tubulointerstitial injury.[13] Osteopontin also contains an arginine-glycine-aspartate cell adhesion sequence, and purified osteopontin has been shown to facilitate adhesion of cultured fibroblasts,[13] which also might be important for the development of interstitial fibrosis.

We, too, have recently observed[13a] that beginning at 4 hours after UUO, there is marked upregulation of renal cortical osteopontin mRNA (Fig 1) and a focal pattern of immunolocalization of this peptide in the cortical tubular epithelium and in the parietal epithelium of Bowman's capsule in obstructed kidneys only. Contralateral unobstructed kidneys only faintly exhibit the peptide in Bowman's capsule. At 96 hours after UUO, persistent upregulated expression of osteopontin mRNA continues, but the pattern of immunolocalization within the cortical tubular epithelium of obstructed kidneys is now diffuse (Fig 2).

The factor(s) causing an obstructed kidney to release a chemoattractant for Møs remains unknown, as does the specific cellular source of this factor, although our immunohistochemical findings of upregulated expression of MCP-1[5] and osteopontin[13a] as well as the findings of Gia-

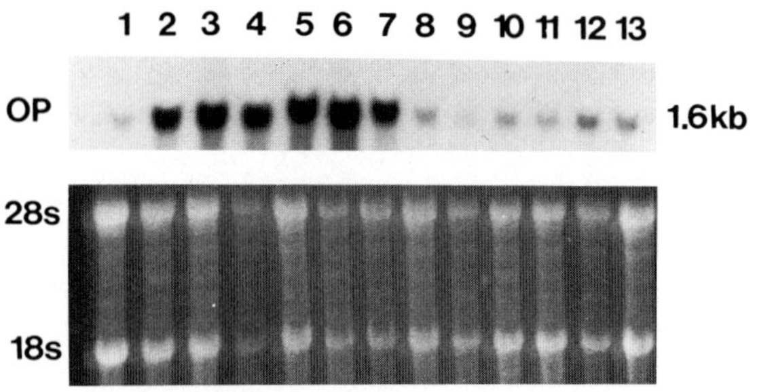

Fig 1. Northern blot analysis of total cortical RNA from a sham-operated rat kidney (lane 1), from obstructed kidneys (lanes 2 to 7), and from contralateral unobstructed kidney specimens of individual rats at 4 hours after UUO (lanes 8 to 13). (Top) Total cortical RNA was probed for rat osteopontin (OP) using the 2B7 cDNA probe (kindly provided by Dr C. Giachelli, University of Washington, Seattle, WA). (Bottom) Intact 28s and 18s ribosomal RNA bands using ethidium bromide staining of the agarose gel. There is markedly increased expression of steady-state mRNA levels of OP in obstructed kidneys compared with either the contralateral unobstructed kidney specimens or the cortex of a normal age-matched rat kidney at this early 4-hour time interval post-UUO.

chelli et al,[13] with regard to osteopontin expression in another model of tubulointerstitial injury, support a cortical tubule epithelial origin. It is possible that an increase in tubular pressure or membrane stretch in response to ureteral obstruction causes the tubular cells to release a chemoattractant.

CORTICAL TRANSFORMING GROWTH FACTOR-β EXPRESSION IN OBSTRUCTIVE NEPHROPATHY

Elimination of the infiltrating Mø burden by prior whole body X-irradiation in rats with bilateral ureteral obstruction markedly attenuated a thromboxane A_2-mediated cortical vasoconstriction in the postobstructed kidney.[2] These data identified the infiltrating interstitial Mø as a potent source of vasoactive (ie, thromboxane A_2) and, perhaps, other proinflammatory mediators. We, among others, have documented upregulation of TGF-β in a variety of models of renal disease.[14-18] The sustained aberrant expression of renal TGF-β results in the pathologic accumulation of extracellular matrix material in both the glomerulus and interstitial compartments.[14-18]

In the UUO model, Kaneto et al[3] demonstrated that a twofold to threefold increase in TGF-β1 mRNA occurred in obstructed kidneys relative to either normal control kidneys or contralateral unobstructed kidney specimens at 3, 5, 7, and 14 days after obstruction. Although a tubular cell origin for the increased mRNA level of TGF-β after obstruction was postulated, these investigators also commented that the Mø could be responsible. Walton et al[4] detected a rapid upregulation of gene expression for TGF-β1 within the renal cortex of obstructed rats. However, the cell type exhibiting the increased TGF-β mRNA

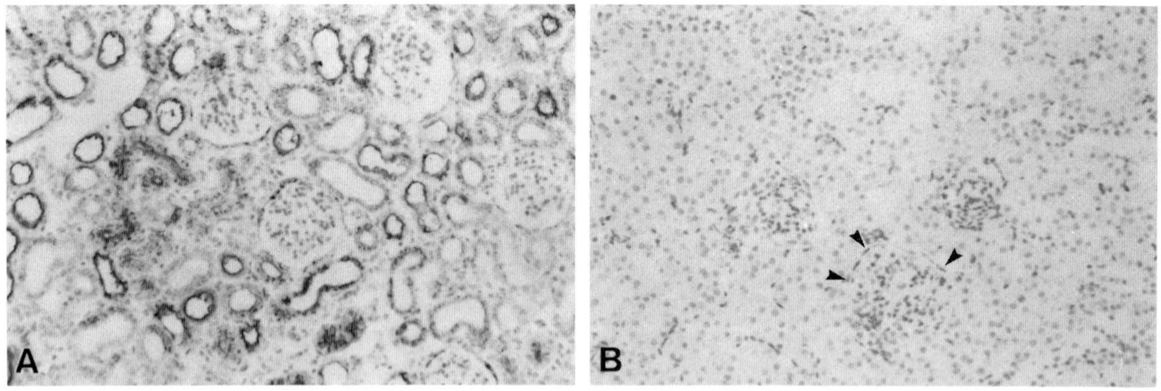

Fig 2. Composite photomicrograph of avidin biotinylated peroxidase immunolabeling for rat osteopontin using a mouse monoclonal IgG antibody, MPI-IIB10 (Developmental Studies Hybridoma Bank, University of Iowa, Iowa City, IA) from the renal cortex of an obstructed kidney (A) and the contralateral unobstructed kidney (B) at 96 hours post-UUO. It is evident in panel A that there is pronounced immunolocalization for osteopontin in the parietal epithelium of Bowman's capsule as well as diffuse staining within the cortical tubular epithelium. In sharp contrast, the contralateral unobstructed kidney specimen only demonstrates faint immunolocalization of osteopontin in Bowman's capsule. (Methyl green counterstain; magnification ×110.)

level was not determined. Recently, we noted highly significant 2.6-, 5.8-, and 7.0-fold increments in renal cortical TGF-β1 mRNA levels at 12, 48, and 96 hours, respectively, in the obstructed kidney versus the contralateral unobstructed kidney specimen.[5] Intracellular TGF-β1, on immunolabeling, was detected only in the obstructed kidneys of UUO rats at all three time points and was confined to peritubular cells of the renal interstitium. We have demonstrated[19] that previous whole body X-irradiation of rats with UUO produced a greater than twofold decrement in steady-state renal cortical TGF-β mRNA levels, further supporting our contention that TGF-β is, in part, Mø derived in this model. In addition, a significant correlation between interstitial Mø number and cortical TGF-β1 mRNA levels was noted,[5] supporting the postulate that the Mø is a source of this peptide growth factor in the UUO model.

Transforming growth factor-β is a peptide growth factor, secreted by many cell types, that has effects on extracellular matrix protein production.[7] The profibrogenic effect of TGF-β is achieved by a combination of inhibition of the degradation of matrix proteins by increased generation of proteinase inhibitors and by decreased expression of degradative proteins, such as collagenase.[7] The net effect of TGF-β on extracellular matrix is one of accumulation.[7] Furthermore, TGF-β is a chemoattractant for fibroblasts and also stimulates fibroblast proliferation.[7]

MYOFIBROBLAST TRANSFORMATION IN OBSTRUCTIVE NEPHROPATHY

Alpers et al[20] have identified accumulation of human renal cortical interstitial cells expressing smooth muscle actin at sites of chronic tubulointerstitial injury. Johnson et al[21] have noted that angiotensin II-infused rats developed focal tubulointerstitial injury that was evident at 14 days postinfusion. In this model,[21] the peritubular space possessed a mononuclear infiltrate and numerous interstitial cells that expressed alpha-smooth muscle actin. Recently, we have observed myofibroblast transformation in the cortex of the obstructed rat kidney.[19] There was evidence of increased alpha-smooth muscle actin mRNA levels in cortical RNA, as well as increased immunolabeling of alpha-smooth muscle actin and desmin in the interstitium of only obstructed kidneys.

Among the smooth muscle cell markers expressed by fibroblast populations undergoing differentiation into myofibroblasts in vivo and in vitro, alpha-smooth muscle actin is the most common, followed by desmin, while myosin is practically always absent.[22,23] The role of the myofibroblast in granulation tissue contraction and in fibrotic disorders is well established,[24] but the regulatory mechanisms of this maladaptive process are not yet fully clarified. Locally liberated cytokines can modulate the phenotypic features of fibroblasts and enhance the expression of smooth muscle markers.[22-26] Several cytokines (ie, interleukin-1, tumor necrosis factor, platelet-derived growth factor), which may contribute to the development of granulation tissue, do not induce the appearance of the alpha-smooth muscle actin-rich myofibroblasts in vivo.[23,25] However, accumulation of Mø clusters (induced by local granulocyte-macrophage colony-stimulating factor application) in rat subcutaneous tissue[25] resulted in abundant expression of alpha-smooth muscle actin by myofibroblasts. Moreover, in transgenic mice expressing granulocyte-macrophage colony-stimulating factor, fibrotic nodules developed in areas where Møs accumulated.[24] Since granulocyte-macrophage colony-stimulating factor does not act directly on cultured fibroblasts to induce alpha-smooth muscle actin synthesis, Vyalov et al[25] concluded that granulocyte macrophage colony-stimulating factor-induced clustered Møs produce a factor(s) capable of stimulating myofibroblast transformation. Desmouliere et al[26] showed that TGF-β1 induced alpha-smooth muscle actin expression in growing and quiescent fibroblasts, and that preincubation of the culture medium with TGF-β1 neutralizing antibodies decreased it.

TISSUE INHIBITORS OF METALLOPROTEINASE

The induction of a profibrogenic state following urinary tract obstruction involves not only the deposition of extracellular matrix but also the dysregulation of degradative proteases, which are involved in extracellular matrix processing and tissue remodeling. A misconception exists that the cellular and molecular perturbations stimulating fibrogenesis develop late after the onset of urinary tract obstruction.

The extracellular matrix exists in a dynamic

state of both synthesis and degradation. This process maintains the integrity of the interstitial space and is responsible for the regulation of a number of cellular events, including adhesion, migration, proliferation, and differentiation. Matrix metalloproteinases (MMPs) are a group of enzymes capable of degrading both the collagenous and noncollagenous components of the extracellular matrix, and thus are intimately involved in the regulation of tissue remodeling.[27,28] These MMPs are secreted as zymogens and their activity is controlled, in part, through cleavage activation or by specific tissue inhibitor of metalloproteinase (TIMP) proteins.[27,28]

The family of mammalian TIMPs includes three proteins that have individual characteristics as well as some common features. Although both TIMP-1 and TIMP-2 are tight-binding inhibitors of all active MMPs, they also form specific complexes with latent 92-kd gelatinase B and 72-kd gelatinase A, respectively.[29,30] Although little is known about the biochemistry of TIMP-3, an important aspect of this inhibitor is that it is found exclusively in the extracellular matrix, in contrast to both TIMP-1 and TIMP-2.[31] Tissue inhibitor of metalloproteinase-3, but not TIMP-1 or TIMP-2, was recently shown to be abundantly expressed in normal adult mouse kidney.[31] Taken together, these observations suggest that TIMPs may be interchangeable in some of their actions, but that each type likely has additional specific physiologic roles.

We recently delineated the kinetics of TIMP-1, TIMP-2, and TIMP-3 mRNA expression within the renal cortex during the early phase of experimental hydronephrosis in the rat[32] since TGF-β could contribute to the fibrosis process by upregulating TIMP expression.[7] We postulated that alterations in the regulation of TIMP expression may contribute to the inception of the fibrogenic response within hours after ureteral obstruction commences, which, if uncorrected, may contribute to interstitial fibrosis after a protracted course.

There was a marked elevation of TIMP-1 mRNA expression following UUO, which was first noted at 12 hours after ureteral ligation.[32] By 96 hours after UUO, there was a 30-fold increment in TIMP-1 mRNA in the obstructed kidneys compared with the contralateral unobstructed kidney or sham-operated rat specimens.[32] In contradistinction to TIMP-1, we noted a decrease in TIMP-3 mRNA levels at 12 hours after ureteral obstruction, which persisted at the 24-, 48-, and 96-hour time intervals.[32] Gene expression of TIMP-2 remained at a relatively constant level during our entire period of study.[32] Intriguingly, in a rabbit UUO model, Sharma et al[6] observed that TIMP-2 mRNA expression appeared to be biphasic with peaks at both days 3 and 16 in post-UUO animals, but no change at day 7. This finding is the first in vivo demonstration in the UUO model of differential mRNA expression for these three members of the TIMP family of proteins.

One profibrogenic effect of TGF-β is achieved by a combination of inhibiting normal extracellular matrix degradative proteases and upregulating TIMP expression.[7] Transforming growth factor-$\beta 1$ also modulates TIMP-1, TIMP-2, and TIMP-3 expression in vitro[31,33] and specifically decreases the expression of collagenase and stromolysin,[7] thereby placing this peptide growth factor as a pivotal moiety in extracellular matrix homeostasis. However, little is known about how growth factors may alter TIMP expression in vivo.

In a variety of cultured cell and tissue types a consensus has emerged indicating that TIMP-1 transcription is highly inducible by diverse cytokines, hormones, and miscellaneous stimuli.[31,33] In contrast TIMP-2 usually is expressed in a constitutive fashion.[33] Our observations in this model of chronic interstitial injury following UUO are consistent with this paradigm. However, the results that we have obtained for expression of the new member of the TIMP family, TIMP-3, raise interesting questions about its participation in normal renal function and responses to injury. The TIMP-3 gene gives rise to a prominent 4.5-kb transcript and exhibits a pattern of expression similar to that of TIMP-1 in mouse and human fibroblasts.[33] Although it is highly inducible by TGF-$\beta 1$ in vitro, key differences in gene expression have been noted, particularly with regard to opposite regulation of TIMP-3 (induction) compared with TIMP-1 (repression) by dexamethasone in fibroblasts, and the low level of expression of TIMP-3 in bone and high renal and brain expression relative to TIMP-1 in adult mice.[33]

Our results demonstrating opposite pattern of expression of TIMP-1 and TIMP-3 in experimental hydronephrosis confirm that the genes probably are separately controlled by tissue-specific mechanisms. In addition, it is important to note that the TIMP-3 protein resides in the extracellular matrix, as opposed to TIMP-1 and TIMP-2, which diffuse freely through interstitial spaces.[33] Our data therefore lead us to suggest that TIMP-3 is a specialized constituent of the renal extracellular matrix that may play an important role in the maintenance of normal tissue architecture through interactions with structural components of the matrix. Alternatively, along the lines of the complexes between TIMP-1 and TIMP-2 and the latent forms of gelatinases, it may interact with and sequester an as yet unidentified MMP that is required for extracellular matrix turnover. Finally, one can speculate that TIMP-3 is derived from tubular epithelium and that its downregulated expression post-UUO is an injurious response to the mechanical disturbance produced by ureteral obstruction. Thus, both the augmented expression of TIMP-1 and the reduced expression of TIMP-3 could contribute to fibrosis in the UUO model by changing the quantity and type of extracellular matrix.

In situ hybridization studies have revealed that tissue localization of TIMP-1 transcripts is present at sites of active remodeling, where its expression significantly overlaps with that of TGF-β1.[34] Our previously documented increase in TGF-β1 expression from 12 to 96 hours in the obstructed kidneys versus the contralateral unobstructed kidney specimens[5] support a relationship between this peptide growth factor and TIMP-1 as a pathobiologic axis for accumulation of extracellular matrix constituents and the development of interstitial fibrosis. Intriguingly, Jones et al[35] noted a strong correlation between interstitial Mø accumulation and TIMP-1 expression in the experimental nephrotic syndrome model produced by puromycin aminonucleoside. One can postulate that either the resident interstitial fibroblast or the infiltrating Mø can represent the responsible cell for TIMP-1 upregulation in our model.

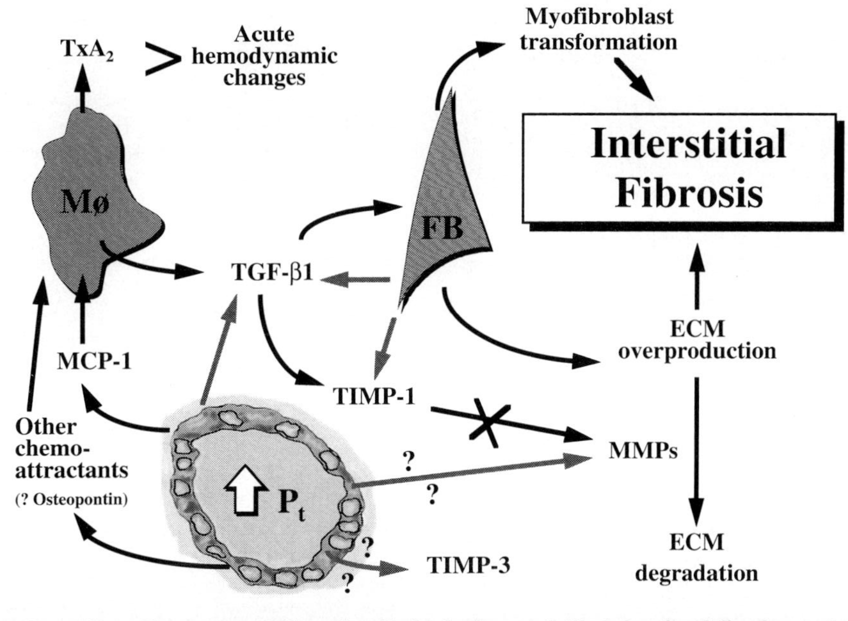

Fig 3. A putative schematic representation of pathobiologic events that develop following ureteral obstruction. In response to the intratubular mechanical disturbance generated by ureteral obstruction, Mø chemoattractant moieties are upregulated and released by the tubular epithelium. Consequently, bone marrow-derived peripheral blood monocytes infiltrate the interstitial space within hours of ureteral obstruction. In addition to vasoactive substances (ie, thromboxane A_2), the Mø releases many peptide growth factors. Our studies have focused on TGF-β1 as a fibrogenic cytokine. Transforming growth factor-β1 upregulates a number of processes, including TIMP-1 expression, extracellular matrix (ECM) production by interstitial fibroblasts, and the modulation of interstitial fibroblasts into myofibroblasts. All these maladaptive processes contribute to the development of interstitial fibrosis.

SUMMARY

As shown in Fig 3, our laboratory investigations have led us to postulate that the tubular epithelium, as a consequence of the mechanical disturbance produced by ureteral obstruction, elaborates a host of Mø chemoattractant moieties. The tubular epithelium also may participate in the dysregulated expression of TIMP moieties and MMPs as well. Many substances can be released by the infiltrating Mø; however, our studies have focused on TGF-β1. Transforming growth factor-β is an important regulator of extracellular matrix[7] through its direct effects and modulation of other growth factors to maintain matrix homeostasis. Its reciprocal effect on extracellular matrix synthesis, downregulation of proteases, and promotion of protease inhibitors place it in a central role during the early development of postobstructive interstitial fibrosis. In addition, as shown in Fig 3, we postulate that TGF-β is, in part, Mø derived. This contention is supported by data from the experimental nephrotic syndrome.[17,18,35]

In addition to the components depicted in Fig 3, we would like to note the recent elegant studies of Kaneto et al,[3] who provided compelling evidence that angiotensin II is important in promoting TGF-β production in the obstructed kidney, perhaps from the tubular epithelium, as well as mediating many profibrogenic effects leading to interstitial fibrosis.

Furthermore, we propose that the markedly increased expression of TGF-β1 following ureteral ligation, detected by a number of laboratories,[3-5] induces a profibrogenic state and initiates a cascade of dysregulatory events, including the upregulation of TIMP-1. The mRNA expression of TIMP-2 appears to be independently regulated from TIMP-1, and TGF-β1 fails to modulate its mRNA level during the early phases of ureteral obstruction. Of interest, we observed a significant downregulation of renal cortical TIMP-3 mRNA levels in the obstructed kidneys; however, the pathophysiologic significance of this finding remains to be elucidated.

In addition, Mø-derived TGF-β1 may serve as a potent stimulus for the modulation of quiescent interstitial fibroblasts into myofibroblasts,[19] as suggested by the elegant studies of Gabbiani and colleagues.[25,26] Further studies in our laboratory are investigating the regulatory mechanisms of this process. Finally, from a therapeutic standpoint, targeting these early cellular and molecular events may be extremely important in interrupting the interstitial fibrotic response to long-term obstructive uropathy.

REFERENCES

1. van Goor H, Ding G, Kees-Folts D, Grond J, Schreiner GF, Diamond JR: Macrophages and renal disease. Lab Invest 71:456-464, 1994

2. Klahr S: New insights into the consequences and mechanisms of renal impairment in obstructive nephropathy. Am J Kidney Dis 29:689-699, 1992

3. Kaneto H, Morrissey J, Klahr S: Increased expression of TGF-β1 mRNA in the obstructed kidney of rats with unilateral ureteral ligation. Kidney Int 44:313-321, 1993

4. Walton G, Buttyan R, Garcia-Montes E, Olsson C, Hensle T, Sawczuk I: Renal growth factor expression during the early phase of experimental hydronephrosis. J Urol 148:510-514, 1992

5. Diamond JR, Kees-Folts D, Ding G, Frye J, Restrepo NC: Macrophages, monocyte chemoattractant peptide-1 and transforming growth factor-β1 in experimental hydronephrosis. Am J Physiol 266:F926-F933, 1994

6. Sharma AK, Mauer SM, Kim Y, Michael A: Interstitial fibrosis in obstructive nephropathy. Kidney Int 44:774-788, 1993

7. Massague JI: The transforming growth factor-β family. Ann Biochem 6:597-641, 1990

8. Harris KPG, Schreiner GF, Purkerson ML, Klahr S: Effect of leukocyte depletion on the post-obstructed rat kidney. Kidney Int 36:210-215, 1989

9. Schreiner GF, Harris KPG, Purkerson ML, Klahr S: Immunological aspects of acute ureteral obstruction. Kidney Int 34:487-493, 1988

10. Rovin BH, Harris KPG, Morrison A, Klahr S, Schreiner GF: Renal cortical release of a specific macrophage chemoattractant in response to ureteral obstruction. Lab Invest 63:213-220, 1990

11. Safirstein R, Megyesi J, Saggi SJ, Price PM, Poon M, Rollins BJ, Taubman MB: Expression of cytokine-like genes JE and KC is increased during renal ischemia. Am J Physiol 261:F1095-F1101, 1991

12. Schmouder RL, Strieter RM, Kunkel SL: Interferon-gamma regulation of human renal cortical epithelial cell-derived monocyte chemoattractant peptide-1. Kidney Int 44:43-49, 1993

13. Giachelli CM, Pichler R, Lombardi D, Denhardt DT, Alpers CE, Schwartz SM, Johnson RJ: Osteopontin expression in angiotensin II-induced tubulointerstitial nephritis. Kidney Int 45:515-524, 1994

13a. Diamond JR, Kees-Folts D, Ricardo SD, Pruzuak A, Eufemio M: Early and persistent up-regulated expression of renal cortical osteopontin in experimental hydronephrosis. Am J Pathol 146: 1995 (in press)

14. Okuda S, Languino LR, Ruoslahti E, Border WA: Elevated expression of transforming growth factor-β and proteoglycan production in experimental glomerulonephritis. Possi-

ble role in expansion of the mesangial extracellular matrix. J Clin Invest 86:453-462, 1990

15. Fukui M, Nakamura T, Ebihara I, Nagaoka I, Tomino Y, Koide H: Low protein diet attenuates increased gene expression of platelet-derived growth factor and transforming growth factor-β in experimental glomerular sclerosis. J Lab Clin Med 121:224-234, 1993

16. Yamamoto T, Noble NA, Miller DE, Border WA: Sustained expression of TGF-$\beta 1$ underlies development of progressive kidney fibrosis. Kidney Int 45:916-927, 1994

17. Ding G, Pesek-Diamond I, Diamond JR: Cholesterol, macrophages and the gene expression of TGF-$\beta 1$ and fibronectin during nephrosis. Am J Physiol 264:F577-F584, 1993

18. Eddy AA: Protein restriction reduces transforming growth factor-β and interstitial fibrosis in nephrotic syndrome. Am J Physiol 266:F884-F893, 1994

19. Diamond JR, van Goor H, Ding G, Englemyer E: Myofibroblasts in experimental hydronephrosis. Am J Pathol 146:121-129, 1995

20. Alpers CE, Hudkins KL, Floege J, Johnson RJ: Human renal cortical interstitial cells with some features of smooth muscle cells participate in tubulointerstitial and crescentic glomerular injury. J Am Soc Nephrol 5:201-210, 1994

21. Johnson RJ, Alpers CE, Yoshimura A, Lombardi D, Pritzl P, Floege J, Schwartz SM: Renal injury from angiotensin II-mediated hypertension. Hypertension 19:464-474, 1992

22. Desmouliere A, Rubbia-Brandt L, Abdiu A, Walz T, Macierira-Coelho A, Gabbiani G: Alpha-smooth muscle actin is expressed in a subpopulation of cultured fibroblasts and is modulated by gamma interferon. Exp Cell Res 201:64-73, 1992

23. Rubbia-Brandt L, Sappino AP, Gabbiani G: Locally applied GM-CSF induces alpha-smooth muscle actin containing fibroblasts. Virchows Arch B Cell Pathol 60:73-82, 1991

24. Gabbiani G: The biology of the fibroblast. Kidney Int 41:530-532, 1992

25. Vyalov S, Desmouliere A, Gabbiani G: GM-CSF-induced granulation tissue formation: Relationships between macrophage and myofibroblast accumulation. Virchows Arch B Cell Pathol 63:231-239, 1993

26. Desmouliere A, Geinoz H, Gabbiani F, Gabbiani G: TGF-$\beta 1$ induces alpha-smooth muscle actin expression in granulation tissue myofibroblasts and in quiescent and growing cultured fibroblasts. J Cell Biol 120:103-11, 1993

27. Matrisian LM: The matrix-degrading metalloproteinases. Bioessays 14:455-463, 1992

28. Murphy G, Reynolds JJ: Current views of collagen degradation. Bioessays 2:55-60, 1985

29. Stetler-Stevenson WG, Krutzsch HC, Liotta LA: Tissue inhibitor of metalloproteinase (TIMP-2). A new member of the metalloproteinase family. J Biol Chem 264:17374-17378, 1989

30. Stetler-Stevenson WG, Brown PD, Onisto M, Levy AT, Liotta LA: Tissue inhibitor of metalloproteinase-2 (TIMP-2) mRNA expression in tumor cell lines and human tumor tissues. J Biol Chem 265:13933-13938, 1990

31. Leco KJ, Khokha R, Pavioff N, Hawkes S, Edwards DR: Tissue inhibitor of metalloproteinase-3 (TIMP-3) is an extracellular matrix-associated protein with a distinctive pattern of expression in mouse cells and tissues. J Biol Chem 269:9352-9360, 1994

32. Englemyer E, van Goor H, Edward DR, Diamond JR: Differential mRNA expression of TIMP-1, -2, and -3 during experimental hydronephrosis. J Am Soc Nephrol 5:1675-1683, 1995

33. Edwards DR, Murphy G, Reynolds JJ, Whitham SE, Docherty JP, Angel P, Heath JK: Transforming growth factor beta modulates the expression of collagenase and metalloproteinase inhibitor. EMBO J 6:1899-1904, 1987

34. Nomura S, Hogan BL, Wills AJ, Heath JK, Edwards DR: Developmental expression of tissue inhibitor of metalloproteinases (TIMP). RNA 105:575-583, 1989

35. Jones CL, Buch S, Post M, McCulloch L, Liu E, Eddy AA: Renal extracellular matrix accumulation in acute puromycin nephrosis in rats. Am J Pathol 141:1381-1396, 1992

Role of Angiotensin II in the Tubulointerstitial Fibrosis of Obstructive Nephropathy

Saulo Klahr, MD, Shigeto Ishidoya, MD, and Jeremiah Morrissey, PhD

● Chronic unilateral ureteral obstruction results in interstitial fibrosis of the affected kidney. Both an angiotensin-converting enzyme inhibitor, enalapril, and an angiotensin II receptor antagonist, SC-51316, ameliorate the increased production of extracellular matrix protein in the tubulointerstitium of the obstructed kidney. Blockade of angiotensin II synthesis or inability of angiotensin II to bind to its receptor lessened the increased levels of mRNA for transforming growth factor-β and collagen IV found in the obstructed kidney of untreated rats. A monocyte/macrophage infiltration was present in the obstructed kidney of untreated rats or rats treated with the angiotensin II receptor antagonists. In contrast, this infiltrate was almost completely absent in the obstructed kidney of rats treated with enalapril. The reason for this different effect of enalapril compared with the angiotensin II receptor antagonist on the macrophage infiltrate seen in obstructive nephropathy has not been elucidated. We conclude that both an angiotensin-converting enzyme inhibitor (enalapril) and a receptor antagonist of angiotensin II ameliorate the tubulointerstitial fibrosis that follows complete unilateral ureteral obstruction in the rat. We suggest that an increased level of angiotensin II has a major role in the development of tubulointerstitial fibrosis following ureteral obstruction.

INDEX WORDS: Transforming growth factor-β; collagen; ureteral obstruction; macrophages.

THE INEXORABLE progression of renal disease to end-stage renal failure after an initial insult in humans is a phenomenon that remains largely unexplained. Evidence from different studies suggests that tubulointerstitial changes, not histologic changes of the glomeruli, correlate better with the decrement in glomerular filtration rate in a variety of renal diseases.[1] In addition, renal tubular cells have been found to produce a diverse array of polypeptide growth factors, vasoactive peptides, and cytokines.[2] Such factors may have an important role in renal damage. These observations suggest that the tubular interstitium and pathology of this space may have an important role in the progression of chronic renal disease.

The tubulointerstitium occupies approximately 80% of total kidney volume. Renal epithelial tubular cells represent the major compartment of the kidney. The interstitium, surrounded by the vascular and tubular compartments and communicating with the glomerular and extraglomerular mesangium, may be particularly susceptible to pathologic events originating in these neighboring areas.[3] Structural derangements of the tubulointerstitial compartment occur with progressive renal disease. These structural changes, regardless of the etiology of the renal disease or compartment in which the disease originates, may represent a specific role of the tubulointerstitial compartment in the progression of renal disease. As mentioned above, histologic tubulointerstitial injury correlates better with renal functional decline in diverse renal diseases than does histologic glomerular injury. It was reported initially by Risdon et al[4] that renal functional impairment in patients with glomerular diseases was closely aligned with tubular atrophy and not with histologic glomerular injury. Subsequently, Schainuck et al[5] correlated histologic changes in the kidney with impairment of renal function and showed the functional significance of structural changes in the tubulointerstitium in this relationship. In the 1970s and 1980s, Bohle and colleagues[6,7] systematically analyzed biopsy material from patients with renal disease in an attempt to relate structure with function and eventual clinical outcome. The data again indicated that structural changes of the tubulointerstitial space correlated significantly with subsequent renal outcome.

A number of entities can result in the development of tubulointerstitial pathology. These structural changes of the tubulointerstitial space generally have been considered secondary to lesions of the glomerular structures. However, some renal diseases are characterized by primary tubulointerstitial pathology, with subsequent glomerular involvement. Obstructive nephropathy, the result of impaired flow of urine in the urinary tract, results in profound changes in the tubulointerstitial compartment of the kidney.[8,9] Renal interstitial fibrosis is a common consequence of longstanding obstruction of the urinary tract. Fibrosis very likely develops because of an imbalance between extracellular matrix synthesis, matrix deposition, and matrix degradation. Several investigators have examined the mechanisms responsible for the fibrogenesis that follows obstruction of the urinary tract. In the 1970s, Nagle and Bulger[8] reported that rabbits with unilateral ureteral obstruction had a widened interstitial space 7 days after the onset of obstruction; these investigators found increased collagen fibers and numerous fibroblasts at this time and by day 16 collagen was greatly increased and was arranged in large bundles. Nagle et al[10] also described a mononuclear cell infiltrate and proliferation of interstitial cells in the renal parenchyma of rabbits with chronic unilateral ureteral obstruction. Sharma et al[9] described increased renal synthesis of several extracellular matrix components (collagen types I, III, and IV, fibronectin, and heparin sulfate proteoglycans) in the renal interstitium of rabbits with ureteral obstruction of 3 and 7 days' duration.

We have described an increase in the relative volume of the cortical interstitium after 3 days of unilateral ureteral obstruction in the obstructed kidney of the rat.[11] The deposition of collagen types I, III, and IV also increased in the tubulointerstitium by the third day of unilateral ureteral obstruction. In addition, the level of mRNA for collagen $\alpha 1$ (IV) was significantly elevated in the obstructed kidney at this time interval. Thus, events leading to interstitial fibrosis are initiated promptly after the onset of obstruction. We also demonstrated using immunofluorescent techniques that the amount of collagen types I, III, and IV did not change in the glomeruli of the obstructed kidney at day 5 after unilateral ureteral obstruction. Additionally, we found that transforming growth factor-$\beta 1$ (TGF-$\beta 1$) mRNA levels did not change in glomeruli of the obstructed kidney but did increase in the tubulointerstitium during unilateral ureteral obstruction.[12] These results are consistent with the finding that glomeruli appear normal by light microscopy through 7 days of obstructive nephropathy.[10,11] The localization of interstitial collagen types I and III in the glomeruli of the normal kidney is controversial.[13-16] However, we found collagen types I and III in the glomeruli of our specimens of rat kidneys when fixed with Histochoice (Amresco, Solon, OH) and when the sections were treated with trypsin to uncover these epitopes.[11] We also reported that both interstitial collagen (types I and III) and the basement membrane collagen (type IV) are deposited in the interstitial space of the obstructed kidney.[11] Collagen types I and III were increased in the interstitial space only, while collagen IV was deposited both in the interstitium of the obstructed kidney and in the tubular basement membrane. Furthermore, our studies showed that collagen IV is the major collagen that increases in the renal cortex of the adult rat during unilateral ureteral obstruction. The increase in collagen IV in both the interstitial space and in the basement membrane of renal tubules may contribute to alterations in tubular function in the obstructed kidney.

Renal tubular cells in culture produce collagen types I, III, and IV.[17,18] We reported that the expression of collagen $\alpha 1$ (IV) mRNA was increased substantially in the tubules of the obstructed kidney. Thus, renal tubules may contribute to the increased production of collagen IV in both tubular basement membrane and interstitium. Nagle and Bulger reported that fibroblasts migrated and proliferated in the interstitium of the obstructed kidney during unilateral ureteral obstruction.[8] In addition, Kuncio et al[19] reported that several cytokines secreted by infiltrating macrophages and T lymphocytes act as chemoattractants and stimulate fibroblast proliferation and that interstitial fibroblasts produce collagen types I, III, and IV. The substantial increase in collagen types I and III that we found in the interstitium of the obstructed kidney at 3 or 5 days after unilateral ureteral obstruction is consistent with the increased cellularity due to fibroblast proliferation and infiltrating mononuclear cells. Thus, the interstitial fibroblasts may contribute to an increase in the production of collagens in the obstructed kidney of rats with unilateral ureteral obstruction.

We also found that TGF-$\beta 1$ mRNA expression is increased in the obstructed kidney and this increase was confined to tubular cells.[12] Transforming growth factor-$\beta 1$ has substantial effects on matrix protein production.[20] It causes (1) an increase in the mRNA of extracellular matrix components, particularly the collagens, (2) a de-

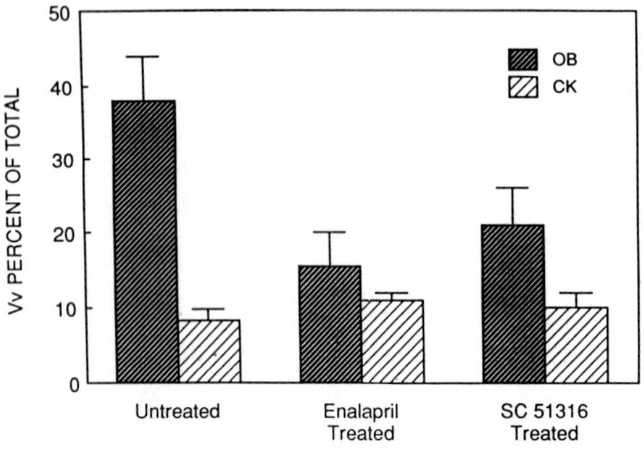

Fig 1. Relative volume (Vv) of the cortical interstitium in the obstructed kidney (OB) and contralateral kidney (CK) of three groups of rats with unilateral ureteral ligation of 5 days' duration. The three groups of rats comprised untreated animals, rats treated with enalapril, and rats treated with a receptor antagonist of angiotensin II (SC-51316).

crease in proteinases degrading these proteins, and (3) an increase in metalloproteinase inhibitors. Thus, an increase in TGF-β1 in the cortical tubules of the obstructed kidney may result in increased collagen α1 IV mRNA. The increase in collagen IV protein is undoubtedly the consequence of the increase in the mRNA. We found that an inhibitor of the angiotensin-converting enzyme, enalapril, significantly blunted the increase in volume of the interstitium that is present in the obstructed kidney of untreated rats at either 3 or 5 days of unilateral ureteral obstruction[11] (Fig 1). Enalapril also decreased the amount of collagen IV present in the obstructed kidney, as assessed by a matrix deposition score and by immunoblotting of the whole renal cortex.[11] The increase in collagen αIV mRNA levels was significantly diminished by enalapril at 5 days but not at 3 days of ureteral obstruction. Thus, the decrease in collagen IV deposition may be due to a decrease in mRNA expression in renal cortex, although this would not account for the reduction in the relative volume of the interstitium at 3 days. It is possible that enalapril administration also decreases the deposition of other types of collagen or other extracellular matrix components.

The histologic features of the kidney after 5 days of unilateral ureteral obstruction in untreated rats and in rats given enalapril are shown in Fig 2. The expansion of the interstitial space and the infiltration of this area by monocytes/macrophages is less in rats treated with enalapril than in control rats.

A monocyte/macrophage infiltration is seen in the obstructed kidney of the rat as early as 4 hours after ureteral ligation.[21] These ED-1–positive cells presumably contribute in part to the expansion of the tubulointerstitial space. In other experiments, we found that enalapril significantly decreased the number of ED-1–positive monocytes infiltrating the interstitium (Fig 3). This would decrease interstitial cellularity and contribute in part to the decreased volume seen in this compartment after treatment with the angiotensin-converting enzyme inhibitor. Enalapril blunts tubulointerstitial fibrosis in the obstructed kidney, whether given intraperitoneally or in the drinking water. Moreover, recent studies have revealed that a non-peptidic receptor antagonist of angiotensin II blunts the relative increase in volume of the interstitium of the obstructed kidney after 5 days of unilateral ureteral obstruction (Fig 1). We also found a decrease in the deposition of collagen in the obstructed kidney of animals treated with this angiotensin II receptor antagonist. However, in contrast to the findings obtained with enalapril, the receptor antagonist did not decrease the number of ED-1–positive monocytes/macrophages present in the interstitium (Fig 3).

The receptor antagonist blunted the increased TGF-β1 mRNA by approximately 75% and collagen IV by 45%, and reduced the expansion of the interstitial space of the obstructed kidney by approximately 45%. The results of this study support an important role of intrarenal angiotensin II in the pathogenesis of the tubulointerstitial fibrosis of obstructive nephropathy.

The hypothesis that progression of renal disease is due to altered regulation of fibrogenesis does not negate a role for hemodynamic factors and glomerular hypertrophy in other models of renal disease, in which the initial pathology is not in the tubulointerstitial space.[22] Although angiotensin II is well recognized for its effects on vascular tone and control of sodium reabsorption in the proximal tubule, it is now evident that angiotensin II also is an important factor in the proliferation of vascular smooth muscle and the

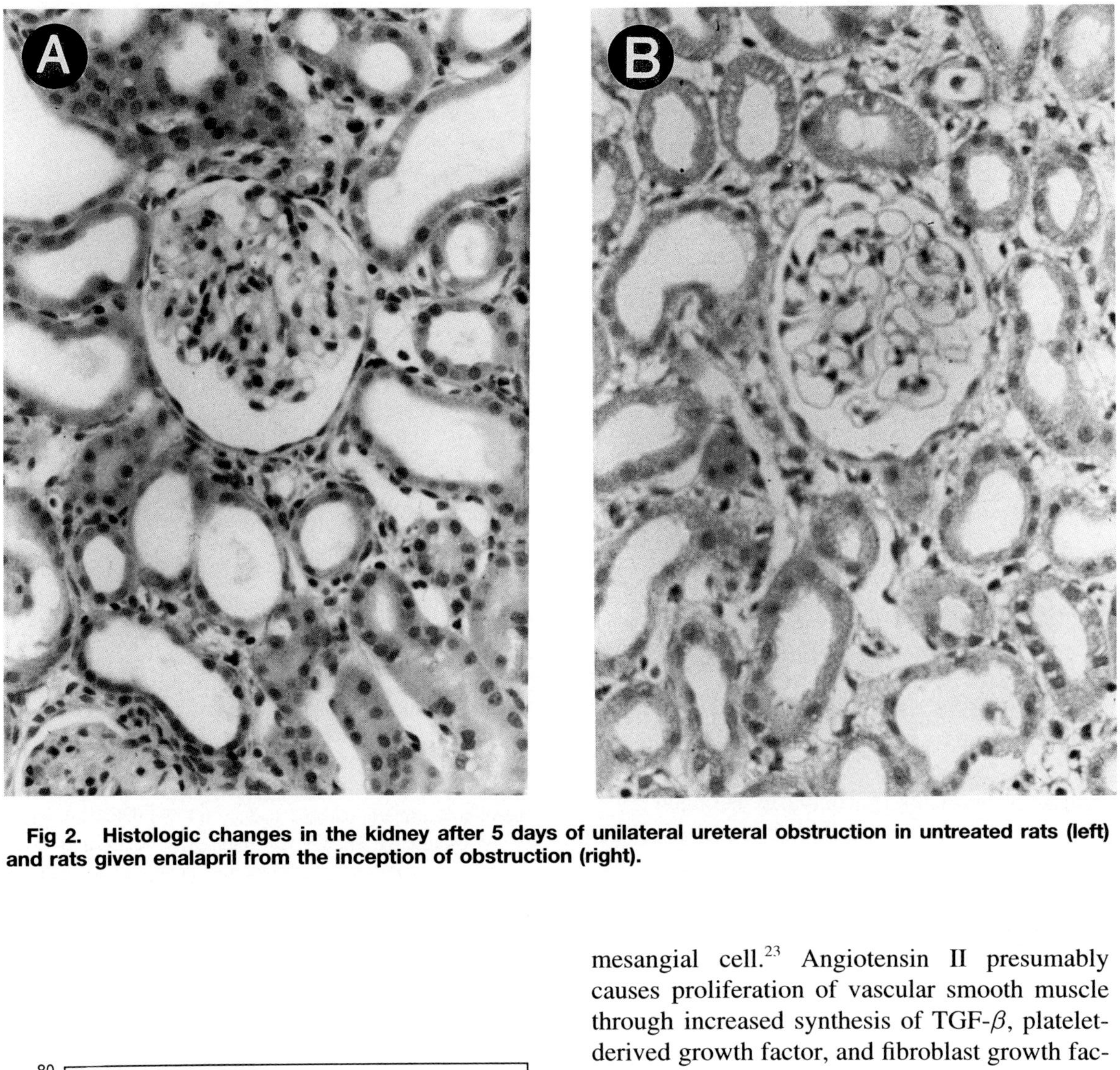

Fig 2. Histologic changes in the kidney after 5 days of unilateral ureteral obstruction in untreated rats (left) and rats given enalapril from the inception of obstruction (right).

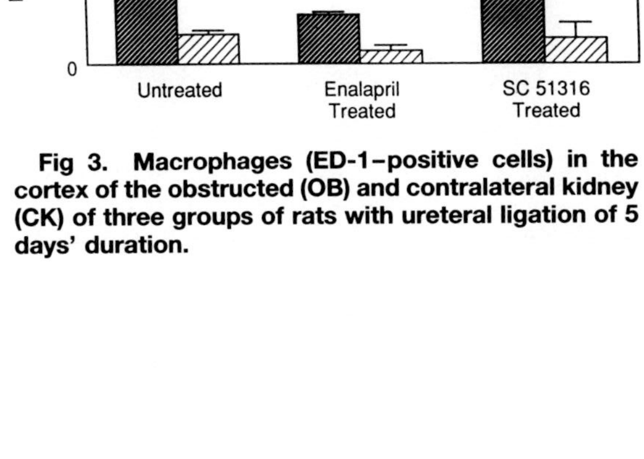

Fig 3. Macrophages (ED-1–positive cells) in the cortex of the obstructed (OB) and contralateral kidney (CK) of three groups of rats with ureteral ligation of 5 days' duration.

mesangial cell.[23] Angiotensin II presumably causes proliferation of vascular smooth muscle through increased synthesis of TGF-β, platelet-derived growth factor, and fibroblast growth factor. Similar events may be involved in the interstitial fibrosis that occurs after ureteral ligation. Angiotensin II also has a direct effect in stimulating the synthesis of osteopontin by renal tubular cells.[24] Osteopontin is a potential growth factor and is strongly chemotactic for macrophages.[25] The role of angiotensin II as a potential growth factor may explain the protective effect of angiotensin-converting enzyme inhibitors or angiotensin II receptor antagonists in the progression of renal disease in humans and also in diverse models of experimental renal disease.

In summary, we suggest that the renin-angiotensin system is activated after ureteral obstruction (Fig 4). Increasing levels of angiotensin II

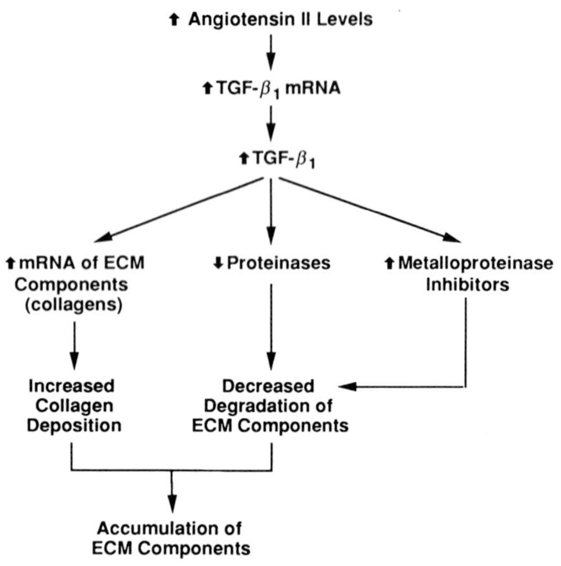

Fig 4. Pathogenesis of interstitial fibrosis in obstructive nephropathy. ↑, increase; ↓, decrease; ECM, extracellular matrix.

stimulate TGF-β1 synthesis in tubular epithelial cells (Fig 4). The increased levels of TGF-β1, in turn, may increase the deposition of extracellular matrix components, particularly collagen IV.[26] These changes, plus the infiltration of the renal parenchyma by macrophages, may cause progressive fibrosis of the interstitial space of the obstructed kidney. Inhibitors of the angiotensin-converting enzyme, such as enalapril, or nonpeptidic receptor-antagonists of angiotensin II, may markedly blunt the pathologic changes described above by interfering with the synthesis or action of angiotensin II.

REFERENCES

1. Nath KA: Tubulointerstitial changes as a major determinant in the progression of renal damage. Am J Kidney Dis 20:1-17, 1992

2. Ong ACM, Fine LG: Tubular-derived growth factors and cytokines in the pathogenesis of tubulointerstitial fibrosis: Implications for human renal disease progression. Am J Kidney Dis 23:205-209, 1994

3. Lemley KV, Kriz W: Anatomy of the renal interstitium. Kidney Int 39:370-381, 1991

4. Risdon RA, Sloper JC, De Wardner HE: Relationship between renal function and histological changes found in renal biopsy specimens from patients with persistent glomerular nephritis. Lancet 1:363-366, 1968

5. Schainuck LI, Striker GE, Cutler RE, Benditt EP: Structural-functional correlations in renal disease. Part II: The correlations. Hum Pathol 1:631-641, 1970

6. Bohle A, Mackensen-Haen S, von Gise H, Grund K-E, Wehrmann M, Batz Ch, Bogenschutz O, Schmitt H, Nagy J, Muller C, Muller G: The consequences of tubulo-interstitial changes for renal function in glomerulopathies. Pathol Res Pract 186:135-144, 1990

7. Mackensen-Haen S, Eissele R, Bohle A: Contribution on the correlation between morphometric parameters gained from the renal cortex and renal function in IgA nephritis. Lab Invest 59:239-244, 1988

8. Nagle RB, Bulger RE: Unilateral obstructive nephropathy in the rabbit. II. Late morphologic changes. Lab Invest 38:270-278, 1978

9. Sharma AK, Mauer SM, Kim Y, Michael AF: Interstitial fibrosis in obstructive nephropathy. Kidney Int 44:774-788, 1993

10. Nagle RB, Bulger RE, Cutler RE, Jervis HR, Benditt EP: Unilateral obstructive nephropathy in the rabbit. I. Early morphologic, physiologic, and histochemical changes. Lab Invest 28:456-467, 1973

11. Kaneto H, Morrissey J, McCracken R, Reyes A, Klahr S: Enalapril reduces collagen type IV synthesis and expansion of the interstitium in the obstructed rat kidney. Kidney Int 45:1637-1647, 1994

12. Kaneto H, Morrissey J, Klahr S: Increased expression of TGF-β1 mRNA in the obstructed kidney of rats with unilateral ureteral ligation. Kidney Int 44:313-321, 1993

13. Jones CL, Buch S, Post M, McCulloch L, Liu E, Eddy AA: Pathogenesis of interstitial fibrosis in chronic purine aminonucleoside nephrosis. Kidney Int 40:1020-1031, 1991

14. Downer G, Phan SH, Wiggins RC: Analysis of renal fibrosis in a rabbit model of crescentic nephritis. J Clin Invest 82:998-1006, 1988

15. Floege J, Johnson RJ, Gordon K, Yoshimura A, Campbell C, Iruela-Arispe L, Alpers CE, Couser WG: Altered glomerular extracellular matrix synthesis in experimental membranous nephropathy. Kidney Int 42:573-585, 1992

16. Yoshioka K, Takemura T, Tohda M, Akano N, Miyamoto H, Ooshima A, Maki S: Glomerular localization of type III collagen in human kidney disease. Kidney Int 35:1203-1211, 1989

17. Haverty TP, Kelly CJ, Hines WH, Amenta PS, Watanabe M, Harper RA, Kefalides NA, Neilson EG: Characterization of a renal tubular epithelial cell line which secretes the autologous target antigen of autoimmune experimental interstitial nephritis. J Cell Biol 107:1359-1368, 1988

18. Creely JJ, Commers PA, Haralson MA: Synthesis of type III collagen by cultured kidney epithelial cells. Connect Tissue Res 18:107-122, 1988

19. Kuncio GS, Neilson EG, Haverty T: Mechanisms of tubulointerstitial fibrosis. Kidney Int 39:550-556, 1991

20. Roberts AB, McCune BK, Sporn MB: TGF-β: Regulation of extracellular matrix. Kidney Int 41:557-559, 1992

21. Schreiner G, Harris K, Purkerson M, Klahr S: Immu-

nologic aspects of acute ureteral obstruction: Immune cell infiltrate in the kidney. Kidney Int 34:487-493, 1988

22. Brenner BM: Nephron adaptation to renal injury or ablation. Am J Physiol 249:F324-F337, 1985

23. Gibbons GH, Pratt RE, Dzau VJ: Vascular smooth muscle cell hypertrophy vs hyperplasia: Autocrine transforming growth factor-β1 expression determines growth response to angiotensin II. J Clin Invest 90:456-461, 1992

24. Johnson RJ, Alpers CE, Yoshimura A, Lombardi D, Pritzl P, Floege J, Schwartz SM: Renal injury from angiotensin II mediated hypertension. Hypertension 19:464-474, 1992

25. Couser WG, Johnson RJ: Mechanisms of progressive renal disease in glomerulonephritis. Am J Kidney Dis 23:193-198, 1994

26. Border WA, Noble NA: Cytokines in renal disease: The role of transforming growth factor-β. Am J Kidney Dis 22:105-113, 1993

LIPIDS AND RENAL DISEASE

Introduction

The mechanisms by which hyperlipidemia may affect the progression of chronic renal disease are incompletely understood. However, both direct and indirect effects of hyperlipidemia may lead to glomerular and perhaps interstitial damage. In addition, it is known that lipoprotein abnormalities are common in patients with renal disease, occurring in most patients with diabetes or nephrotic syndrome and in 30% to 50% of patients with chronic renal failure.

Avram, in a manuscript entitled ''Low-Density Lipoprotein Immunofluorescence at the Site of Renal Injury in Glomerulosclerosis: A Potential Pathogenetic Role for Lipids in Renal Disease,'' links cholesterol with vasoactive responses in animals and humans. He also describes the presence of anti–low-density lipoprotein (LDL) immunofluorescence at the site of renal injury, thus offering immunohistologic evidence of a possible role for this atherogenic lipoprotein in the genesis of renal disease.

A potential cellular mechanism for the ''nephrotoxicity'' of LDL is suggested by Schlondorff, who notes that fenestrated endothelium allows LDL particles access to subendothelial matrix and that mesangial cells closely regulate LDL uptake. Low-density lipoprotein not incorporated by mesangial cells can be trapped in the extracellular matrix. Low-density lipoprotein bound to the matrix can be oxidatively modified, rendering it cytotoxic to mesangial cells. Schlondorff proposes a ''two-hit'' model of lipid-induced injury. First, in dyslipidemic states, LDL accumulates in the mesangial matrix. Expansion or advanced cross-linking of the matrix will further enhance LDL trapping. Second, during oxidative stress from, for example, hypoxia or inflammatory or mechanical injury, the LDL is modified, rendering it cytotoxic and resulting in mesangial and endothelial injury, monocyte influx, and a vicious cycle of matrix expansion and cell injury.

Illingworth presents a comprehensive review of lipoprotein metabolism that outlines the key role of specific apoproteins in the biogenesis, intravascular metabolism, and cellular uptake of lipoproteins in humans. Increases in the plasma concentrations of lipoproteins may result from defects in the synthesis or catabolism of these particles, and genetic defects in lipoprotein metabolism have provided unique insights as to the role of specific lipoproteins in promoting lipid accumulation in tissues. Knowledge of the normal and abnormal pathways of lipoprotein metabolism provides the framework for future studies to delineate, at the cellular and subcellular level, factors that contribute to an enhanced rate of uptake of lipoproteins by specific tissues that may be associated with accelerated rates of glomerular injury or the development of atherosclerosis.

Using rats with dietary-induced hypercholesterolemia, Guijarro et al evaluated the glomerular changes observed before the development of glomerulosclerosis. An early macrophage influx was observed, associated with increased glomerular size, mesangial matrix expansion, lipid deposits, and foam cell formation. Increases in type IV collagen, fibronectin, and laminin were observed, and mRNA expression for transforming growth factor-β (TGF-β) was up-regulated in the glomerulus. The authors note that these early changes are reminiscent of the development of atherosclerosis in arterial walls.

Mulec et al show that the prognosis of diabetic nephropathy has improved remarkably. The disease that was considered to progress relentlessly toward uremia can now be arrested in many patients. In a prospective long-term study of patients with type 1 diabetes and nephropathy, with effective antihypertensive treatment, the cholesterol level was closely correlated to the decline in kidney function. Those patients with low cholesterol levels who were treated with an angiotensin-converting enzyme inhibitor (ACEI) had an especially favorable renal prognosis. This suggests that lipoproteins are harmful to glomerular structures when transported across the damaged glomerular capillary membrane and that ACEI can reduce the deleterious effect of this traffic.

O'Donnell et al demonstrate that the administration of a lipid-lowering agent (lovastatin) beneficially affects the progression of established renal disease. In addition to providing new insights into mechanism of action, these authors show that inhibition with a 3-hydroxy-3-methylglutaryl-coenzyme A (HMG-CoA) reductase inhibitor influences the biology of mesangial cells of obese Zucker rats with established glomerular injury.

Akmal et al report that chronic excess of parathyroid hormone may, in turn, increase the calcium burden of adipose tissue and liver and may impair hepatic and lipoprotein lipases. The reduction of these enzymes may also impair peripheral removal of triglycerides, leading to hypertriglyceridemia. The authors suggest that verapamil may affect these metabolic enzymes.

D'Amico and Gentile report a diet low in protein and cholesterol and rich in polyunsaturated fatty acids showed favorable results in patients suffering from dyslipidemia associated with the nephrotic syndrome and chronic renal insufficiency. Compliance with the diet paralleled improved hypercholesterolemia and, in patients with progressive renal damage, improved hypertriglyceridemia. Proteinuria also improved in nephrotic patients. The authors contend that dietary intervention should be the first-line treatment for the dyslipidemia of these renal diseases.

Low-Density Lipoprotein Immunofluorescence at the Site of Renal Injury in Glomerulosclerosis: A Potential Pathogenetic Role for Lipids in Renal Disease

Morrell M. Avram, MD

● The role of lipids in the genesis of renal disease has received increased attention. We describe the presence of anti–low-density lipoprotein immunofluorescence at the site of renal injury found by light microscopy. This may offer immunohistologic evidence for a potential role of this atherogenic lipid in the genesis of renal disease and glomerulosclerosis. Furthermore, we describe the contribution of cholesterol in early renal disease and markers for malnutrition in the dialytic management of end-stage renal disease. Interventional strategies, including vasoactive agents present and future, are presented.

INDEX WORDS: Cholesterol; low-density lipoprotein immunofluorescence; glomerulosclerosis; vasoactive agents; prealbumin; renal failure malnutrition.

VASCULAR INJURY or dysfunction secondary to hypercholesterolemia is a major factor in the development of atherosclerosis.[1-4] The presence of lipids in vessel walls, especially endothelial cells, at early stages of atherosclerotic injury supports this view.[5,6] We found anti–low-density lipoprotein (LDL) immunofluorescence by light microscopy in a cross section of an area of segmental sclerosis in a human glomerulus (Figs 1 and 2). The presence of this atherogenic fraction of cholesterol in an area of microscopic renal injury supports the concept that glomerulosclerosis and larger vessel atherosclerosis may share common pathogenic mechanisms.[7,8]

Lipid disturbances have effects other than atherogenesis. Low cholesterol predicts morbidity and mortality in humans.[8-11] High cholesterol levels affect vessel function and pathology in animals.[7,12-14] Serum albumin, prealbumin, and serum cholesterol can be used to assess nutritional status. We have recently reported that serum cholesterol and albumin predict survival in patients with end-stage renal disease[15] and we have also reported that prealbumin is an even more sensitive marker of malnutrition and mortality risk in chronic uremia.[16]

Additionally, the discovery of particular subfractions of total cholesterol, such as oxidated LDL and lipoprotein(a), illustrates the difficulties in understanding the role of circulating and tissue lipids in derangements of vessel wall function and structure.[17,18] Lipoprotein(a) is an LDL-like particle that has been linked to atherosclerosis. However, because of its unusual apoprotein, which has strong homology with plasminogen, lipoprotein(a) may directly interfere with the fibrinolytic system.[19,20] and hence may promote thrombosis. Since lipoprotein(a) levels are increased threefold to fourfold in end-stage renal disease.[21,22] we also examined the implications of this lipoprotein in dialysis patients. We found that lipoprotein(a) levels correlated with the incidence of arteriovenous access events over 14 months.[16] Other investigators have found it to predict cardiovascular events over 4 years in dialysis patients.[21] These reports suggest a complex interaction of the effects of serum lipids on renal function, vessel tone, nutrition, hemodynamics, atherosclerosis, and mortality. The obvious challenge with regard to lipids and hypertension is to deduce strategies (exercise,[23] dietary,[24-26] and pharmacologic,[27-29]) for retarding progression to chronic renal failure. In this regard, the most promising pharmacologic strategies involve vasoactive and hypolipidemic agents. A number of vasoactive agents currently in use, such as calcium antagonists, angiotensin-converting enzyme inhibitors, and α blockers, and those of potential use in the future, such as endothelin inhibitors and nitric oxide agonists, are receiving increasing investigative attention.

The interaction of lipids, nutrition (prealbumin), and hemodynamics is also important dur-

Supported in part by grants from The National Kidney Foundation of New York/New Jersey, the Nephrology Foundation of Brooklyn, and The Guild (Gift Shop Division) of The Long Island College Hospital.

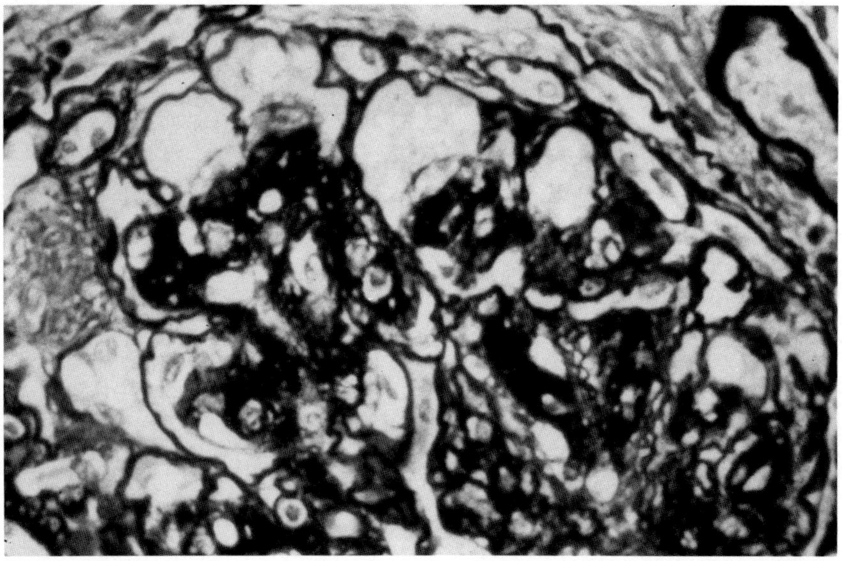

Fig 1. Glomerulus with segmental sclerosis abundant with lipid vacuoles. (Periodic acid silver-methenamine counterstained with hematoxylin-eosin; original magnification ×250, reduced by 30%.)

ing chronic uremia management whether dialytic[10,15,16,30] or associated with transplantation.[31] Vasoactive alterations are especially marked in the diabetic patient at risk for renal failure. Cholesterol may be a major risk factor for diabetic nephropathy.[32] Hypolipidemic agents have been shown to retard progression to renal failure.[6] This new and vital information allows refinement in the prevention and management of renal failure.

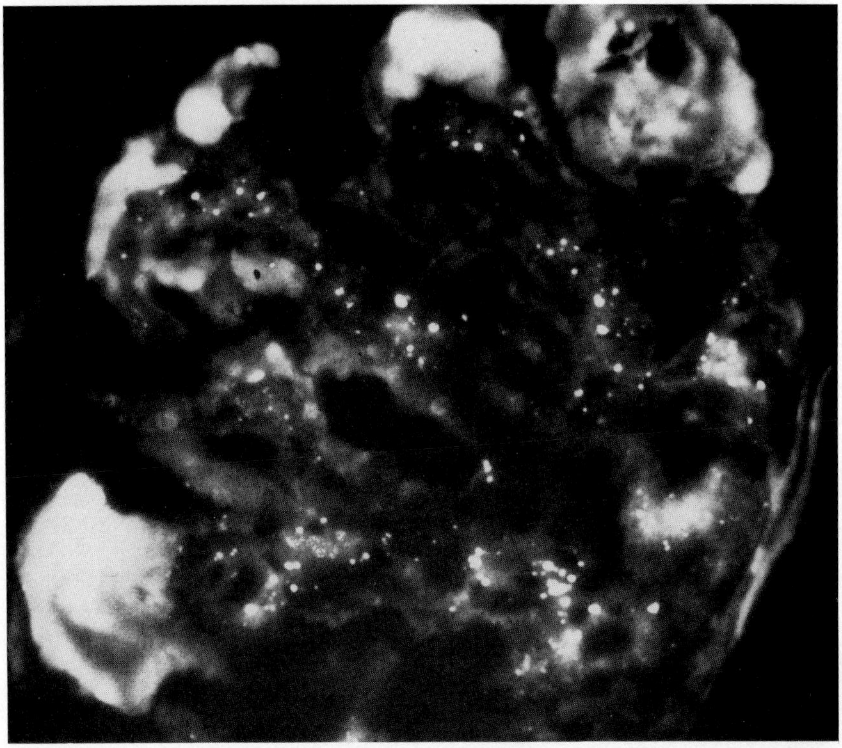

Fig 2. Presence of anti-LDL immunofluorescence staining at the site of renal injury. (Original magnification ×250, reduced by 30%.)

ACKNOWLEDGMENT

The author thanks Dr Gloria Gallo for her expert interpretation of the biopsy material and Marilyn Collins for her technical assistance in preparing this manuscript.

REFERENCES

1. Heistad DD, Armstrong ML, Marcus ML, Pregors DJ, Mark AL: Augmented responses to vasoconstrictor stimuli in hypercholesterolemic and atherosclerotic monkeys. Circulation Res 54:711-718, 1984

2. Creager MA, Cooke JP, Mendelsohn ME, Gallagher SH, Coleman SM, Loscaizo J, Dzau VJ: Impaired vasodilation of forearm resistance vessels in hypercholesterolemic humans. J Clin Invest 86:228-234, 1990

3. Osborne JA, Siegman MJ, Sedar AW, Mooers SU, Lefer AM: Lack of endothelium-dependent relaxation in coronary resistance arteries of cholesterol-fed rabbits. Am J Physiol 256:C591-C597, 1989

4. Luscher TF, Cooke JP, Houston BS, Neves RJ, Vanhoutte PM: Endothelium-dependent relaxations in human arteries. Mayo Clin Proc 62:601-606, 1987

5. Avram MM: Similarities between glomerular sclerosis and atherosclerosis in human renal biopsy specimens: A role for lipoprotein glomerulopathy. Am J Med 87:39-41, 1989

6. Keane WF, Kasiske B, O'Donnell M, Schmitz PG: Therapeutic implications of lipid-lowering agents in the progression of renal disease. Am J Med 87:21-24, 1989

7. Kasiske BL, O'Donnell MP, Schmitz PG, Kim Y, Keane WF: Renal injury of diet-induced hypercholesterolemia in rats. Kidney Int 37:880-891, 1990

8. Jacobs D, Blackburn H, Higgins M, Reed D, Iso H, McMillan G, Neaton J, Nelson J, Potter J, Rifking B, Rossouw J, Shekelle R, Yusuf S: Report of the conference on low blood cholesterol: Mortality associations. Circulation 86:1046-1060, 1992

9. Muldoon MF, Manuck SB, Matthews KA: Lowering cholesterol concentrations and mortality: A quantitative review of primary prevention trials. Br Med J 301:309-314, 1990

10. Avram MM, Goldwasser P, Burrell DE, Antignani A, Fein PA, Mittman N: The uremic dyslipidemia: A cross-sectional and longitudinal study. Am J Kidney Dis 20:324-335, 1992

11. Neaton JD, Blackburn H, Jacobs D, Kuller L, Lee D-J, Sherwin R, Shih J, Stamler J, Wentworth D: Serum cholesterol level and mortality findings for men screened in the multiple risk factor intervention trial. Arch Intern Med 152:1490-1500, 1992

12. Harrison DG, Armstrong ML, Freiman PC, Heistad DD: Restoration of endothelium-dependent relaxation by dietary treatment of atherosclerosis. J Clin Invest 80:1808-1811, 1987

13. Osborne JA, Lento PH, Siegfried MR, Stahl GH, Fushman B, Lefer AM: Cardiovascular effects of acute hypercholesterolemia in rabbits. Reversal with lovastatin treatment. J Clin Invest 83:465-473, 1989

14. Anderson S, King AJ, Brenner BM: Hyperlipidemia and glomerular sclerosis: An alternative viewpoint. Am J Med 87:34-38, 1989

15. Goldwasser P, Mittman N, Antignani A, Burrell D, Michel M-A, Collier J, Avram MM: Predictors of mortality in hemodialysis patients. J Am Soc Nephrol 3:1613-1622, 1993

16. Goldwasser P, Michel M-A, Collier J, Mittman N, Fein PA, Gusik SA, Avram MM: Prealbumin and lipoprotein(a) in hemodialysis: Relationships with patient and vascular access survival. Am J Kidney Dis 21:215-225, 1993

17. Steinberg D, Parthasarathy S, Carew TE, Khoo J, Witzem JL: Modifications of low-density lipoprotein that increase its atherogenicity. N Engl J Med 320:915-924, 1989

18. Ramirez LC, Arauz-Pacheco C, Lackner C, Albright G, Adams BV, Raskin P: Lipoprotein(a) levels in diabetes mellitus: Relationship to metabolic control. Ann Intern Med 117:42-47, 1992

19. Morrisett JD, Guyton JR, Gaubatz JW, Gotto AM, Jr: Lipoprotein(a): Structure, metabolism, and epidemiology, in Gotto AM, Jr (ed): Plasma Lipoproteins. Amsterdam, The Netherlands, Elsevier Science, 1987, pp 129-152

20. McLean JW, Tomlinson JE, Kuang WJ, Eaton DL, Chen EY, Fless GM, Scanu AM. Lawn RM: cDNA sequence of human apolipoprotein(a) is homologous to plasminogen. Nature 330:132-137, 1987

21. Cressman MD, Haykra RJ, Paganini EP, O'Neil J, Skibinski CI, Hoff HF: Lipoprotein(a) is an independent risk factor for cardiovascular disease in hemodialysis patients. Circulation 86:475-482, 1992

22. Parra HJ, Mezdour H, Cachera C, Dracon M, Tacquet A, Fruchart JC: Lp(a) lipoprotein in patients with chronic renal failure treated by hemodialysis. Clin Chem 33:721, 1987

23. Exercise and HDL. Harvard Health Letter 17, No 10, August 1992

24. Kusek JW, Caggiula AW, Williams GW, Klahr S: An overview of the modification of diet in renal disease study. Contrib Nephrol 81:50-60, 1990

25. D'Amico G, Gentile MG: Influence of diet on lipid abnormalities in human renal disease. Am J Kidney Dis 21:151-157, 1993

26. Klahr S: Low-protein diets and angiotensin-converting enzyme inhibition in progressive renal failure. Am J Kidney Dis 21:114-119, 1993

27. Bjorck S, Mulec H, Johnsen SA, Norden G, Aurel M: Renal protective effect of enalapril in diabetic nephropathy. Br Med J 304:339-343, 1992

28. Harris KPG, Purkerson ML, Yates J, Klahr S: Lovastatin ameliorates the development of glomerulosclerosis and uremia in experimental nephrotic syndrome. Am J Kidney Dis 15:16-23, 1990

29. Spitalewitz S, Porush JG, Cattran D, Wright N: Treatment of hyperlipidemia in the nephrotic syndrome: The effects of pravastatin therapy. Am J Kidney Dis 21:143-150, 1993

30. Thillet J, Faucher C, Issad B, Allouache M, Chapman J, Jacobs C: Lipoprotein(a) in patients treated by continuous ambulatory peritoneal dialysis. Am J Kidney Dis 21:226-232, 1993

31. Markell MS, Sumrani N, DiBenedetto A, Friedman EA: Effect of early hyperlipidemia on graft and patient survival in cyclosporine-treated renal transplant patients. Am J Kidney Dis 21:233-239, 1993

32. Mulec H, Johnsen SA, Wiklund O, Björck S. Cholesterol: A major renal risk factor in diabetic nephropathy? Am J Kidney Dis 21:196-201, 1993

Cellular Mechanisms of Lipid Injury in the Glomerulus

Detlef Schlondorff, MD

● Hyperlipidemias may play a role in the progression of various renal diseases, including diabetes mellitus. We therefore examined the characteristics of low-density lipoprotein (LDL) binding and uptake in cultured rat mesangial cells. Mesangial cells bound and took up LDL in a manner consistent with specific receptor mediation. Furthermore, exposure of mesangial cells to LDL enhanced intracellular cholesteryl esterification and decreased de novo cholesterol synthesis. Mesangial cells expressed mRNA for LDL receptor and their expression was downregulated after preloading of cells with LDL. These results are consistent with regulation of cholesterol uptake and metabolism by a specific LDL receptor mechanism. During diabetes the apolipoprotein B of LDL undergoes nonenzymatic glycation, which may alter its affinity for the LDL receptor. Glycation of LDL reduced its affinity for binding to the receptor sites and decreased its uptake by mesangial cells. Thus, during diabetes less LDL may be taken up and more remain extracellularly, where it can be trapped in the matrix. Oxidation of LDL bound to extracellular matrix is believed to be a major factor in the pathobiology of hyperlipidemias. Specific scavenger receptors for oxidized LDL have been described and cloned. We therefore examined whether rat mesangial cells bound and took up oxidized LDL. We demonstrated low-affinity but high-capacity binding sites for oxidized LDL on mesangial cells. In contrast to LDL, which supported mesangial cell proliferation, oxidized LDL was cytotoxic for the cells and resulted in stimulation of mesangial cell prostaglandin E_2 production. Trapping of LDL in the extracellular matrix is considered an initial event in LDL-induced vascular pathology. We therefore evaluated binding of LDL and modified LDL to extracellular matrix produced by cultured mesangial cells. Mesangial matrix had a high capacity to bind LDL and modified LDL (glycated or oxidized) in a nonsaturable manner. These results obtained with cultured mesangial cells and their matrix allow the formulation of a working hypothesis. Under normal eulipemic conditions mesangial cells handle LDL in a regulated manner. During hyperlipidemia or expansion of extracellular matrix LDL accumulates in the matrix. There LDL would be subject to oxidative modifications, especially under conditions of mesangial cell stress, such as inflammatory, mechanical, or ischemic injury. Part of the oxidized LDL could be taken up by scavenger receptors on mesangial cells and monocyte-macrophages, resulting in foam cell formation. Excess oxidized LDL, and specifically the lipid peroxides and lysolipids of oxidized LDL, would act as cytotoxic agents on mesangial, epithelial, and endothelial cells, thereby contributing to a vicious cycle of cell damage and sclerosis.

INDEX WORDS: Low-density lipoprotein; low-density lipoprotein receptors; kidney; mesangial cells; mesangial matrix; lipid injury.

IN THE KIDNEY the glomerulus and renal interstitium may be preferred locations for lipid depositions because of the presence of fenestrated endothelia in glomerular and peritubular capillaries and ascending vasa recta. Furthermore, the glomerular mesangial matrix and mesangial cells are not separated from the capillary stream by an intervening basement membrane. In most other locations plasma lipid particles, such as low-density lipoproteins (LDL), will have limited access to perivascular tissue because of the relative impermeability of the tight endothelium and underlying basement membrane to particles the size of LDL.

Because of these special anatomic features net accumulation of LDL in the mesangium will be determined by the balance between (1) delivery of LDL, (2) binding of LDL to the mesangial matrix, (3) uptake of LDL by mesangial cells and macrophages, and (4) egress of LDL from the mesangium via intermesangial channels and the reverse cholesterol pathway. The delivery of LDL will in turn be determined by (1) the concentration of LDL in plasma, (2) the glomerular plasma flow, (3) the intraglomerular hydrostatic pressure, and (4) the permeability of the endothelial-mesangial interface.

In analogy to the development of atherosclerotic lesions in other vascular beds, deposition and uptake of LDL in the glomerular mesangium and renal interstitium may contribute to the progression of renal disease. The binding and uptake of LDL by mesangial cells and the trapping of LDL in the mesangial matrix are therefore of interest and have been studied during recent years.

BINDING AND UPTAKE OF LOW-DENSITY LIPOPROTEINS BY MESANGIAL CELLS

Uptake of cholesterol-containing lipids is essential for the survival and growth of mammalian

---

Supported by National Institutes of Health Grants No. DK 41566 and DK22036.

cells. In general, uptake and metabolism of LDL is tightly regulated and involves specific LDL receptors.[1] However, receptor-independent uptake of LDL by nonspecific endocytosis also occurs and may account for approximately 30% of LDL clearance.[2] Low-density lipoprotein receptors recognize apolipoprotein B 100 of LDL as well as apolipoprotein E on intermediate-density LDL and beta-very low-density lipoprotein particles.[1,3] Specific binding and uptake of LDL also can be demonstrated with cultured rat and human mesangial cells.[4-6] In initial studies we performed equilibrium binding of radiolabeled LDL to mesangial cells.[4] Binding of LDL is a saturable process with half-maximal binding occurring at LDL protein concentrations of 5 μg/mL. The binding characteristics are similar to those described for other systems.[1] Uptake studies with ^{125}I-labeled LDL were consistent with recycling of LDL receptors.[4] Fluorescent-labeled LDL was taken up by all cultured mesangial cells in a pattern consistent with lysosomal accumulation.[4] Low-density lipoprotein provides cells with cholesterol that is in part esterified with fatty acids such as oleic acid[1] by the acyl-co-enzyme A-cholesterol-acyltransferase. As shown in Fig 1, incubation of mesangial cells with increasing concentrations of LDL and [^{14}C]oleate resulted in enhanced intracellular formation of [^{14}C]oleate cholesteryl esters, indicating that the cells used LDL-cholesterol for the formation of cholesteryl esters. In these studies we also evaluated de novo synthesis of cholesterol by the mesangial cells. Uptake of LDL-cholesterol should decrease cellular synthesis of cholesterol by downregulating the activity of beta-hydroxy-beta-methyl-glutaryl CoA reductase.[1] Preincubation of mesangial cells with increasing concentrations of LDL increased LDL-cholesterol esterification but decreased de novo cholesterol synthesis (Fig 2). To further substantiate the existence and regulation of LDL receptors on mesangial cells we performed Northern blot analysis. Mesangial cells were maintained for 72 hours in medium containing 5% lipoprotein-deficient serum. Cells were then incubated for 24 hours in the same medium or in medium with the addition of 20 or 200 μg/mL of LDL. After 24 hours, total cellular RNA was extracted, separated on agarose gel electrophoresis, transferred to nylon membrane, and hybridized with a cDNA probe for the rat LDL receptor.[7] As shown in Fig 3, mesangial cells contain mRNA for the LDL receptor that has the expected size of 4.8 kb.[7] When mesangial cells had been cholesterol loaded by the addition of LDL to the medium the mRNA levels for the LDL receptor decreased. These results are consistent with downregulation of LDL receptor expression by cholesterol loading.[1]

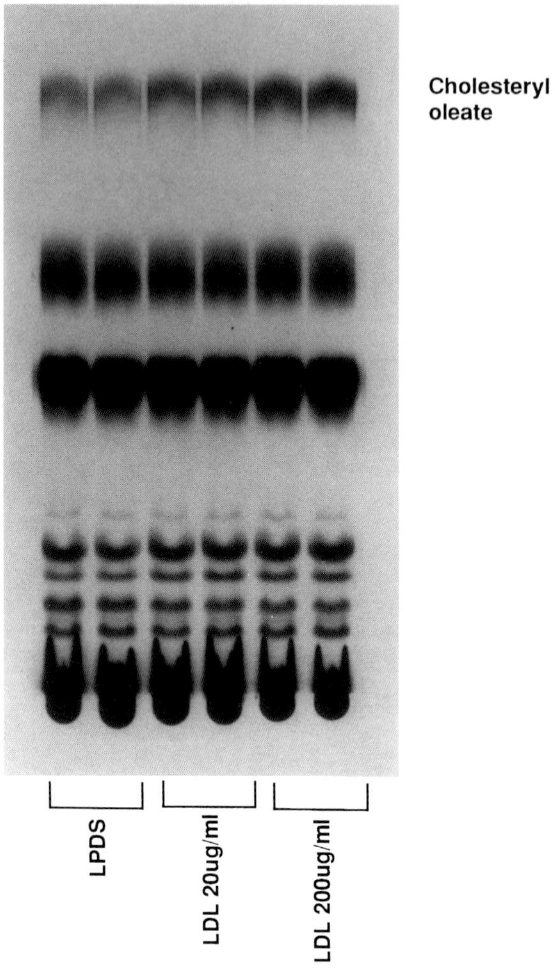

Fig 1. Incubation of mesangial cells with LDL increases [^{14}C]oleate incorporation into intracellular cholesteryl esters. Mesangial cells were incubated for 24 hours with either lipoprotein-deficient serum (LPDS) alone or with the addition of 20 or 200 μg/mL LDL. [^{14}C]oleate was then added for 2 hours before cellular lipids were extracted and separated by thin-layer chromatography. Results are from one experiment, carried out in duplicate. Preincubation with increasing concentrations of LDL enhanced the formation of [^{14}C]cholesteryl oleate, while [^{14}C]oleate uptake into other cellular lipids remained unchanged.

In summary, the experiments with LDL bind-

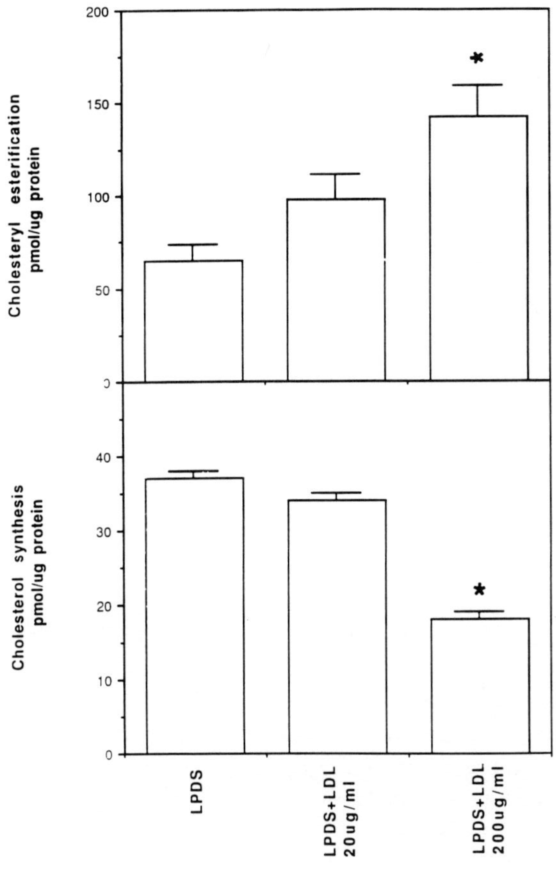

Fig 2. Incubation of mesangial cells with LDL increases [^{14}C]oleate incorporation into cholesteryl esters and decreases de novo cholesterol synthesis. Mesangial cells were incubated in lipoprotein-deficient serum (LPDS) alone or with the addition of 20 or 200 μg/mL of LDL for 24 hours. [^{14}C]oleate was added 2 hours before cellular lipids were extracted and analyzed for [^{14}C]cholesteryl oleate and de novo cholesterol synthesis. Results are means ± SEM from four series of experiments. Asterisks indicate *P* < 0.01 as compared with controls.

ing, uptake, cholesterol esterification, and de novo synthesis and the Northern analysis clearly show that mesangial cells regulate their receptor-mediated uptake of LDL and their cholesterol metabolism in response to changes in extracellular LDL concentrations.

REGULATION OF LOW-DENSITY LIPOPROTEIN UPTAKE BY VASOACTIVE AGENTS AND CYTOKINES

Low-density lipoprotein uptake by mesangial cells may also be influenced by the activity of the cytoskeleton. We recently showed that angiotensin II and a thromboxane analog enhance uptake of macromolecules, including LDL, by cultured mesangial cells.[8] These effects could be mitigated by agents increasing the intracellular cyclic adenisine monophosphate concentrations, such as prostaglandin E_2 (PGE_2).[8] Cyclic adenosine monophosphate is known to influence the cytoskeleton, specifically actin filaments in mesangial cells.[9] Thus, agents increasing mesangial contractility will enhance macromolecular up-

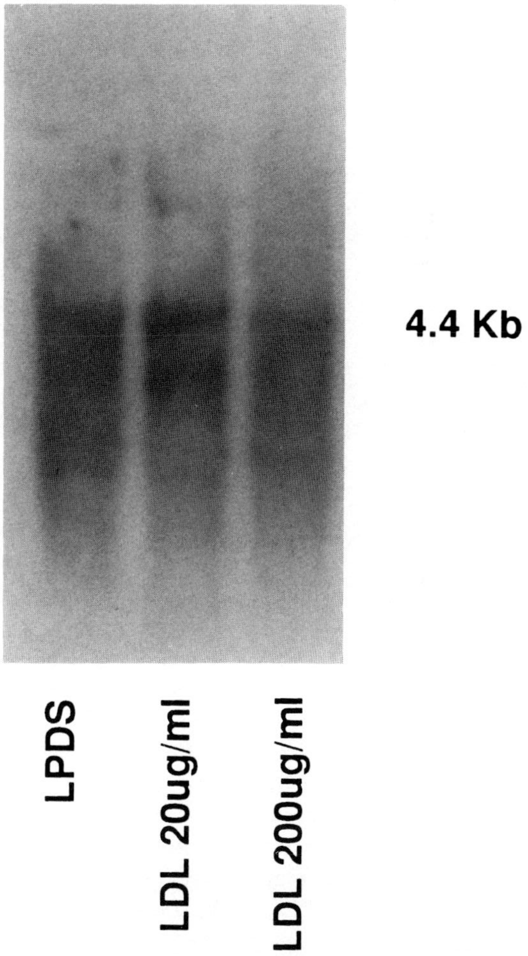

Fig 3. Pretreatment of mesangial cells with LDL decreases mRNA levels for the LDL receptor. Mesangial cells were incubated in lipoprotein-deficient serum (LPDS) alone or with the addition of 20 or 200 μg/mL of LDL. Total RNA was extracted after 24 hours and analyzed by Northern blotting for mRNA of the LDL receptor. Pretreatment with increasing concentrations of LDL decreased the mRNA level for the LDL receptor. No change was observed in mRNA levels for GAPDH, which served as controls for equal RNA loading (results not shown).

take, while vasorelaxant substances may decrease endocytosis. While these effects are only of a modulatory nature, they may be of interest for mesangial handling of LDL during progressive renal diseases, which frequently are associated with increased levels of angiotensin II and thromboxane.

The effects of the vasoactive agents on LDL uptake occurred within an hour and are therefore unlikely to relate to a change in LDL receptor synthesis. However, some cytokines are capable of regulating LDL receptors.[1] Thus, Grone et al reported that a 15-hour preincubation of human mesangial cells with endothelin or platelet-derived growth factor (PDGF) increased LDL uptake approximately twofold.[6] These effects appeared to depend on de novo protein synthesis, as they were abrogated by the protein synthesis inhibitor cycloheximide. The most likely explanation for these findings would be that endothelin and PDGF increase the synthesis of LDL receptors. Both endothelin and PDGF cause proliferation of mesangial cells and LDL synergized with these effects.[6] Thus increased LDL receptor expression during mesangial cell proliferation may serve to provide the cells with cholesterol needed for generation of, for example, new cell membranes.

GLYCATION OF LOW-DENSITY LIPOPROTEIN AND MESANGIAL CELL UPTAKE

Lipid abnormalities are frequently observed in diabetes cases. Hyperglycemia of diabetes mellitus results in nonenzymatic glycation of proteins, including hemoglobulin, albumin, and apolipoprotein B of LDL.[10,11] The extent of LDL glycation correlates with the degree of glycemic control, ranging from 2% to 8%.[12] The nonenzymatic glycation occurs by covalent binding of glucose to the epsilon amino groups of lysine residues of apolipoprotein B.[10,11] As the lysine groups are important for the interaction of LDL with the LDL receptor, it is not surprising that glycation decreases receptor-mediated uptake and metabolism of LDL in intact animals and in cultured cells.[10,13] These considerations may also apply to mesangial cells. We compared binding and uptake of native LDL and of moderately glycated LDL (5% to 8%; ie, as observed in diabetics) by cultured rat mesangial cells.[14] Glycation of LDL decreased total binding to mesangial cells by

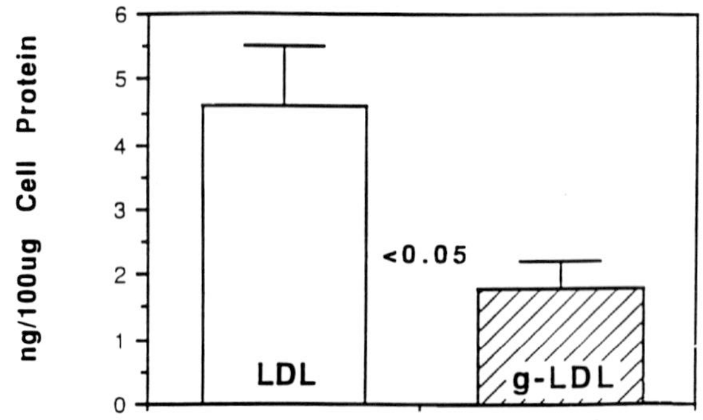

Fig 4. Specific binding of LDL and glycated LDL (g-LDL) to cultured rat mesangial cells. Specific binding of ^{125}I-labeled LDL and g-LDL (2 μg/mL) was determined at a 50-fold excess of the respective unlabeled LDL species. (Data from Gupta et al.[14])

15% to 20% as compared with native LDL.[14] Specific binding (determined to be a 50-fold excess of unlabeled glycateted LDL or LDL, respectively) of glycated LDL was reduced 50% compared with LDL (Fig 4). Competition binding studies were consistent with glycated LDL binding to the LDL receptor, but with a lower affinity than unmodified LDL.[14] The lower binding of glycated LDL also resulted in a decrease in uptake of labeled LDL and the resulting intracellular cholesteryl esterification (Fig 5).[14] Thus, 8% glycation of lysine residues on apolipoprotein B reduces its affinity for the LDL receptor and decreases uptake of glycated LDL by mesangial cells. In diabetes mellitus this modest change in handling of glycated LDL could result in increased accumulation of LDL in the mesangial matrix (see below), which may have consequences for lipid mediated glomerular injury.

BINDING AND UPTAKE OF MODIFIED LOW-DENSITY LIPOPROTEIN BY MESANGIAL CELLS

Chemical alterations of LDL such as oxidative modification reduces its recognition by the LDL receptor.[15] However, a number of cell types (above all, monocyte-macrophages) express specific scavenger receptors for modified LDL.[16] The uptake of modified LDL by scavenger receptors is not downregulated by cellular cholesterol loading and does not result in decreased cellular cholesterol synthesis.[16] This eventually causes cellular lipid overload as demonstrated by the conversion of macrophages into foam cells in,

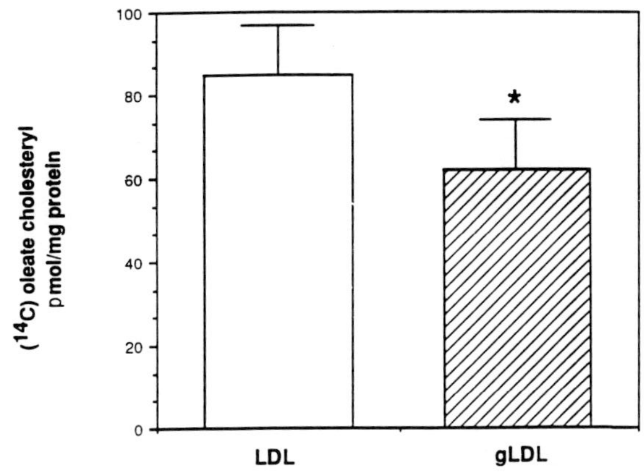

Fig 5. Effects of incubation of mesangial cells with LDL or glycated LDL (gLDL) (100 μg/mL) for 24 hours on [^{14}C]oleate incorporation into cellular cholesteryl esters. Results are means ± SEM from four experiments. (Data from Gupta et al.[14])

for example, atherosclerotic plaques. The modification of the LDL is thought to be initiated by release of reactive oxygen species by activated perivascular cells. This results in peroxidation of lipids in the LDL particles and release of chemically reactive aldehydes, such as malonaldehydes.[17] The aldehydes modify the lysine residues of apolipoprotein B, resulting in decreased positive charge and loss of LDL receptor recognition.[18] The ''oxidized'' LDL is characterized by increased density and negative charge, as demonstrated by altered mobility on agarose gel electrophoresis.[17] The ''oxidized'' LDL also contains cytotoxic lipid-peroxides and lysophospholipids.[17,19] Scavenger receptors for ''oxidized'' LDL have been characterized by binding studies and two related molecular forms have been cloned recently.[16,20,21] They only differ in their C-terminal extracellular domain and both appear to be products of a single gene.[21] The binding site of the scavenger receptors for the modified LDL has a collagenous nature that may be of special interest as LDL and modified LDL also bind to extracellular matrix (see below).

Oxidative modification of LDL can be catalyzed by reactive oxygen species released from a number of cell types, including mesangial cells.[16,17,22,23] It has been proposed that activation of lipoxygenases, which results in free radical formation, may contribute to the lipid oxidation.[24] In addition, LDL undergoes autooxidation under appropriate circumstances, ie, in the absence of antioxidants or other scavengers of free radicals and in the presence of transition metals such as iron.[19] In vivo oxidation of LDL may occur predominantly in the extravascular, interstitial microenvironment, where less protective antioxidants may be available than in the circulation. A major role for oxidative modification of LDL in the generation of atherosclerotic vascular disease has been proposed and is supported by numerous in vitro and in vivo experimental studies and by therapeutic and epidemiologic observations in patients.[17,25] As noted above, uptake of modified LDL results in the formation of foam cells and foam cells are present in the lipid-associated renal disease. We therefore examined the uptake of oxidized LDL by cultured mesangial cells. Oxidative modification of LDL (Ox-LDL) was achieved by incubating LDL in the presence of copper[26] and was verified by the altered mobility on agarose electrophoresis and the presence of thiobartiburic acid-reactive substances.[26] We found that total binding of Ox-LDL to rat mesangial cells exceeded that of native LDL fourfold to fivefold. However, in contrast to the predominant specific LDL binding, approximately 50% of labeled Ox-LDL bound nonspecifically to cultured mesangial cells, ie, they could not be displaced by excess unlabeled Ox-LDL.[26] Competition binding studies showed that LDL and Ox-LDL bound to different binding sites on mesangial cells. This was further supported by experiments with heparin and polyinosinic acid. Heparin should decrease binding of both LDL and Ox-LDL to their respective receptors, while polyinosinic acid should only interfere with Ox-LDL binding.[26] Heparin decreased the binding of both LDL and Ox-LDL, but polyinosinic acid only decreased the Ox-LDL binding. These results are also consistent with the existence of both LDL and Ox-LDL receptors on rat mesangial cells. Furthermore, rat mesangial cells took up more Ox-LDL than native LDL as determined with either labeled LDL species or with [^{14}C]oleate cholesteryl esterification.[26] Finally, Northern blot analysis confirmed the presence of mRNA for both the LDL receptor and for scavenger receptor for LDL in rat mesangial cells.[27] Grone et al recently confirmed the presence of LDL receptors on cultured human mesangial cells.[6] However they failed to detect any binding sites for either acetylated or copper-oxidized LDL on these cells.[6] Using cultured human mesangial cells, however, we were able to detect binding sites for copper-oxidized LDL. The binding characteristics were similar to those reported for rat mesangial cells. At concentrations of 2 μg LDL protein/mL the binding of oxidized LDL (150 ng/mg cell protein) exceeded that of native LDL (40 ng) by fourfold. Also similar to the results with rat mesangial cells,[26] binding of labeled, oxidized LDL to human mesangial cells could only be displaced to 40% by a 50-fold excess of unlabeled oxidized LDL. The discrepancy between our results and those of Grone et al remains unexplained at present, but may relate to differences in, for example, culture conditions. The large amount of nonspecific binding of oxidized LDL to mesangial cells may in part reflect binding of modified LDL to extracellular mesangial matrix (see below). The uptake of oxidatively modified LDL by mesangial cells is of interest as it would result in foam cell formation. Mesangial foam cells are clearly a histologic feature of the kidney in hyperlipidemia and do not correlate with the number of glomerular macrophages.[28]

IN VIVO UPTAKE OF LOW-DENSITY LIPOPROTEINS AND OXIDATIVELY MODIFIED LOW-DENSITY LIPOPROTEINS BY GLOMERULI

To verify the in vitro results on uptake of LDL and oxidized LDL in vivo, we injected radiolabeled LDL or oxidized LDL into the suprarenal aorta of rats. The localization of the LDL preparations was then determined in isolated glomerular and tubular suspensions and compared with the spleen and liver.[26] As expected, the major sites of uptake for LDL and oxidized LDL were the liver and spleen. Low-density lipoprotein localization to glomeruli exceeded that to tubules (expressed per milligram of protein) approximately twofold. A striking 10-fold increase in glomerular localization of oxidized LDL as compared with LDL was observed.[26] These studies do not allow us to determine the exact intraglomerular localization of the oxidized LDL. However, autoradiography suggested that the mesangium may represent a major locus for the intraglomerular localization of oxidized LDL.

EFFECTS OF LIPOPROTEINS ON MESANGIAL CELL PROLIFERATION

Similar to reports for other cell types, LDL enhances proliferation of mesangial cells in culture.[4,6,26] This effect has been observed uniformly at LDL protein concentrations of 10 to 50 μg/mL. The addition of higher concentrations of LDL can result in divergent effects on mesangial cell proliferation, ie, enhancement or inhibition.[4,6,26] These discrepancies most likely are due to some oxidation of LDL during the incubations with formation of cytotoxic, oxidized LDL (see below). While LDL alone only modestly enhances proliferation of cultured mesangial cells, LDL can potentiate the effect of mesangial mitogens, such as endothelin and PDGF.[6] The significance of these proliferative effects of LDL in cell culture to the in vivo situation is questionable. For example, concentrations of LDL enhancing proliferation of cultured mesangial cells (10 to 50 μg/mL) only correspond to 10% of normal plasma LDL concentration. Thus, it is unlikely that under physiologic in vivo conditions LDL ever becomes a rate-limiting factor for mesangial cell growth. The culture situation may simply reflect the need of proliferating cells for adequate lipid and cholesterol supply. Nonetheless, LDL may represent an important co-factor during pathologic situations associated with in vivo glomerular cell proliferation.

EFFECTS OF OXIDATIVELY MODIFIED LOW-DENSITY LIPOPROTEIN ON MESANGIAL CELL VIABILITY

Oxidized LDL is cytotoxic to a large number of cell types.[17] Occasionally noted cytotoxic effects of LDL can be attributed to auto-oxidation that occurs during the preparation of LDL or during incubation with cells.[29] This cytotoxicity can be eliminated by including antioxidants during the preparation of and incubation with LDL.[29] The cytotoxic components of oxidized LDL have been localized to altered lipid components.[29,30] Cytotoxicity correlates with the formation of thiobarbituric acid-reactive substances, which reflect lipid peroxidation.[29,31] The cytotoxicity of oxidized LDL is reversely related to the proliferative state of cells, with nonproliferating cells being the least susceptible.[32] In cultures of mesangial cells, oxidized LDL also decreases [^{3}H]thymidine uptake and cell number.[26] The cytotoxicity of oxidized LDL can also be demonstrated by the direct microscopic observation of cells. These effects of oxidized LDL become apparent at concentrations greater than 25 μg/mL.[26]

Thus, loss of endogenous antioxidants such as vitamin E and or oxidative stress could transform locally deposited LDL into cytotoxic substances and cause damage to endothelial, mesangial, and epithelial cells.

EFFECTS OF LIPOPROTEIN ON PROSTANOID PRODUCTION

Lipoproteins may stimulate eicosanoid synthesis. We compared the effects of native and oxidized LDL on PGE_2 production by cultured rat mesangial cells.[26] Native LDL only slightly increased PGE_2 synthesis. In contrast, oxidized LDL caused a rapid and concentration-dependent increase in PGE_2 synthesis.[26] Thus, oxidized LDL, but not LDL, may activate arachidonic acid release and eicosanoid formation. This is also consistent with our in vivo observations[33] that during experimental hypercholesterolemia oxidation of LDL causes enhanced thromboxane generation and renal vasoconstriction, an effect preventable by the antioxidant drug probucol.

INTERACTIONS OF LIPOPROTEINS WITH MESANGIAL MATRIX

Binding of LDL to the extracellular matrix of arterial walls may be an important factor contributing to the development of atherosclerosis.[17] Only 30% to 40% of the lipids appear to be "trapped" in the extracellular matrix while the rest are bound to collagen and proteoglycans.[34] The binding is mostly by ionic interactions of positive charges on lipoprotein B with negative charges on glycosaminoglycans.[35] Binding is influenced both by the character of the LDL (lipid composition, lipoprotein modification) and by the composition of the proteoglycans.[36] Furthermore, LDL binds to collagens and oxidized LDL may preferentially bind to type 1 collagen.[37] This may relate to the observation that the binding site of the scavenger receptor for LDL contains a collagenous sequence.[20] Alterations of collagen, such as advanced glycation end-product formation in diabetes mellitus, may also influence binding of LDL to extracellular matrix.[38]

Intraglomerular accumulations of lipids are prominent in hyperlipidemias and glomerulosclerosis and are preferentially localized to the extracellular mesangial matrix.[28] We therefore examined the binding of native and modified LDL to extracellular matrix generated by cultured rat

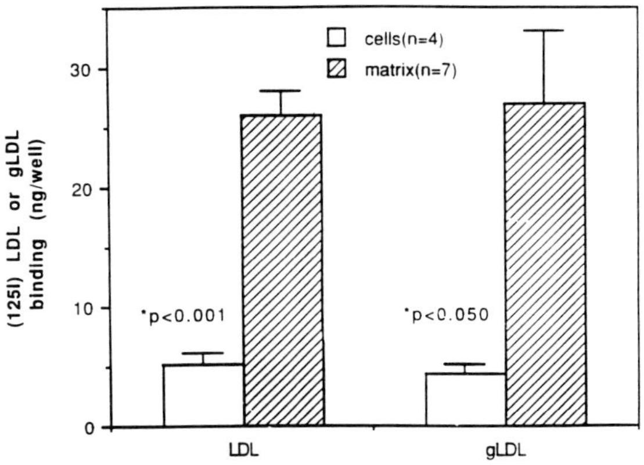

Fig 6. Comparison of binding at 2 μg/mL of LDL or glycated LDL (gLDL) to rat mesangial cells or mesangial matrix. (Used with permission from *Kidney International*, volume 41, page 1166, 1992.[14])

mesangial cells.[14] After 3 weeks of culture the mesangial cells were removed by a detergent-lysis buffer, leaving behind their extracellular matrix. This matrix contains collagens (mostly types I and IV), laminin, fibronectin, and chondroitin and dermatan sulfates.[39] Binding of native LDL, glycated LDL, and oxidized LDL to intact mesangial cells and to the preparation of extracellular mesangial matrix was compared. Both native and modified LDL bound to a considerable extent to the matrix. The binding of LDL to the matrix exceeded that to the cultured mesangial cells, when compared on the basis of area of the culture dish covered by either cells or matrix (Fig 6). However, the binding characteristics of LDL and modified LDL to cells or matrix differed considerably. Binding to cells was a saturable process, consistent with receptor mediation. In contrast, binding to matrix showed no sign of saturability, ie, to appears to not be receptor mediated.[14] The binding to matrix of both LDL and glycated LDL was comparable (26 ± 2 and 27 ± 6 ng bound/1.7 cm^2 matrix for LDL and glycated LDL, respectively, at 2 μg/mL of lipoprotein and 283 ± 44 and 267 ± 44 ng bound/1.7 cm^2, respectively, at 100 μg/mL of lipoprotein). Matrix binding of LDL and Ox-LDL were comparable at 2 μg/mL of the respective lipoprotein preparation, but at higher concentrations more Ox-LDL than LDL bound to the matrix (Fig 7; for details, refer to ref 14). Thus, extracellular mesangial matrix has a large capacity to retain LDL, findings consistent with the in vivo localization

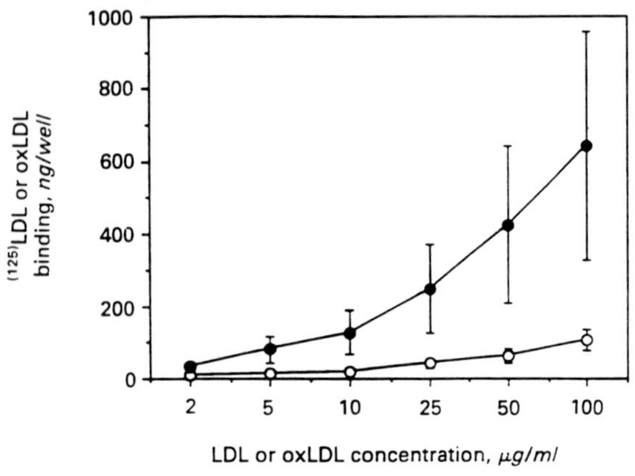

Fig 7. Concentration-dependent binding of [^{125}I]-LDL (○) and [^{125}I]Ox-LDL (●) to mesangial matrix. Results are from four series of experiments. (Used with permission from *Kidney International*, volume 41, page 1166, 1992.[14])

of lipids to glomerular extracellular matrix and to areas of matrix expansion in glomerular diseases.

Besides matrix expansion, changes in matrix characteristics might also influence glomerular trapping of LDL. Cross-linking of matrix components due to the formation of nonenzymatic glycation end products is considered to contribute to extracellular matrix expansion of aging and, in an accelerated fashion, in diabetes mellitus.[40] We therefore also compared binding of LDL and modified LDL to mesangial matrix (prepared as above) and to matrix that was nonenzymatically modified.[14] The modification was performed in vitro by exposure of the matrix to high glucose concentrations (mmol/L) or to glycolaldehyde, a cross-linking agent that may mimic the process of protein cross-linking of advanced diabetes.[39,40] A 2-week exposure of matrix to high glucose did not influence the binding of LDL compared with control matrix.[14] However, cross-linking of matrix components by glycolaldehyde doubled the binding for either LDL or glycated LDL (Fig 8).[14] While the significance of the glycolaldehyde modification to diabetes remains debatable, these results indicate that changes in matrix characteristics could influence LDL accumulation in the mesangial matrix.

HOW COULD LOW-DENSITY LIPOPROTEIN CONTRIBUTE TO THE PROGRESSION OF GLOMERULAR AND RENAL DISEASES?

Under normal, eulipemic conditions a balance exists between delivery, utilization, and removal of LDL from the glomerulus (Fig 9A). Low-density lipoprotein is taken up in a tightly regulated manner by glomerular cells and is used as a source of cholesterol for remodeling of membranes and of fatty acids for metabolism and generation of lipid mediators. In addition, some of the cholesterol may be removed by the reverse cholesterol pathway and some may leave via intermesangial channels to reach lymphatics or reenter blood vessels. Some LDL may remain trapped in the mesangial matrix, but is in equilibrium with the capillary blood stream and cellular uptake. This LDL contains adequate amounts of antioxidants and, in the absence of oxidative stress, does not undergo oxidative modification. Thus, no pathology occurs. The situation may be different with excessive LDL accumulation in the mesangium and or oxidative stress (Fig 9B). During hyperlipidemia, increased amounts of LDL would reach the mesangium exceeding the requirement of the cells. The cells would downregulate their receptor-mediated uptake and the excess LDL would remain trapped in the matrix. Similarly, any process resulting in expansion of mesangial matrix will result in increased accumulation of LDL. In the matrix, LDL-associated antioxidants would slowly be depleted and eventually LDL would be subject to oxidative modification by reactive oxygen species generated by, for example, endothelial and mesangial cells. The modified LDL could be taken up by mesangial cells via scavenger receptors, resulting in their transformation into foam cells. At the same time,

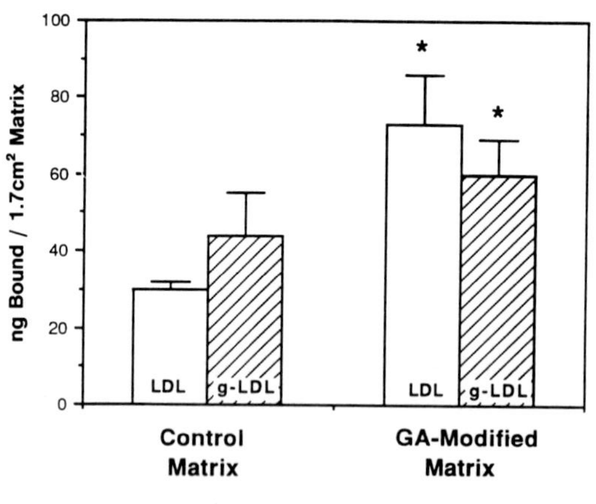

Fig 8. Binding of LDL or glycated LDL (g-LDL) to unmodified mesangial cell matrix or to glycoaldehyde (GA)-modified matrix. (Data from Gupta et al.[14])

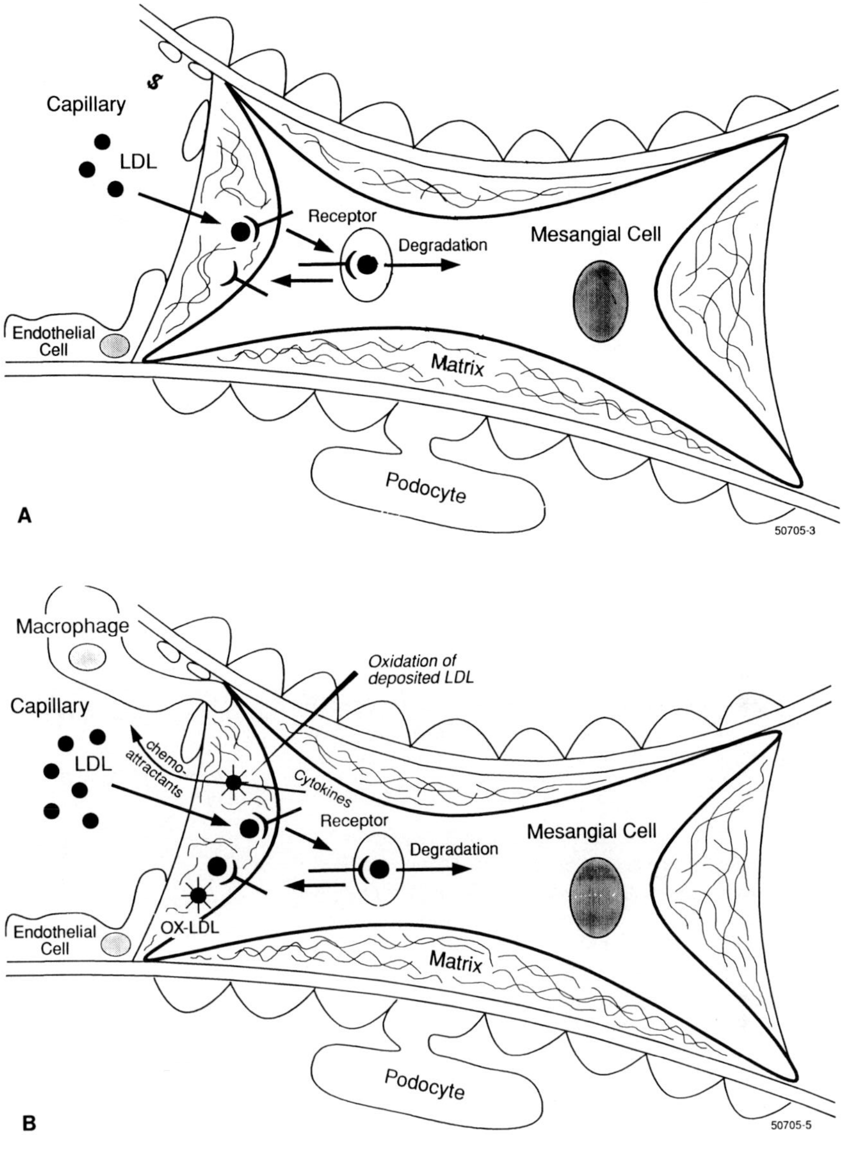

Fig 9. Schematic representation of LDL handling by mesangial cells under (A) control conditions and during (B) hyperlipidemia in the presence of oxidative stress.

monocyte-macrophages would be attracted and also remove the modified LDL. A new steady state might result with excess lipids in the mesangium and formation of foam cells, but without any major further pathology.

During glomerular diseases the above process would be accelerated as generation of reactive oxygen species would be increased. In consequence, excess oxidation of LDL would result and cause build-up of cytotoxic lipid components and activation of endothelial and mesangial cells and of leukocytes and platelets. These, in turn, would release lipid mediators of inflammation and a variety of cytokines, causing a further amplification of the disease process. Thus, two components would have to be involved in order for LDL to participate in glomerular injury: (1) hyperlipidemia and or mesangial expansion resulting in LDL trapping in the extracellular matrix, and (2) modification of the deposited LDL by increased generation of reactive oxygen species.

If this scheme is correct, therapeutic interventions designed to reduce the contribution of hyperlipidemia to the progression of renal disease should include both lowering of lipids and prevention of their oxidation by antioxidants. Antioxidant and lipid-lowering therapy may not only retard the progression of renal disease but also that of the accelerated atherosclerosis for which these patients are at risk.

ADDENDUM

Additional evidence indicates that intracellular glutathione influences collagen generation by mesangial cells.[41] The findings described suggest that the cellular redox state may influence gene transcription in mesangial cells. These observations may explain, in part, injury-associated alterations of matrix generation by mesangial cells.

REFERENCES

1. Brown MS, Goldstein JL: A receptor-mediated pathway for cholesterol homeostasis. Science 232:34-47, 1986

2. Kesaniemi YA, Witzum JL, Steinbreicher UP: Receptor-mediated catabolism of low density lipoprotein in man: Quantitation using glucosylated low density lipoprotein. J Clin Invest 71:950-959, 1983

3. Mahley RW, Innerarity TL, Pitas RE, Weisgraber KH, Brown JH, Gross E: Inhibition of lipoprotein binding to cell surface receptors of fibroblasts following selective modification of arginyl residues in arginine-rich and B apoproteins. J Biol Chem 252:7279-7287, 1977

4. Wasserman J, Santiago A, Rifici V, Holthofer H, Scharschmidt L, Epstein M, Schlondorff D: Interactions of low density lipoprotein with rat mesangial cells. Kidney Int 35:1168-1174, 1989

5. Rayner HC, Horsburgh T, Brown SL, Lavender FL, Winder AF, Walls J: Receptor-mediated endocytosis of low-density lipoprotein by cultured human glomerular cells. Nephron 55:292-299, 1990

6. Grone EF, Abboud HE, Hohne M, Walli AK, Grone H-J, Stuker D, Robenek H, Wieland E, Seidel D: Receptor-mediated uptake and action of lipoproteins in cultured human mesangial cells. Their modulation by mitogenic vasoconstrictors. Am J Physiol 262:F686-F696, 1992

7. Lee LY, Mohler WA, Schafer BL, Freudenherger JS, Connolly Byrne N, Eager KB, Mosley ST, Leighton JK, Thrift RN, Davis RA, Tanaka RD: Nucleotide sequence of the rat low density lipoprotein receptor cDNA. Nucleic Acids Res 17:1259-1260, 1989

8. Singhal PC, Gupta S, Shen Z, Schlondorff D: Effects of PGE_2 and a thromboxne A_2 analogue on uptake of IgG complexes and LDL by mesangial cells. Am J Physiol 261:F537-F544, 1991

9. Singhal PC, Scharschmidt L, Gibbons N, Hays RM: Contraction and relaxation of cultured mesangial cells on a silicone rubber surface. Kidney Int 30:862-873, 1986

10. Witztum JL, Mahoney EM, Branks MJ, Fisher M, Elam R, Steinberg D: Nonenzymatic glucosylation of low-density lipoprotein alters its biologic activity. Diabetes 31:283-291, 1982

11. Schleicher E, Deufel T, Wieland OH: Non-enzymatic glycosylation of human serum lipoproteins. FEBS Lett 129:1-4, 1981

12. Curtiss LK, Witztum JL: Plasma apoliproteins, A1, A2, B, C1 and E are glucosylated in hyperglycemic diabetic subjects. Diabetes 34:452-461, 1985

13. Gonen B, Baenziger J, Schonfeld G, Jacobson D, Farrar P: Nonenzymatic glycosylation of low density lipoproteins in vitro. Effects on cell interactive properties. Diabetes 30:875-878, 1981

14. Gupta S, Rifici V, Crowley S, Brownlee M, Shan Z, Schlondorff D: Interactions of LDL and modified LDL with mesangial cells and matrix. Kidney Int 41:1161-1169, 1992

15. Steinbrecher UP: Oxidation of human low density lipoprotein results in derivatization of lysine residues of apolipoprotein B by lipid peroxide decomposition products. J Biol Chem 262:3603-3608, 1987

16. Brown MS, Goldstein JL: Scavenging for receptors. Nature 343:508-510, 1990

17. Steinberg D, Parthasarathy S, Carew TE, Khoo JC, Witzum JL: Beyond cholesterol: Modifications of low-density lipoprotein that increase its atherogenicity. N Engl J Med 320:915-924, 1989

18. Goldstein JL, Ho YK, Basu SK, Brown MS: Binding site on macrophages that mediates uptake and degradation of acetylated low density lipoprotein, producing massive cholesterol deposition. Proc Natl Acad Sci USA 76:333-337, 1979

19. Steinbrecher UP, Parthasarathy S, Leake DS, Witztum JL, Steinberg D: Modification of low density lipoprotein by endothelial cells involves lipid peroxidation and degradation of low density lipoprotein phospholipids. Proc Natl Acad Sci USA 81:3883-3887, 1984

20. Kodama T, Freeman M, Rohrer L, Zabrecky J, Matsudaira P, Krieger M: Type 1 macrophage scavenger receptor contains alpha-helical and collagen-like coiled coils. Nature 343:531-535, 1990

21. Rohrer L, Freeman M, Kodama T, Penman M, Krieger M: Coiled-coil fibrous domains mediate ligand binding by macrophage scavenger receptor type II. Nature 343:570-572, 1990

22. Morel DW, DiCorleto PE, Chisolm GM: Endothelial and smooth muscle cells alter low density lipoprotein in vitro by free radical oxidation. Arteriosclerosis 4:357-364, 1984

23. Keane WF, Phillips J, Kasiske BL, O'Donnell MP, Kim Y: Injurious effects of low density lipoprotein (LDL) on human mesangial cells (HMC). Kidney Int 37:509, 1990 (abstr)

24. Sparrow CP, Parthasarathy S, Steinberg D: Enzymatic modification of low density lipoprotein by purified lipoxygenase plus phospholipase A_2 mimics cell-mediated oxidative modification. J Lipid Res 29:745-753, 1988

25. Steinberg D: Antioxidants in the prevention of human atherosclerosis. Circulation 85:2337-2344, 1992

26. Coritsidis G, Rifici V, Gupta S, Rie J, Shan Z, Neugarten J, Schlondorff D: Preferential uptake of oxidized LDL to rat glomeruli in vivo and cultured mesangial cells in vitro. Kidney Int 39:858-866, 1991

27. Neugarten J, Schlondorff D: Lipoprotein interactions with glomerular cells and matrix, in, Keane WF, Stein JH (eds): Lipids and Renal Disease. New York, NY, Churchill Livingstone, 1992, pp 173-206

28. Grond J, van Goor H, Erkelens DW, Elema JD: Glomerular sclerotic lesions in the rat. Virchows Arch B Cell Pathol 51:521-534, 1986

29. Hessler JR, Morel DW, Lewis LJ, Chisolm GM: Lipoprotein oxidation and lipoprotein-induced cytotoxicity. Arteriosclerosis 3:215-222, 1983

30. Morel DW, Hessler JR, Chisolm GM: Low density lipoprotein cytotoxicity induced by free radical peroxidation of lipid. J Lipid Res 24:1070-1076, 1983

31. Evensen SA, Sverre K, Nilsen E: LDL-induced cytotoxicity and its inhibition by anti-oxidant treatment in cultured human endothelial cells and fibroblasts. Atherosclerosis 49:23-30, 1983

32. Kosugi K, Morel DW, DiCorleto PE, Chisolm GM: Toxicity of oxidized low-density lipoprotein to cultured fibroblasts is selective for S phase of cell cycle. J Cell Physiol 130:311-320, 1987

33. Kaplan R, Aynedjian HS, Schlondorff D, Bank N: Renal vasoconstriction caused by short-term cholesterol feeding is corrected by thromboxane antagonist or probucol. J Clin Invest 86:1707-1714, 1990

34. Hollander W: Unified concept on the role of acid mucopolysaccharides and connective tissue proteins in the accumulation of lipids, lipoproteins, and calcium in the atherosclerotis plaque. Exp Mol Pathol 25:106-120, 1976

35. Iverius PH: The interaction between human plasma lipoproteins and connective tissue glycosaminoglycans. J Biol Chem 247:2607-2613, 1972

36. Srinivasan SR, Lopez SA, Radhakrishnamurthy B, Berenson GS: Complexing of serum pre-beta and beta-lipoproteins and acid mucopolysaccharides. Atherosclerosis 12:321-334, 1970

37. Hoover GA, McCormick S, Kalant N: Interaction of native and cell-modified low density lipoprotein with collagen gel. Arteriosclerosis 8:525-534, 1988

38. Brownlee M, Vlassara H, Cerami A: Nonenzymatic glycosylation products on collagen covalently trap low-density lipoprotein. Diabetes 34:938-941, 1985

39. Crowley S, Brownlee M, Singhal P, Edelstein D, Schlondorff D: Effects of nonenzymatic glycosylation of mesangial matrix on proliferation of mesangial cells. Diabetes 40:40-47, 1991

40. Brownlee M: Glycosylation products as toxic mediators of diabetic complications. Annu Rev Med 42:159-166, 1991

41. Shan Z, Tan D, Satriano J, Silbiger S, Schlondorff D: Intracellular glutathione influences collagen generation by mesangial cells. Kidney Int 46:388-395, 1994

Lipoprotein Metabolism

D. Roger Illingworth, MD, PhD

● The pathways of cellular synthesis, assembly, and secretion of lipoproteins followed by their subsequent intravascular metabolism and cellular uptake provide an efficient system for the transport of exogenous and endogenous lipids. The present report reviews the pathways of normal lipoprotein metabolism and the roles played by specific apoproteins, transfer proteins, enzymes, and cellular receptors in facilitating the transport of lipids in plasma, as well as in the regulation of cellular cholesterol homeostasis.

INDEX WORDS: Cholesterol; plasma lipoproteins; chylomicrons; lipoprotein receptors; low-density lipoproteins.

THE ABILITY of lipids such as cholesterol, cholesteryl esters, and triglycerides, which are themselves insoluble in aqueous environments, to be transported in plasma is dependant on their incorporation into lipoprotein complexes that contain lipids in association with specific transport proteins termed "apoproteins" (apo). Historically, the separation of lipoproteins has been achieved by two principal techniques, electrophoresis and ultracentrifugation in salt solutions, and the classification of lipoproteins is most commonly expressed on the basis of their separation by ultracentrifugation.[1] Four major classes of lipoproteins are recognized; chylomicrons, very low-density lipoproteins (VLDL), low-density lipoproteins (LDL), and high-density lipoproteins (HDL). Each of these lipoproteins is heterogeneous in terms of size, lipid composition, and apoprotein content, and subfractions of the major lipoprotein classes can be isolated by electrophoresis, gradient ultracentrifugation, or affinity column chromatography. Low-density lipoproteins are often separated into two fractions, LDL1, also referred to as intermediate-density lipoprotein with a density of 1.006 to 1.019 g/mL, and LDL2, which has a density of 1.019 to 1.063 g/mL. A fifth lipoprotein, lipoprotein (a) [Lp (a)], is present in plasma, and the majority of this lipoprotein has a hydrated density between 1.06 and 1.08 g/mL. Lipoprotein (a) consists of an LDL particle to which an additional protein, termed "apoprotein (a)" is covalently bound.[2,3]

Typical values for the composition of the major plasma lipoproteins are shown in Table 1, whereas the apo content is illustrated in Table 2.

Supported in part by National Institutes of Health Research Grant No. HL28399, the General Clinical Research Center's Program RR334, and the Clinical Nutrition Research Unit (P30DK40566).

LIPOPROTEIN COMPOSITION

Chylomicrons are the largest of the lipoprotein particles, with a diameter ranging from 800 Å to 10,000 Å. Following a lipid-rich meal, the fatty acid composition of chylomicron triglycerides resembles that of the consumed dietary fat. Human chylomicrons contain a form of apo B (B-48), which is synthesized in the intestinal mucosal cells. Recent studies[4,5] have indicated that B-48 represents a unique intestinal derived form of apo B, which consists of the amino terminal 2152 amino acids of the normal hepatic apo B-100, which is 4536 amino acids in length. Apoprotein B-48 is produced from the apo B-100 gene by a novel mechanism involving the editing of messenger RNA in the intestine, which results in the insertion of a stop codon (UAA) in place of the normal CAA codon, with the resultant termination of protein synthesis to produce a protein that is 2152 amino acids in length. The reason the intestine has the ability to synthesize this unique form of apo B is unclear; it could be speculated, however, that the smaller size of this protein allows for faster synthesis, which in turn may enable the intestine to rapidly adapt to variations in fat intake and maintain efficient absorption and synthesis of chylomicron particles.

Very low-density lipoproteins constitute the major transport vehicle for endogenous triglycerides in plasma and are synthesized in the liver. Very low-density lipoprotein particles range in diameter from 300 Å to 800 Å, with larger particles being present at times of increased hepatic triglyceride production. These particles contain apo B-100 as their major apoprotein, but also contain the apo C polypeptides and apo E (Table 2).

Low-density lipoproteins constitute the major carrier of cholesterol and cholesteryl esters in plasma (Table 1) and these lipoproteins contain apo B-100 as their major apoprotein (Table 2).

Table 1. Composition of Human Plasma Lipoproteins

	Chylomicrons	VLDL	LDL	HDL
Protein	2	8	21	50
Phospholipid	7	19	22	23
Cholesterol free	2	7	8	4
Cholesteryl ester	5	13	37	18
Triglyceride	84	51	11	4
Non-esterified fatty acid	—	2	1	1

Note. Values are expressed as percentage of total dry weight of the lipoprotein.

High-density lipoproteins are the heaviest (density, 1.063 to 1.21 g/mL) and smallest (particle diameter, 90 Å to 120 Å) of the human lipoproteins and contain apoproteins A-I and A-II as their major protein moieties (Table 2).

Lipoprotein (a) is an LDL-like particle that contains cholesterol, phospholipid, triglycerides, and apo B-100, with the latter linked via a single disulfide bond to a second large protein termed "apoprotein (a)."[3] The structure of apo (a) is very similar to that of plasminogen, and apo (a) contains a number of pretzel-like structures termed "kringles." The molecular weight of apo (a) varies between 450,000 and 750,000; the relationship between molecular weight and plasma concentrations is an inverse one, with the highest plasma concentrations being observed in patients with the smallest molecular weight forms of apo (a). Increased plasma concentrations of Lp (a) are associated with an increased risk of atherosclerosis, but the precise physiologic function of Lp (a) remains unknown.[6]

FUNCTION OF PLASMA APOPROTEINS

The apoprotein moieties of plasma lipoproteins serve unique functions in the biogenesis, transport, and metabolism of plasma lipoproteins. Eleven major apoproteins, A-I, A-II, AIV, B-48, B-100, C-I, C-II, C-III, D, E, and apo (a), have been sequenced, and the genes responsible for their synthesis have been mapped in the human genome.[7,8] With the exception of apo (a), the amino acid sequences of the apoproteins contain domains that result in the formation of an amphipathic helix in which hydrophobic amino acids are arranged on one side and hydrophylic polar amino acids on the other. These properties contribute to the unique ability of the apoproteins to transport lipids in an aqueous environment. With the exception of apo B-48, apo B-100, and apo (a), all the apoproteins appear capable of disassociating from one lipoprotein and moving to another. This movement of apoproteins between lipoproteins not only serves to enhance metabolic processing of a given lipoprotein particle, but also prolongs the residence time of the apoproteins in plasma. With the exception of apo B-48 and probably apo A-IV, which are synthesized exclusively in the intestine, and apo A-II and B-100, which, in humans, are synthesized in the liver, biosynthesis of apo A-I, C-I, C-II, C-III, and E takes place in both the liver and intestine mucosal cells, as well as in certain other tissues, including muscle and macrophages.[9]

Several of the apoproteins play distinct roles in the intravascular metabolism and cellular uptake of lipoproteins in addition to their role in the maintenance of lipoprotein stability (Table 3). Apoprotein C-II serves as a cofactor for lipoprotein lipase, the enzyme that hydrolyzes the triglycerides on plasma chylomicrons and VLDL, and a deficiency of apo C-II is associated with severe hypertriglyceridemia.[10,11] Apoprotein A-I, the major apoprotein of HDL, is a co-factor for lecithin cholesterol-acyltransferase (LCAT), the plasma enzyme that catalyzes the conversion of cholesterol to cholesteryl esters using the fatty acid from the 2 position of phosphatidyl choline.[12] Apoproteins E and B-100 serve unique roles in facilitating the receptor-mediated catabolism of lipoproteins. Apoprotein E

Table 2. Apoprotein Content of Human Plasma Lipoproteins

Chylomicrons	VLDL	LDL	Lp (a)	HDL
Major apoproteins				
Apo B-48	Apo B-100	Apo B-100	Apo B-100	Apo A-I
Apo C-I	Apo C-I		Apo (a)	Apo A-II
Apo C-II	Apo C-II			
Apo C-III	Apo C-III			
Apo E	Apo E			
Minor apoproteins				
Apo A-I	Apo D			Apo C-I
Apo A-II				Apo C-II
Apo A-IV				Apo C-III
Apo D				Apo E

Note. Apoproteins A-I, A-II, and A-IV each constitute 5% to 10% of the apoproteins in lymph chylomicrons but are minor components of the chylomicron particles present in plasma.

Table 3. Metabolic Functions of Plasma Apoproteins

Apoprotein	Molecular Weight	Metabolism Role
A-I	28,000	Activates LCAT
A-II	17,500	Activates hepatic lipase; may inhibit LCAT
A-IV	46,000	Unknown, possibly involved in lipid transfer between lipoproteins
B-48	264,000	Transport of lipids from the gut as chylomicrons
B-100	512,000	Transport of lipids from the liver as VLDL and LDL; recognized by cellular LDL receptors
C-I	7,000	Activates LCAT
C-II	9,000	Activates lipoprotein lipase
C-III	9,000	May inhibit activation of lipoprotein lipase by apo C-II
D	22,000	May be involved in lipid transfer between lipoproteins
E	34,000	Recognized by hepatic apo E receptors and cellular LDL receptors; recognition facilitates hepatic uptake of chylomicron and VLDL remnants
Transfer proteins	Variable	Facilitate the transfer of triglycerides, phospholipids, and cholesteryl esters between lipoproteins

Abbreviation: LCAT, lecithin cholesteryl-acyltransferase.

is the ligand that facilitates the receptor-mediated uptake of chylomicron and VLDL remnant particles by the liver.[13] The hepatic uptake of chylomicron remnants does not require the interaction of apo B-48 with hepatic receptors, but the removal of LDL particles from plasma is facilitated by binding domains present in the C-terminal portion of apo B-100, which are recognized by specific high-affinity LDL receptors.[5] Monoclonal antibodies directed against epitopes on apo B-100 located between amino acids 2980 and 3780 completely block the specific binding of LDL particles to the LDL receptor, and indicate that this region of apo B-100 contains the receptor-binding domain.[5] These studies are also consistent with the observation that patients with familial defective apo B-100, in which the amino acid glutamine is substituted for the normal arginine at position 3500, exhibit increased plasma concentrations of LDL and that the LDL particles isolated from the plasma of these patients show impaired binding to LDL receptors on cultured human cells and, in vivo, show delayed clearance from plasma.[14]

ENZYMES AND TRANSFER PROTEINS INVOLVED IN LIPOPROTEIN METABOLISM

Three enzymes, lipoprotein lipase, hepatic lipase, and LCAT are of physiologic importance in the metabolism of plasma lipoproteins. In addition, a specific transfer protein, cholesteryl ester transfer protein (CETP), facilitates the interchange of cholesteryl esters between HDL and triglyceride-rich lipoproteins and the reciprocal transfer of triglycerides in the reverse direction.

Lipoprotein lipase is a hydrolytic enzyme that is present primarily on endothelial cells in the capillary beds of a number of tissues, including muscle, adipose tissue, and breast tissue.[15] The enzyme is normally present in plasma in very low concentrations, but may be released by the injection of heparin. Physiologically, this enzyme acts to hydrolyze triglycerides present in chylomicron and VLDL particles, and optimal activity of this enzyme necessitates the presence of apo C-II, which acts as a specific activator. Mutations in the gene for lipoprotein lipase that result in an absence of functional enzyme are associated with severe hypertriglyceridemia and the accumulation of chylomicron and, to a lesser extent, VLDL particles in plasma.[16] The activity of lipoprotein lipase in adipose tissue is increased in response to the administration of insulin, and is reduced by fasting and by the presence of uremia.[15]

Hepatic lipase is a distinct hydrolytic enzyme present on hepatocyte cell membranes that can be released into plasma by the intravenous injection of heparin.[17] Deficiency of hepatic lipase has been associated with the accumulation of small triglyceride-rich VLDL particles in plasma, as well as an increase in the concentrations of the lighter HDL subfraction HDL2.[18] Hepatic lipase does not appear to be involved in the initial delipidation of chylomicron and VLDL particles, and its role appears to be primarily to facilitate the further catabolism of chylomicron and VLDL remnants at the hepatocyte cell membrane.

Lecithin cholesterol-acyltransferase is an enzyme present in plasma that catalyzes the transfer of a fatty acid from the 2 position of phosphatidyl choline to cholesterol, with the resultant formation of a cholesteryl ester molecule and lysophosphatidyl choline. The enzyme acts on lipids that are constituents of HDL and results in the formation of most of the esterified cholesterol present in plasma. Lecithin cholesteryl-acyltransferase is activated by apo A-I and apo C-I. Deficiency of LCAT is associated with increased plasma concentrations of non-esterified cholesterol, which results in increased tissue concentrations of free cholesterol and the premature development of atherosclerosis and progressive renal insufficiency.[19]

Cholesterol ester transfer protein is a plasma protein that facilitates the transfer of cholesteryl esters from HDL particles to VLDL, with a reciprocal transfer of triglycerides from VLDL to HDL.[20] Cholesterol ester transfer protein activity has been shown to be increased in hypertriglyceridemia and in patients with diabetes, but is decreased in response to alcohol consumption.[20] A genetic deficiency of CETP has been described in Japan and has been associated with marked increases in the plasma concentrations of HDL cholesterol; this clinical entity lends support to the view that CETP is important in the normal transfer of cholesteryl esters between plasma lipoproteins.[21]

CHYLOMICRON METABOLISM

Chylomicrons are synthesized in the small intestine in response to the absorption of dietary fat. Chylomicron synthesis does not appear to be rate-limiting in the absorption of dietary lipids, and the synthesis and secretion of chylomicron particles is dependant on the intracellular assembly of the constitutive lipids (triglycerides,

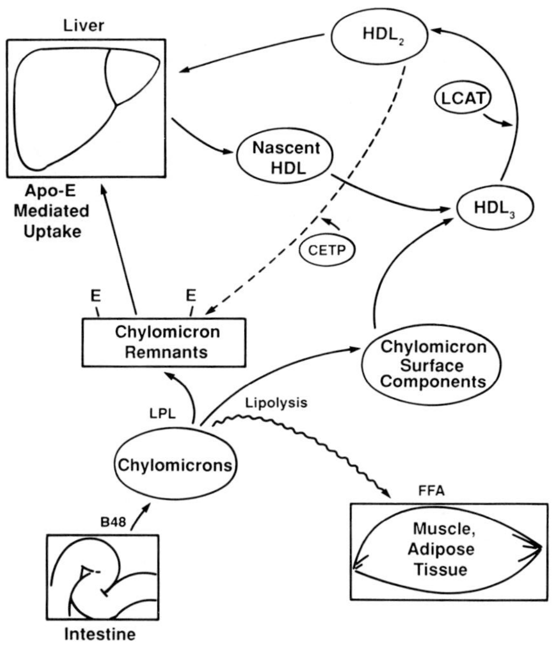

Fig 1. Metabolic transformation of chylomicron particles and the interconversions that occur between chylomicrons and HDL. HDL2, HDL with a density between 1.063 and 1.125 g/mL; HDL3, HDL with a density between 1.125 and 1.21 g/mL; FFA, free fatty acids; LPL, lipoprotein lipase.

cholesteryl esters, retinyl palmitate, and phospholipids) and concurrent synthesis of apo A-I, AIV, B-48, and, possibly, some C and E apoproteins. Following release from the intestinal mucosal cells into the lymph, nascent chylomicrons enter the systemic circulation via the thoracic duct, and are normally rapidly metabolized with a plasma half-life of 5 to 15 minutes. Transfer of apo A-I and apo A-II to HDL and reciprocal transfers of C and E apoproteins from HDL serve to enhance the hydrolysis of chylomicron-triglycerides by the enzyme lipoprotein lipase, and provide a source of chylomicron surface components that act as precursors of nascent HDL particles (Fig 1). Lipolysis of chylomicron-triglycerides by the enzyme lipoprotein lipase occurs predominantly in the capillary beds of muscle and adipose tissue, and results in progress delipidation of the chylomicron particle. Very low-density lipoprotein particles compete with chylomicrons for lipoprotein lipase-mediated catabolism, but chylomicrons appear to be the preferred substrate. Progressive hydrolysis of chylomicron-triglyceride leads to the formation of a smaller chylomicron particle, termed a ''chylomicron remnant,'' which contains almost all the cholesterol originally contained in the nascent particle and several molecules of apo E but which has lost most of the C apoproteins. The uptake of chylomicron remnants is dependant on a specific hepatic receptor that has been termed the ''LDL receptor-related protein,'' and this receptor recognizes the apo E moieties contained on the chylomicron remnant particles and facilitates their uptake from plasma.[22] Receptor-mediated uptake of chylomicron remnant particles by the liver leads to an increased hepatic cholesterol content and is associated with a concurrent decrease in hepatic cholesterol biosynthesis. Genetic or acquired defects in lipoprotein lipase may lead to the abnormal accumulation of chylomicron particles in plasma, whereas abnormalities in chylomicron remnant catabolism lead to the accumulation of potentially atherogenic chylomicron remnant particles. The importance of apo E in facilitating the hepatic clearance of remnant lipoproteins is well-illustrated by the metabolic consequences, which result from substitution of the amino acid cysteine for the normal arginine at position 158 in the apo E molecule; this change leads to impaired receptor binding of apo E and is the most common abnormality in patients with type III hyperlipidemia, in whom VLDL and chylomicron-remnant particles accumulate in plasma.[23]

VERY LOW-DENSITY LIPOPROTEIN METABOLISM

The liver is the major site of synthesis of VLDL, for which apo B-100 is a constitutive apoprotein. Very low-density lipoprotein particles serve to transport endogenous triglycerides from the liver to peripheral tissues, and intravascular hydrolysis of VLDL triglycerides depends on the activity of lipoprotein lipase (Fig 2). The metabolism of VLDL and chylomicron particles show many similarities, but one important difference is that the remnant particles, which result from VLDL lipolysis, can be either taken up by the liver via apo E-mediated catabolism or subsequently converted to LDL. Metabolism of VLDL to LDL is the major source of the latter lipoprotein in human plasma. Many factors, including nutrient intake, plasma concentration of free-fatty acids, and levels of insulin, glucagon, and epinephrine in plasma, appear to modulate the secretion of hepatic VLDL, which in turn influences VLDL concentrations in plasma. The catabolism of VLDL remnant particles by the liver is facilitated by their binding to both high-affinity LDL receptors as well as to the LDL receptor-like protein.[13,22] In normotriglyceridemic human subjects, virtually all the apo B that enters plasma as a constituent of VLDL is preserved as the particle is metabolized to intermediate-density lipoproteins and to LDL. In contrast, in patients with severe hypertriglyceridemia, most of the VLDL particles are removed prior to conversion to LDL, resulting in low plasma concentrations of LDL in this patient population. This precursor-product relationship between VLDL and LDL is seen clinically in patients with moderate hypertriglyceridemia who are treated with either diet or drugs and in whom initial decreases in VLDL are not uncommonly accompanied by reciprocal increases in the plasma concentrations of LDL. Very low-density lipoprotein particles are metabolized slower than chylomicrons and, under normal circumstances, the half-life of VLDL apo B is 6 to 12 hours. Moderate hypertriglyceridemia with plasma triglycerides between 300 and 800 mg/dL usually reflects the accumulation of endogenous VLDL particles in plasma; such an accumulation may result from enhanced rates of VLDL synthesis, genetic or acquired defects in triglyceride hydrolysis, or combinations of both. An accumulation of VLDL remnant particles occurs in the plasma of patients with type III hyperlipidemia or in patients with hepatic lipase deficiency.[18,23]

LOW-DENSITY LIPOPROTEIN METABOLISM

In humans, LDL is the major cholesterol-carrying particle present in plasma and, metabolically, LDL may be regarded as the end product of VLDL metabolism (Fig 2). The catabolism of LDL occurs in both peripheral tissues and the liver, but the liver is responsible for the catabolism of 70% of LDL in normal human subjects. Low-density lipoprotein catabolism is facilitated by both receptor-mediated and non–receptor-mediated pathways, but in normal human subjects, the receptor-mediated pathway predominates and is responsible for the clearance of up to 75% of the plasma LDL pool. The studies of

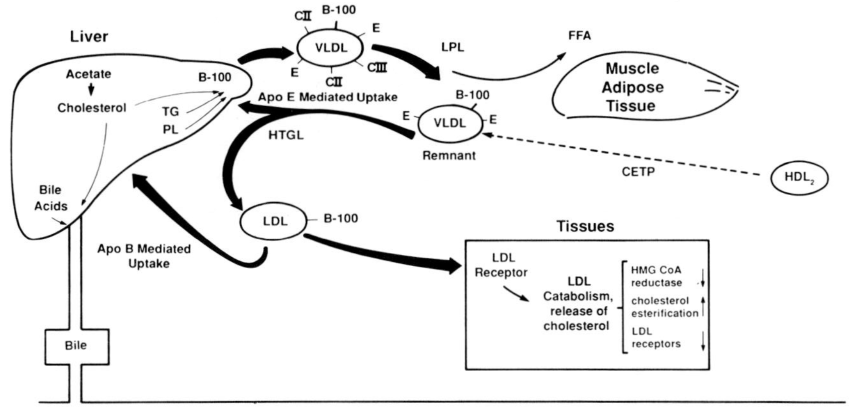

Fig 2. Metabolic interconversions of VLDL and LDL in plasma and the intracellular effects of receptor-mediated uptake of LDL. FFA, free fatty acids; HDL2, HDL with a density between 1.063 and 1.125 g/mL; LPL, lipoprotein lipase; HMG CoA, hydroxymethyl glutacyl coenzyme A; PL, phospholipid; TG, triglyceride; HTGL, hepatic triglyceride lipase.

Russell et al[24] and Hobbs et al[25] have led to a precise understanding of the biochemistry and regulation of specific high-affinity LDL receptors, which appear to be present on virtually all cells, including hepatocytes, mononuclear leukocytes, and cells in steroid hormone-producing tissues. The uptake of LDL by receptor-mediated endocytosis results in the suppression of endogenous cholesterol biosynthesis, an enhanced rate of intracellular cholesteryl esterification, and a reduction in the number of high-affinity LDL receptors expressed on the cell surface (Fig 2). The importance of the LDL receptor in the regulation of LDL concentrations in plasma is exemplified by the severe hypercholesterolemia seen in patients with both heterozygous and homozygous familial hypercholesterolemia, in whom LDL receptors are reduced by 50% (heterozygotes) or are totally absent (receptor-negative homozygotes).[26] Hypercholesterolemia, with increased plasma concentrations of LDL cholesterol, may result from a number of genetic and acquired disorders that lead to either an enhanced rate of VLDL and LDL apo B synthesis, from genetic or acquired defects in LDL catabolism (resulting from impaired expression of high-affinity LDL receptors), from defects in the receptor-binding domain of LDL (which also lead to an impairment in LDL catabolism), or from combined defects resulting in enhanced synthesis and impaired catabolism. The hypercholesterolemia seen in patients with the nephrotic syndrome is an example of an acquired disorder in which high levels of LDL cholesterol appear to result from a combination of increased synthesis and impaired catabolism of LDL.[27]

HIGH-DENSITY LIPOPROTEIN METABOLISM

High-density lipoproteins are derived from both direct synthesis in the liver and from the surface components of chylomicron and VLDL particles, which are generated during intravascular lipolysis (Fig 1). This dual etiology for HDL explains the inverse correlation between plasma triglycerides and HDL as well as the known presence of HDL particles in the plasma of patients with abetalipoproteinemia, a disorder in which chylomicrons, VLDL, and LDL are absent from plasma. Newly synthesized HDL particles appear as disk-shaped structures that contain predominantly protein, free cholesterol, and phospholipid, but which, when exposed to the action of LCAT, are transformed into spherical particles rich in cholesteryl esters.[28] The apoprotein content of individual HDL particles varies and it is apparent that some HDL particles contain both apo A-I and apo A-II, whereas others may only contain apo A-I. The half-life of HDL, as assessed by that of its constituent apoproteins, apo A-I and apo A-II, is from 4 to 6 days and is influenced by both diet and a number of pharmaceutical agents. Thus, diets high in carbohydrate, which raise VLDL, cause a reduction in HDL concentrations and an enhanced rate of HDL turnover, whereas nicotinic acid, which depresses VLDL synthesis, raises the concentrations of HDL and prolongs the half-life of apo A-I in plasma. Epidemiologic studies have shown an inverse correlation between the plasma concentrations of HDL cholesterol and the risk of coronary artery disease[29] and have led to the proposal[30] that one major function of HDL is to transport cholesterol from peripheral tissues back to the liver. Physiologic evidence to support this is not strong. Several factors have been shown to increase the concentrations of HDL in plasma predominantly by affecting concentrations of the lighter HDL2 subfraction. Factors that have been shown to increase HDL concentrations include a moderate consumption of alcohol, sustained regular exercise, and correction of hypertriglyceridemia.[31,32] As previously discussed, a deficiency of CETP also has been associated with increased plasma concentrations of HDL cholesterol.[21] In addition to environmental factors, a number of genetic disorders have been described in which the metabolism and concentrations of HDL particles are profoundly altered; these disorders illustrate the important roles played by apo A-I and A-II in the synthesis and metabolism of HDL particles in humans.[28] With the exception of familial hyperalphalipoproteinemia and CETP deficiency, which are both associated with increased plasma concentrations of HDL cholesterol, other genetic disorders that influence lipoprotein metabolism result in reduced plasma concentrations of HDL cholesterol and its constituent apoproteins. Some, but not all of these disorders are associated with an increased risk of coronary artery disease.

SUMMARY

The physiologic basis of lipid transport in humans is now well-delineated, and it is apparent that a number of factors, both genetic and acquired, can influence this transport system and result in abnormal concentrations of lipoproteins in plasma. Increased plasma concentrations of LDL, Lp (a), and cholesterol-rich VLDL and chylomicron remnants all appear to be highly atherogenic, whereas, on the basis of epidemiologic studies, increased concentrations of HDL cholesterol appear to afford protection from the premature development of atherosclerosis. Modifications in lipoproteins, particularly oxidation or glycosylation of LDL, may also affect the metabolism of these lipoproteins and result in enhanced rates of uptake by ''scavenger receptors'' present on tissue macrophages, with the resultant formation of foam cells.[33,34] It is believed that oxidation of LDL particles occurs in atherosclerotic plaques, but local oxidation of LDL may occur under conditions of endothelial cell injury and potentially under other circumstances in which plasma concentrations of natural antioxidants are reduced. A thorough understanding of the normal and abnormal pathways of lipoprotein metabolism should enable future studies to better define the role, if any, of modified lipoproteins and antioxidant therapy in the pathogenesis of arterial injury and atherosclerosis.

ADDENDUM

Additional information has appeared regarding the drug treatment of dyslipoproteinemia, with emphasis on the appropriate indications for lipid-lowering drugs in adult patients with different lipoprotein disorders.[35] In addition, the mechanisms of action, efficacy, safety profile, and potential uses of lovastatin in patients with hypercholesterolemia have been reviewed.[36] Also, a review of clinical trials of four drugs that act as specific inhibitors of 3-hydroxy-3-methyl coenzyme A (HMG-CoA) has appeared.[37]

REFERENCES

1. Goffman JW, Lindgren FT, Elliot M: Ultracentrifugal studies of lipoproteins of human plasma. J Biol Chem 179:973-980, 1949

2. Alaupovic P: Apoproteins and lipoproteins. Atherosclerosis 13:141-149, 1971

3. Utermann G: The mysteries of lipoprotein (a). Science 246:904-909, 1989

4. Powell LM, Wallace SC, Pease RJ, Edwards YH, Knott TJ, Scott J: A novel form of tissue-specific RNA processing produces apoprotein B-48 in intestine. Cell 50:831-836, 1987

5. Young SG: Recent progress in understanding apolipoprotein B. Circulation 82:1574-1594, 1990

6. Kostner GM, Krempler F: Lipoprotein (a). Curr Opin Lipidol 3:279-284, 1992

7. Schonfeld G: The genetic dyslipidemias: Nosology update 1990. Atherosclerosis 81:81-92, 1990

8. Breslow JL: Lipoprotein transport gene abnormalities underlying coronary heart disease susceptibility. Annu Rev Med 42:357-371, 1991

9. Basu SK, Goldstein JL, Brown MS: Independent pathways for secretion of cholesterol and apolipoprotein E by macrophages. Science 219:871-876, 1983

10. Jackson RL, Pattus F, De Haas G: Mechanism of action of milk lipoprotein lipase at substraight interphases: Effects of apolipoproteins. Biochemistry 19:373-380, 1980

11. Breckenridge WC, Little JA, Steiner G, Chow A, Poapst M: Hypertriglyceridemia associated with a deficiency of apolipoprotein C-II. N Engl J Med 298:1265-1270, 1978

12. Havel RH, Kane JP: Lipoprotein and lipid metabolism disorders, in Scriver CR, Beaudet AL, Sly WS, Valle D (eds): The Metabolic Basis of Inherited Disease (ed 6). New York, NY, McGraw-Hill, 1989, pp 1129-1138

13. Mahley RW, Hussain MM: Chylomicron and chylomicron-remnant catabolism. Curr Opin Lipidol 2:170-175, 1991

14. Innararity TL, Mahley RW, Weisgraber KH, Bersot TP, Krauss RM, Vega GL, Grundy SM, Friedl W, Davignon J, McCarthy BJ: Familial defective apolipoprotein B-100: Mutation of apolipoprotein B that causes hypercholesterolemia. J Lipid Res 31:1337-1349, 1990

15. Eckel RH: Lipoprotein lipase: A multifunctional enzyme relevant to common metabolic diseases. N Engl J Med 320:1060-1067, 1989

16. Santamarina-Fojo S: Genetic dyslipidemias: Role of lipoprotein lipase and apolipoprotein C-II. Curr Opin Lipidol 3:186-195, 1992

17. Olivecrona T, Bengtsson-Olivecrona G: Lipoprotein lipase and hepatic lipase. Curr Opin Lipidol 1:222-230, 1990

18. Breckenridge WC, Little JA, Alaupovic P, Wang CS, Kaksis A, Lindgren F, Gardiner G: Lipoprotein abnormalities associated with a familial deficiency of hepatic lipase. Atherosclerosis 45:161-170, 1982

19. Norum KR, Gjone E, Glomset JA: Familial lecithin cholesterol acyltransferase deficiency including fish eye disease, in Scriver CR, Beaudet AL, Sly WS, Valle D, (eds.) The Metabolic Basis of Inherited Disease (ed 6). New York, NY, McGraw-Hill, 1989, pp 1181-1194

20. Editorial: Cholesterol-ester transfer protein. Lancet 338:666-668, 1991

21. Inazu A, Brown ML, Hesler CB, Agellon LB, Koizumi J, Takata K, Maruhama Y, Mabuchi H, Tall AR: Increased high density lipoprotein levels caused by a common cholesteryl-ester transfer protein gene mutation. N Engl J Med 323:1234-1238, 1990

22. Brown MS, Herz J, Kowal RC, Goldstein JL: The LDL receptor-related protein (LRP): Double agent or decoy? Curr Opin Lipidol 2:65-72, 1991

23. Mahley RW, Rao SC, Jr: Type III hyperlipidemia (dysbetalipoproteinemia): The role of apolipoprotein E in normal and abnormal lipoprotein metabolism, in Scriver CR, Beaudet AL, Sly WS, Valle D (eds): The Metabolic Basis of Inherited Disease (ed 6). New York, NY, McGraw-Hill, 1989, pp 1195-1213

24. Russell DW, Esser V, Hobbs HH: Molecular basis of familial hypercholesterolemia. Arteriosclerosis 9:I-8-I-13, 1989 (suppl)

25. Hobbs HH, Russell DW, Brown MS, Goldstein JL: The LDL receptor locus in familial hypercholesterolemia: Mutational analysis of a membrane protein. Annu Rev Genet 24:133-148, 1990

26. Bilheimer DW, Stone NJ, Grundy SM: Metabolic studies in familial hypercholesterolemia: Evidence for a gene/dosage effect in vivo. J Clin Invest 64:524-532, 1979

27. Warwick GL, Caslake NJ, Boulton-Jones JM, Dagen M, Packard CJ, Shephard J: Low density lipoprotein metabolism in the nephrotic syndrome. Metabolism 39:187-192, 1990

28. Brewer HB, Jr, Raider DJ: HDL: Structure, function and metabolism. Prog Lipid Res 30:139-144, 1991

29. Abbott RD, Wilson BWF, Kanel WB, Castelli WP: High density lipoprotein cholesterol, total cholesterol screening and myocardial infarction. Arteriosclerosis 8:207-211, 1988

30. Glomset JA, Norum KR: The metabolic role of lecithin cholesterol acyltransferase: Perspectives from pathology. Adv Lipid Res 11:1-18, 1973

31. Krauss RM: Regulation of high density lipoprotein levels. Med Clin North Am 66:403-417, 1982

32. Williams PJ, Krauss RM, Wood PD, Albers JJ, Dreon D, Ellsworth N: Association of diet and alcohol intake with high density lipoprotein subclasses. Metabolism 34:524-529, 1985

33. Steinberg D, Parthasarathy S, Carew TE, Khoo JC, Witztum JL: Beyond cholesterol: Modifications of low density lipoprotein that increases its atherogenecity. N Engl J Med 320:915-924, 1989

34. Gaziano JM, Hennekens CH: Vitamin antioxidants and cardiovascular disease. Curr Opin Lipidol 3:291-294, 1992

35. Larsen ML, Illingworth DR: Drug treatment of dyslipoproteinemia. Med Clin North Am 78:225-245, 1994

36. Illingworth DR, Stein EA, Mitchel YB, Dujovne CA, Frost PH, Knopp RH, Tun P, Zupkis RV, Greguski RA: Comparative effects of lovastatin and niacin in primary hypercholesterolemia. A prospective trial. Arch Intern Med 154:1585-1595, 1994

37. Illingworth DR, Tobert JA: A review of clinical trials comparing HMG-CoA reductase inhibitors. Clin Ther 16:366-385, 1994

Early Glomerular Changes in Rats With Dietary-Induced Hypercholesterolemia

Carlos Guijarro, MD, Bertram L. Kasiske, MD, Youngki Kim, MD, Michael P. O'Donnell, PhD, Hyun Soon Lee, MD, and William F. Keane, MD

● Increasing evidence suggests that lipids may be important modulators of progressive glomerular injury. We previously reported the long-term glomerular changes in rats with dietary-induced hypercholesterolemia. In this work, we evaluated the early glomerular changes induced by hypercholesterolemia that precede the development of glomerulosclerosis. In cholesterol-fed rats, an early macrophage influx was observed. This was associated with an increase in glomerular size, mesangial matrix expansion, lipid deposits, and foam cell formation. Immunohistochemical techniques showed that type IV collagen, fibronectin, and laminin were increased in cholesterol-fed rats. The mRNA expression for the α_1 chain of type IV collagen and an inhibitor of type IV collagenase were increased, suggesting that both increased synthesis and reduced degradation may be involved in cholesterol-induced mesangial matrix accumulation. The glomerular mRNA expression of transforming growth factor-β1 was also upregulated, suggesting that transforming growth factor-β1 could be an important mediator for mesangial matrix accumulation in hypercholesterolemic states. The early cholesterol-induced changes in the glomerulus are reminiscent in many respects to the process leading to glomerulosclerosis in the vessel wall.

INDEX WORDS: Hypercholesterolemia; glomerular injury; macrophages; mesangial matrix.

IT IS GENERALLY accepted that after major renal damage has occurred, there often is a progressive deterioration in function even when the initial cause of renal injury is no longer evident.[1] The final pathologic picture (ie, glomerulosclerosis) is remarkably similar in different diseases, suggesting that there is a final common pathway of progressive renal injury.[1] A number of different mechanisms have been suggested for this relentless decline in renal function. Compensatory increases in glomerular pressure, abnormalities in coagulation, and metabolic disorders have been implicated in the progression of renal injury.[1]

The potential role of lipids in the pathogenesis of progressive glomerulosclerosis has received considerable attention in recent years.[2-4] Although increasing evidence suggests a role for lipids in human progressive renal insufficiency, most of our understanding concerning lipids and progressive glomerular injury comes from experimental studies.[5] Endogenous and exogenous hyperlipidemia have been found to promote progressive renal injury in different animal models.[5] In addition, cholesterol feeding has been shown to aggravate the renal lesions in animals with another underlying cause of renal injury, such as puromycin nephrosis,[6] hypertension,[7] or reduced renal mass.[8,9]

We have previously reported the long-term effects of dietary-induced hypercholesterolemia.[9] In this model, we have found that long-term (18 weeks) cholesterol feeding was associated with glomerular lipid deposition, increased mesangial matrix and cellularity, and a modest degree of glomerulosclerosis.[9] The pathologic changes seen in cholesterol-fed rats were associated with increased urinary albumin excretion and a trend toward increased serum creatinine. In the same study, preliminary data suggested that glomerular abnormalities were already present as early as 4 weeks after the initiation of the cholesterol diet and preceded the development of glomerulosclerosis and functional changes. In the present study, therefore, we further characterized the early glomerular changes associated with diet-induced hypercholesterolemia.

MATERIALS AND METHODS

Animals and Diets

Normal, 8-week-old, Sprague-Dawley rats (Charles River, Wilmington, MA) were fed with either standard rodent chow (5001; Ralston Purina, Richmond, IN) or standard chow supplemented with 4% cholesterol and 2% cholic acid for 4 weeks. There were 10 rats in each of the two experimental groups, and all rats were allowed free access to food and water. In a parallel experiment, six rats per dietary group were killed after 3, 7, 14, and 28 days to determine macrophage influx at earlier times and glomerular mRNA expression at 4 weeks (see below).

Supported in part by a grant from the American Heart Association, Dallas, TX. C. Guijarro is the recipient of grants from Fondo de Investigación Sanitaria (Nos. 92/5510, 93/5439), Spanish Ministry of Health, Madrid, Spain.

Laboratory Measurements

After 4 weeks of cholesterol feeding, rats were individually housed in metabolic cages for a 24-hour urine collection. During the collection rats were allowed free access to water, but food was withdrawn to prevent contamination of the urine. Urine albumin was measured using a monoclonal antibody to rat albumin (Cappel Laboratories, West Chester, PA) and a laser nephelometer (Hyland, Deerfield, IL). After the 24-hour urine collection had been completed, the rats were anesthetized with ether and killed by aortic puncture. Blood was used to determine (fasting) levels of serum cholesterol and creatinine. Cholesterol and creatinine were measured on an autoanalyzer using standard colorimetric techniques. Kidney tissue sections for immunofluorescence studies were flash-frozen using precooled isopentane and liquid nitrogen (see below). Other kidney sections were fixed in glutaraldehyde for electron microscopy or in Zenker's solution for light microscopic determination of the glomerular area (see below).

Immunofluorescence Studies

All immunofluorescence studies were carried out using tissue that had been snap-frozen using isopentane and liquid nitrogen. Glomerular macrophages were identified with the monoclonal antibody ED-1 (Accurate Chemical and Scientific Corp, Westbury, NY) and epifluorescence microscopy as previously described.[9] The number of positive cells per glomerulus was determined by examining a minimum of 10 glomeruli for each tissue specimen. Frozen tissue also was stained with goat anti-type IV collagen (Southern Biotechnology, Birmingham, AL), rabbit anti-fibronectin (Cappel, Malvern, PA), and rabbit antilaminin (gift from Dr A Charonis, University of Minnesota, Minneapolis, MN). Secondary FITC-conjugated rabbit anti-goat IgG (Kallestadt, Austin, TX) and FITC-conjugated goat anti-rabbit IgG (Tago, Burlingame, CA) were used. For each antibody the degree of immunofluorescence was graded on a scale of 0 to 4.

Glomerular Morphometric Measurements

Coronal sections fixed in Zenker's solution were imbedded in paraffin and stained using periodic acid with Schiff's reagent. Glomerular areas were determined using a point counting technique.[10] For each specimen, 25 glomeruli, randomly encountered on a serpentine course between cortex and medulla, were measured using a 100-point eyepiece grid. The area of each glomerulus was determined by multiplying the fraction of points falling on the glomerular tuft by the calibrated area of the grid. The glomerular area for each specimen was calculated as the mean of the 25 measurements. The fractional mesangial area was calculated based on the number of points that fell on mesangial matrix as a percentage of the total glomerular points as previously described.[10]

Electron Microscopy

Tissue was fixed in 2.5% glutaraldehyde and sodium cacodylate buffer for 4 hours, postfixed in 1% osmium tetroxide, and then embedded in epon. Thick sections were cut and stained with toluidine blue to facilitate the selection of the centermost glomerulus. Ultrathin sections were stained with uranyl acetate and lead citrate prior to examination. Two glomeruli from each animal were assessed. A Hitachi H-600 electron microscope (Hitachi Scientific Instruments, Mountain View, CA) was used to photograph the sections. To be nonselective, the photographs were taken in the four corners of a grid square randomly positioned over the most central area of a glomerulus at a magnification of ×1,500. Micrographs were printed at a final magnification of approximately ×3,500 with a calibration grid (1134 lines/mm) to monitor the exact magnification. The number of lipid-laden foam cells over the reference glomerular area also was determined for each micrograph. The mean number of foam cells per glomerulus was calculated by adding the number of foam cells for all the micrographs from two glomeruli per animal. The presence of extracellular fat vacuoles in the mesangial matrix also was evaluated. Fat vacuoles appeared as either empty vacuoles or homogeneously electron-dense globules.

cDNA Probes

A cDNA probe for the α_1 chain of type IV collagen was kindly supplied by Dr Y. Yamada (National Institute of Dental Research, Bethesda, MD). The probe encompasses nucleotides 145-981 of the cDNA for murine α_1(IV) collagen and

Table 1. Effects of Cholesterol Diet on Body Weight, Kidney Weight, Serum Cholesterol, and Renal Function

Variable	Diet: Normal	Diet: Cholesterol	Effect*	Probability Value
Serum cholesterol (mg/dL)	44 ± 9	169 ± 108	↑	<0.01
Body weight (g)	340 ± 15	295 ± 35	↓	<0.01
Kidney weight (g)	1.42 ± 0.11	1.18 ± 0.14	↓	<0.001
KW × 100/BW	0.42 ± 0.02	0.40 ± 0.02		NS
Serum creatinine (mg/dL)	0.38 ± 0.04	0.40 ± 0.05		NS
Urine albumin excretion (mg/24 hr)	0.62 ± 0.04	0.92 ± 0.03		NS

NOTE. Values given are mean ± SD.
Abbreviations: KW, kidney weight; BW, body weight.
* The significance of effects was tested by Student's *t*-test.

detects a major transcript of approximately 6.7 kb and a minor one of approximately 5.4 kb.[11] We found that this probe detects two similar transcripts in rat mesangial cells.[12] A cDNA probe for human 72 kd collagenase was generously provided by Dr G.I. Goldberg (Washington University, St Louis, MO).[13] A NcoI fragment of the insert of approximately 0.8 kb was subcloned by Dr A. Sharma (McGill University, Montreal, Quebec, Canada), and we found this to recognize a 3.1 kb transcript in rat mesangial cells.[12,14] A cDNA probe for tissue inhibitor of metalloproteinases-2 (TIMP-2) was kindly provided by Dr W.G. Stetler-Stevenson (National Cancer Institute, Bethesda, MD).[15] This human cDNA insert is 0.75 kb in length and has been shown to recognize a major transcript of approximately 3.5 kb and a minor one of approximately 1.0 kb in different human cell lines and tissues.[15] We found that this probe also detects two transcripts of similar sizes in rat mesangial cells.[12] A cDNA probe for rat transforming growth factor-β1 (TGF-β1) was obtained from American Type Culture Collection (Rockville, MD).[16] The 0.985 kb insert was excised with HindIII/XbaI from the original pBluescript 2KS+ vector and was shown to recognize a transcript of approximately 2.5 kb. A cDNA probe for 28s ribosomal RNA was kindly provided by Dr ML Iruela Arispe (University of Washington, Seattle, WA).[17] The 280 bp fragment between two EcoRI sites was used. Between 10 and 50 μg of a cDNA template was labeled with 50 μCi of ^{32}[P]-2′-deoxycytidine-5′-triphosphate using Prime It II, a random primer DNA labeling system (Stratagene Cloning System, La Jolla, CA). The cDNAs were purified on a Nuctrap probe purification column (Stratagene Cloning System). The specific activity varied between 1 and 2 $\times$ 10^8 cpm/μg cDNA.

Isolation of Glomerular RNA and Northern Blot Analysis

In a separate experiment two groups of six rats fed standard chow or standard chow supplemented with 4% cholesterol and 2% cholic acid for 4 weeks, as described above, were used for the evaluation of glomerular mRNA expression. Glomeruli were isolated and pooled from three animals of each group at 4°C by standard sieving techniques. The preparation of isolated glomeruli contained more than 90% glomeruli with minimal tubular fragments. The glomerular preparation was homogenized and total RNA was isolated using a modification of the single step guanidinium-thiocyanate-phenol-chloroform extraction method.[18] The isolated RNA was quantified by absorbance at 260 nm and its purity was determined by a 260:280 absorbance ratio greater than 1.8 to 2.0. Ten to twenty microgram samples of denatured RNA together with 10 μg of an RNA ladder (BRL Inc, Gaithersburg, MD) were electrophoresed in 1% agarose gel containing 2.2 mol/L formaldehyde, 20 mmol/L 3-[N-morpholino]propanesulfonic acid (MOPS), 8 mmol/L sodium acetate, and 1 mmol/L ethylene diaminetetraacetic acid (EDTA). The gel was stained with ethidium bromide to assess degradation and molecular size. The electrophoresed RNA was then transferred to a Zeta Probe membrane (BioRad, Richmond, CA). Examination of the gel and the filter by UV light confirmed similar amounts of RNA in each lane. The membrane was dried, baked at 80°C for 30 to 60 minutes in a vacuum oven, and stored at room temperature. Blotted membranes were incubated for 12 to 24 hours with 1.5 $\times$ 10^6 cpm/mL of a ^{32}P-labeled cDNA probe in standard hybridization solution, subjected to stringency washes, and exposed on Kodak X-OMAT XAR5 film (Rochester, NY) at −70°C. To assess that equivalent amounts of RNA were loaded, the membranes were stripped and reprobed for 28s ribosomal RNA. Autoradiograms of the probed RNA were scanned by densitometry and normalized to the respective 28s values.

Reverse Transcription and Polymerase Chain Reaction Analysis

For reverse transcription-polymerase chain reaction (PCR) analysis, 1 μg of glomerular RNA was subjected to reverse transcription at 42°C for 1 hour in a reaction containing 15 U of avian myeloblastosis virus reverse transcriptase and oligo dT as a primer under the conditions specified by the provider (Promega, Madison, WI). Aliquots of this reaction

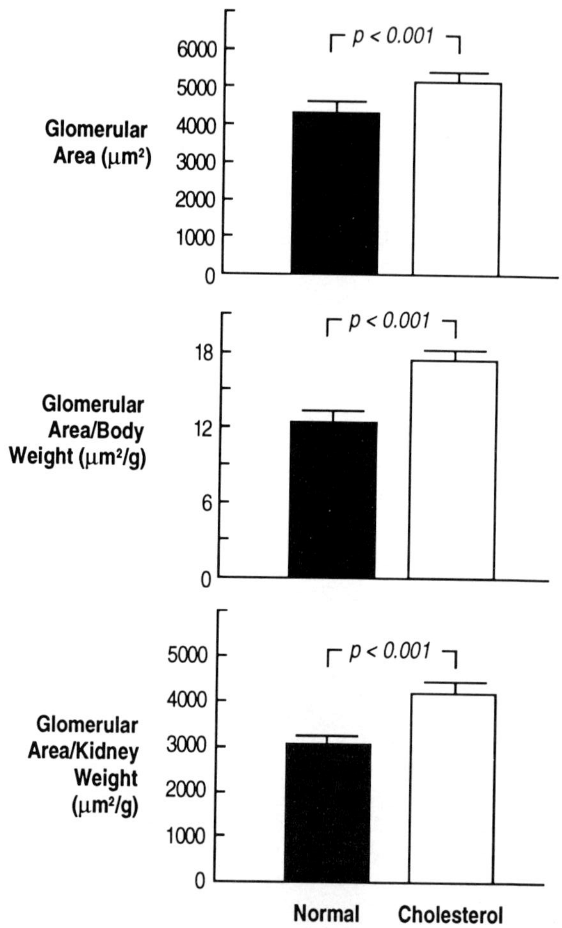

Fig 1. Effect of cholesterol feeding on glomerular area.

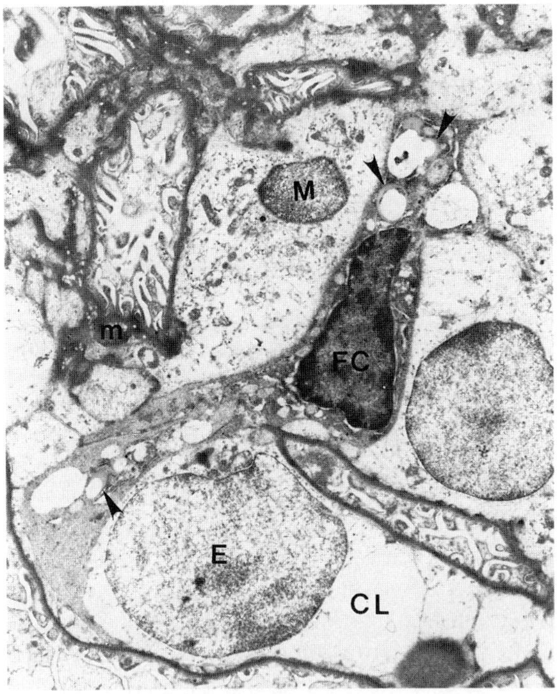

Fig 2. Electron micrograph of a glomerulus from a cholesterol-fed rat. A foam cell (FC) with cytoplasmic lipid droplets (arrowheads) is diapedesing from the capillary lumen (CL) to the mesangium. Fine lipid vacuoles also are seen in mesangial matrix (m). An endothelial cell nucleus (E) and a mesangial cell nucleus (M) also are evident. (Original magnification ×7,500.)

were subjected to PCR amplification in a reaction containing 1.25 U of Taq DNA polymerase, 50 mmol/L KCl, 10 mmol/L Tris-HCl, pH 9, 2 mmol/L $MgCl_2$, 0.8 mmol/L deoxynucleotide triphosphates, 0.1% Triton X-100, and 1 μmol/L of forward and reverse primers. The primers for 72 kd collagenase were designed with a computer program (PRIMER, kindly provided by the Whitehead Institute for Biomedical Research, Cambridge, MA) on the basis of the GenBank-deposited cDNA sequence for the rat 72 kd collagenase (GenBank accession number X71466).[14] The selected primers comprised the bases (5′ to 3′) 1265-1287 (forward) and 1759-1737 (reverse) of the GenBank 72 kd collagenase cDNA sequence. The PCR product had the expected molecular size (0.495 kb) and its specificity was confirmed by hybridization with a ^{32}P-labeled internal oligonucleotide (bases 1537-1509, 5′ to 3′, of the GenBank 72 kd collagenase sequence). The cycle parameters were (94°C 5 min/60°C 5 min/72°C 90 sec) ×1 followed by (94°C 45 sec/60°C 45 sec/72°C 90 sec) ×25 to 40. Aliquots of the reaction were sampled every two to four cycles, slot-blotted onto nylon filters, and probed with the specific internal ^{32}P-labeled oligonucleotide. After hybridization, the filters were cut and the amount of bound probe from each sample was determined by liquid scintillation spectrometry. The results were plotted in a semilogarithmic scale against the number of PCR cycles. Only those samples within the exponential phase of the PCR were used for quantitation.

Statistical Analysis

Differences in the means of parametric data from the experimental groups were tested for significance using Student's *t*-test. Differences in nonparametric data were tested using chi-squared contingency tables and the Kruskal-Wallis test. Analysis was carried out using the Statistical Package for the Social Sciences software package.[19] Differences were considered significant for $P < 0.05$. All results are reported as mean ± SD.

RESULTS

As expected, the cholesterol diet caused a marked increase in serum cholesterol levels (Table 1). Changes in renal function were not expected during the short, 4-week experimental feeding period. There were no differences in serum creatinine or urine albumin excretion between rats fed a high cholesterol diet and rats fed standard chow (Table 1).

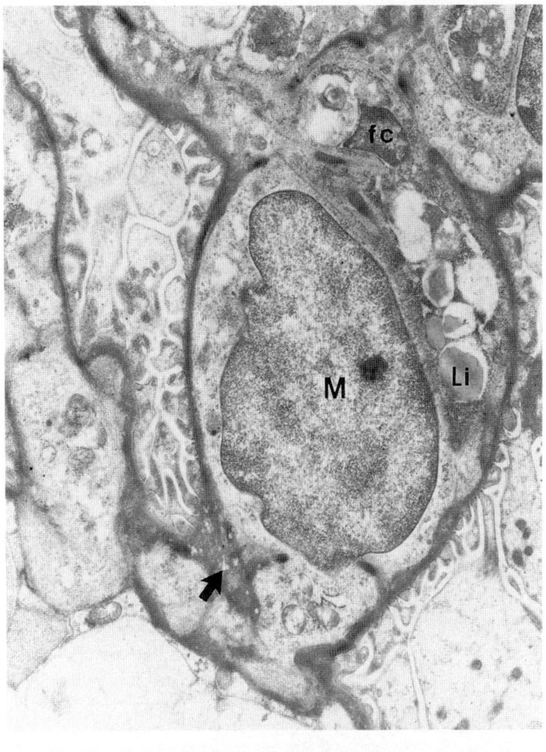

Fig 3. Electron micrograph from a glomerulus of a cholesterol-fed rat showing a lipid (Li)-laden foam cell (fc) in the mesangium. In the mesangial matrix, patchy deposition of tiny fat vacuoles (arrow) is present. A mesangial cell nucleus (M) is present. (Original magnification ×12,000.)

Rats in both diet groups appeared healthy and grew well. Rats fed the high cholesterol diet, however, weighed 13% less than rats fed the standard chow (Table 1), findings similar to those in our previous study.[9] Kidney weights also were slightly lower in the cholesterol-fed rats (Table 1). However, there was a close correlation between kidney weight and body weight ($r = 0.88$, $P < 0.01$), and cholesterol feeding had no effect on kidney weight that was normalized to body weight (Table 1).

Although kidney weight was lower, glomerular area was increased by 20% in rats fed cholesterol compared with rats fed standard chow (Fig 1). The cholesterol-induced increase in glomerular area was even more striking when glomerular area was factored by body weight or kidney weight (Fig 1). Thus, cholesterol had a specific trophic effect on the glomeruli of rats that was independent of changes in kidney weight and body weight.

Extracellular lipid deposits and glomerular foam cells were frequently seen in the mesangial matrix of cholesterol-fed rats (Figs 2 to 4). There were no lipid deposits or glomerular foam cells in rats fed standard chow. ED-1–positive cells were more frequently seen in the glomeruli of cholesterol-fed rats than in rats fed standard chow (Fig 4). Ultrastructurally, macrophages and mesangial cells were morphologically distinguishable, since the nuclei of the former exhibited more condensed and darker chromatin patterns with more ragged contours than those of the latter (Figs 2 and 3). Rarely, mesangial cells exhibited a small amount of intracellular lipid deposition, but never showed foam cell changes comparable to those of macrophages. As macrophages have been considered potential mediators of cholesterol-induced injury, macrophage influx

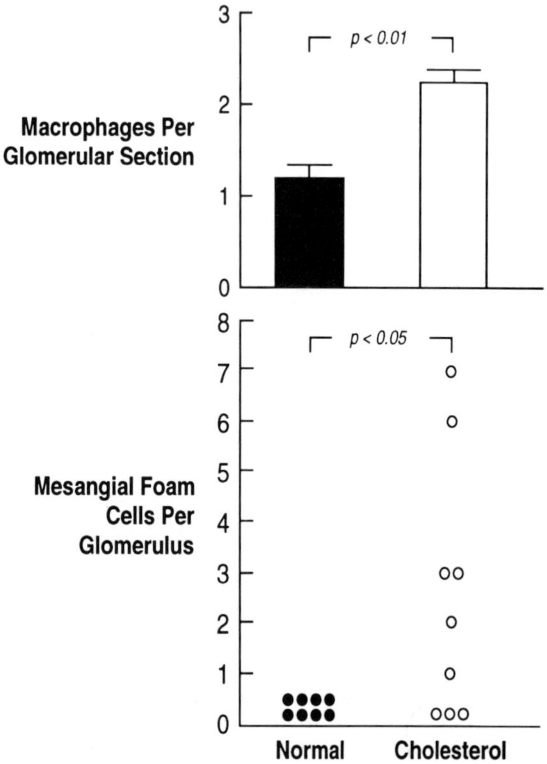

Fig 4. Effects of cholesterol diet on glomerular macrophages and foam cells.

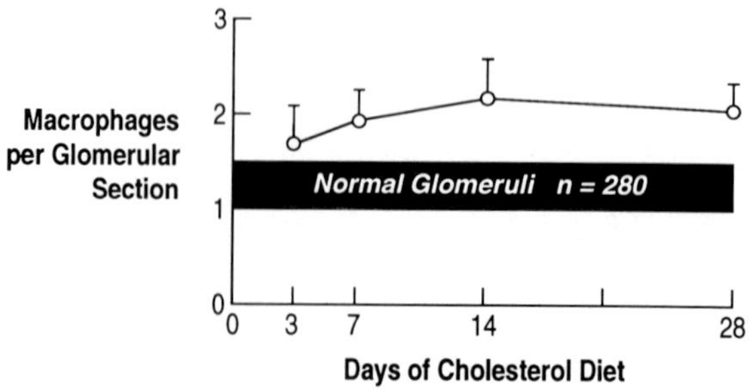

Fig 5. Time course of macrophage glomerular infiltration following the initiation of cholesterol diet. Cholesterol-fed rats versus rats fed standard chow: $P < 0.05$ at 7, 14, and 28 days.

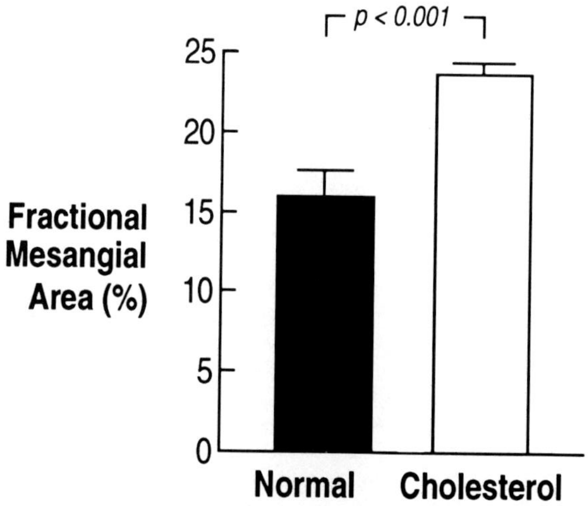

Fig 6. Effects of hypercholesterolemia on fractional mesangial area. Mesangial area is expressed as a percentage of total glomerular area.

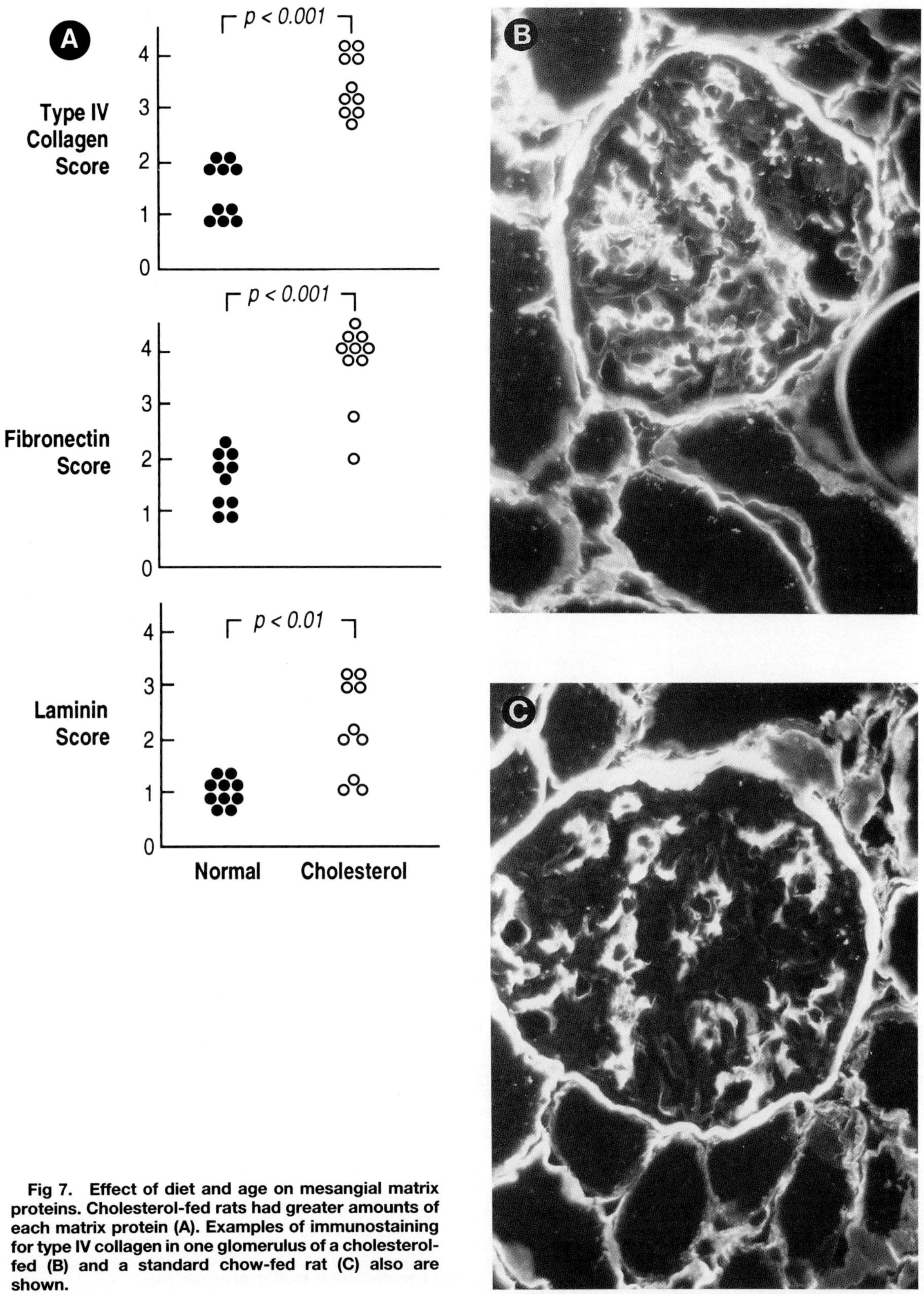

Fig 7. Effect of diet and age on mesangial matrix proteins. Cholesterol-fed rats had greater amounts of each matrix protein (A). Examples of immunostaining for type IV collagen in one glomerulus of a cholesterol-fed (B) and a standard chow-fed rat (C) also are shown.

was determined at earlier times. An influx of macrophages was seen as early as 3 days after the initiation of cholesterol feeding, peaked at 2 weeks, and remained stable thereafter (Fig 5).

In addition to increased glomerular size, cholesterol feeding was associated with mesangial matrix expansion (Fig 6). To further characterize the components responsible for the increased mesangial matrix, three different constituents of the mesangial matrix were assessed by semiquantitative immunohistochemistry. Cholesterol feeding was associated with increases in mesangial collagen (type IV), fibronectin, and laminin (Fig 7). To assess whether the accumulation of type IV collagen was related to increased synthesis or reduced degradation, the mRNA expression of different genes involved in type IV collagen metabolism was assessed by Northern analysis. Cholesterol feeding was associated with an increase in glomerular expression for the α_1 chain of type IV collagen (Fig 8). Northern analysis did not detect mRNA expression for 72 kd collagenase, specific for type IV collagen. However, by reverse transcription and PCR amplification it was shown that mRNA for this collagenase was expressed, albeit at a low level. Cholesterol feeding did not appear to affect the level of expression of 72 kd collagenase (not shown). By contrast, the glomerular mRNA expression for TIMP-2, the major inhibitor of 72 kd collagenase, was found to be increased in association with cholesterol feeding (Fig 8). To further characterize the mechanism of increased matrix deposition, the mRNA for TGF-β1, a major cytokine involved in matrix accumulation, also was evaluated. Cholesterol feeding was associated with increased glomerular TGF-β1 mRNA expression (Fig 8).

DISCUSSION

Increasing experimental evidence suggests that lipids can be important modulators of progressive renal injury.[2-4] Different animal models

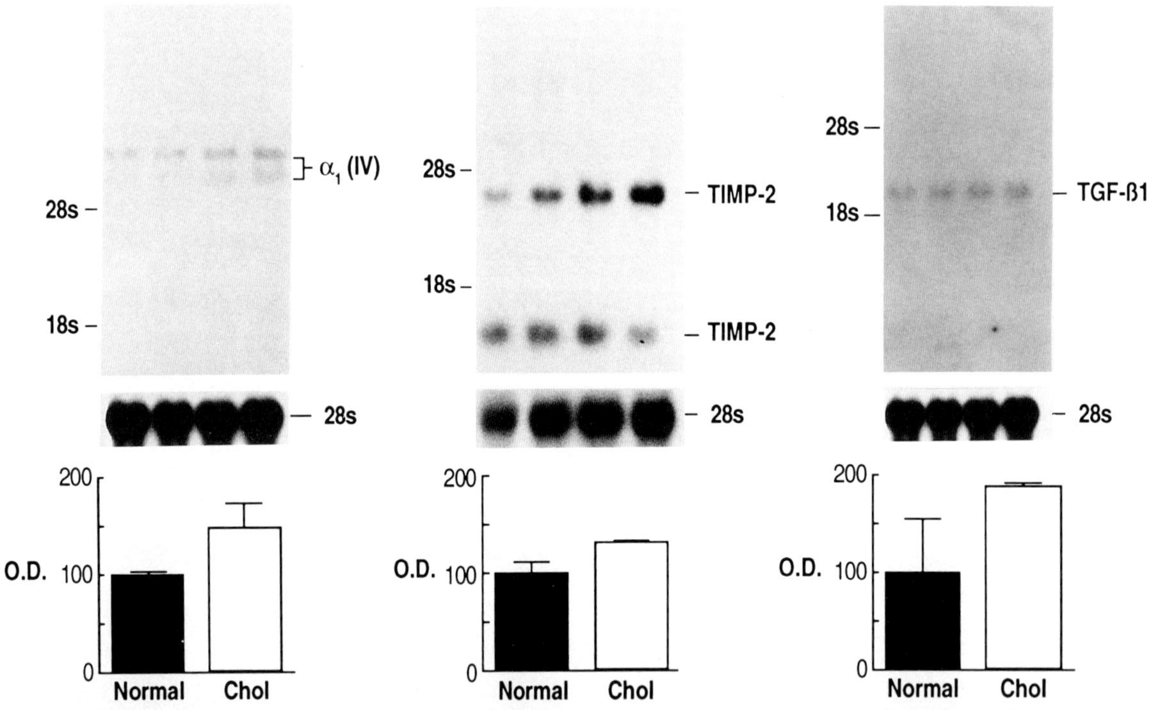

Fig 8. **Northern blot analysis of the effects of cholesterol feeding on glomerular mRNA expression of the α_1 chain of type IV collagen [α_1(IV)], TIMP-2, and TGF-β1 in rats fed standard chow (Normal) or standard chow supplemented with 4% cholesterol (Chol). α_1(IV) and TIMP-2 presented two major transcripts, as indicated. Markers of the ribosomal RNA (28s and 18s) are shown on the left. The reprobed membranes for 28s ribosomal RNA also are shown. The densitometric analysis of the Northern blots is shown at the bottom. The OD (optical density, arbitrary units) of all the transcripts of each gene were added and normalized to the respective 28s values. The results represent the mean ± SD of each experimental group.**

of spontaneous or dietary-induced hypercholesterolemia have been found to develop progressive renal injury.[5] Similarly, cholesterol feeding has been shown to aggravate the renal lesions in animals with a variety of nephropathies of different etiologies.[6-9] We previously reported the long-term effects of dietary-induced hypercholesterolemia on glomerular structure and renal function in otherwise normal rats.[9] We present here the earlier glomerular changes associated with short-term cholesterol feeding. As expected, cholesterol feeding for 4 weeks resulted in marked elevation of serum cholesterol, without significant changes in renal function and without development of glomerular sclerosis.

The results of several studies have suggested that macrophages play a central role in mediating immune and non-immune glomerular injury.[20-22] In both humans and in animal models of renal disease, hyperlipidemia and glomerular injury are frequently associated with an increase in the number of glomerular macrophages.[6,9,23,24] In the present study, an increase in glomerular macrophages was detected as early as 3 days after the initiation of cholesterol feeding, peaked at approximately 2 weeks, and remained stable thereafter. The mechanisms leading to macrophage recruitment are not completely understood and were not addressed by the present work. It has been reported, however, that oxidized lipoproteins can promote monocyte chemotaxis by themselves[25] and through the induction of specific chemoattractants.[26-28] Our data demonstrate that glomerular lipid deposition follows cholesterol feeding. It also has been shown that mesangial cells can oxidize lipoproteins and endocytose these modified lipoproteins through a scavenger receptor.[29-33] In addition, circulating oxidized lipoproteins can be trapped by glomeruli with an efficiency comparable to liver and spleen[34] and remain preferentially bound to the mesangial matrix, where further oxidization may take place.[33,35] Recruited macrophages may also oxidize lipoproteins, ingest them, and become foam cells.[36] Our results showing that all the mesangial foam cells were of macrophage origin are in agreement with this capability.

We and others have previously noted that diet-induced hypercholesterolemia caused an increase in glomerular size.[8,9] It is possible that the greater increase in glomerular size was, in part, the result of one or more products secreted by glomerular macrophages. Macrophages produce a number of cytokines and growth factors that may have stimulated growth and proliferation of glomerular cells.[20] Alternatively, cytokines and growth factors released by other glomerular cells (eg, mesangial cells) may have caused or contributed to the larger glomeruli.[37]

Mesangial matrix constituents (eg, type IV collagen, laminin, and fibronectin) were all increased in cholesterol-fed rats. The increased mRNA expression of the α_1 chain of type IV collagen and the inhibitor of collagen degradation TIMP-2, without any major changes in the 72 kd collagenase for type IV collagen, suggests that both increased synthesis and reduced degradation of type IV collagen may play a role in the mesangial matrix accumulation associated with cholesterol feeding. We have previously reported that rat mesangial cells exposed in vitro to lipoproteins exhibit an increased mRNA expression of type IV collagen and TIMP-2 without a significant change in 72 kd collagenase.[12] Other investigators also have found an increased expression of fibronectin in cholesterol-fed rats.[24] Similarly, lipoproteins enhance the mesangial cell production of fibronectin.[27] Together, these data suggest a role for cholesterol in modulating expansion of mesangial matrix.

Transforming growth factor-β1 has been considered a major cytokine involved in matrix accumulation.[38] Our data showing an increased glomerular TGF-β1 mRNA expression are consistent with a role for TGF-β1 in the matrix expansion associated with hypercholesterolemia. Although initial reports suggested that TGF-β1 might not have a relevant role in type IV collagen accumulation,[39] Isaka et al have reported increased glomerular type IV collagen in rats transfected in vivo with TGF-β1.[40] In addition, high glucose concentrations have been reported to increase type IV collagen expression and production by mesangial cells.[41] The increased type IV collagen production was paralleled by increased TGF-β1 expression and could be prevented by antibodies against TGF-β1.[41] Exogenous TGF-β1 has been shown to activate α_1(IV) collagen expression at the transcriptional level in cultured rat mesangial cells.[42] Finally, TGF-β1 also may play a role in matrix accumulation by promoting the synthesis of inhibitors of proteases involved in matrix degradation.[43,44] Although a direct role of lipoproteins in modulating mesangial cell matrix turnover seems likely, macrophages also may play an important role. Macrophage infiltration and expression of TGF-β1 have been reported to be increased in puromycin nephrosis and exacerbated by cholesterol feeding.[24] Our study was not designed to address the cellular source of TGF-β1. However, although both mesangial cells[45] and macrophages can secrete TGF-β1, it has been suggested that infiltrating macrophages are the major source.[24]

In summary, our findings regarding the early events of glomerular damage induced by hypercholesterolemia, as well as abundant information from other in vivo and in vitro studies, suggest that the process leading to glomerulosclerosis is reminiscent in many respects of the process leading to atherosclerosis in the blood vessel wall.[2-4,33,46] Local lipoprotein accumulation, monocyte recruitment, the formation of foam cells, and the subsequent release of mediators promoting growth and matrix accumulation appear to be key features of both processes.[2-4,33,46]

REFERENCES

1. Klahr S, Schreiner G, Ichikawa I: The progression of renal disease. N Engl J Med 318:1657-1666, 1988

2. Guijarro C, Keane WF: Lipid-induced glomerular injury. Nephron 67:1-6, 1994

3. Diamond JR, Karnovsky MJ: A putative role of hypercholesterolemia in progressive glomerular injury. Annu Rev Med 43:83-92, 1992

4. Gröne EF, Walli AK, Gröne HJ, Miller B, Seidel D: The role of lipids in nephrosclerosis and glomerulosclerosis. Atherosclerosis 107:1-13, 1994

5. Keane WF, Kasiske BL, O'Donnell MP, Kim Y: The role of altered lipid metabolism in the progression of renal disease: Experimental evidence. Am J Kidney Dis 17:38-42, 1991

6. Pesek-Diamond I, Ding GH, Frye J, Diamond JR: Macrophages mediate adverse effects of cholesterol feeding in experimental nephrosis. Am J Physiol 263:F776-F783, 1992

7. Tolins JP, Stone BG, Raij L: Interactions of hypercholesterolemia and hypertension in initiation of glomerular injury. Kidney Int 41:1254-1261, 1992

8. Rayner HC, Ward L, Walls J: Cholesterol feeding following unilateral nephrectomy in the rat leads to glomerular hypertrophy. Nephron 57:453-459, 1991

9. Kasiske BL, O'Donnell MP, Schmitz PG, Kim Y, Keane WF: Renal injury of diet-induced hypercholesterolemia in rats. Kidney Int 37:880-891, 1990

10. Weibel ER, Gomez DM: A principle for counting tissue structures on random section. J Appl Physiol 17:343-348, 1962

11. Laurie GW, Horikoshi S, Killen PD, Segui-Real B, Yamada Y: In situ hybridization reveals temporal and spacial changes in cellular expression of mRNA for a laminin receptor, laminin, and basement membrane (type IV) collagen in the developing kidney. J Cell Biol 109:1351-1362, 1989

12. O'Donnell MP, Guijarro C, Kasiske BL, Kim Y, Keane WF: Independent and interactive effects of IGF-1 and LDL on mesangial cell DNA synthesis and expression of collagen mRNA. J Lab Clin Med 1995 (in press)

13. Collier IE, Wilhelm SM, Eisenz A, Marmer BL, Grant GA, Seltzer JL, Kronberger A, He C, Bauer EA, Goldberg GI: H-*ras* oncogene-transformed human bronchial epithelial cells (TBE-1) secrete a single metalloproteinase capable of degrading basement membrane collagen. J Biol Chem 263:6579-6587, 1988

14. Marti HP, Mcneil L, Davies M, Martin J, Lovett DH: Homology cloning of rat 72 kDa type-IV collagenase-cytokine and 2nd-messenger inducibility in glomerular mesangial cells. Biochem J 291:441-446, 1993

15. Stetler-Stevenson WG, Brown PD, Onisto M, Levy AT, Liotta LA: Tissue inhibitor of metalloproteinases-2 (TIMP-2) mRNA expression in tumor cell lines and human tumor tissues. J Biol Chem 265:13933-13938, 1990

16. Qian SW, Kondaiah P, Roberts AB, Sporn MB: cDNA cloning by PCR of rat transforming growth factor β-1. Nucleic Acids Res 18:3059, 1990

17. Iruela-Arispe ML, Diglio CA, Sage EH: Modulation of extracellular matrix proteins by endothelial cells undergoing angiogenesis in vitro. Arterioscler Thromb 11:805-815, 1991

18. Chomczynski P, Sacchi N: Single-step method of RNA isolation by acid guanidinium thiocyanate-phenol-chloroform extraction. Anal Biochem 162:156-159, 1987

19. Norusis MJ: Statistical Package for the Social Sciences. (SPSS/PC+™ V2.0): Base Manual. Chicago, SPSS Inc, 1988

20. Schreiner GF: The role of the macrophage in glomerular injury. Semin Nephrol 11:268-275, 1991

21. Saito T, Atkins: Contribution of mononuclear leucocytes to the progression of experimental focal glomerular sclerosis. Kidney Int 37:1076-1083, 1990

22. van Goor H, Fidler V, Weening JJ, Grond J: Determinants of focal and segmental glomerulosclerosis in the rat after renal ablation. Lab Invest 64:754-765, 1991

23. Magil AB, Cohen AH: Monocytes and focal glomerulosclerosis. Lab Invest 61:404-409, 1989

24. Ding GH, Pesek-Diamond I, Diamond JR: Cholesterol, macrophages, and gene expression of TGF-beta-1 and fibronectin during nephrosis. Am J Physiol 264:F577-F584, 1993

25. Quinn MT, Parthasarathy S, Fong LG, Steinberg D: Oxidatively modified low density lipoproteins: A potential role in recruitment and retention of monocyte/macrophages during atherogenesis. Proc Natl Acad Sci U S A 84:2995-2998, 1987

26. Yu X, Dluz S, Graves DT, Zhang L, Antoniades HN, Hollander W, Prusty S, Valente AJ, Schwartz CJ, Sonenshein GE: Elevated expression of monocyte chemoattractant protein 1 by vascular smooth muscle cells in hypercholesterolemic primates. Proc Natl Acad Sci U S A 89:6953-6957, 1992

27. Rovin BH, Tan LC: LDL stimulates mesangial fibronectin production and chemoattractant expression. Kidney Int 43:218-225, 1993

28. Navab M, Imes SS, Hama SY, Hough GP, Ross LA, Bork RW, Valente AJ, Berliner JA, Drinkwater DC, Laks H: Monocyte transmigration induced by modification of low density lipoprotein in cocultures of human aortic wall cells is due to induction of monocyte chemotactic protein 1 synthesis and is abolished by high density lipoprotein. J Clin Invest 88:2039-2046, 1991

29. Gupta S, Rifici V, Crowley S, Brownlee M, Zihe S, Schlöndorff D: Interactions of LDL and modified LDL with mesangial cells and matrix. Kidney Int 41:1161-1169, 1992

30. Wheeler DC, Fernando RL, Gillett MP, Zaruba J, Persaud J, Kingstone D, Varghese Z, Moorhead JF: Characterisation of the binding of low-density lipoproteins to cultured rat mesangial cells. Nephrol Dial Transplant 6:701-708, 1991

31. Wheeler DC, Chana RS, Topley N, Petersen MM, Davies M, Williams JD: Oxidation of low density lipoprotein by mesangial cells may promote glomerular injury. Kidney Int 45:1628-1636, 1994

32. Keane WF, O'Donnell MP, Kasiske BL, Kim YK: Oxidative modification of low-density lipoproteins by mesangial cells. J Am Soc Nephrol 4:187-194, 1993

33. Schlöndorff D: Cellular mechanisms of lipid injury in the glomerulus. Am J Kidney Dis 22:72-82, 1993

34. Coritsidis G, Rifici V, Gupta S, Rie J, Shan ZH, Neugarten J, Schlöndorff D: Preferential binding of oxidized LDL to rat glomeruli in vivo and cultured mesangial cells in vitro. Kidney Int 39:858-866, 1991

35. Magil AB, Frohlich JJ, Innis SM, Steinbrecher UP: Oxidized low-density lipoprotein in experimental focal glomerulosclerosis. Kidney Int 43:1243-1250, 1993

36. Schönholzer KW, Waldron M, Magil AB: Intraglomerular foam cells and human focal glomerulosclerosis. Nephron 62:130-136, 1992

37. Sedor JR, Konieczkowski M, Huang S, Gronich JH, Nakazato Y, Gordon G, King CH: Cytokines, mesangial cell activation and glomerular injury. Kidney Int 39:S65-S70, 1993

38. Border WA, Noble NA: Cytokines in kidney disease: The role of transforming growth factor-β. Am J Kidney Dis 22:105-113, 1993

39. Border WA, Okuda S, Languino LR, Ruoslahti E: Transforming growth factor-β regulates production of proteoglycans by mesangial cells. Kidney Int 37:689-695, 1990

40. Isaka Y, Fujiwara Y, Ueda N, Kaneda Y, Kamada T, Imai E: Glomerulosclerosis induced by in vivo transfection of transforming growth factor-beta or platelet-derived growth factor gene into the rat kidney. J Clin Invest 92:2597-2601, 1993

41. Ziyadeh FN, Sharma K, Eriksen M, Wolf G: Stimulation of collagen gene expression and protein synthesis in murine mesangial cells by high glucose is mediated by autocrine activation of transforming growth factor-β. J Clin Invest 93:536-542, 1994

42. Suzuki S, Ebihara I, Tomino Y, Koide H: Transcriptional activation of matrix genes by transforming growth factor $\beta 1$ in mesangial cells. Exp Nephrol 1:229-237, 1993

43. Overall CM, Wrana JL, Sodek J: Independent regulation of collagenase, 72 kDa progelatinase, and metalloendoproteinase inhibitor expression in human fibroblasts by transforming growth factor-β. J Biol Chem 264:1860-1869, 1989

44. Tomooka S, Border WA, Marshall BC, Noble NA: Glomerular matrix accumulation is linked to inhibition of the plasmin protease system. Kidney Int 42:1462-1469, 1992

45. Kaname S, Uchida S, Ogata E, Kurokawa K: Autocrine secretion of transforming growth factor-β in cultured rat mesangial cells. Kidney Int 42:1319-1327, 1992

46. Ross R: The pathogenesis of atherosclerosis: A perspective for the 1990s. Nature 362:801-809, 1993

Cholesterol: A Renal Risk Factor in Diabetic Nephropathy?

Henrik Mulec, MD, Svend Aage Johnsen, MD, Olle Wiklund, MD, and Staffan Björck, MD

● In a prospective follow-up of 30 patients with type 1 diabetes and nephropathy, serum cholesterol, triglycerides, apolipoprotein AI and B, and lipoprotein(a) were determined to study their relationship to the rate of decline in glomerular filtration rate. The patients had proteinuria and advanced nephropathy with a mean ± SD glomerular filtration rate of 39 mL/min/1.73 m^2. The decline in glomerular filtration rate was determined during 2.5 ± 0.5 years. High serum cholesterol, triglycerides, and apolipoprotein B were correlated to a more rapid deterioration in kidney function. The rate of decline in glomerular filtration rate was 1.0 ± 2.5 mL/min/yr in the 10 patients with the lowest cholesterol level, compared with 4.5 ± 3.2 mL/min/yr in the patients with the highest serum cholesterol ($P = 0.015$). The combined effect of the measured lipids, blood pressure, type of antihypertensive treatment, protein intake, proteinuria, and hemoglobin A_{1C} on the rate of decline in glomerular filtration rate was assessed by multiple regression analysis. The measured factors together had a high explanatory power for the rate of decline in glomerular filtration rate. In this model, 73% of the variation in decline in glomerular filtration rate was explained by the measured variables (multiple $r^2 = 0.73$). Low cholesterol and treatment with an angiotensin-converting enzyme inhibitor were the strongest predictors of a favorable renal prognosis. This suggests that hypercholesterolemia is an important risk factor for diabetic nephropathy.

INDEX WORDS: Diuabetes; diabetic nephropathy; lipids; cholesterol; apolipoproteins; angiotensin-converting enzyme inhibition.

MORTALITY in diabetic patients with nephropathy has decreased dramatically during the last few years[1] and the decline in kidney function that previously was regarded as inevitable can be arrested in many patients.[2] However, some patients will still lose kidney function rapidly despite satisfactory control of the known risk factors. Other mechanisms that lead to destruction of kidney function, therefore, have to be sought.

Experimental results indicate that hyperlipidemia can accelerate the loss of renal function in renal diseases.[3-5] Similarities may exist between the process that leads to destruction of glomerular structures and atherosclerosis.[6,7] Furthermore, a synergistic harmful renal effect in renal diseases of hypertension and high cholesterol has been suggested.[8-11] As the relevance of these animal data in humans is unknown, we studied the relationship between hyperlipidemia and the decline in glomerular filtration rate in a population of patients with type 1 diabetes and nephropathy.

PATIENTS AND METHODS

Patients

The glomerular filtration rate was prospectively studied in 30 patients with type 1 diabetes and nephropathy during 2.5 years (range, 1.5 to 3.0 years). They had type 1 diabetes, diabetic nephropathy, reduced renal function, and other diabetic complications such as retinopathy. The patients had a mean age of 44 years (range, 23 to 59 years) and mean age of onset of diabetes of 17 years (3 to 38 years). The mean duration of diabetes was 28 years (range, 16 to 46 years). All patients had retinopathy and three patients were blind. The onset and development of the kidney disease were typical of diabetic nephropathy in all patients. All patients were on antihypertensive treatment and at the start of the prospective monitoring of renal function they were randomized to angiotensin-converting enzyme inhibitor or beta-blocker treatment. Seventeen patients were given enalapril and 13 were given metoprolol. The effect of the antihypertensive treatment on kidney function has been previously reported.[2] The study was performed after obtaining the patients' informed consent and approval by the local ethical committee.

Methods

We measured blood pressure, urinary albumin excretion, serum electrolytes, hemoglobin, and hemoglobinA_{1C} at baseline and at 2-month intervals, and urinary nitrogen and glomerular filtration rate at 6-month intervals.

The glomerular filtration rate was measured as the rate of disappearance of chromium-51 edetic acid in plasma after a single injection. Albumin excretion was measured in 24-hour urine samples by immunochemical turbidimetric assay, electrophoresis, or immunoprecipitation assay, depending on the routine of hospitals. Dietary protein intake was calculated from urinary nitrogen excretion.[12]

Lipid Determinations

At baseline and at 6-month intervals, nonfasting serum samples were analyzed for cholesterol and triglycerides using fully enzymatic methods. These values are listed in the Results section. For further analysis of the lipid profile, fasting samples were obtained on one occasion in all patients for analysis of apolipoprotein AI (ApoAI), apolipoprotein B (ApoB), and lipoprotein(a) (Lp(a)). Apolipoproteins AI and B

Supported by grants from the Swedish Medical Research Council (projects 4531 and 05230), the Swedish Heart and Lung Foundation, and the Ericsson Medical Research Fund.

were determined with immunoturbidometric methods (UniKit LaRoche, catalog nos. 07 2995 7 and 07 2994 9, Hoffmann LaRoche, Basel, Switzerland) in a Cobas Fara Autoanalyser (Hoffmann LaRoche); between assay variations were 4.4% and 3.4% respectively. For the determination of Lp(a) a radioimmunoassay was used (catalog no. 10-6497-01, Pharmacia Diagnostics AB, Uppsala, Sweden). Reference values for serum cholesterol, triglycerides, apo AI, and apo B were obtained from the Göteborg sample of the MONICA study.[13] A value of Lp(a) above 200 mg/L was considered elevated (population data not available).

Statistics

Results are presented as means ± SD. Due to their skewed distribution, urinary albumin excretion, cholesterol, triglycerides, and Lp(a) are given as geometric means (anti-log 95% confidence interval of the logarithms). In Tables 1 to 4, the results obtained during the observation period are summarized by one mean value for each patient; these values are used to calculate the means and geometric means. However, ApoAI, ApoB, and Lp(a) were only measured once in each patient. Serum cholesterol determined at this occasion showed a strong correlation ($r = 0.8$) to the average cholesterol level. The rate of deterioration of renal function was analyzed by regression lines for chromium-51 edetic acid clearance over time, determined for each patient over the whole period for that patient.

One- and two-factor analysis of variance was used for comparisons between groups and $P < 0.05$ was considered significant. Data were analyzed after logarithmic transformation of urinary albumin excretion, serum cholesterol, triglycerides, ApoAI, ApoB, and Lp(a). Forward stepwise linear regression analysis was carried out to assess the influence of possible explanatory variables on the rate of decline in glomerular filtration rate. Statistical software was Statview SE–Graphics (Abacus Concepts Inc, Berkeley CA).

RESULTS

The clinical data and results of the serum analyses for the patients are given in Table 1. Fourteen patients had serum cholesterol and 12 patients had serum triglycerides above the 90th percentile of the population for their age group. Eighteen patients had elevated Lp(a). It was recently shown that angiotensin-converting enzyme inhibitor treatment can reduce proteinuria and the rate of the deterioration of glomerular filtration rate in diabetic nephropathy.[2] The differences in the results presented in Table 1 between angiotensin-converting enzyme inhibitor- and non–angiotensin-converting enzyme inhibitor-treated patients were rate of decline in glomerular filtration rate −1.6 ± 1.9 mL/min/yr versus −4.3 ± 3.5 mL/min/yr ($P = 0.01$), serum triglycerides 1.6 mmol/L (1.2 to 2.2) versus 3.4 mmol/L (2.4 to 4.9) ($P = 0.001$), and albuminuria

Table 1. Clinical Data and Laboratory Results During the Observation Period for 30 Patients With Diabetic Nephropathy

Female/male	18/12
Age (yr)	45.3 ± 9.1 SD
Duration of diabetes (yr)	29 ± 8.0 SD
GFR (mL/min)	39 ± 14 SD
Hemoglobin A_{1c} (%)	8.8 ± 1.7 SD
Cholesterol (mmol/L)	6.8 (6.3-7.4)
Triglycerides (mmol/L)	2.0 (1.7-2.5)
ApoAI (g/L)	1.9 ± 0.3 SD
ApoB (g/L)	1.8 ± 0.5 SD
Lp(a) (mg/L)	180 (109-295)
Change in GFR (mL/min/yr)	−2.8 ± 3.0 SD
Albuminuria (g/24 hr)	0.8 (0.5-1.2)
Serum albumin (g/L)	38.6 ± 4 SD
Protein intake (g/24 hr)	1.0 ± 0.3 SD
Blood pressure (mm Hg)	138/84 ± 11/5 SD

Note. Each patient is summarized by one mean value. These values are used to calculate the means and geometric means.

Abbreviation: GFR, glomerular filtration rate.

0.5 g/24 hr (0.3 to 0.9) versus 1.4 g/24 hr (0.9 to 2.1) ($P = 0.007$), respectively. The differences in albuminuria and triglyceride levels are not due to differences before allocation to the two treatments since there were no differences before randomization. The serum triglyceride level was 1.8 mmol/L (1.3 to 2.4) in the angiotensin-converting enzyme inhibitor-treated patients and 2.0 mmol/L (1.5 to 2.5) in the beta-blocker–treated patients; urinary albumin excretion was 1.5 g/24 hr (0.9 to 2.5) and 1.4 g/24 hr (0.8 to 2.4), respectively.

The rate of decline in glomerular filtration rate was negatively correlated to serum cholesterol, triglycerides, and ApoB and positively correlated to ApoAI. Coefficients are given in Table 2. Mean arterial blood pressure, hemoglobin A_{1C}, and protein intake were not correlated to the decline in glomerular filtration rate.

The relative importance of the different variables listed in Table 1 for the decline in glomerular filtration rate, assessed by stepwise regression analysis, is shown in Table 3. When all variables are entered into the equation, the multiple correlation coefficicent is 0.86. With this model, the variation in the rate of decline in glomerular filtration rate is 73% determined by the variables used (multiple $r^2 = 0.73$). The highest significances are found for angiotensin-converting and

Table 2. Correlations Between Explanatory Variables and the Rate of Change in Glomerular Filtration Rate in 30 Patients With Diabetic Nephropathy

Variable	*r* (n = 30)
Cholesterol	−0.61*
Triglycerides (0.81)	−0.48*
Albuminuria (0.23)	−0.12
ApoB (0.78)	−0.39†
Lp(a) (0.1)	−0.11
HemoglobinA1 (0.24)	−0.26
Mean arterial pressure (0.51)	−0.29
Protein intake (−0.3)	0.28
ApoAI (−0.34)	0.43†

Note. The correlations between cholesterol and the other variables are given in parentheses.
*$P < 0.01$.
†$P < 0.05$.

non–angiotensin-converting enzyme inhibitor treatment and serum cholesterol level ($P \leq 0.002$).

Since the rate of decline in glomerular filtration rate is best predicted by the cholesterol level, the patients have been divided into three equal groups according to cholesterol level (Table 4). Diastolic blood pressure differed between these groups. The rate of decline in glomerular filtration rate differed significantly between the three groups and increased in proportion to serum cholesterol.

The strongest explanatory factors for the decline in glomerular filtration rate were serum cholesterol and type of treatment (angiotensin-converting enzyme inhibitors *v* beta-blockade). The relationship between these two variables is shown in Fig 1. The patients in the enalapril and the metoprolol group are divided into three groups, as equal in size as possible, depending on cholesterol. These two factors (type of treatment and cholesterol) are both independently correlated to the decline in glomerular filtration rate ($P < 0.03$ and $P < 0.009$, respectively; two-factor analysis of variance).

DISCUSSION

Hypertension is the most important factor known that accelerates the progressive decline in kidney function in diabetic nephropathy.[1] Careful attention to, and good control of, the blood pressure in most of our patients gives an opportunity to assess the importance of other risk factors by minimizing the influence of blood pressure.

The progression of diabetic nephropathy is a multifactorial process. The interrelationship between many risk factors confounds any attempt to assess the importance of individual risk factors, but the strong association between cholesterol level and the decrease in glomerular filtration rate in our patients supports the hypothesis of a nephrotoxic effect of hypercholesterolemia in renal disease in humans.

Lipid abnormalities secondary to proteinuria, reduced renal function, or dietary intake have been pointed out as one of the possible mediators in the progression of initial glomerular injury to glomerulosclerosis.[3] Glomerulosclerosis and atherosclerosis share several features, as recently reviewed.[14] Similarity to atherosclerosis is also suggested by the association between ApoAI and rate of progression. The specific lipid fraction responsible for progressive nephron destruction has not been identified. Kasiske et al[8] suggest that alterations in serum cholesterol may be more closely associated with glomerular injury than alterations in serum triglycerides, which is in agreement with our findings.

The serum triglyceride level was clearly elevated in patients treated with metoprolol, whereas it was only moderately increased in those treated with enalapril. This is not explained by such factors as degree of renal failure, metabolic control, and proteinuria. A higher serum triglyceride level during treatment with beta-blockers has been shown in several studies.[15]

Table 3. Result of Forward Stepwise Multiple Regression Analysis of Different Variables on the Rate of Decline in Glomerular Filtration Rate in 30 Patients With Diabetic Nephropathy

Variable	F Value to Enter	*P*
Cholesterol	14.4	<0.001
Enalapril/metoprolol treatment	6.1	<0.01

Note. The stepwise procedure selects the best subset of predictor variables and stops adding variables when the contribution to the result is small. Two variables were selected. The variables not in the equation and their F values are ApoA, 2.5; albuminuria, 1.8; hemoglobinA1, 1.7; triglycerides, 1.6; ApoB, 0.9; mean arterial blood pressure, 0.05; Lp(a), 0.3; and protein intake, 0.03.

Table 4. Clinical and Laboratory Characteristics in 30 Patients With Diabetic Nephropathy Divided Into Three Groups According to Their Serum Cholesterol Value

	Cholesterol Level (mmol/L)			
	<6.0	6.0-7.7	>7.7	*P**
No. of patients	10	10	10	
ACE inhibitor treatment	6	7	4	0.41
Male/Female	4/6	5/5	9/1	0.05
HemoglobinA$_1$ (%)	8.1 ± 1.3	9.4 ± 1.8	9.0 ± 2.0	0.27
Blood pressure	134/80 ± 9/6	138/86 ± 11/4	143/85 ± 11/5	0.20/<u>0.023</u>
GFR (mL/min)	44.8 ± 10.3	33 ± 12.8	40.9 ± 16.8	0.16
ΔGFR (mL/min/yr)	−0.9 ± 1.9	−2.9 ± 3.0	−4.5 ± 3.2	<u>0.027</u>
Protein intake (g/kg/d)	1.2 ± 0.3	1.0 ± 0.3	1.0 ± 0.4	0.21
Albuminuria (g/24 hr)	0.6 ± 0.3-1.1	0.8 ± 0.3-1.8	1.1 ± 0.5-2.3	0.45

Abbreviations: ACE, angiotensin-converting enzyme; GFR, glomerular filtration rate; ΔGFR, change in GFR.

* Probability value for between-group differences were analyzed with one factor analysis of variance. The significances are underscored.

Our patients had high cholesterol, triglyceride, and ApoB levels. This can be partly explained by poor metabolic control of the diabetes. Hemoglobin A_{1C} was 9.1% ± 2.7%, which is similar to what is usually described in this type of patient.[1] Most of our patients were treated with four daily injections of insulin, adjusted after self-measurement of blood glucose. However, the impact of metabolic control on lipids is relatively small. In a recent study, a 1% decrease in hemoglobin A_{1C} was associated with a decrease in total cholesterol of only 0.17 mmol/L and a decrease in triglycerides of 0.13 mmol/L.[16] Proteinuria appears to be more important. Even with proteinuria within the microalbuminuric range, an atherogenic lipid profile is present,[17-19] and it is further exaggerated in the presence of increasing proteinuria and decreasing renal function.[20]

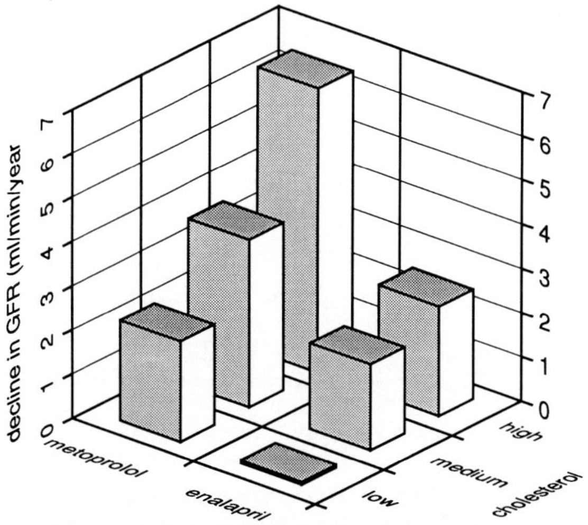

Fig 1. Relationship between the rate of decline in glomerular filtration rate, enalapril/metoprolol treatment, and cholesterol level. Metoprolol- and enalapril-treated patients are both divided into three categories depending on cholesterol level.

Lipoprotein(a), considered to be an independent risk factor for ischemic heart disease,[21] was elevated in 18 of the 30 patients, in agreement with findings in microalbuminuric patients.[22] There was no correlation between Lp(a) and rate of decline in glomerular filtration rate.

The interrelationship between risk factors is shown in Table 4. When the patients are grouped according to cholesterol level, the rate of decline in glomerular filtration rate increases linearly between the groups. However, there is a significant difference in blood pressure between the groups. When further analyzed by multiple regression analysis, serum cholesterol and type of antihypertensive treatment are found to be the most important explanatory variables for the variation in the rate of decline in glomerular filtration rate. In our analysis of the present data we found a clear-cut difference between the effect of the two main factors (angiotensin-converting enzyme inhibitor treatment and cholesterol level) and the remaining variables (Table 3) on the rate of decline in glomerular filtration rate.

It could be speculated that lipid nephrotoxicity

is enhanced by an increased passage of macromolecules, including lipids, into the mesangial area and that reduction of this traffic by angiotensin-converting enzyme inhibitor treatment could be one explanation for the beneficial renal effect of angiotensin-converting enzyme inhibition. A reduction in cholesterol secondary to a reduction in proteinuria could therefore further enhance this effect.[2,23] This view is supported by the biphasic antiproteinuric response to angiotensin-converting enzyme inhibitors. There is a decrease in proteinuria within weeks and a continued progressive decline in proteinuria over up to 3 years.[2] Experimental studies have shown that hyperlipidemia may interact with hypertension and pre-existing renal damage to increase the glomerular damage dramatically.[3-5,8-11]

Dietary protein intake was the same in the three groups and does not correlate with the decline in glomerular filtration rate. Interestingly, in a recent study showing a beneficial renal effect of dietary protein restriction, low-density lipoprotein cholesterol was reduced by 21%.[24]

In glomerular diseases, progression to renal failure is rare in the absence of proteinuria and interventions designed to reduce proteinuria seem to have a beneficial effect on progression of chronic renal disease.[25] Therefore, reactive mechanisms triggered by an increased protein traffic across the glomerular capillary have been suggested to be a key factor in the development of glomerulosclerosis.[26] However, our data indicate that hypercholesterolemia, which is linked to proteinuria, is the important factor contributing to glomerular injury.

Thus, serum cholesterol might be one of the major risk factors in the multifactorial process of progression of renal failure in patients with diabetic nephropathy. If the importance of cholesterol is established by prospective studies aiming at normalization of cholesterol, this introduces the possibility of arresting the progression in many patients, considering the greatly improved prognosis that has already been achieved in this group of patients.[1,2]

REFERENCES

1. Parving HH, Hommel E: Prognosis in diabetic nephropathy. Br Med J 299:230-233, 1989

2. Björck S, Mulec H, Johnsen SA, Norden G, Aurell M: Renal protective effect of enalapril in diabetic nephropathy. Br Med J 304:339-343, 1992

3. Moorhead JF, Chang MK, El-Nahas M, Varghese Z: Lipid nephrotoxicity in chronic progressive glomerular and tubulointerstitial disease. Lancet 1:1309-1311, 1982

4. Moorhead JF: Lipids and progressive kidney disease. Kidney Int 39:35-40, 1991 (suppl 31)

5. Keane WF, Mulcahy S, Kasiske BL, Youngki K, O'Donnell MP: Hyperlipidemia and progressive renal disease. Kidney Int 39:41-48, 1991 (suppl 31)

6. El Nahas AM: Glomerulosclerosis: A form of atherosclerosis. Proceedings of the Xth International Congress of Nephrology 2:1206-1220, 1987

7. Diamond JR, Karnovsky MJ: Focal and segmental glomerulosclerosis: Analogies to atherosclerosis. Kidney Int 33:917-924, 1988

8. Kasiske BL, O Donnell MP, Cowardin W, Keane WF: Lipids and the kidney. Hypertension 15:443-450, 1990

9. Kasiske BL, O'Donell MP, Garvis WJ, Keane WF: Pharmacologic treatment of hyperlipidemia reduces glomerular injury in rat 5/6 nephrectomy model of chronic renal failure. Circulation Res 62:367-374, 1988

10. Kasiske BL, O Donell MP, Schmitz PG, Kim Y, Keane WF: Renal injury of diet-induced hypercholesterolemia in rats. Kidney Int 37:880-891, 1990

11. Kasiske BL, O'Donell MP, Clearly MP, Keane WF: Effects of reduced renal mass on the tissue lipids and renal injury in hyperlipidemic rats. Kidney Int 35:40-47, 1989

12. Nyberg G, Norden G, Attman PO, Aurell M, Uddebom G, Arvidsson R, Isaksson B: Diabetic nephropathy: Is dietary protein harmful? J Diabet Complications 1:37-40, 1987

13. Keil U, Kuulasma K: WHO MONICA Project: Risk factors. Int J Epidemiol 18:S46-S65, 1989 (suppl 1)

14. Diamond JR: Analogous pathobiologic mechanism in glomerulosclerosis and atherosclerosis. Kidney Int 39:S-29-S-34, 1991 (suppl 31)

15. Weinberger MH: Antihypertensive therapy and lipids. Paradoxical influence on cardiovascular disease risk. Am J Med 80:64-70, 1986 (suppl 2A)

16. Semenkovich CF, Ostlund RE, Schechtman KB: Plasma lipids in patients with type I diabetes mellitus: Influence of race, gender and plasma glucose control in black women. Arch Intern Med 149:51-56, 1989

17. Jensen T, Stender S, Deckert T: Abnormalities in plasma concentration of lipoproteins and fibrinogen in type 1 (insulin-dependent) diabetic patients with increased urinary albumin excretion. Diabetologia 31:142-145, 1988

18. Vannini P, Ciavarella A, Flammini M, Bargossi AM, Forlani G, Borgnino LC, Orsoni G: Lipid abnormalities in insulin-dependent diabetic patients with albuminuria. Diabetes Care 7:151-154, 1984

19. Jones SL, Close CF, Mattock MB, Jarrett RJ, Keen H, Viberti GC: Plasma lipid and coagulation factor concentrations in insulin dependent diabetics with microalbuminuria. Br Med J 298:487-490, 1989

20. Attman P-O, Nyberg G, William-Olsson T, Knight-Gibson C, Alaupovic P: Lipid and apolipoprotein profile in diabetic chronic renal failure. Abstracts of the 17th Congress of the EDTA, Wienna, Austria, 1990, p 71 (abstr)

21. Scanu AM: Update on lipoprotein(a). Curr Opin Lipidol 2:253-258, 1991

22. Kapelrud H, Bangstad H-J, Dahl-Jörgensen K, Berg K, Hansen KF: Serum Lp(a) lipoprotein concentrations in

insulin dependent diabetic patients with microalbuminuria. Br Med J 303:675-678, 1991

23. Keilani T, Schlueter W, Levin M, Battle DC: Reduction of serum total cholesterol and proteinuria with fosinopril, a new converting enzyme inhibitor. J Am Soc Nephrol 2:231, 1991 (abstr)

24. Walker JD, Bending JJ, Dodds RA, Mattock MB, Murrells TJ, Keen H, Viberti GC: Restriction of dietary protein and progression of renal failure in diabetic nephropathy. Lancet 86771:1411-1415, 1989

25. Björck S, Mulec H, Johnsen SA, Nyberg G, Aurell M: Contrasting effects of enalapril and metoprolol on proteinuria in diabetic nephropathy. Br Med J 300:904-907, 1990

26. Remuzzi G, Bertani T: Editorial review: Is glomerulosclerosis a consequence of altered glomerular permeability to macromolecules? Kidney Int 38:384-394, 1989

Lovastatin Retards the Progression of Established Glomerular Disease in Obese Zucker Rats

Michael P. O'Donnell, PhD, Bertram L. Kasiske, MD, Youngki Kim, MD, Paul G. Schmitz, MD,* and William F. Keane, MD

● Considerable experimental evidence indicates that hyperlipidemia can induce glomerular injury. The importance of lipids in the progression of established glomerular disease has not been established and is of clinical relevance because of the frequent association of lipid abnormalities with human renal disease. In the present study, 26-week-old hyperlipidemic obese Zucker rats (OZRs) with established nephropathy were treated for a period of 18 weeks with daily injections of the cholesterol synthesis inhibitor lovastatin (4 mg/kg). Compared with control OZRs treated with vehicle, lovastatin-treated OZRs had significantly ($P < 0.05$) lower serum cholesterol and triglyceride levels throughout the treatment period. Blood pressure and urine albumin excretion in lovastatin-treated OZRs were reduced over the first 12 weeks of therapy, but increased toward the levels in the control OZRs at the end of the protocol. After 18 weeks of therapy, the incidence of glomerulosclerosis in lovastatin-treated OZRs (23.2% ± 5.8%) was approximately half of that in vehicle-treated OZRs (44.6% ± 7.7%) ($P < 0.05$). The reduction in glomerular injury in lovastatin-treated OZRs was not associated with changes in either glomerular area or glomerular macrophage content. In separate experiments, mesangial cells were cultured from glomeruli isolated from 26-week-old proteinuric OZRs. Lovastatin (5 to 40 μmol/L) caused a significant dose-dependent inhibition of serum-stimulated mesangial cell DNA synthesis. The inhibitory effects of lovastatin were completely prevented in the presence of exogenous mevalonate (100 μmol/L). Thus, lovastatin retarded the progression of established glomerular disease in OZRs. This may have resulted from beneficial effects of lowering of serum lipids and/or from direct effects of lovastatin to inhibit mesangial cell proliferation.

INDEX WORDS: Glomerulosclerosis; albuminuria; hyperlipidemia; mevalonate; macrophages.

SEVERAL experimental studies have provided evidence that lipid abnormalities can initiate glomerular injury. Feeding laboratory animals high-fat or cholesterol-rich diets has been shown to cause hyperlipidemia, proteinuria, and glomerular structural injury.[1-5] In some experimental models of renal disease, early initiation of therapy with lipid-lowering drugs was found to markedly ameliorate glomerular injury.[6-8] In this regard, hyperlipidemic obese Zucker rats (OZRs) given daily clofibric acid or lovastatin beginning at 8 weeks of age had substantially less albuminuria and focal glomerulosclerosis (FGS) at 40 weeks of age compared with untreated obese rats.[6]

While it seems clear from these previous studies that lipid alterations can induce glomerular injury, the importance of lipids in the progression of established glomerular disease has not been defined. In the present study, therefore, 26-week-old hyperlipidemic OZRs with established nephropathy were treated for 18 weeks with daily injections of the cholesterol synthesis inhibitor lovastatin. The effects of this intervention on blood pressure, serum lipids, and the course of glomerular disease were evaluated.

We have recently found that lovastatin inhibits proliferation of rat mesangial cells isolated from young OZRs. Moreover, it was suggested that lovastatin might reduce glomerular injury, at least in part, through this effect.[9] In the present study, therefore, we also evaluated the effect of lovastatin on proliferation of cultured mesangial cells obtained from 26-week-old proteinuric OZRs.

METHODS

In Vivo Study

Sixteen male OZRs (Charles River Breeding Laboratories, Wilmington, MA) were entered into the study at 8 weeks of age. All experiments were conducted in accord with the National Institutes of Health Guide for the Care and Use of Laboratory Animals. Rats were fed standard laboratory chow (Ralston Purina #5001, St Louis, MO) ad libitum and were allowed free access to tap water. Body weights were recorded weekly. Fasting serum cholesterol and triglycerides and urine albumin excretion (UalbV) were measured at 14, 20, and 26 weeks of age. Awake, systolic blood pressure (BP) was measured at 20 and 26 weeks of age, and creatinine clearance was measured at 26 weeks.

At 26 weeks of age the obese rats were divided into two groups matched for blood pressure, serum lipid levels, and UalbV. Together, these variables were used as an index of the degree of established nephropathy in each group. One group of obese rats (n = 8) then received daily subcutaneous injections of lovastatin (4 mg/kg body weight) for a period

Supported in part by a grant from Merck, Sharp and Dohme, Inc, and the Baxter Extramural Grant Program.

of 18 weeks. The other group of obese rats (n = 8) received daily injections of vehicle (propylene glycolethanol; diluted 1:1). Dosages were adjusted weekly for changes in body weight. Measurements of BP, UalbV, and fasting serum lipids were repeated in all rats at 32, 38, and 44 weeks of age. Creatinine clearance was measured at 44 weeks of age. At 44 weeks, rats were anesthetized with ether and the kidneys were removed, blotted, and weighed. Coronal tissue sections were obtained and processed for light microscopy. A piece of cortical tissue was snap-frozen in isopentane pre-cooled with liquid nitrogen, and was stored at −70°C until processed for immunohistochemistry.

Measurements of blood pressure, serum lipids, and urine albumin. Systolic blood pressure in awake, quietly restrained rats was measured on two consecutive mornings using the tail-cuff method as we have previously described.[6,7] Individual readings were averaged. Twenty-four–hour urine collections were obtained from rats that were individually housed in metabolic cages. Rats were fasted during the collection period, but were allowed free access to water. Urine albumin concentration was measured with a nephelometer using a monospecific antibody to rat serum albumin (Cappel Laboratories, West Chester, PA) as we have previously described.[6,7] After the urine collection, fasting tail vein blood samples were obtained from rats lightly anesthetized with ether. Serum cholesterol and triglycerides were measured using an autoanalyzer (ASTRA, Beckman Instruments, Brea, CA).

Histology and immunohistochemistry. Coronal tissue sections were fixed in Zenker's solution and stained with periodic acid-Schiff. All tissue was examined without knowledge of the group from which it originated. Light microscopy (×400) was used to determine the percentage of glomeruli with any evidence of glomerulosclerosis. At least 100 glomeruli in each tissue specimen were examined for the presence of glomerulosclerosis, as previously described.[5-7] Areas of nonsclerotic glomeruli were estimated by measuring the glomerular tuft circumferences using a video-displayed, morphometric computer program (Microcomp DS and PM-2, Southern Micro Instruments, Atlanta, GA).

Identification of glomerular Ia-positive monocyte/macrophages was done in nonsclerotic glomeruli using a monoclonal antibody directed against cell surface antigen (OX4), as previously described.[5] After incubation and washing, tissue was reacted with FITC-conjugated rabbit anti-mouse IgG $F(ab')_2$ followed by FITC-conjugated goat anti-rabbit IgG $F(ab')_2$ (Pel-Freeze Biologicals, Rogers, AR). Epifluorescence microscopy was used to determine the number of positive cells in each glomerulus examined. Ten glomeruli in each tissue specimen were examined.

In Vitro Study

Mesangial cell culture. The OZRs (n = 3) used for this study were the same age (26 weeks) as the obese rats of the in vivo study at the time lovastatin treatment was initiated. Moreover, UalbV in the obese rats used for the in vitro study was similar to that in the obese rats of the in vivo study. Glomeruli were isolated by sieving of renal cortical tissue through stainless steel screens. Mesangial cells were grown in culture from the glomerular isolates using previously described techniques.[9] For the present experiments, cells between the ninth and 15th passages were used.

Measurement of DNA synthesis. Mesangial cell DNA replication was assessed using cellular ^{3}H-thymidine incorporation as we have previously described.[9] Briefly, confluent mesangial cells were synchronized to quiescence (G_0) by incubation in serum-free culture medium. After 48 hours, the cells were exposed to medium containing 10% fetal bovine serum to stimulate proliferation. Some cells were also exposed to either lovastatin alone (5 to 40 μmol/L) or lovastatin plus mevalonate (100 μmol/L). The exogenous mevalonate was added to override the inhibition of intracellular mevalonate production caused by lovastatin. Incorporation of ^{3}H-thymidine was measured over a 42-hour period.

Statistics

All results are expressed as mean ± SEM. Differences between means of two groups were analyzed using two-tailed Student's *t*-test for unpaired data. One-way analysis of variance with the Duncan multiple range test was used to analyze differences between means of more than two groups. When group variances were unequal, logarithmic transformation of data was performed prior to analysis. All analyses were performed using the Statistical Package for the Social Sciences.[10] Differences were considered significant at $P < 0.05$.

RESULTS

In Vivo Study

At 26 weeks of age, when the OZRs were assigned to either the lovastatin or vehicle treatment groups, there were no differences in body weight, BP, fasting serum lipids, or creatinine clearance between the two groups (Table 1; Figs 1 and 2). Urine albumin excretion at 26 weeks was also not different between the two groups (Table 1; Fig 3). Moreover, the increase in UalbV between 14 and 26 weeks of age was similar in both groups (Fig 3). Together, the comparable values of BP, serum lipids, and UalbV in the two groups of obese rats was taken as evidence that the degree of established nephropathy was similar in the two groups at the time treatment was begun.

There were no differences in body weight between the two groups of OZRs after the initiation of treatment (Fig 1; Table 1). Blood pressure in the vehicle-treated obese rats increased between 26 and 38 weeks of age and then remained essentially constant over the last 6 weeks of the protocol (Fig 1). In contrast, BP in the lovastatin-treated obese rats remained constant between 26 and 38 weeks of age. At 38 weeks (after 12 weeks of treatment), BP in the lovastatin-treated obese rats (127 ± 7 mm Hg) was significantly lower

Table 1. Characteristics of Obese Zucker Rats at the Initiation of Treatment (26 Weeks of Age) and at the End of the Experimental Period (44 Weeks of Age)

	26 Weeks of Age		44 Weeks of Age	
	Lovastatin	Vehicle	Lovastatin	Vehicle
Body weight (g)	649 ± 24	660 ± 24	700 ± 31	732 ± 30
Systolic BP (mm Hg)	123 ± 4	123 ± 3	138 ± 6	144 ± 7
CHOL (mg/100 mL)	148 ± 24	178 ± 24	156 ± 19*	252 ± 28
TG (mg/100 mL)	822 ± 165	718 ± 147	347 ± 30*	736 ± 132
UalbV (mg/24 hr)	116 ± 27	127 ± 21	158 ± 37	214 ± 36
Creatinine clearance (mL/min)	1.26 ± 0.17	1.15 ± 0.11	1.27 ± 0.16	1.53 ± 0.33
Kidney weight (g)	—	—	4.01 ± 0.68	4.21 ± 1.02
Glomerular area (μ^2)	—	—	5,363 ± 399	4,861 ± 362

NOTE. The results are expressed as means ± SE.

Abbreviations: CHOL, fasting serum cholesterol; TG, fasting serum triglycerides; BP, blood pressure; UalbV, urine albumin excretion.

* $P < 0.05$ *v* vehicle group at the same age.

than that in the vehicle-treated obese rats (146 ± 4 mm Hg) ($P < 0.05$). Blood pressure in the lovastatin-treated rats increased over the last 6 weeks of the protocol and, at 44 weeks of age, was not different from that in the vehicle-treated obese rats (Fig 1; Table 1).

Serum cholesterol in the vehicle-treated obese rats increased throughout the treatment period (Fig 2). In the lovastatin-treated obese rats, serum cholesterol during the treatment period remained similar to that at the time treatment was begun. Thus, lovastatin did not reduce serum cholesterol from the pretreatment level, but was effective in preventing a further increase. At 44 weeks of age, serum cholesterol in the lovastatin-treated rats was 41% less than that in the vehicle-treated rats (Fig 2; Table 1).

Serum triglycerides in the lovastatin-treated OZRs were reduced at all measurement times in the treatment period compared with triglycerides in the vehicle-treated obese rats (Fig 2). At 44 weeks of age, serum triglycerides in the lovastatin-treated obese rats were 53% lower than serum triglycerides in the vehicle-treated obese rats (Fig 2; Table 1).

After treatment was begun, UalbV in the vehicle-treated obese rats continued to increase (Fig 3). In contrast, UalbV in the lovastatin-treated obese rats decreased significantly over the first 12 weeks of treatment to a value of 78 ± 17 mg/24 hr at 38 weeks of age. This was 62% less than UalbV in the vehicle-treated obese rats (208 ± 41 mg/24 hr) at the same age ($P < 0.05$). Urine albumin excretion in the lovastatin-treated rats increased over the last 6 weeks of treatment so that, at 44 weeks of age, the value was not significantly different from that in the vehicle-treated obese rats (Fig 3; Table 1).

Lovastatin treatment in OZRs reduced the incidence of FGS at 44 weeks of age by nearly half (Fig 3). Approximately 23% of glomeruli in tissue of the lovastatin-treated obese rats exhibited FGS compared with 45% in tissue of the vehicle-treated obese rats. Creatinine clearance, kidney weight, and glomerular area at 44 weeks were each not different between the two groups of obese rats (Table 1). The glomerular content of Ia-positive macrophages at 44 weeks of age was not different between the lovastatin-treated OZRs (1.53 ± 0.16 cells/glomerular profile) and the vehicle-treated obese rats (1.65 ± 0.18 cells/glomerular profile).

In Vitro Study

Lovastatin caused a dose-dependent decrease in mesangial cell DNA synthesis (Fig 4). At a concentration of 20 μmol/L, lovastatin reduced serum-stimulated ^{3}H-thymidine incorporation by 78%. The inhibitory effects of lovastatin on mesangial cell DNA replication were completely prevented in the presence of exogenous mevalonate.

DISCUSSION

Several studies have indicated that lipid abnormalities, either caused by dietary maneuvers or secondary to experimental renal disease, can par-

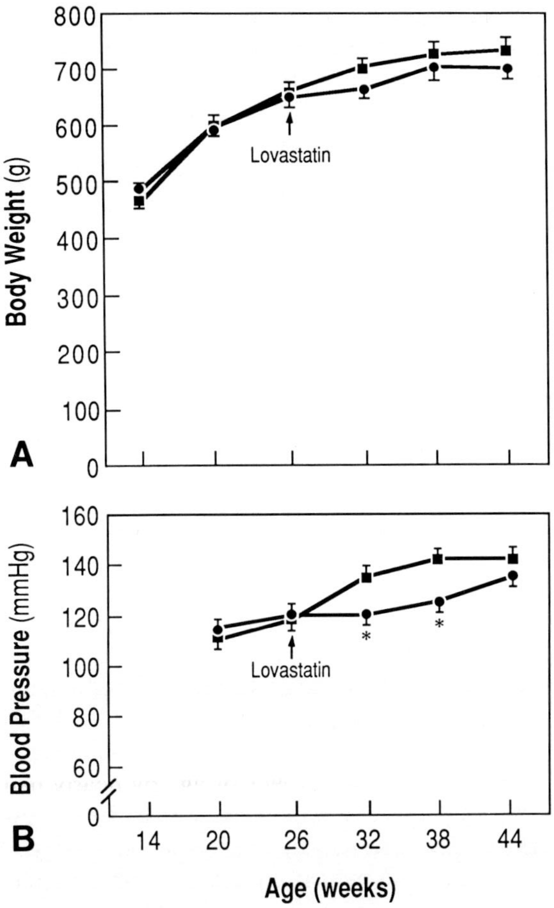

Fig 1. **Body weights (A) and systolic BPs (B) in vehicle-treated (squares) and lovastatin-treated (circles) OZRs. Treatments were initiated at 26 weeks of age, as indicated. *P < 0.05.**

ticipate in the development of glomerular injury characterized by lipid deposition, albuminuria, progressive mesangial matrix expansion, macrophage infiltration, and, ultimately, FGS.[1-8] By their design, these studies have provided a wealth of evidence that lipid alterations can potentially initiate the process of glomerular structural injury. The significance of lipids in the progression of glomerular disease, however, has not been defined. One important finding of the present study, therefore, was that the lipid-lowering agent lovastatin significantly retarded the progression of established glomerulopathy in OZRs. The present results, together with results of previous studies,[1-8] suggest that lipid abnormalities can both initiate glomerular injury and contribute to the progression of glomerular disease.

One mechanism by which lovastatin reduced glomerular injury in OZRs may have involved lowering of serum lipid levels. Recent studies have demonstrated lipoprotein binding and uptake by glomerular epithelial and mesangial cells.[11-15] Moreover, mesangial cells oxidized low-density lipoprotein (LDL), and oxidized LDL was cytotoxic and stimulated expression of type IV collagen mRNA.[16-19] It also has been suggested that glomerular lipoprotein accumulation may stimulate macrophage infiltration, foam cell formation, and release of potentially injurious cytokines and growth factors.[20] Thus, by lowering serum lipids, lovastatin may have attenuated the potentially harmful effects of lipoprotein accumulation and subsequent oxidation within the glomerulus.

An alternate mechanism by which lovastatin retarded the progression of glomerular disease may have involved direct effects of lovastatin on mesangial cell proliferation or turnover. Lovastatin significantly inhibited DNA synthesis in cultured mesangial cells obtained from OZRs

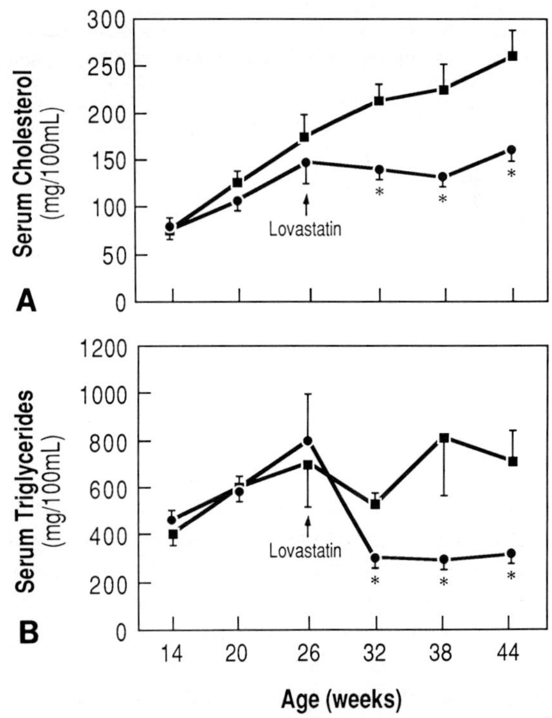

Fig 2. **Fasting serum cholesterol (A) and triglycerides (B) in vehicle-treated (squares) and lovastatin-treated (circles) OZRs. Treatments were initiated at 26 weeks of age, as indicated. *P < 0.05.**

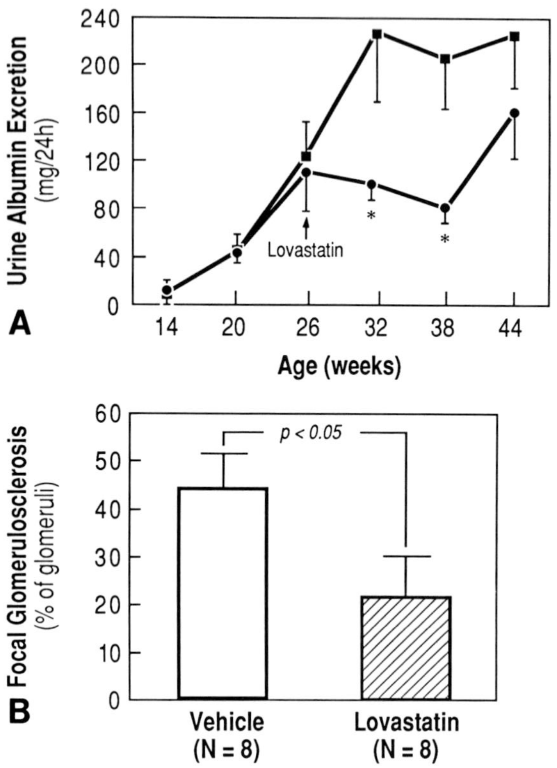

Fig 3. (A) Urine albumin excretion in vehicle-treated (squares) and lovastatin-treated (circles) OZRs. Treatments were initiated at 26 weeks of age, as indicated. *$P < 0.05$. (B) Incidence of glomerulosclerosis at 44 weeks of age (18 weeks of treatment) in vehicle-treated and lovastatin-treated OZRs.

with established glomerular injury. These results were qualitatively similar to our recent finding that lovastatin inhibited proliferation of cultured mesangial cells obtained from young OZRs.[9] In that study,[9] it was suggested that lovastatin inhibited mesangial cell proliferation by blocking the production of mevalonate and subsequent metabolism of mevalonate to isoprenoid intermediates, such as farnesol, which are necessary for cell proliferation. As we previously found,[9] lovastatin inhibition of mesangial cell DNA synthesis in the present study was completely prevented by the addition of exogenous mevalonate.

To our knowledge, there are no pharmacokinetic data regarding lovastatin disposition in rats. Thus, it is difficult to relate the concentrations of lovastatin that inhibited mesangial cell proliferation in vitro to the in vivo plasma concentrations achieved with a dose of 4 mg/kg body weight. Using human pharmacokinetic data, we previously estimated that in vitro lovastatin concentrations of 1 to 20 μmol/L are probably somewhat higher than the in vivo concentrations that might be expected with a lovastatin dose of 4 mg/kg.[9]

There is evidence that glomerular macrophage infiltration may play an important role in both immune-mediated and nonimmune-mediated glomerular injury. Increased glomerular cells exhibiting macrophage surface or cytosol markers have been found in several experimental models of glomerular disease.[3,5,21-23] Moreover, maneuvers that deplete glomerular macrophages have been found to ameliorate glomerular injury.[24,25] In the present study, lovastatin did not exert its beneficial effects in OZRs through a reduction in glomerular macrophages. It cannot be ruled out, however, that lovastatin altered glomerular macrophage function and, in this way, affected the course of glomerular disease.

Glomerular growth has been shown to be an important factor in the pathogenesis of glomerular disease.[26-29] Lovastatin did not affect the glomerular area in OZRs, suggesting that attenuation of glomerular growth was not the mechanism by which lovastatin exerted its beneficial effects. These results are consistent with our previous study in which lovastatin, administered from 8 weeks of age, did not affect the glomerular area in OZRs despite causing a marked reduction in glomerular injury.[6]

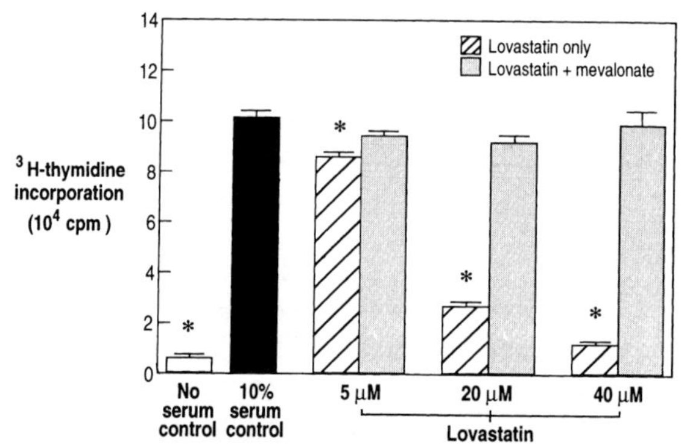

Fig 4. DNA synthesis (^{3}H-thymidine incorporation) in confluent mesangial cells stimulated to proliferate by exposure to 10% fetal bovine serum. Data represent means ± SE of quadruplicate samples; each sample was the total counts per minute obtained from four wells of a 96-well culture plate. Mevalonate concentration was 100 μmol/L. *$P < 0.05$ versus 10% serum control.

The salutary effects of lovastatin on the progression of glomerular injury in OZRs appeared to decline over the last 6 weeks of treatment. Albuminuria and blood pressure in the lovastatin-treated obese rats were each significantly reduced after 12 weeks of treatment (38 weeks of age), but each subsequently increased such that, at 44 weeks of age, the values of each were not significantly different from those in the vehicle-treated obese rats. This was likely not due to reduced bioavailability of lovastatin, since serum triglycerides, which we have previously shown to be particularly sensitive to lovastatin treatment,[6] were still reduced at 44 weeks. Moreover, serum cholesterol in the lovastatin-treated obese rats at 44 weeks of age was similar to that in rats at earlier ages in the treatment period.

There are at least two possible explanations for the apparent decline in lovastatin effects in the last 6 weeks of treatment. First, throughout the treatment period, lovastatin did not reduce serum cholesterol in OZRs from the level at the time treatment was begun. Thus, although lovastatin was effective in preventing a further increase in serum cholesterol, as occurred in the vehicle-treated obese rats, serum cholesterol levels in the lovastatin-treated rats remained approximately twice those normally found in age-matched, lean Zucker rats.[6] Lipid-mediated glomerular injury may therefore have persisted in the lovastatin-treated rats, albeit at a slower rate than in the vehicle-treated obese rats, in which serum lipid levels were substantially higher.

Alternatively, reduced lovastatin efficacy at the end of the in vivo study may have reflected declining effects of lovastatin on mesangial cell proliferation or turnover. Compared with mesangial cells from young OZRs,[9] mesangial cells from the 26-week-old obese rats in the present experiments appeared to be less sensitive to lovastatin. In the present study, a lovastatin dose of 5 μmol/L inhibited DNA synthesis by only 16%, while this same dose inhibited thymidine incorporation by mesangial cells from young obese rats by nearly 80%.[9] Thus, it is possible that with increasing age or increasing extent of glomerular injury, mesangial cells become less responsive to inhibitory actions of lovastatin on DNA synthesis and proliferation.

Alterations in circulating lipid and lipoprotein levels are commonly associated with human renal disease, and there are many clinical studies that have examined the effects of lipid-lowering agents on serum lipids in patients with renal disease.[30-32] In general, these studies were short-term, and no effects of lipid-lowering therapy on proteinuria were observed. In one recent report, however, Rabelink et al demonstrated that simvastatin administered to nephrotic patients for 48 weeks reduced the magnitude of proteinuria.[33] In another study, hypercholesterolemic diabetic patients with nephropathy were administered pravastatin for a period of 12 weeks.[34] Pravastatin significantly reduced albuminuria in diabetic patients with either dipstick-positive proteinuria or microalbuminuria while having no effects on either glycemic control or blood pressure. It should be noted that these were not controlled studies and that assessments of renal histology and glomerular filtration rate were not reported. Nevertheless, these results are consistent with our experimental findings in OZRs and suggest that lipids may be important in the progression of clinical renal disease.

ADDENDUM

The beneficial effects of 3-hydroxy-3 methylglutaryl-coenzyme A (HMG-CoA) reductase inhibitors, such as lovastatin, in models of progressive glomerular injury may not all be due to reduction in circulating lipoproteins and decreases in glomerular lipoprotein deposition. These drugs may have direct effects on glomerular mesangial cells that could explain the amelioration of renal injury. Specifically, HMG-CoA reductase inhibitors may block the synthesis of isoprenoids necessary for mesangial cell proliferation. It has been suggested[35] that isoprenylation plays a role in the pathogenesis and treatment of induced glomerular injury.

ACKNOWLEDGMENT

The authors wish to thank Ellen Davis and Deanna Gunderson for their assistance in the preparation of this manuscript. The authors also recognize the expert technical assistance of Frank Daniels, Bonnie Stesin, and Gregory Holden.

REFERENCES

1. Wellmann KF, Volk BW: Renal lesions in experimental hypercholesterolemia in normal and in subdiabetic rabbits. II. Long term studies. Lab Invest 24:144-155, 1971

2. Peric-Golia L, Peric-Golia M: Aortic and renal lesions

in hypercholesterolemic adult, male, virgin Sprague-Dawley rats. Atherosclerosis 46:57-65, 1983

3. Al-Shebeb T, Frohlich J, Magil AB: Glomerular disease in hypercholesterolemic guinea pigs: A pathogenetic study. Kidney Int 33:498-507, 1988

4. Gröne HJ, Walli A, Gröne E, Niedmann P, Thiery J, Seidel D, Helmchen U: Induction of glomerulosclerosis by dietary lipids: A functional and morphological study in the rat. Lab Invest 60:433-446, 1989

5. Kasiske BL, O'Donnell MP, Schmitz PG, Kim Y, Keane WF: Renal injury of diet-induced hypercholesterolemia in rats. Kidney Int 37:880-891, 1990

6. Kasiske BL, O'Donnell MP, Cleary MP, Keane WF: Treatment of hyperlipidemia reduces glomerular injury in obese Zucker rats. Kidney Int 33:667-672, 1988

7. Kasiske BL, O'Donnell MP, Garvis WJ, Keane WF: Pharmacologic treatment of hyperlipidemia reduces glomerular injury in rat 5/6 nephrectomy model of chronic renal failure. Circ Res 62:367-374, 1988

8. Harris KPG, Purkerson ML, Yates J, Klahr S: Lovastatin ameliorates the development of glomerulosclerosis and uremia in experimental nephrotic syndrome. Am J Kidney Dis 15:16-23, 1990

9. O'Donnell MP, Kasiske BL, Kim Y, Atluru D, Keane WF: Lovastatin inhibits proliferation of rat mesangial cells. J Clin Invest 91:83-87, 1993

10. Norusis MJ: Statistical Package for the Social Sciences (SPSS/PC+ V2.0): Base Manual. Chicago, IL, SPSS, Inc, 1988

11. Wasserman J, Santiago A, Rifici V, Holthofer H, Scharschmidt L, Epstein M, Schlondorff D: Interactions of low density lipoproteins with rat mesangial cells. Kidney Int 35:1168-1174, 1989

12. Rayner HC, Horsburgh T, Brown SL, Lavender FL, Winder AF, Walls J: Receptor-mediated endocytosis of low-density lipoprotein by cultured human glomerular cells. Nephron 55:292-299, 1990

13. Wheeler DC, Persaud JW, Fernando R, Sweny P, Varghese Z, Moorhead JF: Effects of low-density lipoproteins on mesangial cell growth and viability in vitro. Nephrol Dial Transplant 5:185-191, 1990

14. Gröne HJ, Walli AK, Gröne E, Krämer A, Clemens MR, Seidel D: Receptor mediated uptake of apo B and apo E rich lipoproteins by human glomerular epithelial cells. Kidney Int 37:1449-1459, 1990

15. Singhal PC, Gupta S, Shan Z, Schlondorff D: Effects of PGE_2 and a thromboxane A_2 analogue on uptake of IgG complexes and LDL by mesangial cells. Am J Physiol 261:F537-F544, 1991

16. Mulcahy WS, Hetzel CA, Mills DCB, Smith JB, Krishna GG: Lysophosphatidylcholine is the major cytotoxic component of oxidized LDL in proliferating rat mesangial cells. J Am Soc Nephrol 1:636, 1990 (abstr)

17. Keane WF, Phillips J, Kasiske BL, O'Donnell MP, Kim Y: Injurious effects of low density lipoproteins on human mesangial cells. Kidney Int 37:509, 1990 (abstr)

18. Coritsides G, Rifici V, Gupta S, Rie J, Shan Z, Neugarten J, Schlondorff D: Preferential binding of oxidized LDL to rat glomeruli in vivo and cultured mesangial cells in vitro. Kidney Int 39:858-866, 1991

19. Keane WF, Kasiske BL, O'Donnell MP, Kim Y: Oxidized low density lipoprotein increases mesangial cell expression of type IV collagen mRNA. J Am Soc Nephrol 1993 (in press)

20. Kasiske BL, O'Donnell MP, Schmitz PG, Keane WF: The role of lipid abnormalities in the pathogenesis of chronic, progressive renal disease, in Grünfeld J-P, Bach JF, Funck-Brentano J-L, Maxwell MH (eds): Advances in Nephrology, vol 20. St Louis, MO, Mosby-Year Book, 1991, pp 117-118

21. Schreiner GF, Cotran RS, Unanue ER: Modulation of Ia and leukocyte common antigen expression in rat glomeruli during the course of glomerulonephritis and aminonucleoside nephrosis. Lab Invest 51:524-533, 1984

22. Matsumoto K, Atkins RC: Glomerular cells and macrophages in the progression of experimental focal and segmental glomerulosclerosis. Am J Pathol 134:933-945, 1989

23. Magil AB, Cohen AH: Monocytes and focal glomerulosclerosis. Lab Invest 61:404-409, 1989

24. Diamond JR, Pesek I, Ruggieri S, Karnovsky MJ: Essential fatty acid deficiency during acute puromycin nephrosis ameliorates late renal injury. Am J Physiol 257:F798-F807, 1989

25. Diamond JR, Pesek-Diamond I: Sublethal x-irradiation during acute puromycin nephrosis prevents late renal injury: role of glomerular macrophages. Am J Physiol 260:F779-F786, 1991

26. Fries JU, Sandstrom DS, Meyer TW, Rennke HG: Glomerular hypertrophy and epithelial cell injury modulate progressive glomerulosclerosis in the rat. Lab Invest 60:205-218, 1989

27. Yoshida Y, Fogo A, Ichikawa I: Glomerular hemodynamic changes vs. hypertrophy in experimental glomerular sclerosis. Kidney Int 35:654-660, 1989

28. Daniels BS, Hostetter TH: Adverse effects of growth in the glomerular microcirculation. Am J Physiol 258:F1409-F1416, 1990

29. Fogo A, Ichikawa I: Evidence for a pathogenic linkage between glomerular hypertrophy and sclerosis. Am J Kidney Dis 17:666-669, 1991

30. Groggel GC, Cheung AK, Ellis-Benigni K, Wilson DE: Treatment of nephrotic hyperlipoproteinemia with gemfibrozil. Kidney Int 36:266-271, 1989

31. Valeri A, Gelfaud J, Blum C, Appel GB: Treatment of the hyperlipidemia of the nephrotic syndrome: A controlled trial. Am J Kidney Dis 8:388-396, 1986

32. Iida H, Izumino K, Asaka M, Fujita M, Nishino A, Sasayama S: Effect of probucol on hyperlipidemia in patients with nephrotic syndrome. Nephron 47:280-283, 1987

33. Rabelink AJ, Hené RJ, Erkelens DW, Joles JA, Koomans HA: Partial remission of nephrotic syndrome in patients on long-term simvastatin. Lancet 335:1045-1046, 1990

34. Sasaki T, Kurata H, Nomura K, Utsunomiya K, Ikeda Y: Amelioration of proteinuria with pravastatin in hypercholesterolemic patients with diabetes mellitus. Jpn J Med 29:156-163, 1990

35. Kasiske BL, O'Donnell MP, Kim Y, Atluru D, Keane WF: Cholesterol synthesis inhibitors inhibit more than cholesterol synthesis. Kidney Int 45:S51-S53, 1994 (suppl 45)

Verapamil Prevents Chronic Renal Failure-Induced Abnormalities in Lipid Metabolism

Mohammad Akmal, MD, Stephen Perkins, MD, Sidika E. Kasim, MD, Ha-Young Oh, MD, Miroslaw Smogorzewski, MD, and Shaul G. Massry, MD

● Hypertriglyceridemia is common in chronic renal failure (CRF); this derangement is due to decreased peripheral removal of triglycerides. Certain data indicate that the state of secondary hyperparathyroidism of CRF is, at least in part, responsible for derangements in lipid metabolism. It has been proposed that chronic excess of parathyroid hormone exerts its deleterious effects on many organs through its ability to raise basal levels of cytosolic calcium. Prevention of the latter by a calcium channel blocker is followed by the correction of organ dysfunctions. The present study examined the effect of treatment of CRF rats with verapamil on several parameters of lipid metabolism. Chronic renal failure rats displayed hypertriglyceridemia, fat intolerance, reduced postheparin plasma lipoprotein and hepatic lipase activities, decreased hepatic lipase in liver homogenate, and elevated calcium content in liver and epididymal fat. Treatment of the CRF rats with verapamil prevented all these derangements in lipid metabolism. These effects of verapamil were similar to those produced by parathyroidectomy of CRF rats. The data are consistent with the formulation that chronic excess of parathyroid hormone increases the calcium burden of liver and adipose tissue and consequently impairs the synthesis and/or release of lipoprotein and hepatic lipases. Reduced availability of these enzymes in plasma results in impared peripheral removal of triglycerides, leading to hypertriglyceridemia.

INDEX WORDS: Chronic renal failure; rats; verapamil; hyperlipidemia; epididymal fat; calcium; parathyroid hormone.

CHRONIC renal failure (CRF) is associated with hyperlipidemia[1-3] due in major part to impaired removal of triglycerides from plasma.[3,4] Indeed, the postheparin lipolytic activity is reduced[3,4] and removal of the intravenous lipid load is impaired[4,5] in CRF. Previous studies in dogs with CRF demonstrated that the state of secondary hyperparathyroidism of CRF[6-8] plays a paramount role in the genesis of the derangements of lipid metabolism in CRF.[4] Indeed, CRF parathyroidectomized (PTX) dogs maintained normocalcemic have normal plasma triglyceride levels, postheparin lipolytic activity, and intravenous lipid tolerance.[4]

Chronic excess of parathyroid hormone (PTH) in CRF exerts adverse effects on the function of many cells[9]; and these effects are most likely mediated by the ability of the hormone to increase calcium influx into the cells, consequently increasing their cytosolic calcium ($[Ca^{2+}]$) levels.[8,10,11] Indeed, the calcium channel blocker, verapamil, by blocking the PTH-induced calcium entry into cells, prevents the increase in $[Ca^{2+}]_i$ of cells as well as the derangements in cell function in CRF[10-13] despite the presence of chronic excess of PTH.

It is possible that the elevated blood levels of PTH are associated with increased calcium burden in cells that generate lipases, which are responsible for the peripheral removal of triglycerides. If this is indeed the case, one may propose that the prevention of such a calcium burden by verapamil should prevent the CRF-induced abnormalities in lipid metabolism. The present study examined this issue.

METHODS

Male Sprague-Dawley rats weighing 260 to 500 g were studied. They were fed normal chow diet (ICN Nutritional Biochemical, Cleveland, OH) throughout the study and were allowed to drink at libitum. Experiments were performed in five groups: (1) normal rats (normal), (2) normal rats treated with verapamil for 6 weeks (normal-Ver), (3) rats with CRF of 6 weeks' duration (CRF), (4) CRF rats treated with verapamil for 6 weeks (CRF-Ver), and (5) parathyroidectomized-CRF rats maintained normocalcemic for 6 weeks (CRF-PTX).

Chronic renal failure was produced by two stage 5/6 nephrectomy. The animals underwent right partial nephrectomy through a flank incision; 1 week later, a left nephrectomy was performed. Parathyroidectomy was done by electrocautery and the success of the procedure was confirmed by a decrease in serum levels of calcium of at least 2 mg/dL. The PTX rats were allowed to freely drink water containing 5% calcium gluconate. This procedure is adequate to normalize serum calcium in PTX rats. Seven days after PTX, the animals underwent 5/6 nephrectomy as described above. Groups of CRF and normal rats received verapamil (Isoptin; Knoll AG, Ludwigshafen, Germany) in a dose of 0.1 μg/g body weight given twice daily by subcutaneous injections. The normal CRF and CRF-PTX rats received subcutaneous injections of vehicle only.

Supported by Grant No. DK-29955 from the National Institute of Diabetes, Digestive and Kidney Diseases.

On day 42 of the study, the following investigations were performed in rats from all five groups. After an overnight fast, blood samples were obtained from the tail vein for measurements of serum triglycerides. The blood samples were collected in EDTA-containing tubes, centrifuged immediately at 4°C, and kept frozen at −70°C. Serum triglycerides were measured enzymatically.

An intravenous fat tolerance test was performed after an overnight fast. The rats received a rapid intravenous injection of 20% intralipid (Kabi Vitrum, Alameda, CA) in a dose of 0.5 mL/kg body weight; this is equivalent to 0.1 g triglyceride/kg body weight. Blood samples were obtained prior to and at 5, 15, 30, and 45 minutes after the injection of the intralipid. The blood samples were processed as described above for the measurements of triglycerides.

Measurements of postheparin plasma lipolytic activity were done. Each animal received a bolus injection of 100 U heparin/kg body weight. Blood samples were obtained at 5, 15, and 30 minutes after the injection of heparin. The samples were collected in EDTA-containing tubes, centrifuged immediately at 4°C, and stored at −70°C until the assay was made. Both lipoprotein lipase and hepatic lipase activity in plasma were measured in duplicate as described by Nilsson-Ehle and Ekman[14] using specific substrate prepared by sonicating [^{3}H]trioleolglyceride with lysophosphatidylcholine.

Hepatic lipase activity was determined in liver homogenate prepared in 5 mmol/L sodium barbital buffer. The lipase activity was assayed using a specific substrate[14] as described above.

Calcium contents of liver and epididymal fat were measured. Approximately 0.5 to 1.0 g of liver or epididymal fat was placed in tared porcelain crucibles and weighed to 0.01 mg. All samples were dried at 105°C for 48 hours and then re-weighed to determine water content. Samples were then ashed for 12 hours in an oven with 700°C. The samples were extracted in 0.75 HNO_3 for 24 hours and calcium concentration was determined.

The concentrations of calcium in serum and in hepatic and epididymal fat extract were measured with atomic absorption spectrophotometer model 503 (Perkin-Elmer, Corp, Norwalk, CT), and the concentrations of phosphorus and creatinine in serum were measured with an autoanalyzer (Technicon Instrument Corp, Tarrytown, NY). Data are expressed as mean values ± SE. Statistic analysis were made with one-way analysis of variance and Turkey's honest statistical difference for multiple comparison between groups.

RESULTS

The biochemical data of the various groups of rats are presented in Table 1. The 5/6 nephrectomy resulted in a significant ($P < 0.01$) increase in the concentration of serum creatinine. The serum creatinine levels in CRF, CRF-PTX, and CRF-Ver rats are not different, but they are three times higher than those in normal and normal-Ver animals. There were no significant differences in the concentrations of serum calcium and phosphorus among the five groups of animals.

Chronic renal failure animals have significantly ($P < 0.01$) elevated serum levels of triglycerides (114 ± 8.3 mg/dL) as compared with normal animals (65 ± 3.6 mg/dL) (Fig 1). The hypertriglyceridemia in CRF is prevented by PTX or verapamil treatment, and blood levels of triglycerides in CRF-PTX (69 ± 5.6 mg/dL) and CRF-Ver (71 ± 5.0 mg/dL) rats are not different from normal. Verapamil treatment of normal rats did not affect serum levels of triglycerides.

The changes in the serum levels of triglycerides during the IVFTT in the five groups of rats are given in Fig 2. The only group of animals that display fat intolerance is CRF rats. Fat tolerance is normal in the CRF-PTX and CRF-Ver rats despite the CRF. Verapamil treatment of normal rats did not affect fat tolerance.

Figure 3 depicts the postheparin plasma levels of lipoprotein lipase and hepatic lipase activity in all groups of animals. Since there are no significant differences in the values at 5, 15, or 30 minutes after heparin injection, only data at 15 minutes are presented. Both lipoprotein lipase and hepatic lipase activity are significantly ($P < 0.01$) lower in CRF rats than in normal, CRF-PTX, CRF-Ver, and normal-Ver animals. The values in the latter four groups of animals are not different.

Lipase activity of liver homogenate obtained from CRF animals (31 ± 3.7 μmol fatty acids/g liver/min) is significantly ($P < 0.01$) lower than those found in normal (53 ± 3.2 μmol fatty acids/g liver/min), CRF-PTX, CRF-Ver, and normal-Ver rats. The values in the latter four groups of animals are not different (Fig 4).

Chronic renal failure is associated with a significant ($P < 0.01$) increase in the calcium content of the liver (401 ± 32 mg/kg dry weight) and epididymal fat (163 ± 15.5 mg/kg dry weight) as compared with values in normal rats (liver, 189 ± 15 mg/kg dry weight; epididymal fat, 81 ± 7.8 mg/kg dry weight) (Fig 5). The calcium contents of these tissues in CRF-PTX and CRF-Ver animals are not different from normal rats, and verapamil did not affect liver calcium content in normal rats.

DISCUSSION

The results of the present study demonstrate that CRF in the rat, as in humans[3] and dogs,[4] is associated with hypertriglyceridemia and fat

Table 1. Biochemical Data of the Five Groups of Animals Studied

Rat Group	Weight (g)	Serum (mg/dL) Creatinine	Calcium	Phosphorus
Normal	365 ± 17.9	0.40 ± 0.03	10.3 ± 0.13	7.4 ± 0.19
CRF	373 ± 14.8	1.35 ± 0.02*	9.8 ± 0.22	7.3 ± 0.20
CRF-PTX	402 ± 23.0	1.37 ± 0.01*	10.0 ± 0.21	6.7 ± 0.41
CRF-Ver	402 ± 19.5	1.38 ± 0.01*	9.7 ± 0.38	6.9 ± 0.30
Normal-Ver	359 ± 13.7	0.41 ± 0.04	10.1 ± 0.15	7.0 ± 0.30

Note. Data presented as means ± SE.
* $P < 0.01$ versus normal and normal-ver rats.

intolerance. This is due, in large part, to impaired peripheral removal of triglycerides since the activity of the enzymes responsible for this process is impaired. Indeed, the postheparin plasma activity of lipoprotein lipase and hepatic lipase as well as the lipase activity of liver homogenate are impaired. This finding is in agreement with other observations.[3-5]

Again, our results show that the derangements in lipid metabolism in CRF rats, as in CRF dogs,[4] are largely mediated by the state of secondary hyperparathyroidism. This conclusion is supported by our finding that CRF-PTX rats maintained normocalcemic had normal serum levels of triglycerides, fat tolerance test, postheparin plasma lipolytic activity, and lipase activity of liver homogenate. Shoji et al[15] also found that a certain aspect of the deranged lipid metabolism in CRF patients is also related to the elevated blood levels of PTH; these investigators found an association between reduced hepatic triglyceride lipase activity and high blood levels of PTH.

Chronic excess of PTH in the absence or presence of CRF is associated with an increase in $[Ca^{2+}]_i$ of many cells.[8,10,11,16] This is due to increased PTH-induced calcium influx and decreased calcium extrusion out of cells.[17] Such chronic and sustained elevation in $[Ca^{2+}]_i$ causes cellular dysfunction and participates in the genesis of many manifestations of the uremic syndrome.[8-13,16] It is plausible that a similar phenomenon occurs in the cells responsible for the synthesis and release of lipoprotein lipase (adipose tissue and muscle,[18,19] and hepatic lipase) that are responsible for the peripheral clearance of triglycerides.

Although we did not measure the $[Ca^{2+}]_i$ of these cells, we found that the calcium contents of the liver and epididymal fat are significantly elevated in CRF rats. This finding suggests that the $[Ca^{2+}]$ in liver and fat cells is increased in CRF animals since an elevation of calcium con-

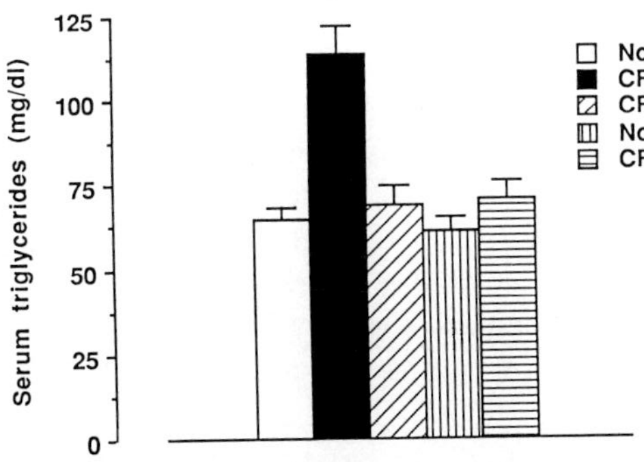

Fig 1. Serum levels of triglycerides in the five groups of animals studied. Each column represents the mean values obtained in six to 13 rats and the brackets denote ±1 SE. *$P < 0.01$ versus all other groups.

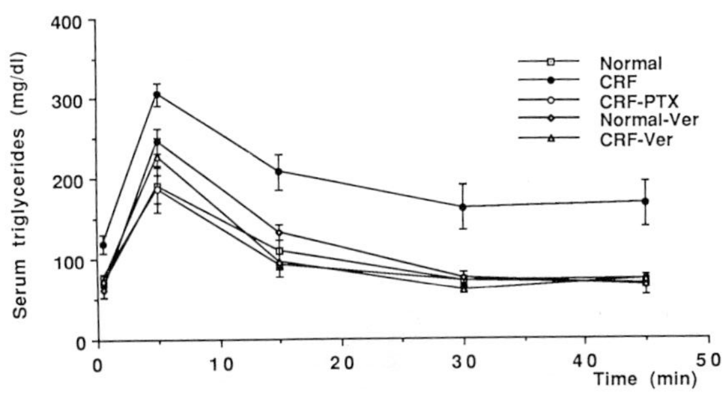

Fig 2. The changes in the serum levels of triglycerides during the intravenous fat tolerance test in the five groups of rats studied. Each datum point represents the mean value from studies performed in five to six rats. Brackets denote ±1 SE.

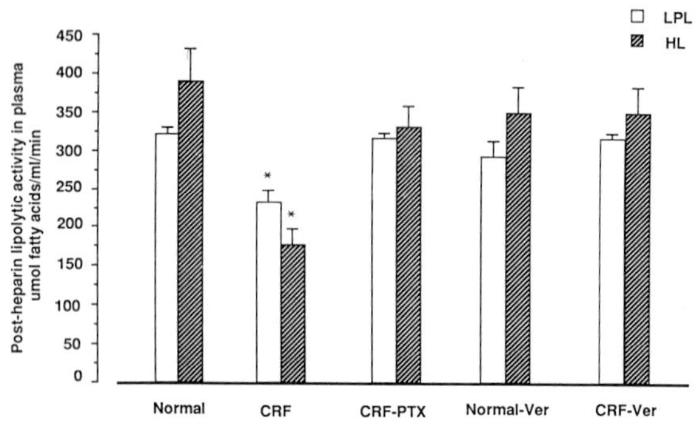

Fig 3. The postheparin plasma lipoprotein lipase (open bars) and hepatic lipase (shaded bars) in the five groups of animals studied. Each column represents the mean value of studies performed in five to eight rats. Brackets denote ±1 SE. *$P < 0.01$ versus all other groups.

tent of other tissues, such as brain[20] and pancreas,[21] is associated with elevated $[Ca^{2+}]_i$ of cells of these organs.[8,10]

The treatment of CRF rats with the calcium channel blocker verapamil prevented the increase in $[Ca^{2+}]_i$ of many cells, including pancreatic islets,[13] brain synaptosomes,[10] and polymorphonuclear leucocytes,[11] and corrected the dysfunction of these cells[10,11,13] despite CRF and chronic excess of PTH. Again, the data of the present study show that treatment of CRF rats with verapamil prevented the increase in the calcium content of the liver and epididymal fat and corrected both postheparin plasma lipoprotein lipase and hepatic lipase as well as hepatic lipase of liver homogenate.

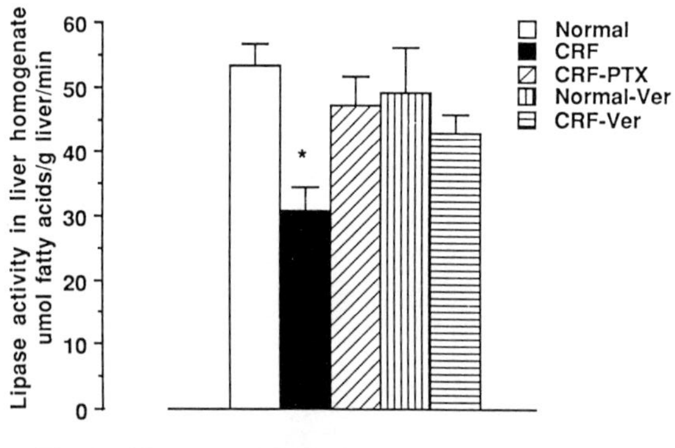

Fig 4. Lipase activity in liver homogenate in the five groups of rats studied. Each column represents the mean value of studies performed in five to nine rats. Brackets denote ±1 SE. *$P < 0.01$ versus all other groups.

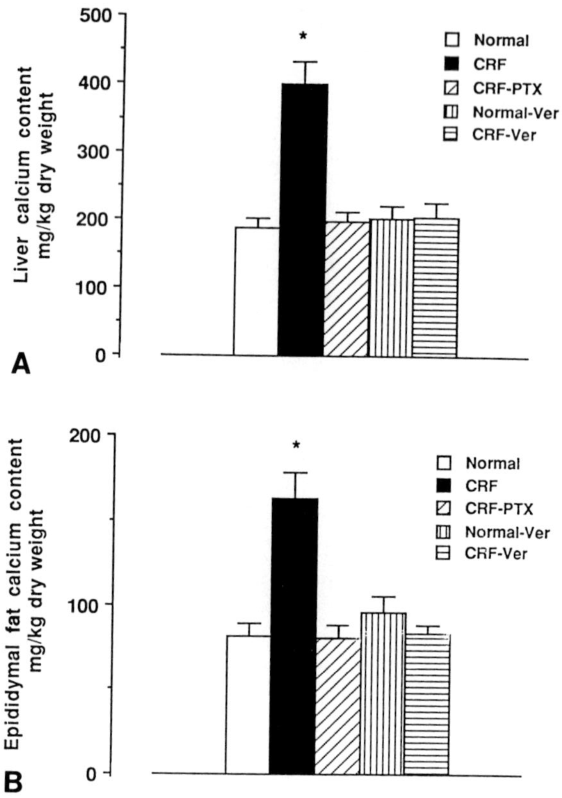

Fig 5. Calcium content of liver (top) and of epididymal fat (bottom) in the five groups of rats studied. Each column represents the mean value of studies performed in eight to 10 rats. Brackets denote ±1 SE. *$P < 0.01$ versus all groups.

Consequently, triglyceride removal became normal, resulting in the correction of fat tolerance and of hypertriglyceridemia. Thus, our data are consistent with the proposition that verapamil blocks the PTH-induced influx of calcium into the cells that are responsible for the synthesis and secretion of the lipoprotein lipase and hepatic lipase. Consequently, calcium does not accumulate in these cells and therefore their function is not impaired. It is theoretically possible that verapamil reduced the blood levels of PTH in the CRF rats and that such a reduction contributes to the effect of verapamil on lipid metabolism. Although we did not measure blood levels of PTH in this study, we have already shown that the treatment of CRF rats with verapamil has no effect on other blood levels of PTH.[11,13] Marotta et al[22] found that treatment of hypertensive subjects (who presumably have increased calcium burden of cells) with nifedipine resulted in enhancement of exogenous triglyceride removal. Furthermore, Fain and Garcia-Sainz[23] found that an increase in calcium burden of liver cells by calcium inophore lowered hepatic lipase secretion. The observations of Marotta et al[22] and of Fain and Garcia-Sainz[23] are consistent with our results.

A second possibility for the effect of verapamil on lipid metabolism in CRF should also be considered. Chronic renal failure is associated with impaired insulin secretion by pancreatic islets[8]; this defect is prevented by treatment with verapamil.[13] Insulin is essential for the synthesis of lipoprotein lipase,[24] and insulin deficiency may cause a deficiency in lipoprotein lipase. Indeed, infusion of insulin to CRF rats reversed the abnormalities in lipoprotein lipase in lipid metabolism.[25] It is therefore plausible that the correction of impaired insulin secretion of pancreatic islets of CRF rats by verapamil treatment[13] contributes to the normalization of the abnormalities in lipid metabolism in CRF. Similar reasoning applies to the effect of PTX, since the latter procedure also normalizes insulin secretion[8] and lipid metabolism in CRF rats.

The observations of the present study may provide a therapeutic approach for the control of the hypertriglyceridemia of CRF. However, it must be mentioned that in our study verapamil was given from day 1 of CRF. It is possible that verapamil may not be able to reverse these derangements in the case of pre-existing CRF. However, we have found that verapamil reversed the abnormalities in insulin secretion of CRF when the drug was given to rats with pre-existing CRF.[26] It seems reasonable to suggest that a similar effect could be obtained with regard to lipid metabolism in CRF.

ADDENDUM

Available data indicate that adipocytes are targets for PTH action, and chronic excess of PTH increases calcium burden of fat tissue, suggesting that PTH increases entry of calcium into adipocytes. A recent study[27] has shown that (1) PTH−1-84 increases $[Ca^{2+}]i$ of adipocytes, (2) this action of the hormone is receptor mediated, (3) the hormone uses a G protein activation of calcium channels and the phospholipase C pathway in mediating its action on $[Ca^{2+}]i$, and (4) the increase in $[Ca^{2+}]i$ is due to both increased calcium influx into the adipocytes and mobilization of calcium from intracellular stores.

REFERENCES

1. Bagdade J, Casaretto A, Albers J: Effects of chronic uremia, hemodialysis and renal transplantation on plasma lipids and lipoproteins in man. J Lab Clin Med 87:37-48, 1976

2. Norbeck HE, Oro L, Calson LA: Serum lipid and lipoprotein concentrations in chronic uremia. Acta Med Scand 200:487-492, 1976

3. Chan MK, Varghese Z, Moorhead JF: Lipid abnormalities in uremia, dialysis and transplantation. Kidney Int 19:625-637, 1981

4. Akmal M, Kasim SE, Soliman AR, Massry SG: Excess parathyroid hormone adversely affects lipid metabolism in chronic renal failure. Kidney Int 37:854-858, 1990

5. Russel GI, Davies JG, Walls J: Evaluation of the intravenous fat tolerance test in chronic renal disease. Clin Nephrol 13:282-286, 1980

6. Berson SA, Yallow RS: Parathyroid hormone in plasma in adenomatous hyperparathyroidism, uremia, and bronchogenic carcinoma. Science 154:907-909, 1966

7. Massry SG, Coburn JW, Peacock M, Kleeman CR: Turnover of endogenous parathyroid hormone in uremic patients and those undergoing hemodialysis. ASAIO Trans 8:410-421, 1972

8. Fadda GZ, Hajjar SM, Perna AF, Zhou X-J, Lipson LG, Massry SG: On the mechanisms of impaired insulin secretion in chronic renal failure. J Clin Invest 87:255-261, 1991

9. Massry SG: The toxic effect of parathyroid hormone in uremia. Semin Nephrol 3:306-328, 1983

10. Smogorzewski M, Koureta P, Fadda GZ, Perna AF, Massry SG: Chronic parathyroid excess in vivo increases resting levels of cytosolic calcium in brain synaptosomes: Studies in the presence and absence of chronic renal failure. J Am Soc Nephrol 1:1162-1168, 1991

11. Chervu I, Kiersztejn M, Alexiewicz JM, Fadda GZ, Smogorzewski M, Massry SG: Impaired phagocytosis in chronic renal failure is mediated by secondary hyperparathyroidism. Kidney Int 41:1501-1505, 1992

12. Smogorzewski M, Islam A, Minasian R, Soliman AR, Massry SG: Verapamil corrects abnormalities in norepinephrine metabolism of brain synaptosomes in CRF. Am J Physiol 258:F1036-F1041, 1990

13. Thanakitcharu P, Fadda GZ, Hajjar SM, Massry SG: Verapamil prevents the metabolic and functional derangements in pancreatic islets of chronic renal failure. Endocrinology 129:1749-1754, 1991

14. Nilsson-Ehle P, Ekman R: Rapid simple and specific assays for lipoprotein lipase and hepatic lipase. Artery 3:194-209, 1977

15. Shoji T, Nishizawa Y, Nishitani H, Yamakawa M, Morii H: Impaired metabolism of high density lipoprotein in uremic patients. Kidney Int 41:1653-1661, 1992

16. Perna AF, Fadda GZ, Zhou X-J, Massry SG: Mechanisms of impaired insulin secretion after chronic excess of parathyroid hormone. Am J Physiol 259:F210-F216, 1990

17. Massry SG, Fadda GZ: Chronic renal failure is a state of cellular calcium toxicity. Am J Kidney Dis 21:81-86, 1992

18. Rossner S: Studies on an intravenous fat tolerance test. Methodological, experimental and clinical experiences with intralipid. Acta Med Scand Suppl 564:1-24, 1974

19. Lithell H, Orlander J, Schele R, Sjodin B, Karlsson J: Lipoproteins, lipoprotein lipase activity and lipid stores in human skeletal muscle with prolonged heavy exercise. Acta Physiol Scand 107:257-261, 1979

20. Akmal M, Goldstein DA, Multani S, Massry SG: Role of uremia, brain calcium and parathyroid hormone on changes in electroencephalogram in chronic renal failure. Am J Physiol 246:F575-F579, 1984

21. Fadda GZ, Akmal M, Premdas FH, Lipson LG, Massry SG: Insulin release from pancreatic islets: Effects of chronic renal failure and excess parathyroid hormone. Kidney Int 33:1066-1072, 1988

22. Marotta T, Farrara LA, Pasanisi F, Rubba P, Iovine C, Mancini M: Enhancement of exogenous triglyceride removal following calcium channel blockade. Artery 16:312-326, 1989

23. Fain JN, Garcia-Sainz JA: Adrenergic regulation of adipocyte metabolism. J Lipid Res 24:946-966, 1983

24. Cryer A: Tissue lipoprotein lipase activity and its action in lipoprotein metabolism. Int J Biochem 13:525-542, 1981

25. Roullet JB, Lacour B, Drueke T: Partial correction of lipid disturbances by insulin in experimental renal failure. Contrib Nephrol 50:203-210, 1986

26. Thanakitcharu P, Fadda GZ, Hajjar SM, Levi E, Stojecva-Taneva O, Massry SG: Verapamil reverses glucose intolerance in pre-existing chronic renal failure: Studies on mechanisms. Am J Nephrol 12:179-187, 1992

27. Ni Z, Smogorzewski M, Massry SG: Effects of parathyroid hormone on cytosolic calcium of rat adipocytes. Endocrinology 135:1837-1844, 1994

Influence of Diet on Lipid Abnormalities in Human Renal Disease

Giuseppe D'Amico, MD, and Maria Gabriella Gentile, MD

● The scarce literature on dietary manipulation of dyslipidemia in patients with nephrotic syndrome and in patients with chronic renal insufficiency is reviewed. Our favorable personal experience in both clinical conditions is illustrated as well. A special low-protein soy diet given for 2 or 4 months partially corrected hypercholesterolemia in nephrotic patients, and a low-protein diet also low in cholesterol and rich in polyunsaturated fatty acids corrected hypertriglyceridemia and hypercholesterolemia in patients with progressive renal damage. The soy diet had an additional favorable effect on proteinuria of nephrotic patients that might have been a direct consequence of the partial correction of the hypercholesterolemia. The addition of 5 g/d of fish oil to the soy diet did not modify the effects of the soy diet on proteinuria nor was it able to correct the hypertriglyceridemia of nephrotic patients. Dietary intervention should be the first-line treatment for the dyslipidemia of these renal diseases, since it can be used for long periods of time and is devoid of side effects so long as good nutritional status is maintained.

INDEX WORDS: Dietary treatment; vegetarian soy diet; dyslipidemia in renal diseases; nephrotic syndrome; chronic renal failure.

OUR PRESENT knowledge of the lipid abnormalities commonly associated with two pathologic conditions of interest to the nephrologist, the nephrotic syndrome and chronic renal failure deriving from many types of progressive renal diseases, recently has been reviewed exhaustively.[1-4] It is universally accepted that in both conditions these abnormalities might favor the development of atherosclerotic complications. Moreover, evidence is accumulating, at least in animal models, that some of these alterations might also have a more direct adverse effect on the progression of the renal damage, since they may promote mesangial damage and favor glomerular sclerosis.[5-9]

Therefore, correction of lipid abnormalities, or their prevention when possible, is becoming accepted as a prominent goal in the management of the above-mentioned pathologic conditions. Many old and new lipid-lowering agents are available and have been used with promising results, especially in animal models of renal diseases.[4,10-12] However, none is without toxic effects in humans, particularly when there is renal functional impairment and long-term administration is necessary. On theoretical grounds, there is little doubt that the most physiologic and harmless approach to the problem of correcting hyperlipidemia or preventing its occurrence, which could be an alternative to the use of lipid-lowering drugs or complementary to it, is dietary intervention. Unlike lipid-lowering drugs, dietary manipulation can also help to correct associated risk factors, such as arterial hypertension and obesity.

Unfortunately, however, very few studies have systematically tested the efficacy of dietary therapy for controlling hypercholesterolemia and/or hypertriglyceridemia in nephrotic and uremic patients. The aim of our review is to discuss the existing evidence on the effects of dietary intervention, mainly in human renal diseases (others will deal in this issue with the more numerous and more convincing data from animal models of renal disease), and to comment on our personal experience in this field.

DIETARY INTERVENTION IN PATIENTS WITH NEPHROTIC SYNDROME

All investigators seem to agree on the importance of prescribing low-cholesterol diets high in polyunsaturated fatty acids (PUFAs) as first-line treatment for all nephrotic patients, although Grundy and Vega[13] have recently warned against the use of diets with a low-fat content since these could accentuate hypertriglyceridemia while correcting the hypercholesterolemia. However, until a few years ago, the only study systematically testing the efficacy of dietary therapy alone was that of Kasiske et al,[14] who prescribed a low-cholesterol diet for 4 weeks to seven nephrotic patients before starting a treatment with lovastatin; these investigators reported nonstatistically significant (6%) reductions of both serum total cholesterol and low-density lipoprotein cholesterol levels without any change in triglycerides and apolipoproteins.

We first became aware of the possible benefi-

Supported by the National Research Council, targeted project "Prevention and Control of Disease Factors."

cial effects of dietary intervention on hypercholesterolemia while conducting a multicenter trial on 24 untreated patients with nephrotic syndrome due to membranous nephropathy to ascertain whether long-term reduction of protein intake reduces urinary protein loss.[15] In a randomized cross-over design, the patients ate sequentially (each for 3 months) (1) a normal-protein diet with a calculated intake of 1.1 ± 0.3 g/kg/d of proteins and (2) a low-protein diet containing vegetable proteins supplemented with a mixture of essential amino acids and their ketoanalogues with a total calculated protein intake of 0.7 ± 0.1 g/kg/d. Both diets were low in fat (<30% of calories) and cholesterol (<200 mg/d) and rich in PUFAs and in linoleic acid (10% of energy). Neither urinary protein excretion nor serum albumin concentration were significantly different at the end of the low-protein diet period from those after the normal-protein diet period (whatever the sequence of the two diets). However, at the end of the 6 months of dietary manipulation, regardless of the sequence of the two diet periods for the individual patient, serum total cholesterol and low-density lipoprotein cholesterol were reduced 24% and 27%, respectively, from the values at the beginning of the run-in period, when all the patients had unrestricted fat intake.[15]

In a subsequent experiment,[16] we evaluated the effects of a more sophisticated vegetarian diet based on the use of soy. The choice was based on previous findings that vegetarians have lower plasma lipid and lipoprotein concentrations than omnivorous individuals[17] and that soy protein significantly reduces plasma cholesterol concentrations.[18-20] The diet we studied (Table 1) was low in fat (28% of total calories) and protein (0.70 g/kg/d), very low in saturated fatty acids, rich in PUFAs (especially linoleic acid) and monounsaturated fatty acids (unsaturated/saturated ratio = 2.5), and had almost no cholesterol. The content of complex carbohydrates and insoluble and soluble fiber was also high; the effect of fiber on serum concentrations of total cholesterol and low-density lipoprotein cholesterol is well known.[21]

This diet was prescribed for 2 months to 20 untreated patients with chronic glomerular diseases, stable longlasting severe proteinuria, and hypercholesterolemia after a baseline control period of 2 months on free diet. At the end of the dietary period, all patients were asked to resume eating the same free diet as in the baseline period for 2 more months (washout period). During the soy diet period there were significant decreases in total serum cholesterol, low-density lipoprotein cholesterol, and apolipoprotein B concentrations (Fig 1A-C); at the end of the second month of dietary intervention these concentrations had decreased by 28%, 33%, and 19%, respectively, changes quantitatively comparable to those recently achieved after 6 weeks of treatment with 40 mg/d of lovastatin.[14] Serum triglyceride concentrations did not change during the experiment. Interestingly, during the soy diet period there was a moderate but highly significant reduction of urinary protein excretion (Fig 1D). On discontinuation of the soy diet, the values of total cholesterol, low-density lipoprotein cholesterol, apolipoprotein B, and urinary proteins reversed toward pre-diet values, but remained lower than in the run-in period. Although a tendency-to-the-mean effect cannot be excluded, we think that the failure to reach pre-diet levels during the washout period was due, in part, to the resistance of some of the patients in resuming their previous free diets once they had become aware of the favorable effects of their special diet. However, the mean values for the four parameters during the washout period were significantly different from those during the soy diet period (Fig 1). It is unlikely that the decrease in proteinuria was due

Table 1. Composition of the Low-Protein Vegetarian Soy Diet Prescribed to Patients With the Nephrotic Syndrome

Protein (% of total calories)	11% (0.7 g/kg of ideal body weight)
Carbohydrates	61% of total calories
Complex	46% of total calories
Simple	15% of total calories
Total fat	28% of total calories
Saturated fatty acids	4.3% of total calories
Monounsaturated fatty acids	12.8% of total calories
PUFAs	10.9% of total calories
Linoleic acid	8.2% of total calories
P/S ratio	2.5%
Cholesterol (mg/d)	0
Fiber (mg/d)	43
Sodium (mg/d)	930
Total calories (amount necessary to maintain or obtain ideal body weight)	

Abbreviation: P/S, unsaturated/saturated.

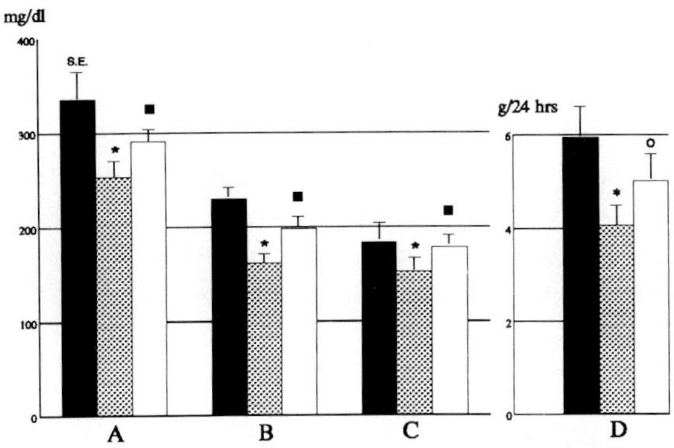

Fig 1. Serum levels of total cholesterol (A), low-density lipoprotein cholesterol (B), and apolipoprotein B (C) and daily urinary protein excretion (D) during the three periods of the study. Mean values of all measurements during a period for each of the 20 patients were used to calculate the overall period mean values (columns) ± standard errors. ■, Baseline; ▨, soy diet; □, washout. The asterisks indicate $P < 0.01$ from baseline (paired *t*-test), the solid boxes indicate $P < 0.01$ in comparison with the soy diet period, and the open circle indicates $P = 0.02$ in comparison with the soy diet period. (Modified and reprinted with permission from D'Amico G, Gentile MG, Manna G, Fellin G, Ciceri R, Cofano F, Petrini C, Lavarda F, Perolini S, Porrini M: Effect of vegetarian soy diet on hyperlipidaemia in nephrotic syndrome, 1:1131-1134, © by The Lancet Ltd, 1992.[16])

to the quantitative restriction of dietary protein intake because of our previous experiment which showed that a quantitatively very similar restriction, protracted for a longer period of time (3 months instead of 2), did not modify urinary protein loss. However, the quality of the plant proteins varied in this second study, in which soy protein was used, and we cannot rule out the possibility that the quality of ingested proteins influences urinary protein loss: Kaysen et al[22] have recently demonstrated that some amino acids in the diet may be more important than others in altering the glomerular permselectivity in nephrotic rats. The alternative possibility that the reduced urinary loss of proteins was a direct consequence of the quantitative and qualitative manipulation of dietary lipid intake must also be taken into consideration. Indeed, evidence is accumulating that such manipulation, as well as the administration of lipid-lowering agents, is able to reduce the glomerular damage and proteinuria in several experimental models of immunologically and nonimmunologically mediated renal disease,[5-10,23] even though such drugs have never induced significant changes of proteinuria in nephrotic patients.[12]

Compliance to the diet was good in our patients, as judged by the significant reductions in urinary urea nitrogen and phosphate.[16] Good nutritional status was confirmed by the values of body mass index and by the stability of serum albumin and transferrin concentrations during the diet period.[16] Systolic and diastolic blood pressure remained unchanged during the diet period.

We recently completed a third experiment of dietary intervention. Twenty nephrotic patients were given the same vegetarian soy diet described above for a longer period of time (4 months instead of 2), but we added for 2 months, in a randomized cross-over design, a moderate oral amount of fish oil. We wanted to ascertain whether (1) longer-term dietary restriction causes difficulties with compliance and nutritional adequacy and whether (2) better control of dyslipidemia (particularly hypertriglyceridemia) could be achieved with the additional administration of n-3 PUFAs, as suggested by many studies in experimental renal disease.[24-29]

After an initial observation period on the free diet, the patients were randomly allocated either to 2 months on the soy diet alone or to 2 months on the same diet plus 5 g of an oral fish oil preparation that supplied 0.9 g/d eicosapentaenoic acid (EPA) and 0.6 g/d docosahexaenoic acid (DHA), integrated with butylhydroxytoluene as antioxidant. At the end of this first study period, all patients crossed over to the alternative dietary regimen for 2 additional months. Finally, all patients resumed eating the same free diet as in the initial run-in period for 2 months. We chose a moderate dose of fish oil in our protocol, since we were looking for a treatment that, if beneficial, could be prescribed to nephrotic patients for very long periods of time without any risk. Even the combination of diet and fish oil was unable to significantly reduce the hypertriglyceridemia of our nephrotic patients. (It has been shown[30] that dietary fish oil has a greater hypotriglyceridemic effect in individuals eating diets high in saturated fats than in those eating mainly polyunsaturated vegetable oils rich in n-6 fatty acids.) As for total cholesterol, low-density lipoprotein cholesterol, and apolipoprotein B, the addition of fish oil to the vegetarian soy diet had no further beneficial effects (Fig 2A-C). On the

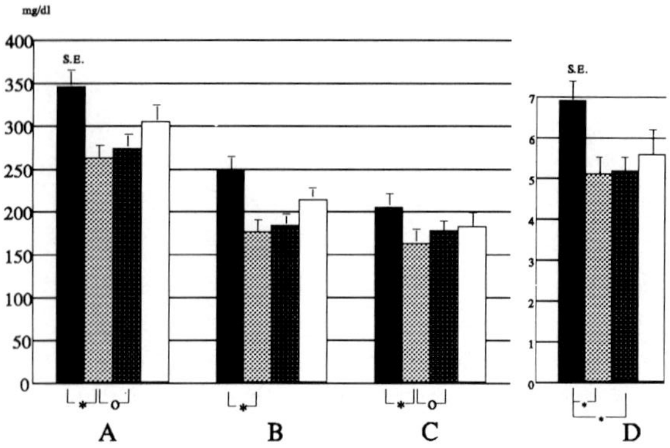

Fig 2. Serum levels of total cholesterol (A), low-density lipoprotein-cholesterol (B), and apolipoprotein B (C) and daily urinary protein excretion (D) during the washout period. Mean values of the two last measurements during a period for each of the 20 patients were used to calculate overall period mean values (colum) ± standard errors. ■, Baseline; ▒, soy diet; ▓, soy diet; + fish oil; □, washout. The asterisks indicate *P* < 0.01 for differences from baseline and the open circles indicate *P* < 0.01 for differences between soy diet plus fish oil and soy diet alone (paired *t*-test).

contrary, fish oil induced a slight but significant elevation of the serum concentrations of total cholesterol and of apolipoprotein B over those on the soy diet alone. (These paradoxic effects had already been described[31-33] in both normotriglyceridemic and hypertriglyceridemic subjects after consumption of moderate amounts of fish oils rich in n-3 fatty acids.) Urinary protein and albumin excretion decreased significantly from baseline at the end of both periods of dietary manipulation. During the subsequent washout period, the mean values of total cholesterol, low-density lipoprotein cholesterol, apolipoprotein B, and urinary proteins tended to climb toward baseline values, without reaching them. The values of total cholesterol, low-density lipoprotein cholesterol, and apolipoprotein B during the washout period were still significantly higher than in both diet periods, while those of proteinuria were not. Therefore, a tendency-to-the-mean effect for proteinuria cannot be excluded as an explanation for the effects of the soy diet on urinary protein excretion. The addition of fish oil to the soy diet did not change mean levels of proteinuria (Fig 2D).

Systolic blood pressure did not change during the study, while diastolic blood pressure was significantly lower during the period when fish oil was added to the soy diet.

After 4 months on the special diet, nutritional status, as evaluated from the stability of the body mass index and serum albumin and transferrin concentrations, was unmodified.

The temporal sequence of the mean levels for the end of the baseline period, the end of the first diet period, the end of the second diet period (whichever the sequence of addition of the fish oil to the soy diet for an individual patient), and the end of the washout period is shown in Fig 3 for two serum lipid parameters (low-density lipoprotein cholesterol and apolipoprotein B) and for two urinary parameters (urea nitrogen and total proteins). Sequential values for nitrogen excretion indicate that compliance to the dietary nutrition was good for the entire period of its prescription. Sequential values for low-density lipoprotein cholesterol and apolipoprotein B serum levels as well as for protein urinary excretion document a progressive decrease over the entire 4-months of the soy diet. These data suggest that even a rather protracted dietary restriction can be accepted and well tolerated by nephrotic patients, with partial correction of dyslipidemia and reduction of urinary protein loss.

DIETARY INTERVENTION IN PATIENTS WITH CHRONIC RENAL FAILURE

In 1977, Sanfelippo et al[34] showed that simple dietary restriction of carbohydrate and choles-

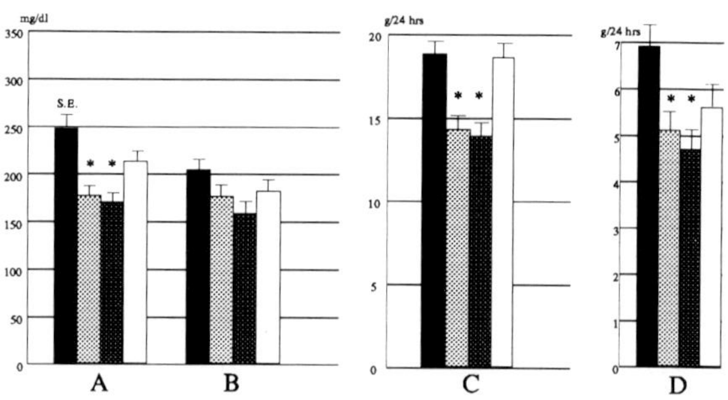

Fig 3. Serum levels of low-density lipoprotein-cholesterol (A), apolipoprotein B (B) and daily urinary excretion of urea nitrogen (C), and total proteins (D) are shown in chronologic sequence at the end of the baseline period, the first diet period, the second diet period (whichever the sequence of adition of the fish oil to the soy diet for an individual patient), and the washout period. Mean values of the two last measurements during each period for each of the 20 patients were used to calculate the overall mean values for the period (colums) ± standard errors. ■, Run in; ▒, 1 diet period; ▓, 2_0 diet period; □, washout. The asterisks indicate *P* < 0.01 from baseline (paired *t*-test).

terol, with no change in protein intake, may result in significant reduction of fasting serum triglycerides and the triglyceride production rate in patients with chronic renal failure (CRF). In this last decade, since treatment with protein-reduced diets has been increasingly used to slow the progression of renal damage, the amount of energy-containing nutrients such as carbohydrates and fats has been increased in dietary regimens, disregarding the frequent existence of the alterations of lipid metabolism, mainly hypertriglyceridemia, in patients with CRF. This may explain the lack of effects on lipid or apolipoprotein levels in patients during long-term treatment with a severely protein-restricted diet, which has been documented by Swedish[35,36] and German[37] investigators. More encouraging results have been reported by Italian and French investigators,[38-43] documenting a correction of hypertriglyceridemia in patients on low-protein diets also low in cholesterol and rich in nonsaturated fatty acids.

We have obtained similar results in patients who participated in a trial studying the effects of protein restriction on the progression of CRF. The low-protein diet (mean protein intake of 0.6 g/kg body weight/d) to which they had been randomly assigned was also low in cholesterol and rich in PUFAs and monounsaturated fatty acids (Table 2), to also correct the associated risk factors such as obesity, arterial hypertension, and hyperparathyroidism.

Table 2. Daily Nutrient Composition of the Low-Protein Diet Prescribed to Patients With Chronic Renal Insufficiency

Protein*	0.6 g/kg body weight
Total fat	32% of total calories
Saturated fat	4% of total calories
Monounsaturated fat	14% of total calories
Linoleic acid	8.6% of total calories
P/S ratio	1
Cholesterol (mg/d)	200
Sugar	18% of total calories
Complex carbohydrates	42% of total calories
Sodium (mg/d)†	325
Phosphate (mg/kg/body weight)	9.6
Calcium (mg/d)‡	250
Total calories suitable to maintain or promote ideal body weight	

Abbreviation: P/S, unsaturated/saturated.
* Protein of high biologic value = 0.5 g/kg body weight.
† Additional salt (usually 2 g/d) was prescribed.
‡ Calcium carbonate supplements were prescribed.

Table 3. Serum Concentration Changes After 2 Years of a Low-Protein Diet in 88 Patients With Chronic Renal Insufficiency (Mean values ± SE)

	At the Time of Enrollment	28 mo After Enrollment	*P*
Total cholesterol (mg/dL)	217.0 ± 4.0	202.6 ± 4.2	0.002
HDL cholesterol (mg/dL)	42.6 ± 1.0	43.0 ± 1.1	NS
Triglycerides (mg/dL)	182.7 ± 8.9	157.9 ± 7.8	0.002
Creatinine clearance (mL/min)	27.0 ± 1.1	21.7 ± 1.3	0.001

Abbreviations: HDL, high-density lipoprotein; NS, not significant.

In a group of 88 patients after 28 ± 23 months on the controlled diet, both triglycerides and total cholesterol were significantly lower than at the time of enrollment, when the patients had been eating a free diet, while creatinine clearance had deteriorated further (Table 3).

In conclusion, we believe that dietary intervention can be of value for partially controlling lipid alterations in both nephrotic patients and in patients with chronic renal insufficiency. Since such alterations are important risk factors, not only because they favor atherosclerotic complications but also because they can probably directly influence the renal damage, the dietary approach cannot be neglected. Its advantages in comparison with the pharmacologic approach are obvious, especially considering that in both clinical conditions the treatment of dyslipidemia must be pursued for long periods of time to be effective.

We have demonstrated, probably favored by the dietary habits of Italian patients, that an effective dietary approach is possible for both nephrotic patients and patients with CRF. Even though the existing evidence does not firmly establish the ideal dietary rules to be recommended to patients with longlasting severe protein loss and dyslipidemia, we think that the administration of a nonvegetarian diet low in cholesterol and fat and rich in PUFAs and fiber can produce a 20% to 25% reduction of total cholesterol and low-density lipoprotein cholesterol. A better correction of dyslipidemia can be achieved with a vegetarian diet based on soy, but this is certainly more difficult to adhere to. Both these suggested diets should be low in proteins (0.7 g/kg of ideal body weight/d) and supplementation with aminoacids and their ketoanalogues is not necessary. The low intake in proteins per se does not seem to reduce proteinuria, but when soy proteins are used a moderate reduction in urinary protein loss can be obtained, the mechanism of which is still obscure. The nonvegetarian, low-protein, low-fat diet we recommend is definitely compatible with a good nutritional status, as demonstrated by several long-term studies in patients with chronic renal insufficiency. We do not yet have such long-term experience for the vegetarian soy diet, although the evidence in countries in which such a diet is commonly eaten by the majority of the population suggests that it is adequate.

However, we admit that dietary management in renal disease is not easy. To achieve good results, a dedicated and experienced staff is of fundamental importance. But, to establish such a staff, it is first essential that nephrologists be convinced about the feasibility and the usefulness of dietary treatment. This is not a common attitude among the physicians in the industrialized countries, who are trained mainly to give drugs to their patients. (It is easier and more immediately satisfying to prescribe medications than to convince patients to change their dietary habits.)

REFERENCES

1. Avram MM: Role of Cholesterol and Lipids in Renal Disease. Am J Med 87:1-75, 1989 (suppl 5N)

2. D'Amico G, Sanna G (eds): Lipid Abnormalities in Renal Disease. Kidney Int 39:S1-S71, 1991 (suppl 21)

3. Keane WF, Stein JH (eds): Lipids and Renal Disease. Contempory Issues in Nephrology, vol 24. New York, NY, Churchill Livingstone, 1991

4. Appel GB: Lipid abnormalities in renal disease. Kidney Int 39:169-183, 1991

5. Moorhead JF, El-Nahas M, Chan Mk, Vargese Z: Lipid nephrotoxicity in chronic progressive glomerular and tubulo-interstitial disease. Lancet 2:1309-1312, 1982

6. Keane WF, Kasiske BL, O'Donnel MP: Lipids and progressive glomerulosclerosis. A model analogous to atherosclerosis. Am J Nephrol 8:261-271, 1988

7. Diamond JR, Karnovsky MJ: Focal and segmental glomerulosclerosis: Analogies to atherosclerosis. Kidney Int 33:917-924, 1988

8. Moorhead JF: Lipids and progressive kidney disease. Kidney Int 39:35-40, 1991 (suppl 31)

9. Keane FW, Mulcahy WS, Kasiske BL, Kim J, O'Donnel M: Hyperlipidemia and progressive renal disease. Kidney Int 39:41-48, 1991 (suppl 31)

10. Grundy SM: Management of hyperlipidemia of kidney disease. Kidney Int 37:847-853, 1990

11. O'Donnell MP, Schmitz PG: Dietary and pharmacologic manipulation of lipids. Impact on progression of experimental renal disease, in Keane WF (ed): Lipids and Renal Disease. New York, NY, Churchill Livingstone, 1991, pp 127-147

12. D'Amico G, Gentile MG: Pharmacological and dietary treatment of lipid abnormalities in nephrotic patients. Kidney Int 39:65-69, 1991 (suppl 31)

13. Grundy SM, Vega GL: Rationale and management of hyperlipidemia of the nephrotic syndrome. Am J Med 5-12, 1989 (suppl 5A)

14. Kasiske BL, Velosa JA, Halstenson CE, La Belle P, Langerdorf A, Keaane WF: The effects of lovastatin in hyperlipidemic patients with nephrotic syndrome. Am J Kidney Dis 15:8-15, 1990

15. D'Amico G, Remuzzi G, Maschio G, Gentile MG, Gotti E, Oldrizzi L, Manna G, Mecca G, Rugiu G, Fellin G: Effect of dietary proteins and lipids in patients with membranous nephropathy and nephrotic syndrome. Clin Nephrol 35:237-242, 1991

16. D'Amico G, Gentile MG, Manna G, Fellin G, Ciceri R, Cofano F, Petrini C, Lavarda F, Perolini S, Porrini M: Effect of vegetarian soy diet on hyperlipidaemia in nephrotic syndrome. Lancet 1:1131-1134, 1992

17. Sacks FM, Castelli WP, Donner A, Kass EH: Plasma lipids and lipoproteins in vegetarians and controls. N Engl J Med 292:1148-1151, 1975

18. Sirtori CR, Agradi E, Conti F, Mantero O, Gatti E: Soyabean protein diet in the treatment of type II hyperlipoproteinemia. Lancet 1:275-277, 1977

19. Goldberg AP, Lim A, Kolar JB, Grundhauser JJ, Steinke F, Schonfeld G: Soybean protein independently lowers plasma cholesterol levels in primary hypercholesterolemia. Atherosclerosis 43:355-368, 1982

20. Lovati MR, Manzoni C, Canavesi A, Sirtori M, Vaccarini V, Marchi M, Gaddi G, Sirtori R: Soyabean protein diet increases low density lipoprotein receptor activity in mononuclear cells from hypercholesterolemie patients. J Clin Invest 80:1498-1502, 1987

21. Connor WE: Dietary fiber-nostrum or critical nutrient? N Engl J Med 322:193-195, 1990

22. Kaysen GA, Al Bander H, Martin V, Joins HJR, Hutchinson F: Branched-chain amino acids augment neither albumin synthesis nor albuminuria in nephrotic rats. Am J Physiol 260:F177-F184, 1991

23. Schreiner GF: Dietary treatment of immunologically mediated renal disease. Kidney Int 39:49-56, 1991 (suppl 31)

24. Robinson DR, Pricket JD, Makoul GT: Dietary fish oil reduces progression of established renal disease in NZBxNZW f1 mice and delays renal disease in BXSB and MRL/1 strains. Arthritis Rheum 29:539-546, 1986

25. Heifets M, Morissey JJ, Purkerson ML, Morrison AR, Klahr S: Effect of dietary lipids on renal function in rats with subtotal nephrectomy. Kidney Int 32:335-341, 1987

26. Ito Y, Barcelli U, Yamashita W, Weiss M, Glas-Greenwalt P, Pollak V: Fish oil has beneficial effects on lipids and renal disease of nephrotic rats. Metabolism 37:352-357, 1988

27. Clark FW, Pabtani A, Philbrick DJ, Holub BJ, Huff

MW: Chronic effects of n-3 fatty acids (fish oil) in a rat 5/6 renal ablation model. J Am Soc Nephrol 12:1343-1353, 1991

28. Barcelli U: Effect of dietary prostaglandin precursors on the progression of renal disease in animals. Kidney Int 39:57-64, 1991 (suppl 31)

29. Kasiske BL, O'Donnell MP, Lee H, Kim J, Keane W: Impact of dietary fatty acid supplementation on renal injury in obese Zucker rats. Kidney Int 39:1125-1134, 1991

30. Garg ML, Thomson ABR, Clandinin MT: Hipotriglyceridemic effect of dietary n-3 fatty acids in rats fed low versus high levels of linoleic acid. Biochim Biophys Acta 1006:127-130, 1989

31. Harris WS: Fish oils and plasma lipid and lipoprotein metabolism in humans: A critical review. J Lipid Res 30:785-807, 1989

32. Rogers S, James KS, Butland BK, Etherington MD, O'Brien JR, Jones JG: Effects of a fish oil supplement on serum lipids, blood pressure, bleeding time, haemostatic and rheological variables. Atherosclerosis 63:137-143, 1987

33. Kestin M, Clifton P, Belling GB, Nestel P: n-3 Fatty acids of marine origin lower systolic blood pressure and triglycerides but raise LDL cholesterol compared with n-3 and n-6 fatty acids from plants. Am J Clin Nutr 51:1028-1034, 1990

34. Sanfelippo ML, Swenson RS, Reaven GM: Reduction of plasma triglycedides by diets in subjects with chronic renal failure. Kidney Int 11:54-61, 1977

35. Attman P-O, Gustafson A, Alaupovic P, Wang C-S: Effect of protein-reduced diet on plasma lipids, apolipoproteins and lipolytic activities in patients with chronic renal failure. Am J Nephrol 4:92-98, 1984

36. Attman P-O, Gustafson A: Lipid and carbohydrate metabolism in uremia. Influence of treatment with protein reduced diet and essential amino acids. Nutr Metab 24:261-280, 1980

37. Schafer B, Kluthe R: Fettstoffwechselstorungen bei chronischen Niereninsuffizienz unter konservative Behandlung. Med Klin 69:577-581, 1974

38. Barsotti G, Ciardella F, Moretti E, Fioretti P, Melis GB, Paoletti A, Niosi F, Caprioli R, Fosso A, Carbone C, Giovannetti S: Restoration of blood levels of testosterone in male uremics following a low protein diet supplemented with essential aminoacids and ketoanalogues. Contrib Nephrol 49:63-69, 1985

39. Ciardella F, Morelli E, Niosi F, Caprioli R, Baldi R, Cupisti A, Petronio G, Carbone C, Barsotti G: Effects of a low phosphorus, low nitrogen diet supplemented with essential aminoacids and ketoanalogues on serum triglycerides of chronic uremic patients. Nephron 42:196-199, 1986

40. Aparicio M, Bouchet JL, Gin H, Potaux L, Horsl D, De Precigont V, Lipermann F, Gonzalez R: Effects of a low-protein diet on urinary albumin excretion in uremic patients. Nephron 50:288-291, 1988

41. Loschiavo C, Ferrari S, Panebianco R, Bedogna V, Oldrizzi L, Bonazzi L, Maschio G: Effect of protein-restricted diet on serum lipids and atherosclerosis risk factors in patients with chronic renal failure. Clin Nephrol 29:113-118, 1988

42. Maschio G, Oldrizzi L, Rugiu C, Lo Schiavo C: Serum lipids in patients with chronic renal failure on long-term, protein-restricted diets. Am J Med 87:51N-54N, 1989

43. Maschio G, Oldrizzi L, Rugiu C, De Biase V, Lo Schiavo C: Effect of dietary manipulation on the lipid abnormalities in patients with chronic renal failure. Kidney Int 39:70-72, 1991 (suppl 31)

DYSLIPIDEMIA AND PROTEINURIA

Introduction

The Nephrotic syndrome is a clinical entity characterized by several renal and extrarenal abnormalities. The most characteristic features include proteinuria, hypoalbuminuria, hyperlipidemia, and hypercoagulability. Although the presence of hyperlipidemia is not essential for the diagnosis of nephrotic syndrome, it is present in most cases. Most serum lipids and lipoprotein fractions are elevated in the patient with the nephrotic syndrome. The main concern is that these changes may carry a risk of ischemic heart disease.

In the first paper of this section, Kaysen et al emphasize that the hyperlipidemia of the nephrotic syndrome is characterized both by increased lipogenesis and decreased lipid catabolism. Whether decreased lipolysis occurs only as a consequence of the increase in blood lipids caused by augmented lipogenesis is controversial. To establish whether decreased lipolysis occurs independently from elevated blood lipid levels and in the absence of lipoproteins in an isolated organ of a nephrotic animal, the authors measured chylomicron lipolysis by isolated perfused hearts from rats with passive Heymann nephritis. They found reduced lipolysis of chylomicron by isolated hearts in the absence of other rat lipoproteins and in the absence of increased lipid levels associated with reduced activity of lipoprotein lipase on the cardiac endothelium, providing a potential mechanism for reduced chylomicron clearance in the nephrotic syndrome.

In another paper, Kaysen et al describe their investigation of the cause of elevated apolipoprotein (apo) A-I in nephrotic rats and in rats with hereditary analbuminemia, conditions associated with reduced plasma albumin and colloid oncotic pressure. Apo A-I clearance was reduced and total apo A-I turnover (apo A-I synthesis rate) was increased in rats with passive Heymann nephritis and in analbuminemic rats. Infusion of albumin or ficoll into rats with Heymann nephritis in quantities sufficient to normalize and maintain plasma oncotic pressure for days resulted in normal cholesterol and apo A-I levels despite ongoing proteinuria. This suggests that apo A-I levels are increased in both conditions as a result of both increased synthesis and reduced catabolism in response to reduced plasma oncotic pressure.

Radhakrishnan et al report on investigations of cholesteryl ester transfer protein, which may play an important role in the genesis of the abnormal lipid profile of nephrotic patients. These patients have a high level of cholesteryl ester transfer protein, which is responsible for the exchange of cholesteryl esters from high-density lipoprotein (HDL) to very low-density lipoprotein (LDL), and may account for the low or normal HDL cholesterol levels found despite very high total and LDL cholesterol levels. The authors studied 100 patients with either membranous nephropathy or focal sclerosis, two common forms of idiopathic nephrotic syndrome in which remission of proteinuria is unlikely. They found very high levels of total and LDL cholesterol and high total cholesterol to HDL cholesterol ratios. Most patients had more than one risk factor for atherosclerotic heart disease. The small number of documented ischemic cardiac events during the follow-up period and the effects of treatment on risk factors precluded an analysis of the true incidence of cardiovascular disease. However, correlates with progression to renal failure and remission of proteinuria were analyzed.

Spitalewitz et al note that the hyperlipidemia of the nephrotic syndrome is characterized by elevated levels of total and LDL cholesterol, a normal or low level of HDL cholesterol, and increased triglyceride levels later in the course of the disease. The authors describe a double-blind, placebo-controlled trial investigating the efficacy and safety of pravastatin in the nephrotic syndrome. Although levels of total cholesterol and LDL declined 20% to 30%, they did not reach normal range, indicating the need for combination drug therapy in many patients. Renal function and protein excretion were unaffected in this 24-week study. A more recent study by a different group is also described; although the follow-up was longer (2 years), it yielded similarly promising results, with some components of the lipid profile nearing normal in some patients.

Hemmelder et al retrospectively analyzed the effects of pregnancy on progressive renal function decline in women with biopsy-proven glomerular disease who were observed for 11 years. Pregnancy and the degree of proteinuria, but not histologic diagnosis, age, blood pressure, or renal function, were independently related to renal function loss.

Markell et al found no correlation between dyslipidemia and heart disease in renal transplant recipients. Although hyperlipidemia is now recognized as a common consequence of renal transplantation, questions about the natural history of the disorder and its clinical significance have arisen. The authors follow longitudinal measurement of cholesterol, starting in the pretransplant period, and demonstrate that early hypercholesterolemia does persist in the untreated patient. Patients who do not develop hypercholesterolemia in the absence of chronic rejection by 3 months posttransplant remain normolipidemic, at least over the 4-year follow-up period. The question as to whether prolonged hypercholesterolemia impacts on loss of renal allografts was also addressed. Early hyperlipidemia alone does not result in increased graft loss when 4-year actual survival data are examined. The observations about hypercholesterolemia suggest that early hyperlipidemia does not remit despite reduction in the dose of immunosuppressive drugs, and that treatment regimens may be initiated early. The observation that graft survival is not significantly different for patients stratified into groups based on early cholesterol values suggests that other factors are necessary and that if hypercholesterolemia plays a role in exacerbating renal dysfunction, it does so after another factor serves as the initiating event (eg, immunologic injury).

Sehgal et al report on risk factors for progressive renal insufficiency in cardiac transplant recipients, suggesting that, in the patients they studied, age at transplant, dyslipidemia, and severity of hypertension were risk factors.

Defective Lipolysis Persists in Hearts of Rats With Heymann Nephritis in the Absence of Nephrotic Plasma

George A. Kaysen, MD, PhD, X-M. Pan, MD, William G. Couser, MD, and Ilona Staprans, PhD

• Catabolism of triglyceride-rich lipoproteins, including chylomicrons (CM), is reduced in the nephrotic syndrome. It has been suggested that hyperlipidemia per se might lead to reduced CM catabolism by saturating catabolic sites. Evidence also implicates disordered high-density lipoprotein function as reducing the activity of lipoprotein lipase (LPL), the final effector of CM lipolysis. To establish whether CM lipolysis would be abnormal in the absence of either abnormal rat lipoproteins or hyperlipidemia, we measured CM lipolysis by isolated perfused hearts of rats with passive Heymann nephritis. We found that lipolysis was significantly reduced by 30% at 30 minutes (246 ± 40 μmol *v* 164 ± 10 μmol fatty acid released/hr, $P < 0.05$). Uptake of fatty acids was also significantly less in nephrotic hearts than in control hearts (7.25% ± 0.93% of dose *v* 3.32% ± 0.011% of dose, $P < 0.01$). Total heart LPL activity was reduced by 40% in hearts of nephrotic animals (368.5 ± 39.4 μmol *v* 210.6 ± 25.9 μmol free fatty acid released/hr/g heart, $P < 0.01$). The heparin-releasable LPL pool is that pool bound to the vascular endothelium and represents the biologically active fraction. We perfused hearts with heparin and found that heparin-releasable LPL was reduced by an order of magnitude in hearts from nephrotic rats (173 ± 33 μmol *v* 19.4 ± 11.7 μmol free fatty acid released/hr/heart, $P < 0.001$). The decrease in this pool represented nearly entirely the difference in total heart LPL in the two groups. Thus, Heymann nephritis causes reduced lipolysis of CM by isolated hearts in the absence of other rat lipoproteins and in the absence of increased lipid levels. Decreased lipolysis is associated with reduced activity of LPL on the cardiac endothelium, providing a potential mechanism for the reduced CM clearance in the nephrotic syndrome.

INDEX WORDS: Lipoproteins; lipoprotein lipase; chylomicrons; nephrotic syndrome; vascular endothelium.

HYPERLIPIDEMIA in the nephrotic syndrome is a consequence both of increased synthesis and decreased clearance of lipoproteins.[1-3] While there is general agreement that lipogenesis is increased,[1] the relationship between increased production of lipoproteins, their decreased catabolism, and hyperlipidemia in this syndrome has been an area of controversy.[4] It has been argued that one mechanism causing defective lipid catabolism is one of saturation of catabolic sites by the persistent hyperlipidemia caused by primary overproduction of lipids.[4] Indeed, unlike the situation for many other plasma proteins,[5,6] the fractional clearance of lipoproteins decreases as the plasma concentration increases. It has been hypothesized that this effect is in part a consequence of steric interaction between lipoprotein molecules at the receptor site.[7] We previously reported that the absolute rate of chylomicron (CM) catabolism, whether measured kinetically or by direct tissue uptake of triglycerides (TG), was reduced to approximately 25% of normal in nephrotic rats when measured in the fasting state.[8] This observation was compatible with the existence of a defect in CM catabolism that was not a consequence of hyperlipidemia, but instead a cause of increased lipid levels in the nephrotic syndrome. Thus, defective lipoprotein catabolism would appear to be at least in part independent of an increased rate of lipogenesis.

While the enzyme lipoprotein lipase (LPL) is the final effector of CM lipolysis, the biologic activity of this enzyme can only be indirectly determined by measuring its total activity in tissue. Interaction between CM and this enzyme is dependent on steric factors. Hydrolysis of CM is so rapid in vivo that to account for their short half-life Olivecrona and Bengstsson-Olivecrona[9] suggested that many LPL molecules must react simultaneously with these large particles during their period of attachment to the vascular endothelium. These investigators suggested that CM must be bound to the vascular endothelium for considerable periods of time to allow their hydrolysis to proceed as rapidly as observed,[2,4,10,11] consistent with the low turnover number of LPL (10^4 sec^{-1}) in comparison to the large number of acyl bonds in a single CM.

Lipoprotein lipase activity is dependent on the presence of apolipoproteins that may either inhibit the activity of this enzyme (apolipoprotein C-III [apo C-III]) or be required for its activity (apo-C II).[12] These small apolipoproteins in turn are shuttled between high-density lipoprotein (HDL) and both CM and very low-density lipo-

Supported in part by the research service of the United States Department of Veterans Affairs and in part by National Institutes of Health Grants No. 1-RO1 DK 42297 and DK 39198. Dr Pan was supported by The Pacific Vascular Research Foundation.

protein (VLDL). Thus, interaction between apolipoproteins plays an important role in regulating their rate of catabolism. High-density lipoprotein composition is altered in the nephrotic syndrome.[13] Apolipoprotein A-I is increased,[14,15] while the concentration of other apolipoproteins is decreased, including apo C-II and apo A-IV, a lipoprotein recently discovered to be necessary for transfer of apo C-II from HDL to other lipoproteins.[16] Indeed, Furukawa[17] found that lipolysis of rat VLDL by LPL in vitro was significantly greater when incubated in the presence of HDL from normal rats when compared with HDL isolated from nephrotic rats.

To determine the effect of the nephrotic syndrome on CM lipolysis in the absence of hyperlipidemia and independently of other lipoproteins, we measured CM lipolysis by isolated perfused hearts of nephrotic rats compared with hearts from normal animals. We chose to study lipoprotein catabolism in the heart in part because this tissue actively metabolized fatty acids and also because LPL has been reported to be normal in this tissue.[4] We had previously reported that fatty acid uptake was reduced in the heart to the same extent as it was in adipose tissue,[10] a tissue in which LPL activity was reduced significantly in the nephrotic syndrome. Our observations, taken in conjunction with those of Levy et al,[4] that cardiac LPL was not reduced suggested that lipoprotein-lipoprotein interaction might contribute to defective lipolysis in the nephrotic syndrome.

While LPL is synthesized by mesenchymal cells, it is only that pool bound to the vascular endothelium that is able to make effective contact with CM. It might be possible that the LPL pool associated with the endothelium might be decreased, specifically in the nephrotic syndrome, without a change in total cardiac LPL. For this reason we also measured total cardiac LPL activity and that pool of LPL released from isolated perfused hearts by heparin.

METHODS

Protocol No. 1: Measurement of Chylomicron Catabolism by Isolated Perfused Hearts

Male Sprague Dawley rats were maintained on purina rat chow with free access to water. Four were injected intraperitoneally with the sheep anti-FX1A serum[18,19] to induce passive Heymann nephritis (HN); four served as controls. Fifteen days following injection with antiserum, each animal was placed in a metabolic cage for 24-hour urine collection to measure urinary albumin excretion. The animals were fasted overnight, then anesthetized with ether. Their hearts were excised and perfused as described below. Terminal blood was collected for measurement of cholesterol, TGs, albumin, and total protein.

Protocol No. 2: Determination of Cardiac Lipoprotein Lipase Activity in Nephrotic Rats

A total of 10 HN and nine control animals were studied. Nephrotic rats were each placed in a metabolic cage for 24 hours for urine collection. All animals were fasted overnight prior to study. Four controls and five HN animals were anesthetized with ether as in protocol no. 1 and their hearts were perfused with heparin as described below. Terminal blood was collected for measurement of TGs, cholesterol, and albumin. Lipoprotein lipase activity was determined both in the perfusate and in the heparin-perfused heart as described below. Total LPL activity was the sum of LPL activity obtained from assay of the perfusate and activity obtained from assay of the heparin-perfused heart. Total LPL activity was also measured in five hearts from HN animals and from five control hearts without prior heparin perfusion to determine whether the perfusion procedure artifactually reduced LPL activity. These hearts were frozen in liquid N_2 without prior perfusion for analysis of LPL in tissues that had not been either subjected to postmortem warming or exposed to heparin.

Heart Perfusion

Retrograde aortic perfusion of isolated rat hearts was carried out by the method of Langendorff as described by Fielding.[20] Hearts were rapidly removed. They were initially perfused without recirculation with buffered Krebs-bicarbonate (0.118 mol/L NaCl, 0.025 mol/L $NaHCO_3$, 0.0035 mol/L $CaCl_2$, 0.005 mol/L KCl, 0.001 mol/L KH_2PO_4, 0.001 mol/L $MgSO_4$, pH 7.4), gassed with 95% O_2 and 5% CO_2, at a flow rate of 6 mL/min for 15 minutes to establish viability. The hearts were then perfused with medium containing human serum albumin (1%) and glucose (1 mg/mL). The total perfusion volume of 30 mL was used when we measured CM catabolism, but the volume of perfusate was reduced to 15 mL when the hearts were perfused with heparin in order to release LPL.

When CM catabolism was measured perfusion was carried out with a recirculating system at 6 mL/min and duplicate 0.2-mL samples were withdrawn every 5 minutes for analysis. Lipids were then extracted from each blood sample by the Dole method, as modified by Trout et al.[21] The samples were each extracted with the Dole method (acid-heptane) to determine residual activity in unhydrolyzed TGs. After extraction, the heptane phase was mixed with 0.5 mL of ethanolic thymol blue solution and made alkaline with 0.05 mL of 0.01 mol/L NaOH. The heptane phase containing nonhydrolyzed CM was counted in a scintillation counter (Beckman Instruments, Palo Alto, CA) for 10 minutes and the dose remaining in the perfusate was calculated. The aqueous phase was acidified and re-extracted with Dole's mixture and counted to examine the generation of free fatty acids. Individual CM clearance curves were calculated from the slopes of serum counts per minute using the method of least squares. The rate constant for CM clearance was determined for each animal as $\ln_2/t_{1/2}$. A mean CM disappearance curve was determined for each group of animals by regression analysis using the means of each time point (based on the percentage of remaining counts) from all animals within each group.

To verify that labeled CM were not lost due to sticking to the apparatus, leakage, or other nonspecific causes, the perfusion was also carried out as described above, but without the heart.

Tissue Extraction

Hearts were extracted with chloroform/methanol in a dilution of 2:1. Tissues were homogenized with a polytron tissue homogenizer (Brinkman Instruments, Westbury, NY) so that the ratio of organic phase (chloroform/methanol) to aqueous phase was 20:1. The clear organic phase was then filtered through glass wool. Five milliliters of the filtrate was allowed to evaporate to dryness and was then dissolved in heptane and counted in a liquid scintillation counter for 20 minutes.[10]

In protocol no. 2, heparin (50 U/15 mL perfusate) was added to the perfusate after the 15-minute period of initial stabilization. The entire 15 mL of perfusate was allowed to pass through the heart a single time and was collected for analysis. Both the heart and perfusate were rapidly frozen on dry ice and stored overnight at −70°C until analysis the following day.

Preparation of Chylomicrons

Labeled CMs were obtained from a thoracic duct cannula by a modification of the technique of Bollman et al[22] as previously described.[2] The rats were gavage fed with a 2-mL mixture of corn oil/milk (1:2 dilution) emulsion sonicated together with 0.15 mCi of glycerol tri-(9-10[^{3}H])-oleate (Amersham Searle Corp, Arlington Heights, IL). The chyle was collected in iced tubes for 18 hours and CMs were isolated by layering the chyle under 0.15 mol/L NaCl and by flotation in a SW-40 rotor (Beckman Instruments) at 5×10^6 g/min at 16°C for 1 hour.

Lipoprotein Lipase

To assay LPL in heart perfusate a total reaction mixture of 3.5 mL was prepared using 1.55 mL of the 15 mL of perfusate, to which was added 0.32 mL of 1.3 mol/L Tris-HCl (Sigma Chemical Co, St Louis, MO), pH 8.6; 0.50 mL of 0.025 mol/L NH_4OH, pH 8.6; 0.1 mL of 10% Intralipid (Vitrum, Stockholm Sweden); 0.03 mL VLDL (0.8 mg protein/mL); and 1.00 mL 15% (w/v) crystalline bovine serum albumin (Sigma). The reaction mixture was then incubated at 37°C. One milliliter was removed at time 0, and duplicate 1.0-mL samples were removed from the reaction mixture at 45 minutes. Samples were analyzed for free fatty acids (FFAs) as described below. Free fatty acids were extracted and their content determined by titration with tetrabutyl ammonium hydroxide. Lipoprotein lipase activity was defined in units as micromoles of FFA released per hour per gram of tissue.

For measurement of total cardiac LPL activity, 0.4 g of heart was first homogenized in 0.025 mol/L ammonia, adjusted to pH 8.2 with HCl, containing 5 mmol/L ethylenediaminotetraacetic acid (EDTA) and 0.8 mg Triton X-100, 0.4 mg sodium dodecyl sulfate, 1 μg pepstatin, 10 μg leupeptin, 25 KIE Trasylol, and 50 U heparin/mL.[23] Total volume of the extract was 4.0 mL. To assay LPL in heart extract, a total reaction mixture of 3.5 mL was prepared using 0.2 mL of the 4 mL of cardiac extract, to which was added 0.375 mL of 1.3 mol/L Tris-HCl, pH 8.6; 0.5 mL of 0.025 mol/L NH_4OH, pH 8.6; 0.1 mL of 10% Intralipid (Uppsala, Sweden); 0.03 mL VLDL (0.8 μg protein/mL); 1.125 mL of 15% (w/v) crystalline bovine serum albumin; and 1.17 mL of 0.154 mol/L NaCl. The reaction mixture was then incubated as described for the heart perfusate samples.

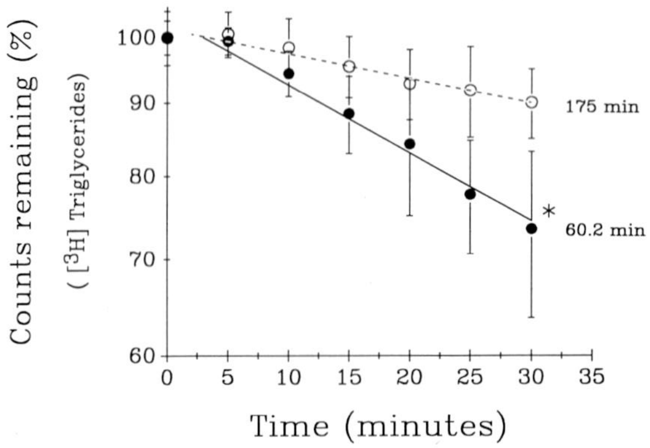

Fig 1. **^{3}H remaining in unhydrolyzed CM in the perfusate of isolated hearts from HN (open circles, broken line) or SD (closed circles, solid line) rats (n = 4 for each group). *$P < 0.05$, (v nephrotic. Data points represent the means ± SEM.**

Analytic Methods

Albumin was measured by electroimmunodiffusion as described previously.[11] Both TGs and cholesterol in plasma were determined using kits obtained from Sigma (Cholesterin 50, catalog #352-50; triglycerides-GPO-TRINDER 20, catalog #339-20). Total protein was measured by the method of Lowry et al.[24] Statistical analysis was performed using a one-way analysis of variance.[25] $P < 0.05$ was considered to be statistically significant.

RESULTS

The rate of hydrolysis of TGs from CM was reduced in hearts from nephrotic animals. Both the $t_{1/2}$ of TG removal from CM (Fig 1, Table 1) and the release of FFA into the perfusate (Fig 2) were reduced to approximately 40% of control. Chylomicron hydrolysis by the hearts of nephrotic animals was proportional to the fasting premortem serum TG concentration ($r = 0.9696$, $P < 0.05$). The uptake of fatty acids by normal hearts was also significantly greater than the uptake by hearts from nephrotic animals (Table 1).

Table 1. Characteristics of Rats in Which Cardiac Chylomicron Lipolysis Was Determined

Group	Weight (g)	Heart Weight (g)	TG (mg/dL)	Chol	Alb (mg/mL)	TP (mg/mL)	UalbV (mg/24 hr)	CM β ($ln_2/t_{1/2}$)	FFA Uptake (% of Dose)
Control animals (n = 4)	220 ± 3.7	1.005 ± 0.0039	63 ± 5	102 ± 12	33 ± 1.7	59 ± 3.7	NM	$1.2 \times 10^{-2} \pm 0.4 \times 10^{-2}$	7.25 ± 0.93
HN animals (n = 4)	194 ± 5	0.9325 ± 0.0236	388 ± 85*	452 ± 53*	13 ± 1.9*	49 ± 7	440 ± 53	$4.36 \times 10^{-3} \pm 1.24 \times 10^{-3}$*	3.32 ± 0.11*

Note. Comparison of animals used to measure CM catabolism in isolated perfused hearts. Weight refers to total body weight on the day of study. Data are presented as the means ± SEM.

Abbreviations: TG, serum triglycerides measured in terminal blood; Chol, serum cholesterol measured in terminal blood; Alb, serum albumin measured in terminal blood; TP, total protein measured in terminal blood; UalbV, 24-hour urinary albumin excretion determined in the 24-hour period preceding the experiment; CM β, the rate constant of TG removal from CMs in the perfusion system; FFA uptake, the percentage of counts in the perfusate that is present in hearts at the end of the 30-minute perfusion period.

* $P < 0.05$ versus control.

The sum of [^{3}H]oleate remaining in CM, released as FFA and taken up in the hearts, remained unchanged throughout the period of perfusion in both normal control Sprague Dawley (SD) and HN hearts, demonstrating that [^{3}H]-oleate hydrolyzed from CM was not bound nonspecifically to the perfusion apparatus and that disappearance of counts from CM was a consequence of lipolysis.

Total LPL activity was reduced by less than 50% in the hearts of nephrotic rats when compared with controls (Fig 3). Both total LPL activity and heparin releasable LPL activity were significantly less in hearts of HN rats (Table 2, Fig 3). However, there was no significant difference in the fraction of LPL activity extracted from the hearts after perfusion with heparin.

Total cardiac LPL activity was also significantly less in HN rats than in controls when hearts were not subjected to perfusion with heparin prior to extraction (Table 3). Indeed, total cardiac LPL activity was not affected by prior perfusion with heparin, suggesting that perfusion at 37°C did not inactivate the enzyme.

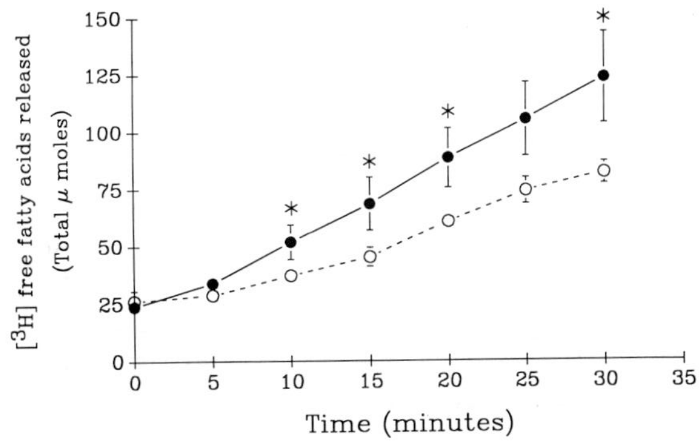

Fig 2. The appearance of ^{3}H in FFAs from CM during perfusion of hearts isolated from HN (open circles, broken line) or SD (closed circles, solid line) rats (n = 4 for each group). *$P < 0.05$ *v* nephrotic. Data points represent the means ± SEM.

DISCUSSION

The hydrolysis and clearance of plasma CM is regulated by the endothelium-bound enzyme

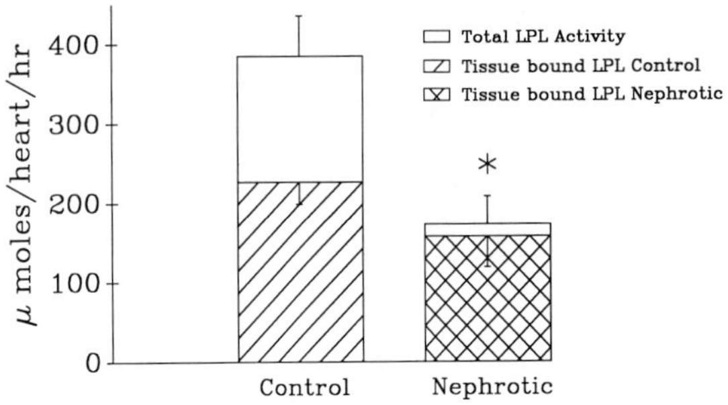

Fig 3. Lipoprotein lipase activity solubalized by heparin in the solution used to perfuse isolated hearts of HN and control rats (open area of bars) and LPL activity remaining in the perfused heart (cross-hatched area of bar, hearts from HN rats; diagonal-shaded area of bar, hearts from control animals). The upward-pointing error bars are the SEM of measurement of LPL activity in the perfusate and the differences are significant at $P < 0.01$. The downward-pointing error bars are the SEM of measurement of LPL activity in the residual myocardium and the differences between these measurements are not significantly different. Total cardiac LPL activity for each of these two groups is the sum of these two values and is represented by the total height of the bars. n = 5 for nephrotic animals and n = 4 for control animals. *$P < 0.05$ *v* control.

Table 2. Characteristics of Rats in Which Heparin Releasable Lipoprotein Lipase Activity Was Determined

						Heparin-releasable LPL (μmol FFA Released/hr)		Tissue-bound LPL (μmol/hr)		Total LPL Activity (μmol FFA Released/hr)	
Group	Heart Weight (g)	TG (mg/dL)	Chol	Alb (mg/mL)	UalbV (mg/24 hr)	Per Gram of Heart	Per Heart	Per Gram Heart	Per Heart	Per Gram Heart	Per Heart
Control (n = 4)	0.925 ± 0.028	64 ± 7	69 ± 3	36.6 ± 0.4	NM	173 ± 33	159 ± 29	226 ± 28	207.7 ± 23	385 ± 51	353.5 ± 43.4
HN (n = 5)	0.82 ± 0.026	434 ± 40*	434 ± 39*	12.6 ± 0.15*	377 ± 20	19.4 ± 11.7*	15.6 ± 9.8*	156.8 ± 38.6	129.4 ± 32.5	172.4 ± 36*	142.0 ± 30.4*

Note. Comparison of animals used to measure heparin-labile LPL activity in isolated perfused hearts. Data are presented as means ± SEM.

Abbreviations: TG, serum triglycerides measured in terminal blood; Chol, serum cholesterol measured in terminal blood; Alb, serum albumin measured in terminal blood; UalbV, 24-hour urinary albumin excretion determined in the 24-hour period preceding the experiment; NM, not measured. Total LPL activity is the sum of LPL activity released by heparin during infusion and LPL activity extracted from the perfused heart.

* $P < 0.05$ versus control.

LPL.[26] Lipoprotein lipase is synthesized in parenchymal cells, but its biologic activity is expressed only by that fraction that is bound on the vascular endothelium and has access to circulating lipoproteins. Lipoprotein lipase is tethered to the vascular endothelium by the glycosaminoglycan heparan sulfate.[27] It is predominantly this fraction that is solubilized when heparin is administered or added to the perfusate. It has been reported that the activity of this enzyme is reduced in nephrosis.[3,4,10,11,28] Our findings that the activity of this enzyme is reduced in hearts of HN rats, specifically and only in the heparin labile compartment, are compatible with the hypothesis that depletion of LPL from the vascular endothelium contributes to reduced clearance of CM in the nephrotic syndrome. Reduced LPL activity alone, however, may not be sufficient to cause reduced CM lipolysis.

Chylomicron and VLDL clearance is normal in rats with hereditary analbuminemia,[11] even though LPL activity is also greatly reduced in postheparin plasma in these animals. Lipoprotein clearance only becomes abnormal on the development of proteinuria in these animals, suggesting that urinary protein loss plays a necessary role in the pathogenesis of the abnormality in lipoprotein clearance, independent of any effect on serum albumin concentration or in postheparin LPL activity. Although LPL activity is re-

Table 3. Lipoprotein Lipase Activity in Hearts Obtained From Rats With Heymann Nephritis

						LPL Activity (μmol FFA Released/hr)	
Group	Weight (g)	Heart Weight (g)	TG (mg/dL)	Chol (mg/dL)	Alb (mg/mL)	Per Gram Heart	Per Heart
Control (n = 5)	215 ± 7	0.882 ± 0.049	34.6 ± 8.7	68.2 ± 11.5	33.1 ± 2.4	368.5 ± 39.4	323.9 ± 35.3
HN (n = 5)	187 ± 7*	0.75 ± 0.052	274.0 ± 54.5*	369.2 ± 77.6*	11.0 ± 1.04*	210.6 ± 25.9*	154.7 ± 14.9*

Note. Comparison of animals used to measure LPL activity in unperfused hearts. Data are presented as the means ± SEM.

Abbreviations: Weight, total body weight on the day the animals were killed; TG, serum triglycerides measured in terminal blood; Chol, serum cholesterol measured in terminal blood; Alb, serum albumin measured in terminal blood; UalbV, 24-hour urinary albumin excretion determined in the 24-hour period preceding the experiment; LPL is lipoprotein lipase activity; NM, signifies not measured.

* $P < 0.05$ versus control.

duced in the nephrotic syndrome, this may therefore not be the sole cause of defective lipoprotein catabolism in vivo.

The ratio of protein to lipid is reduced in nephrotic lipoproteins,[4,29] and the relative concentration of specific apolipoproteins within each lipoprotein class is also abnormal.[30] While plasma apo A-I levels are increased in proportion to HDL levels in nephrosis, the concentration of virtually all other apolipoproteins (A-II, A-IV, E, and C-II) is reduced in proportion to HDL.[13,14] While total plasma apo C-II is normal in both nephrotic rats[13,14] and patients,[31,32] the concentration of this important LPL activator is reduced per CM or VLDL particle[32] and the concentration of the competitive inhibitor of LPL, apo C-III, is increased.[33] Apolipoprotein C-II is a necessary LPL co-factor and apo A-IV is required for efficient release of apo C-II from either HDL or VLDL,[16] a process necessary for LPL-mediated hydrolysis of TG in nascent CMs. Thus, abnormalities in the apolipoprotein composition of nephrotic lipoproteins could contribute in their decreased rate of catabolism.

Furukawa et al[17] reported that VLDL was hydrolyzed by LPL at a lower rate in vitro in the presence of HDL from nephrotic rats compared with HDL from normal rats, suggesting that LPL might perform suboptimally in vivo because of an abnormality in HDL and not because of a reduction in LPL.

We initiated these studies because we had previously found that the rate of fatty acid uptake was similarly decreased in heart and adipose tissue.[10] The decrease in TG uptake was not only a consequence of dilution of labeled TGs in a large unlabeled pool since absolute uptake of fatty acids was decreased. We found this especially interesting in light of the report of Levy et al,[4] which indicated that LPL activity in the heart was normal in nephrotic rats. This finding, were it verified, would exclude a role for decreased LPL per se as being responsible for decreased CM lipolysis in the nephrotic syndrome and would support Furakawa et al's[17] observations that HDL may be dysfunctional in nephrotic animals. The finding that decreased lipolysis occurred in the isolated perfused heart despite the absence of plasma from nephrotic animals is direct evidence that local endothelial factors necessary for CM lipolysis are abnormal in the nephrotic rat, but do not exclude abnormalities in lipoprotein-lipoprotein interactions as well. Indeed, the difference in CM lipolysis by isolated hearts for nephrotic animals compared with controls was much less than the differences in cardiac TG uptake observed in vivo.[10]

The difference between our observations and those of Levy et al may be explained by the differences in methods used to determine LPL activity. Levy et al[4] extracted LPL from an acetone powder, while we used a more gentle detergent extraction from frozen hearts. It is possible that Levy et al extracted an especially tightly bound LPL pool that we did not, or that their method inactivated LPL while ours did not. Nevertheless, the relatively small, but biologically important LPL pool releasable by heparin is reduced by nearly an order of magnitude in hearts from nephrotic animals and the methods used by Levy et al could not have revealed the differences that we observed, even if total LPL activity is indeed nearly identical in nephrotic and normal myocardium.

It is not known why the heparin labile pool of LPL is so reduced in the nephrotic syndrome. Karpe et al[34] recently established that plasma LPL activity increased in normal human subjects after an oral fat load. They suggested that this response might be a consequence of release of LPL mediated by its interaction with either TGs or FFAs. They did not measure postheparin LPL activity in these patients to establish whether any depletion of the heparin labile pool also occurred. Saxena et al[35] found that LPL bound to endothelial cells in tissue culture could be released by exposure to the TG lipoproteins VLDL and CM. Thus, hyperlipidemia, as occurs in both the nephrotic syndrome and in the condition of hereditary analbuminemia, might be in part responsible for reduced heparin labile LPL activity.

ACKNOWLEDGMENT

The authors acknowledge the expert assistance of Agnes Frank.

REFERENCES

1. Marsh JB: Lipoprotein metabolism in experimental nephrosis. J Lipid Res 25:1619-1623, 1984

2. Staprans I, Felts JM, Couser WG: Glycosaminoglycans and chylomicron metabolism in control and nephrotic rats. Metabolism 36:496-501, 1987

3. Garber DW, Gottlieb BA, Marsh JB, Sparks CE: Catabolism of very low density lipo-proteins in experimental nephrosis. J Clin Invest 74:1375-1383, 1984

4. Levy E, Ziv E, Bar-On H, Shafrir E: Experimental nephrotic syndrome: Removal and tissue distribution of chylomicrons and very-low-density lipoproteins of normal and nephrotic origin. Biochim Biophys Acta 1043:259-266, 1990

5. Hoffenberg R: Control of albumin degradation in vivo and in the perfused liver, in Rothschild MA, Waldmann T (eds): Plasma Protein Metabolism Regulation of Synthesis, Distribution, and Degradation. New York, NY, Academic Press, 1970, pp 239-255

6. Waldmann TA: Albumin catabolism, in Rosemoer M, Oratz M, Rothschild A (eds): Albumin Structure, Function and Uses. New York, NY, Pergamon, 1977, pp 255-273

7. Chappell DA, Fry GL, Waknitz MA, Berns JJ: Ligand size as a determinant for catabolism by the low density lipoprotein (LDL) receptor pathway. J Biol Chem 266:19296-19302, 1991

8. Kaysen GA: Nephrotic hyperlipidemia: Primary abnormalities in both lipoprotein catabolism and synthesis. Miner Electrolyte Metab 18:212-216, 1992

9. Olivecrona T, Bengtsson-Olivecrona G: Lipoprotein lipase from milk—The model enzyme in lipoprotein lipase research, in Borensztajn J (ed): Lipoprotein Lipase. Chicago, IL, Evener Publishers, 1987, pp 15-58

10. Kaysen GA, Mehendru L, Pan X-M, Staprans I: Both peripheral chylomicron and hepatic uptake of remnants are defective in nephrosis. Am J Physiol 263:F335-F341, 1992

11. Davies RW, Staprans I, Hutchison FN, Kaysen GA: Proteinuria, not altered albumin metabolism, effects hyperlipidemia in the nephrotic rat. J Clin Invest 86:600-605, 1990

12. Garfinkel AS, Schotz MC: Lipoprotein lipase, in Gotto AM, Jr (ed): Plasma Lipoproteins. New York, NY, Elsevier Scientific, 1987, pp 335-357

13. Michaeli J, Bar-On H, Shafrir E: Lipoprotein profiles in a heterogeneous group of patients with nephrotic syndrome. Isr J Med Sci 17:1001-1008, 1981

14. Marshall JF, Apostolopoulos JJ, Brack CM, Howlett GJ: Regulation of apolipoprotein gene expression and plasma high-density lipoprotein composition in experimental nephrosis. Biochim Biophys Acta 1042:271-279, 1990

15. Sparks CE, Tennenberg SD, Marsh JB: Catabolism of the apolipoproteins of HDL in control and nephrotic rats. Bioch Biophys Acta 665:8-12, 1981

16. Goldberg IJ, Scheraldi CA, Yacoub LK, Saxena U, Bisgaier CL: Lipoprotein apo C-II activation of lipoprotein lipase. Modulation by apolipoproteins A-IV. J Biol Chem 265:4266-4272, 1990

17. Furukawa S, Hirano T, Mamo JCL, Nagano S, Takahashi T: Catabolic defect of TG is associated with abnormal very-low-density lipoprotein in experimental nephrosis. Metabolism 39:101-107, 1990

18. McFarlane AS: Catabolism of plasma proteins. Lancet 1:131-132, 1963

19. Couser WG, Steinmuller DR, Stilmant MM, Salant DJ, Lowenstein LM: Experimental glomerulonephritis in the isolated perfused rat kidney. J Clin Invest 62:1275-1287, 1985

20. Fielding CJ: Metabolism of cholesterol-rich chylomicrons. J Clin Invest 62:141-151, 1978

21. Trout DL, Estes EH, Jr, Freidberg SJ: Titration of free fatty acids of plasma: A study of current methods and a new modification. J Lipid Res 1:199-202, 1960

22. Bollman JL, Cain JL, Grindlay JA: Techniques for the collection of lymph from the liver, small intestine or thoracic duct of the rat. J Lab Clin Med 33:1349-1352, 1948

23. Semb H, Olivecrona T: Lipoprotein lipase in guinea pig tissues: Molecular size and rates of synthesis. Biochim Biophys Acta 878:330-337, 1986

24. Lowry OH, Rosebrough NJ, Farr AL, Randall RJ: Protein measurement with the Folin phenol reagent. J Biol Chem 193:265-275, 1951

25. Matthews DE, Farewell W: Using and Understanding Medical Statistics. New York, Karger, 1985

26. Eckel RH: Lipoprotein lipase. A multifunctional enzyme relevant to common metabolic diseases. N Engl J Med 320:1044-1047, 1989

27. Williams MP, Streeter HB, Wusteman FS, Cryer A: Heparan sulfate and the binding of lipoprotein lipase to porcine thoracic aorta endothelium. Biochim Biophys Acta 756:83-91, 1983

28. Yamada M, Matsuda I: Lipoprotein lipase in clinical and experimental nephrosis. Clin Chim Acta 30:787-794, 1970

29. Marsh JB, Sparks CE: Hepatic secretion of lipoproteins in the rat and the effect of experimental nephrosis. J Clin Invest 64:1229-1237, 1979

30. Gherardi E, Rota E, Calandra S, Genova R, Tamborino A: Relationship among the concentrations of serum lipoproteins and changes in their chemical composition in patients with untreated nephrotic syndrome. Eur J Clin Invest 7:563-570, 1977

31. Kashyap ML, Srivastava LS, Hynd BA, Brady D, Perisutti F, Glueck CJ, Gartside PS: Apolipoprotein CII and lipoprotein lipase in human nephrotic syndrome. Atherosclerosis 35:29-40, 1980

32. Joven J, Villabona C, Vilella E, Masana L, Albertí R, Vallés M: Abnormalities of lipoprotein metabolism in patients with the nephrotic syndrome. N Engl J Med 323:579-584, 1990

33. Brown WV, Baginsky ML: Inhibition of lipoprotein lipase by an apoprotein of human very low density lipoprotein. Biochem Biophys Res Commun 46:375-382, 1972

34. Karpe F, Olivecrona T, Walldius G, Hamsten A: Lipoprotein lipase in plasma after an oral fat load: Relation to free fatty acids. J Lipid Res 33:975-984, 1992

35. Saxena U, Witte LD, Goldberg IJ: Release of endothelial cell lipoprotein lipase by plasma lipoproteins and free fatty acids. J Biol Chem 264:4349-4355, 1989

Effect of Oncotic Pressure on Apolipoprotein A-I Metabolism in the Rat

George A. Kaysen, MD, PhD, Elaine Hoye, BS, Hardin Jones, Jr, PhD, Arie van Tol, PhD, and Jaap A. Joles, DVM, PhD

● **The nephrotic syndrome is characterized by reduced plasma albumin and colloid osmotic pressure (π), urinary protein loss and hyperlipidemia. High-density lipoprotein (HDL) and the level of apo A-I, the principal apolipoprotein in HDL, is increased in nephrotic rats and rats with hereditary analbuminemia (NAR)—animals with virtually no albumin in plasma and reduced plasma π, but without proteinuria, suggesting that urinary protein loss is not responsible for increased plasma apo A-I levels. We conducted these studies to determine the mechanism responsible for increased plasma apo A-I levels in the nephrotic syndrome and NAR and to determine whether reduced plasma π or albumin was responsible for increased apo A-I. We first measured the clearance of ^{125}I apo A-I HDL in NAR and rats with passive Heymann nephritis (HN) compared with normal Sprague Dawley (SD) control. Both the clearance of apo A-I and fractional apo A-I turnover rate (FTR) were significantly reduced both in HN (7.40 ± 2.18% plasma pool/hr) and NAR (5.63 ± 1.12) compared with SD (9.87 ± 0.75). Total apo A-I turnover rate, which in steady state equals apo A-I synthesis rate, was also significantly increased in both HN (487 ± 127 μg/100 g body weight/hr) and NAR (253 ± 16), compared with SD (216 ± 19). Thus decreased apo A-I catabolism and increased synthesis both contributed to increased apo A-I levels in HN and NAR. We then infused either hyperoncotic human albumin or ficoll into two additional groups of HN for days in quantities sufficient to maintain plasma π within the normal range. Both cholesterol and apo A-I levels decreased to normal, even though proteinuria persisted. Thus apo A-I levels were increased both in HN and NAR as a result of both increased synthesis and reduced catabolism in response to reduced plasma π. Neither hypoalbuminemia nor proteinuria were necessary.**

INDEX WORDS: Nephrotic syndrome; analbuminemia, proteinuria; protein synthesis; protein catabolism.

THE NEPHROTIC syndrome is characterized by proteinuria, hypoalbuminemia, with a consequent decrease in plasma colloid osmotic pressure (π), and hyperlipidemia.[1] Hyperlipidemia is a consequence both of increased synthesis of lipids and apolipoproteins[2,3] and of their decreased catabolism.[4] Decreased lipolysis of triglyceride-bearing lipoproteins is not a consequence of decreased plasma albumin concentration because lipolysis is not decreased in rats with hereditary analbuminemia (the Nagase analbuminemic rat [NAR]),[5] animals with a reduced plasma π and essentially no albumin in plasma. Defective lipolysis of triglycerides contained in chylomicrons and in very-low-density lipoprotein (VLDL) follows the onset of proteinuria, is probably a consequence of proteinuria and is unrelated to hypoalbuminemia per se.

Lipoprotein levels are nevertheless increased in NAR,[6,7] suggesting that decreased plasma albumin concentration or π also plays a role in establishing lipid levels in the nephrotic syndrome. Infusion of either dextran or albumin reduces lipid levels in the nephrotic syndrome,[8] providing evidence that reduced plasma π rather than hypoalbuminemia is at least partially responsible for the increased level of cholesterol and triglycerides in plasma in addition to any effect contributed by urinary albumin loss.

The principal cholesterol-bearing lipoprotein in the rat is high-density lipoprotein (HDL),[9] and apolipoprotein (apo) A-I constitutes 50% or more of total protein found in HDL. Plasma levels of apo A-I are increased in the plasma of both nephrotic[10,11] and analbuminemic rats.[6,7,12] Apo A-I synthesis by perfused livers isolated from rats rendered nephrotic with puromycin aminonucleoside (PAN) is increased.[3] Apo A-I mRNA levels are increased as is the rate of transcription of apo A-I in the liver in both nephrotic and analbuminemic rats,[10,11] suggesting that increased hepatic synthesis of this apolipoprotein is in part responsible for the increased plasma levels and that increased synthesis is transcriptionally regulated. In contrast there is no change in apo A-I mRNA in the gut of nephrotic rats,[10] the only other organ that synthesizes significant amounts of this protein.

We first performed two experiments that further established the relationship between plasma albumin concentration or π and plasma apo A-I

Supported in part by the research service of the United States Department of Veterans Affairs, Washington, DC, and in part by the National Institutes of Health, Bethesda, MD, grant no. RO1 DK 42297. Dr Joles was supported by the Netherlands Kidney Foundation, Bussum, the Netherlands, grant no. C92.1244.

levels. We determined that both increased synthesis and decreased catabolism of apo A-I contributed to increased plasma apo A-I levels in both rats with Heymann nephritis (HN) and rats with hereditary analbuminemia. Lipoprotein lipase (LPL) is reduced in both the nephrotic syndrome[13,14] and in hereditary analbuminemia.[5] Apo A-I levels correlate inversely with postheparin LPL activity in humans[15] and in the monkey.[16] LPL inhibition increases apo A-I fractional catabolic rate (FCR) specifically by increasing the renal catabolism of apo A-I.[16] We previously found that renal catabolism of HDL was not increased in rats with either adriamycin-induced nephrotic syndrome or in rats with HN,[17] in contrast to what would be predicted by Goldberg et al[16]; however, in both cases renal dysfunction might prevent increased catabolism of filtered proteins. We therefore measured renal apo A-I catabolism in analbuminemic rats because analbuminemic rats have normal kidneys.

MATERIALS AND METHODS

Protocol 1: Kinetics of [^{125}I] apo A-I HDL in NAR and in Rats With Passive Heymann Nephritis

All animals were maintained in a 12-hour light-dark cycled room and fed Purina rat chow (Ralston Purina, Richmond, IN) throughout the study. Thirteen male Sprague Dawley (SD) rats (180 to 210 g) were obtained from Bantin Kingman Farms (Freemont, CA). Seven of these were rendered nephrotic with an intraperitoneal injection of sheep antibodies prepared against fraction FX1A (Courtesy of Dr William Couser, Seattle, WA) to induce passive HN, as described previously.[18] Five NAR were obtained from our own breeding colony. Six normal SD rats were not injected with antiserum and served as controls for the other two groups. Eleven days after injection with antiserum, all rats with HN were placed in individual metabolic cages for collection of two sequential 24-hour urine specimens for measurement of both urinary albumin and apo A-I excretion.

Apo A-I was prepared, iodinated, and used to reconstitute HDL as described below. Tracer apo A-I and HDL was always prepared from normal male SD rats. After urine collection, approximately 7 mg of reconstituted HDL labeled with ^{125}I in the apo A-I moiety, containing approximately 2.5×10^7 cpm of ^{125}I, was injected into the tail vein of each animal as a bolus. The animals were lightly restrained but were not anesthetized. Blood samples of approximately 200 μL were obtained from a tail vein at 5, 15, 30, 60, and 120 minutes, and at 5, 10, 24, 36, 48, 72, and 78 hours. Three 10-μL aliquots were counted in a gamma counter (Searle Analytics, Des Plaines, IL) for 10 minutes.

The plasma-specific radioactivity curve was integrated by the method of trapezoids using the log trapezoidal rule.[19,20] The dose injected (D) divided by the area under the plasma specific radioactivity curve (AUC) yields a result in mass turnover/unit time,[17] where D is the total number of counts injected at time = 0, A-I is the serum apo A-I concentration in mg/mL measured at each time point, and C is the trichloroacetic acid (TCA) precipitable counts/mL of serum. Specific radioactivity is counts per milligram of apo A-I at each time point. The advantage of this method is that it allows for calculation of catabolic rate in the presence of a varying plasma concentration throughout the period of observation.

$$\text{Total apo A-I turnover} = D/\int_0^{\infty} (1/\text{A-I}) \cdot (C \cdot dt) \quad \text{(Eq. 1)}$$

In the absence of extracorporeal loss of intact apo A-I, apo A-I turnover is also equal to its catabolic rate. If measurable extracorporeal loss of a protein occurs, then its catabolic rate is its turnover rate minus measurable losses.

To determine apo A-I clearance we integrated TCA preciptable counts in plasma at each time point. Total counts injected (D) divided by this integral represents apo A-I clearance, as reported by us for other proteins.[18,19,21] Plasma π was measured on the initial plasma samples obtained from the nephrotic and analbuminemic rats in this protocol.

Protocol 2: The Effect of Plasma Albumin Concentration or π on Apo A-I Levels in Rats With Heymann Nephritis

The effect of plasma π and albumin concentration on plasma apo A-I levels was determined by experiments designed to establish separately the effect of plasma albumin concentration and plasma π, by infusing either hyperoncotic human albumin or a nonprotein carbohydrate polymer ficoll, as an oncotic support agent. HN was induced by intraperitoneal administration of anti FX 1-A antibodies as previously described.[18] Shortly after the onset of proteinuria (5 days after injection), nephrotic rats were anesthetized by intraperitoneal administration of sodium pentobarbital, and transjugular catheters were inserted. The neck was shaved and prepared using sterile technique. The jugular vein was exposed through a lateral incision. A second incision was made on the back of the neck, and a tunnel was created extending from the back of the neck around the subscapular area, under the front leg to the site of the lateral incision. The catheter was inserted into the vein, which was then ligated, and the catheter was secured to surrounding muscle. The catheter was then fed through a coiled spring and then through a swivel to allow the rat free mobility within the cage. The animals were allowed to recover from anesthesia and surgery for at least 24 hours before infusion of solute.

After surgery nephrotic rats were divided into three groups. Hyperoncotic (25%) human serum albumin (Baxter Health Care Corp, Glendale, CA) was infused into one group of five animals, hyperoncotic (25%) ficoll was infused in five, and saline was infused in the remaining five nephrotic animals for a period of 90 to 96 hours. Plasma was obtained twice daily for measurement of albumin and π to allow for adjustment of the infusion rate to maintain plasma π within the target range. Terminal blood was obtained at the end of the infusion period for measurement of albumin, π, cholesterol, and apo A-I. Urine was collected during each of the days of infusion for measurement of albumin. Plasma albumin was measured on samples obtained each morning used to monitor plasma π. If plasma albumin concentration decreases and urinary albumin excretion does not, it is possible not to detect a change in glomerular permselectivity. For this reason we monitored the effect of ficoll and albumin infusion on the renal clearance of rat albumin. The renal clearance of albumin was calculated daily as 24-hour urinary albumin excretion/plasma albumin concentration/hr. The last three measurements for each animals were averaged, and the average value for each animal was used to express a mean renal albumin clearance for each animal.

Nonnephrotic rats (n = 15) were also studied in three groups, although in this case when solute was infused it was by repeated tail injections, because plasma π did not decrease rapidly after bolus injection because animals had no urinary losses of injected solute. As in the nephrotic animals, one group of five animals was infused with hyperoncotic human albumin, one group with ficoll (n = 5), and the third group with saline (n = 5).

Protocol 3: Renal and Hepatic Catabolism of HDL in Analbuminemic Rats

Tyramine cellobiose is a ligand that can be labeled with ^{125}I, covalently bound to proteins, and is retained within lysosomes at the site of protein catabolism.[22] It is thus possible to quantify the fraction of a protein catabolized at a specific site. Free tyramine cellobiose is shed into the bile by the liver and into the urine by the kidney. To quantify catabolism by these organs it is necessary therefore to collect stool and urine and to measure counts found in gut contents. To determine whether there were changes in the principal sites of apo A-I catabolism in NAR compared with normal SD rats, we first reconstituted HDL with apo A-I labeled with ^{125}I tyramine cellobiose.[22]

Six normal male control SD rats and three male analbuminemic rats were studied in the fed state. Approximately 5 mg HDL protein reconstituted with apo A-I ^{125}I tyramine cellobiose was injected into a tail vein. Blood was obtained at 5 and 15 minutes to determine apo A-I levels. The animals were returned to individual metabolic cages with urine and stool separators. All urine and stool was collected for 24 hours, after which the animals were removed from the cage, and preterminal blood was obtained for measurement of remaining counts and apo A-I levels. The animals were anesthetized with sodium pentobarbital (20 mg/kg intraperitoneally) and exsanguinated by aortic puncture. After removal of approximately 10 mL blood, the aorta was perfused with approximately 300 mL isotonic saline with 0.01% ethylenediaminetetra-acetic acid. The vena cava was incised for removal of perfusate.

After perfusion, the liver, intestines, and bowel were removed. The liver was further perfused after removal using an additional 60 mL perfusion solution. The bowel contents were removed, weighed, and homogenized. Four pieces of tissue weighing between 200 mg and 1 g were excised from each of the above tissues, and each individually counted in a gamma counter as above. Tissues were then homogenized in phosphate-buffered saline, 0.5% deoxycholic acid using a polytron (Brinkmann Instruments, Westbury NY), and then centrifuged at 3,000*g*. The supernatant was filtered through gauze and then centrifuged at 17,000*g* twice. The high-speed supernatant was then subjected to gel permeation chromatography using Sephadex G 25.[22] Counts were determined in the void volume (apo A-I) and in later eluting fractions (catabolized apo A-I). Between 85% and 90% of counts recovered represented catabolized apo A-I. Plasma π was measured in all animals studied in this protocol.

Laboratory Methods

Purification of apo A-I. Rat apo A-I was purified from serum harvested from normal male SD rats according to the method of Dallinga-Thie et al.[23] Purity was assessed to be at least 99% apo A-I by Coomassie-stained 4% to 15% polyacrylamide gel electrophoresis. The purified apo A-I was stored at −80°C after extensive dialysis against 0.15 mol/L NaCl containing 1 mmol/L ethylenediaminetetra-acetic acid.

We were concerned that even the mild conditions used for iodination might oxidize the lipid components of the lipoprotein. Therefore HDL used to measure catabolic rates and distribution was prepared by incorporating previously [^{125}I]-labeled apo A-I into nonradioactive HDL.[24]

Apo A-I was iodinated with 3 mCi ^{125}I, using 1,3,4,6-Tetrachloro-3α,6α-diphenylglycouril, a solid phase oxidant (Iodogen; Pierce Chemical Co, Rockford, IL) as described previously.[16]

For this experiment, approximately 0.75 mg labeled apo A-I was combined with 36 mg (protein) HDL in a volume of 12 mL. HDL was then isolated by ultracentrifugation, harvesting the 1.050 to 1.22 g/mL density fraction. Twenty-five percent of the counts were subsequently found in the HDL fraction at the top of the tube. Virtually all of the counts in this fraction were preciptable with 10% trichloroacetic acid. Before injection into the rats, labeled HDL was dialyzed extensively and diluted in 0.15 mol/L NaCl so that it had 4.4 $\times 10^7$ cpm/mL. Rats were injected with 0.6 mL/250 g body weight.

Apo A-I concentration was determined in the urine both of nephrotic and of normal rats by radioimmunoassay.[17] Urinary apo A-I losses were subtracted from apo A-I turnover rate to determine apo A-I catabolic rate when urinary losses of this protein were detected.

Apolipoprotein A-I radioimmunoassay. For the radioimmunoassay, antibodies to rat apo A-I were raised in New Zealand white rabbits. One hundred micrograms purified protein was combined with complete Freund's adjuvant and injected in multiple intramuscular sites for the first injection. Incomplete Freund's adjuvant was used for subsequent injections. Apo A-I used as the standard in the assay and for iodination was purified and stored as above. For the radioimmunoassay, 35 μg apo A-I was iodinated with 1.0 mCi ^{125}I, using 15 μg iodogen as a catalyst.

Purified apo A-I was used as a standard. Protein concentration in the apo A-I standard was determined by the method of Lowry et al,[25] using a weighed bovine serum albumin standard (Fraction V, Sigma Chemical, St. Louis, MO). Standards and unknowns were diluted in phosphate-buffered saline 0.02% sodium azide, 0.1% bovine serum albumin, and 0.1 mol/L sodium dodecyl sulfate. Fifteen microliters was used for the assay.

Measurements of plasma and urine albumin in all protocols

Table 1. Characteristics of Nephrotic, Analbuminemic, and Normal Control Rats in Which Apo A-I Clearance and Synthesis Was Determined

Group	Weight (g)	SAlb (mg/mL)	$U_{alb}V$ (mg/d)	$U_{a\text{-}I}V$ (μg/d)	Chol (mmol/L)	Tg (mmol/L)	PVol (% BW)	Apo A-I (mg/dL)	π (mm Hg)
SD (n = 6)	233 ± 10	37.8 ± 2.03	NM	0	1.89 ± 0.24	1.12 ± 0.50	5.13 ± 0.53	45.9 ± 2.3	NM
HN (n = 7)	225 ± 21	10.13* ± 2.68	372 ± 84	2373 ± 742	8.17* ± 2.01	8.76* ± 5.46	5.15 ± 0.58	130.9* ± 12.9	11.67 ± 2.73
NAR (n = 5)	264*† ± 10	0.018*† ± 0.007	NM	NM	6.13* ± 1.31	1.39 ± 0.47	4.52 ± 0.56	77.1*† ± 8.78	17.33† ± 2.93

NOTE. Values are expressed as means ± SD. Weight is body weight in grams.

Abbreviations: S_{Alb}, serum albumin concentration at the time of apo A-I injection (T_0) in mg/mL; $U_{alb}V$, average of two consecutive measurements of albumin excreted in the two 24-hour periods immediately preceeding T_0; Chol, serum cholesterol; TG, serum triglycerides in mmol/L at T_0; PVol, initial volume of distribution of [^{125}I]apo A-I; Apo A-I concentration in mg/dL, average plasma apo A-I concentration for all time points measured; $U_{a\text{-}I}V$, urinary apo A-I in μg/day; NAR, Nagase analbuminemic rat; NM, not measured.

* $P < 0.05$ v SD (control).

† $P < 0.05$ v HN (nephrotic).

was performed using electroimmunodiffusion as described previously.[18] When human albumin was infused, both rat and human albumin concentrations were each measured both in urine and plasma separately by the same method. There is no cross-reaction between either the anti-rat albumin and human albumin or the anti-human albumin and rat albumin. Total protein was measured by the method of Lowry et al.[25]

Plasma π was measured with a micromembrane oncometer using an Amicon YM10 semipermeable membrane (W.R. Grace & Co, Danvers, MA) and a Viggo-Spectramed transducer Model P 10 EZ (Viggo-Spectramed, Oxnard, CA) using 10-μL samples. These measurements were made immediately on obtaining plasma samples so that solute infusion could be appropriately adjusted.

Enzymatic methods were used for the determination of total plasma cholesterol using a kit obtained from Boehringer (Mannheim, Germany). Plasma apo A-I was measured by electroimmunoassay as described previously[18] in protocol 2.

Statistical analysis was performed using a one-way analysis of variance[26] with post hoc Student Newman Keuls comparison. A P value of <0.05 was considered to be statistically significant.

RESULTS

Apo A-I levels were increased significantly both in HN and in NAR studied in protocol 1 (Table 1). Apo A-I clearance was significantly reduced in both HN and NAR (Fig 1, Table 2). Fractional catabolic rate (FCR) was reduced significantly in both HN and NAR and was not different between the two experimental groups (Table 2). Absolute apo A-I turnover was increased significantly in both NAR and HN (Table 2), suggesting that increased synthesis of apo A-I contributed to increased plasma levels, in addition to the contribution by a decreased FCR. Thus decreased plasma albumin concentration or π led to increased apo A-I synthesis and decreased apo A-I FCR. These observations also suggested that urinary protein excretion was not an important factor in establishing apo A-I levels.

Urinary apo A-I losses were approximately 10% of total apo A-I turnover in HN and contributed to apo A-I FTR. However, even including urinary loss of apo A-I, apo A-I FTR was still significantly less in HN than in control animals.

Apo A-I turnover rate equals apo A-I synthesis under these conditions. In HN apo A-I synthesis was increased more than twofold, and plasma concentration was increased approximately threefold. Thus increased synthesis was the predominant mechanism responsible for increased apo A-I levels in nephrotic rats. Apo A-I synthesis was only increased by about 20% in NAR studied in this protocol, and plasma apo A-I levels were increased by 67%. Thus, decreased FCR played a greater role in establishing increased plasma apo A-I levels in these animals.

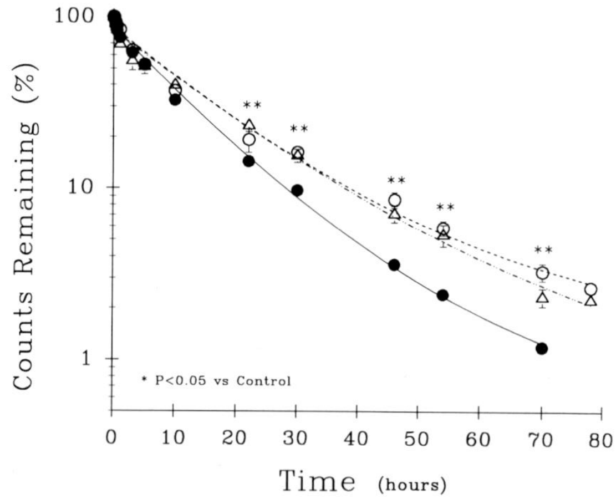

Fig 1. Disappearance of [^{125}I] from plasma of normal control rats (solid circle, solid line), rats with passive HN (open circles, broken line), and Nagase analbuminemic rats (open triangles, dashed double dotted line), during study of apo A-I turnover. Apo A-I was iodinated using iodogen, and HDL was reconstituted.

Table 2. Apo A-I Clearance and Synthesis Rate in Normal Rats, Rats With Heymann Nephritis, and Rats With Hereditary Analbuminemia

Group	Apo A-I Clearance (mL/100 g/hr)	Apo A-I Turnover (μg/100 g BW/hr)	FTR (% plasma pool/hr)	FCR (% plasma pool/hr)
SD (n = 6)	0.476 ± 0.028	216 ± 19	9.87 ± 0.75	9.87 ± 0.75
HN (n = 7)	0.353* ± 0.066	487* ± 127	7.40* ± 2.18	6.65* ± 1.56
NAR (n = 5)	0.325* ± 0.049	253*† ± 16	5.63* ± 1.12	5.63* ± 1.12

* $P < 0.05$ *v* SD (control).
† $P < 0.05$ *v* HN.

Infusion of both ficoll and human serum albumin caused an increase in plasma π into the normal range in both nephrotic groups studied in protocol 2 (Table 3) and was sustained throughout the period of infusion. Plasma π remained significantly greater in both the ficoll-infused and the albumin-infused animals throughout the period of study compared with saline-infused controls. Plasma π was not significantly different between the ficoll- and albumin-infused nephrotic animals. Similarly, both ficoll and albumin infusion increased plasma π above the normal range in the nonnephrotic animals (Table 3).

Urinary excretion of rat albumin was the same in all three groups of nephrotic animals studied in protocol 2, irrespective of whether they were infused with albumin, ficoll, or saline (Table 3). Furthermore the renal clearance of albumin was also the same in all three groups of animals.

Plasma cholesterol and apo A-I levels were significantly increased in nephrotic rats infused with saline (Table 3); however, both albumin and ficoll infusion normalized these values in nephrotic rats (Table 3). In contrast, infusion of neither albumin nor ficoll had any significant effect on apolipoprotein A-I or cholesterol in control animals (Table 3).

Total removal of apo A-I from the plasma compartment was significantly reduced in analbuminemic rats as judged by residual labeled apo A-I 24 hours after injection of ^{125}I tyramine cellobiose, consistent with our kinetic data (Table 4). There was, however, no difference in catabolism of apo A-I by either the liver or the kidney between the two groups, suggesting that reduced catabolism of apo A-I by organs other than kidney or liver are responsible for the reduction in the fractional apo A-I catabolic rate in analbuminemic rats, as we have shown for nephrotic animals[17] (Table 4).

Table 3. The Effect of Ficoll or Human Albumin Infusion on Plasma Apo A-I Level in Normal Rats and in Rats With Heymann Nephritis

Group	Apo A-I (mg/dL)	Chol (mmol/L)	π (mm Hg)	Alb (mg/mL)	$U_{alb}V$ (mg/24 hr)	C_{alb} (mL/hr)
HN Sal (n = 5)	127* ± 4	5.8* ± 1.7	11* ± 1	11* ± 1	402 ± 50	2.08 ± 0.35
HN Alb (n = 5)	50.4 ± 11	2.6 ± 1.2	24 ± 0.6	34Σ ± 2	336 ± 76	2.52 ± 0.87
HN Fic (n = 5)	48.1 ± 2.8	2.1 ± 0.1	20 ± 2	6* ± 2	316 ± 50	3.45 ± 2.27
Con Sal (n = 5)	49.7 ± 1	1.9 ± 0.2	25 ± 1	30 ± 5	NM	NM
Con Alb (n = 5)	48.1 ± 4	1.7 ± 0.1	31* ± 2	46*Σ ± 3	NM	NM
Con Fic (n = 5)	43.1 ± 6	1.6 ± 0.3	29* ± 3	23* ± 4	NM	NM

NOTE. Data are expressed as means ± SD.

Abbreviations: Σ, sum of human + rat albumin; HN Fic or Con Fic, HN or control rats (nonnephrotic) infused with hyperoncotic ficoll; HN Alb or Con Alb, HN or control rats infused with hyperoncotic human albumin; HN Sal or Con Sal, HN or control rats infused with isotonic saline; Chol, plasma cholesterol level; Alb, plasma albumin concentration; $U_{alb}V$, 24-hour urinary albumin excretion on the final day of infusion; C_{alb}, renal clearance of albumin (urinary albumin/plasma albumin/hr), using the mean clearance calculated for the last 3 days of solute infusion in each animal; NM, not measured.

* $P < 0.05$ *v* Con Sal.

Table 4. Sites of Uptake of Apo A-I in Normal and Analbuminemic Rats

Group	Control (n = 6)	NAR (n = 3)
Body weight (g)	251 ± 13	241 ± 5.5
Plasma apo A-I (mg/dL)	77.3 ± 11.8	177 ± 21.8*
Plasma cholesterol (mmol/L)	3.22 ± 0.27	6.43 ± 0.73*
Plasma π (mm Hg)	24.0 ± 0.9	19.0 ± 0.5*
Plasma (%)	12.2 ± 1.6	19.5 ± 2.5*
Kidney (%)	26.0 ± 1.8	21.7 ± 10.2
Urine (%)	3.5 ± 0.4	4.0 ± 1.1
Kidney + urine (%)	29.5 ± 2.2	25.7 ± 10.4
Liver (%)	11.2 ± 0.9	11.2 ± 0.5
Feces (%)	2.9 ± 0.4	1.0 ± 1.3
Gut contents (%)	1.4 ± 0.7	1.2 ± 0.1
Liver + feces + gut contents + large intestine (%)	18.9 ± 1.3	19.5 ± 2.4

NOTE. Data are expressed as means ± SD. Distribution of total ^{125}I recovered from plasma and tissues of normal and analbuminemic rats 20 hours after injection of [^{125}I] HDL reconstituted with apo A-I labeled using tyramine cellobiose. Values represent percent of total counts injected. Plasma cholesterol, apo A-I level, and π (colloid osmotic pressure) were measured 15 minutes after injection and on the terminal blood sample. Values presented for these variables represent an average of these two measurements.

* $P < 0.05$ *v* control.

Plasma π was greatest in normal control animals, was significantly less in all analbuminemic rats studied (Tables 1 and 4), and was lowest in rats with HN (Tables 1 and 3).

DISCUSSION

Plasma cholesterol and apo A-I levels are increased both in the nephrotic syndrome[3,10,11] and NAR,[6,7,12] suggesting that reduced plasma albumin concentration or π is responsible for their increased levels. The observation in nephrotic rats that infusion of either albumin or ficoll are equally effective in reducing apo A-I levels and cholesterol, even though urinary protein losses are unabated and the renal clearance of albumin unchanged, is consistent with a hypothesis that reduced plasma π is necessary for the occurrence of increased levels of apo A-I and that reduced plasma albumin does not play a specific role in affecting plasma apo A-I levels. Proteinuria also clearly plays no obvious role in causing the increase in apo A-I levels, because apo A-I was increased in NAR in the absence of urinary protein loss, and was normalized in nephrotic rats when plasma π was increased to normal, despite prodigious urinary protein losses.

Urinary apo A-I excretion has been long recognized in the nephrotic syndrome. In the current study we found that approximately 10% of total apo A-I removal, by catabolism and direct urinary loss, was by urinary loss. Thus urinary apo A-I losses could potentially lead to a decrease in plasma apo A-I levels in the nephrotic syndrome if these additional losses were not counterbalanced by an increase in apo A-I synthesis or a decrease in apo A-I catabolism elsewhere. Indeed it has been proposed that urinary apo A-I losses are responsible for decreased apo A-I levels in the nephrotic syndrome in patients,[27] although plasma apo A-I levels are not consistently found to be decreased in nephrotic syndrome in humans.[28]

Apo A-I is a 28-kd protein and circulates both bound to HDL and unbound to lipoprotein in plasma. The kidney is a major site of apo A-I catabolism,[17,29,30] being responsible for approximately 30% of total apo A-I removal. Unbound apo A-I is of small enough size (28 kd) to be filtered extensively by the normal glomerulus. Presentation of apo A-I for renal catabolism is normally dependent on the size of its free fraction, because filtration of a 28-kd protein should not be encumbered by the normal glomerulus, whereas HDL particles of >200 kd[9] should be excluded entirely from normal glomerular ultrafiltrate. Although altered permselectivity, as seen here in HN, should vastly increase clearance of HDL-sized particles, the clearance of a 200-kd macromolecule should still remain several orders of magnitude less than that of free apo A-I, a molecule only sightly larger than inulin. By directly measuring renal apo A-I catabolism and urinary apo A-I excretion separately, we found that urinary excretion of intact apo A-I was mirrored by a reciprocal decrease in renal apo A-I catabolism.[17] Thus total renal losses, ie, intact apo A-I and catabolized apo A-I were not increased, suggesting that total filtration of apo A-I was not increased, and that changes in renal apo A-I catabolism may be a consequence of changes in the fraction of filtered apo A-I that is reabsorbed in the kidney and catabolized there.

Our previous studies, however, were carried out in animals with renal injury, and our failure to find increased renal catabolism could also have been a result of the renal lesions.

Decreased apo A-I FCR may be peculiar to the rat with decreased plasma π. In a very limited study, Saku et al[31] reported an increase in Apo A-I FCR in two nephrotic patients. LPL is reduced both in the nephrotic and in the analbuminemic rat[5]; yet apo A-I as well as apo A-I FCR is decreased in both, in contrast to both the human[15] and monkey.[16] Goldberg et al[16] postulated that HDL composition was altered as a consequence of hypertriglyceridemia resulting from LPL inhibition, so that the affinity of apo A-I for HDL was reduced and the free apo A-I pool increased. The increased free apo A-I pool would then lead to increased renal apo A-I catabolism. We have previously shown that renal apo A-I catabolism does not increase in nephrotic rats,[17] and now have shown the same to be true in analbuminemic rats.

One important difference between HDL metabolism in the rat and in primates is the presence of cholesterol ester transfer protein in primates and its absence in the rat.[32] As a result the rat does not transfer the cholesterol ester–laden core of HDL_2 to VLDL and as a consequence the fraction of the smaller HDL_3 is reduced. The affinity of HDL_3 for apo A-I is less than the affinity of HDL_2 for apo A-I.[33] Thus, the absence of cholesterol ester transfer protein in the rat might provide an explanation for the observation that renal apo A-I catabolism is not increased in either nephrotic[17] or analbuminemic rats despite the decrease in LPL in both the nephrotic syndrome[13,14] and in analbuminemia.[5] This is especially important because cholesterol ester transfer protein activity is increased in the nephrotic syndrome in humans,[34] and this increase may play a role in establishing plasma apo A-I levels in patients with the nephrotic syndrome.

Nephrotic syndrome in the rat is accompanied by hepatic hypertrophy[35-37] and in increased levels of mRNAs encoding specific secreted proteins, including albumin,[38,39] fibrinogen,[35,40] and apo A-I.[10,11] Synthesis of all of these proteins is regulated transcriptionally.[10,11,35,38,39] Increased transcription is restricted only to genes encoding a few proteins. Synthesis of nonsecreted proteins is not increased,[40] and transcription of genes encoding other secreted proteins, including apo B and E, is also unaffected,[11] although synthesis of these proteins is increased.[3]

Many of the changes in hepatic gene expression that occur in the nephrotic rat also occur in the liver of NAR,[11,35,41] suggesting that it is not the loss of protein in the urine that directly affects hepatic gene expression. The data presented here suggest, at least with regard to apo A-I, that reduction in plasma π causes increased apo A-I synthesis, most likely acting transcriptionally, although it has not yet been established that increasing plasma π into the normal range reverses increased apo A-I mRNA levels.

HDL levels are increased both as a consequence of increased synthesis and decreased catabolism in rats with the nephrotic syndrome and in rats with hereditary analbuminemia. Increased apo A-I synthesis and decreased apo A-I FCR both then are a consequence of decreased plasma π, or of another physical chemical change in plasma such as increased viscosity,[42] but are not dependent on the presence of urinary protein loss nor are they much influenced by plasma albumin concentration specifically. The rate of apo A-I synthesis in NAR, although significantly greater than in SD, was also significantly less than in nephrotic animals. Plasma π was also intermediate in NAR, falling between SD and nephrotic animals, suggesting that plasma π may quantitatively regulate the rate of apo A-I synthesis in the rat. It is not known how reduced plasma π or the increased viscosity that should also be present under these conditions affects hepatic gene expression, nor is it known by what mechanism apo A-I catabolism is reduced under these circumstances.

ACKNOWLEDGMENT

FX1A antiserum was a gift from Dr William Couser, Seattle, WA.

REFERENCES

1. Earley LE, Farland M: Nephrotic syndrome, in Strauss MB, Welt LG (eds): Diseases of the Kidney (ed 3). pp 765-813 Boston, MA, Little Brown, 1979, pp 765-813

2. Radding CM, Steinberg D: Studies on the synthesis and secretion of serum lipoproteins by rat liver slices. J Clin Invest 39:1560-1569, 1960

3. Marsh JB: Lipoprotein metabolism in experimental nephrosis. J Lipid Res 25:1619-1623, 1984

4. Chan MK, Persaud JW, Ramdial L, Varghese Z, Seveny

P, Moorhead JF: Hyperlipidemia in untreated nephrotic syndrome, increased production or decreased removal? Clin Chim Acta 117:317-323, 1981

5. Davies RW, Staprans I, Hutchison FN, Kaysen GA: Proteinuria, not altered albumin metabolism, affects hyperlipidemia in the nephrotic rat. J Clin Invest 86:600-605, 1990

6. Joles JA, Willekes-Koolschijn N, van Tol A, Geelhoed-Mieras MM, Danse LH, van Garderen E, Kortlandt W, Erkelens DW, Koomans HA: Hyperlipoproteinemia in one-year-old analbuminemic rats. Atherosclerosis 88:35-47, 1991

7. Van Tol A, Jansen EH, Koomans HA, Joles JA: Hyperlipoproteinemia in Nagase analbuminemic rats: Effects of pravastatin on plasma (apo)lipoproteins and lecithin:cholesterol acyltransferase activity. J Lipid Res 32:1719-1728, 1991

8. Baxter JH, Goodman HC, Allen JC: Effects of infusions of serum albumin on serum lipids and lipoproteins in nephrosis. J Clin Invest 40:490-498, 1961

9. Dallinga-Thie GM, Schneÿderberg VLM, van Tol A: Identification and characterization of rat serum lipoprotein subclasses. J Lipid Res 27:1035-1043, 1986

10. Marshall JF, Apostolopoulos JJ, Brack CM, Howlett GJ: Regulation of apolipoprotein gene expression and plasma high-density lipoprotein composition in experimental nephrosis. Biochim Biophys Acta 1042:271-279, 1990

11. Sun X, Jones H Jr, Joles JA, van Tol A, Kaysen GA: Apolipoprotein gene expression in analbuminemic rats and in rats with Heymann nephritis. Am J Physiol 262:F755-F761, 1992

12. Joles JA, Feingold KR, Van Tol A, Cohen LH, Sun X, Jones H Jr, Davies RW, Kaysen GA: Extrahepatic lipogenesis contributes to hyperlipidemia in the analbuminemic rat. Am J Physiol 265):F70-F76, 1993

13. Yamada M, Matsuda I: Lipoprotein lipase in clinical and experimental nephrosis. Clin Chim Acta 30:787-794, 1970

14. Garber DW, Gottlieb BA, Marsh JB, Sparks CE: Catabolism of very low density lipo-proteins in experimental nephrosis. J Clin Invest 74:1375-1383, 1984

15. Brinton EA, Eisenberg S, Breslow JL: Increased Apo A-I and Apo A-II fractional catabolic rate in patients with low high density lipoprotein-cholesterol levels with or without hypertriglyceridemia. J Clin Invest 87:536-544, 1991

16. Goldberg IJ, Blaner WS, Vanni TM, Moukides M, Ramakrishnan R: Role of lipoprotein lipase in the regulation of high density lipoprotein apolipoprotein metabolism. J Clin Invest 86:463-473, 1990

17. Kaysen GA, Hoye E, Jones H Jr: Apolipoprotein A-I levels are increased in part as a consequence of reduced catabolism in nephrotic rats. Am J Physiol 268:F532-F540, 1995

18. Kaysen GA, Kirkpatrick WG, Couser WG: Albumin homeostasis in the nephrotic rat: Nutritional considerations. Am J Physiol 247:F192-F202, 1984

19. Kaysen GA, Schoenfeld PY: Albumin homeostasis in patients undergoing continuous ambulatory peritoneal dialysis. Kidney Int 25:107-114, 1984

20. Riegelman S, Collier P: The application of statistical moment theory to the evaluation of in vivo dissolution time and adsorption time. J Pharmacokinet Biopharm 8:509-534, 1980

21. Al-Bander H, Martin VI, Kaysen GA: Plasma IgG levels are not defended when urinary protein loss occurs. Am J Physiol 262:F333-F337, 1992

22. Glass CK, Pittman RC, Keller GA, Steinberg D: Tissue sites of degradation of apoprotein A-I in the rat. J Biol Chem 258:7161-7167, 1983

23. Dallinga-Thie GM, Groot PHE, van Tol A: Distribution of apolipoprotein A-IV among lipoprotein subclasses in rat serum. J Lipid Res 26:970-976, 1985

24. Chen Y-DI, Sheu WH-H, Swislocki ALM, Reaven GM: High density lipoprotein turnover in patients with hypertension. Hypertension 17:386-393, 1991

25. Lowry OH, Rosebrough NJ, Farr AL, Randall RJ: Protein measurement with the Folin reagent. J Biol Chem 193:265-275, 1951

26. Matthews DE, Farewell W: Using and Understanding Medical Statistics. New York, NY, Karger, 1985.

27. Short CD, Durrington PN, Mallick NP, Hunt LP, Tetlow L, Ishola M: Serum and urinary high density lipoproteins in glomerular disease with proteinuria. Kidney Int 29:1224-1228, 1986

28. Dullaart RP, Gansevoort RT, Dikkeschei BD, de Zeeuw D, de Jong PE, Van Tol A: Role of elevated lecithin: Cholesterol acyltransferase and cholesteryl ester transfer protein activities in abnormal lipoproteins from proteinuric patients. Kidney Int 44:91-7, 1993

29. Glass CK, Pittman RC, Keller GA, Steinberg D: Tissue sites of degradation of apoprotein A-I in the rat. J Biol Chem 258:7161-7167, 1983

30. Van't Hooft FM, van Tol A: The sites of degradation of purified rat low density lipoprotein and high density lipoprotein in the rat. Biochim Biophys Acta 836:344-353, 1985

31. Saku K, Mendoza SG, Laver M, Hynd BA, Gartside PS, Kashyap ML: High-density lipoprotein apolipoprotein A I and A II turnover in moderate and severe proteinuria. Nephron 50:112-115, 1988

32. Oschry Y, Eisenberg S: Rat plasma lipoproteins: Re-evaluation of a lipoprotein system in an animal devoid of cholesteryl ester transfer activity. J Lipid Res 23:1099-1106, 1982

33. Tall AR: Plasma high density lipoproteins: Metabolism and relationship to atherogenesis. J Clin Invest 86:379-384, 1990

34. Moulin P, Appel GB, Ginsberg HN, Tall AR: Increased concentration of plasma cholesteryl ester transfer protein in nephrotic syndrome: Role in dyslipidemia. J Lipid Res 33:1817-1822, 1992

35. Sun X, Martin V, Weiss RH, Kaysen GA: Selective transcriptional augmentation of hepatic gene expression in the rat with Heymann nephritis. Am J Physiol 264:F441-F447, 1993

36. Goldberg ACRK, Oliveira HCF, Quintao ECR, McNamara DJ: Increased hepatic cholesterol production due to liver hypertrophy in rat experimental nephrosis. Biochim Biophys Acta 710:71-75, 1982

37. Marsh JB, Drabkin DL: Experimental reconstruction

of metabolic pattern of lipid nephrosis: Key role of hepatic protein synthesis in hyperlipemia. Metabolism 9:946-955, 1960

38. Yamauchi A, Imai E, Noguchi T, Tanaka T, Yamamoto S, Mikami H, Fukuhara Y, Fujii M, Orita Y, Kamada T: Albumin gene transcription is enhanced in liver of nephrotic rats. Am J Physiol 254:E676-E679, 1988

39. Kaysen GA, Jones H Jr, Martin V, Hutchison FN: A low protein diet restricts albumin synthesis in nephrotic rats. J Clin Invest 83:1623-1629, 1989

40. Lewandowski AE, Liao WSL, Stinson-Fisher CA, Kent JD, Jefferson LS: Effects of experimentally induced nephrosis on protein synthesis in rat liver. Am J Physiol 254:C634-C642, 1988

41. Esumi H, Sato S, Okui M, Sugimura T, Nagase S: Turnover of serum proteins in rats with analbuminemia. Biochem Biophys Res Commun 87:1191-1199, 1979

42. McGinley E, Lowe GDO, Boulton-Jones M, Forbes CD, Prentice CRM: Blood viscosity and haemostasis in the nephrotic syndrome. Thromb Haemost 49:155-157, 1983

The Nephrotic Syndrome, Lipids, and Risk Factors for Cardiovascular Disease

J. Radhakrishnan, MD, A.S. Appel, PhD, A. Valeri, MD, and Gerald B. Appel, MD

● The hyperlipidemia associated with the nephrotic syndrome is well characterized. There is, however, a paucity of data in humans on the risk factors for atherosclerotic heart disease and the role of hyperlipidemia on the risk of progression of renal disease in this population. In our study, we retrospectively evaluated a large uniform population of patients (mean creatinine, 1.78 mg/dL; mean 24-hour proteinuria, 7.1 g) with idiopathic nephrotic syndrome for the presence of risk factors for coronary artery disease. One hundred patients with either focal segmental glomerulosclerosis (n = 56) or membranous nephropathy (n = 44) were assessed for the following cardiovascular risk factors: male sex or postmenopausal female, hyperlipidemia, hypertension, smoking history, and left ventricular hypertrophy. Sixty-six percent of the patients were either male or postmenopausal females; 35% were smokers. Hypertension and left ventricular hypertrophy were present in 53% and 13% of patients, respectively. Eighty-seven percent, 53%, and 25% of patients had a total cholesterol of more than 200 mg/dL, more than 300 mg/dL, and more than 400 mg/dL, respectively. Low-density lipoprotein cholesterol was greater than 130 mg/dL and greater than 160 mg/dL in 77.2% and 64.9% of patients, respectively. Virtually all patients (99%) had at least one risk factor for cardiovascular disease; over two thirds (68%) had two risk factors and over one quarter (26%) had three risk factors. In comparing the group that progressed to renal failure with the groups that did not, the initial mean serum cholesterol was lower in the group that progressed (292 mg/dL *v* 388 mg/dL, $P < 0.01$). There was no difference in the cholesterol to high-density lipoprotein ratio, 24-hour protein excretion, or presence of hypertension between the two groups. In analyzing the group that went into remission from the nephrotic syndrome, patients who remitted had a lower serum creatinine at presentation (1.21 mg/dL *v* 1.64 mg/dL, $P < 0.02$). However, there was no statistical difference between the two groups when serum cholesterol, cholesterol to high-density lipoprotein ratio, presence of hypertension, and 24-hour urine protein levels were compared. Thus, this nephrotic population had a high prevalence of risk factors for coronary artery disease. Many patients had multiple risk factors. An elevated cholesterol level at onset did not predict progression to renal failure. The patients who experienced a remission of the nephrotic syndrome had lower serum creatinine levels at onset as compared with those that remained nephrotic.

INDEX WORDS: Hyperlipidemia; nephrotic; cardiovascular risk.

THE PROTEINURIA of the nephrotic syndrome is typically associated with edema, hypoproteinemia, and hyperlipidemia.[1] In recent years the pattern of lipoprotein abnormalities in the nephrotic syndrome has been clarified, and there has been considerable progress in understanding the potential pathogenesis of these lipid abnormalities.[1-5] We recently investigated the role of cholesteryl ester transfer protein (CETP) in the pathogenesis of the characteristic lipid patterns seen in the nephrotic syndrome.[6] Clinically, two major concerns of nephrologists dealing with hyperlipidemic nephrotic patients are the risk of atherosclerotic complications and the risk of enhanced progression of the renal disease.[4] In animal models considerable data have accumulated on the role of hyperlipidemia in promoting the progression of renal disease.[7] In humans there is only scanty information on this important area.[8,9] Moreover, there are still little data regarding the overriding question of the risk for atherosclerotic complications to individual nephrotic patients. Indeed, while there are many studies dealing with risk factors for atherosclerotic complications in the general population, in uremic patients, in patients on hemodialysis and peritoneal dialysis, and after renal transplantation, there are no similar studies in the nephrotic population.[10-22] In this paper we have evaluated a large, uniform nephrotic population for the presence of the most common risk factors for atherosclerotic complications.

Supported in part by National Institutes of Health Grant No. RR00645.

LIPOPROTEIN PATTERNS IN THE NEPHROTIC SYNDROME

Virtually all studies of patients with the nephrotic syndrome have found high levels of total serum cholesterol. Moreover, the majority of studies have found elevated levels of low-density lipoprotein (LDL) cholesterol.[4] Very low-density lipoprotein (VLDL) cholesterol has often been elevated in those patients with the lowest serum albumin concentrations. Recently, we and others have documented the abnormal composition of the lipoprotein components in patients with the nephrotic syndrome.[6] There has been greater controversy over the levels of high-density lipoprotein (HDL) cholesterol in patients with the nephrotic syndrome. While some studies have found high levels, the majority have found normal or low levels.[2,3] In our initial study of lipids in the nephrotic syndrome we found elevated levels of total, LDL, and VLDL cholesterol in most patients.[3] High-density lipoprotein cholesterol was elevated in only one of 20 patients; moreover, HDL cholesterol was low in six of the 20 patients studied. A subsequent study found that children with minimal-change pattern nephrotic syndrome had higher levels of HDL cholesterol than we had reported.[23] In an adult population of patients with minimal-change nephrotic syndrome we were unable to confirm those results, and we found values for this pattern of nephrotic syndrome similar to those for patients with focal segmental glomerulosclerosis and membranous nephropathy.[2] Regardless, the pattern of lipid abnormalities is clearly of less concern in patients with minimal-change nephrotic syndrome who are likely to undergo remission and who are therefore not at long-term cardiovascular risk from hyperlipidemia. We have now analyzed the data from a population of 100 patients with either focal glomerulosclerosis or membranous nephropathy who may indeed be at long-term risk for atherosclerotic complications.

MECHANISM OF HYPERLIPIDEMIA IN THE NEPHROTIC SYNDROME

The precise mechanism(s) involved in the hyperlipidemia of the nephrotic syndrome are clearly complex.[3-5] There is considerable support for a major role of increased lipid-lipoprotein synthesis by the liver. This includes animal data showing (1) isolated perfused livers from nephrotic animals produce more lipoproteins and lipids than do controls, (2) liver slices and homogenates from nephrotic animals secrete a greater quantity of lipoproteins, and (3) increased activity of rate-limiting enzymes such as hydroxy-methylglutaryl CoA reductase. Studies on humans of lipid kinetics have also documented increased synthesis of lipoproteins, and turnover studies with labeled glycerol and mevalonate have documented increased synthesis of triglycerides and cholesterol. The signal to the liver for increased lipoprotein synthesis has been debated, but probably involves the sensing of decreased plasma oncotic pressure perhaps influenced by the loss of urinary regulatory substances.[4] A role for impaired clearance of circulating lipoproteins due to impaired lipoprotein lipase or lecithin cholesterol acyltransferase activity, and urinary loss of HDL cholesterol have also been implicated as influencing lipid abnormalities in the nephrotic syndrome.

We recently documented an abnormality of CETP in nephrotic patients.[6] Cholesteryl ester transfer protein is a glycoprotein synthesized in the liver that influences the distribution and levels of cholesteryl esters among plasma lipoproteins. It mediates the transfer of cholesteryl esters from HDL into apolipoprotein B-containing lipoproteins. Patients with the nephrotic syndrome have higher levels of cholesteryl esters and free cholesterol in VLDL and LDL fractions than do control populations.[6] Patients with genetic deficiencies of CETP have increased HDL cholesteryl esters and depleted cholesteryl esters in their other lipoprotein fractions. In a group of 21 consecutive patients with the nephrotic syndrome we found increased concentrations of plasma CETP compared with an age- and sex-matched control population (3.6 mg/L *v* 2.3 mg/L, $P < 0.001$). This was positively correlated with the cholesteryl ester concentration in VLDL ($r = +0.69$, $P = 0.004$) and with plasma apolipoprotein B concentration ($r = +0.68$, $P = 0.007$). Of interest, those patients receiving corticosteroid therapy, but who were still nephrotic had normalization of plasma CETP levels and of the cholesteryl ester to triglyceride ratio in VLDL. In hypertriglyceridemic nephrotic patients there was an inverse correlation between plasma CETP and HDL cholesterol. Thus, the high levels of CETP found in the nephrotic syndrome may play a role in the enrichment of VLDL and, hence, LDL with cholesteryl esters while decreasing the HDL cholesterol levels.[6]

THE RISK OF ATHEROSCLEROTIC CARDIOVASCULAR DISEASE

Over the years a number of studies have tried to define the risk of cardiovascular disease in patients with the nephrotic syndrome.[4] At least seven studies have examined the course of nephrotic patients and the incidence of ischemic cardiovascular events.[24-30] These have produced conflicting results. Many studies were flawed by small sample size and the inclusion of patients with minimal-change nephrotic syndrome who experienced a remission of the nephrotic syndrome, as well as diabetics and other patients with unique risk factors. The only histologic study of the coronary arteries of patients with the nephrotic syndrome concluded that they exhibited greater coronary luminal narrowing than did age- and sex-matched controls.[31] The study did not, however, control for the fact that some of the nephrotic patients had diabetes or systemic lupus, diseases known to be associated with vascular lesions. Nor did this study control for steroid use, hypertension, or the presence of renal failure. A recent abstract concluded that in 157 nondiabetic nephrotic patients over a greater than 5-year follow-up period, the relative risk of death from coronary artery disease compared with a control population was 5.5, the risk of myocardial infarct was 5.3, and the risk of all coronary artery disease was 2.5.[30]

In the general population without renal disease the risk of ischemic heart disease has been shown to be related to a number of risk factors,[10] including the presence of hypertension, hyperlipidemia (hypercholesterolemia, a high LDL cholesterol, and a low HDL cholesterol), glucose intolerance, smoking, a positive family history for atherosclerotic cardiovascular disease (ASCVD), and left ventricular hypertrophy. The risk of ischemic heart disease increases markedly as a patient develops a greater number of risk factors. The dialysis and renal transplant populations have been extensively studied for the presence of these risk factors and their contribution to ischemic heart disease.[13-22] Similar studies have not been performed to evaluate these data in the nephrotic population. Moreover, no study has examined the cardiovascular risk factors in the nephrotic population at highest risk for cardiovascular complications, those patients in whom a remission of proteinuria is less likely and in whom a prolonged course of hyperlipidemia and renal disease may be expected.

PATIENTS AND METHODS

To elucidate the cardiovascular risk profile of such nephrotic patients we analyzed the data from 100 adult nephrotic patients with either focal segmental glomerulosclerosis (N = 56) or membranous nephropathy (N = 44) chosen from the office files of the Columbia-Presbyterian Renal Group. These patients represent all the patients with these diagnoses actively followed by the senior author as well as a small additional group actively followed by colleagues. It was felt that these patients were representative of the most common patterns of adult idiopathic nephrotic syndrome who are at long-term risk from their hyperlipidemia and other cardiovascular risk factors. We retrospectively reviewed the records of these patients at the time of their presentation to Columbia Presbyterian Medical Center or at the time of renal biopsy by our group for the following risk factors for atherosclerotic heart disease: male sex or postmenopausal female, hyperlipidemia (vide infra), hypertension, smoking history, and left ventricular hypertrophy. Four of the patients had concurrent glucose intolerance, but no patient with diabetic retinopathy or biopsy evidence of diabetic nephropathy was included. Full data on lipid profiles were not available on all patients; hence, data are reported on the percentage tested. Family history for atherosclerotic heart disease could not be adequately assessed from the records and therefore was not analyzed. Because of inaccuracies in the history it was felt that it was reasonable to arbitrarily consider all women older than 48 years to be in the postmenopausal range. This is clearly a conservative estimate since some patients with renal disease will have an early menopause.

The prevalence of hyperlipidemia was analyzed at various cut-off levels, including a total serum cholesterol greater than 200 mg/dL, greater than 300 mg/dL, or greater than 400 mg/dL. The prevalence of an elevated LDL cholesterol was determined at levels greater than 130 mg/dL or 160 mg/dL. The prevalence of an elevated total cholesterol to HDL cholesterol ratio was determined at values greater than 6.5, greater than 10, or greater than 15. Hypertension was defined as a diastolic blood pressure greater than 90 mm Hg or the requirement for antihypertensive medications. Smoking history was considered positive in patients who currently smoked cigarettes or who had given up smoking cigarettes less than 5 years prior to presentation. Left ventricular hypertrophy was judged from its presence on electrocardiograms since echocardiograms were not routinely done in this population. Statistical analysis was performed using the *t*-test or Chi-square analysis as appropriate.

RESULTS

Of the entire group of 100 nephrotic patients 55% were male and 45% were female (Table 1). The mean age was 42.1 years (range, 15 to 82 years). The mean serum creatinine was 1.78 mg/dL. The mean 24-hour urinary protein excretion was 7.1 g/d. The values for those subpopulations with membranous and focal sclerosis are also shown in Table 1.

Lipid profiles are depicted in Figs 1 through 4. The majority of patients had elevated serum total cholesterol greater than 200 mg/dL (87%) and LDL cholesterol greater than 130 mg/dL (77.2%) (Figs 1 and 2). The mean total choles-

Table 1. Population Characteristics

	No. of Patients	No. of Males (%)	No. of Females (%)	Mean Age (yr)	Creatinine (mg/dL)	24-hr Protein (g/d)
Membranous	44	26 (59)	18 (41)	45.9	1.5	7.4
FSGS	56	29 (52)	27 (48)	39.1	2.0	6.9
Total	100	55 (55)	45 (45)	42.1	1.78	7.1

Abbreviation: FSGS, focal segmental glomerulosclerosis.

terol to HDL cholesterol ratio was 7.8 (Fig 3). Plasma triglycerides were greater than 200 mg/dL in 71% and greater than 300 mg/dL in 33% of the patients (Fig 4). Of the entire group 66% of the patients were either male or postmenopausal females. Thirty-five percent of the patients had a positive smoking history. Hypertension was present in 53% and left ventricular hypertrophy was documented in 13% (Fig 5).

Since the risk of atherosclerotic coronary vascular disease is increased not only by each risk factor but by the concurrent number of multiple risk factors, we analyzed the population for the number of patients with either hypercholesterolemia (cholesterol >200 mg/dL), smoking history, the presence of hypertension, or left ventricular hypertrophy. Of the membranous patients 100% had at least one risk factor for atherosclerotic heart disease; 72% had two risk factors and 33% had three risk factors. When the group of patients with focal sclerosis was analyzed, 98%, 65%, and 21% of the patients had one, two, and three risk factors, respectively. For the entire nephrotic population, 98.8%, 68%, and 26% of patients had one, two, and three risk factors, respectively.

In this retrospective analysis we had available the final outcome of many of the patients. Thirty-four percent of the membranous patients and 44% of the focal sclerosis patients progressed to end-stage renal disease (ESRD) (defined by a serum creatinine >6 mg/dL or the need for dialysis or transplantation). For the membranous group the mean length of follow-up was 4.3 years for those who progressed to ESRD and 4.7 years for those who did not (P = NS). For the group with focal sclerosis the mean length of follow-up was 4.1 years for the group that progressed to ESRD and 3.8 years for the group that did not (P = NS). The mean cholesterol at presentation of those patients who progressed to ESRD (292 mg/dL) was significantly lower than that of those patients who did not progress to ESRD (388 mg/dL, $P < 0.01$) (Fig 6). The mean creatinine at presentation of those patients who progressed to ESRD (1.96 mg/dL) was significantly higher than that of those patients who did not (1.29 mg/dL, $P < 0.02$). There was no significant correla-

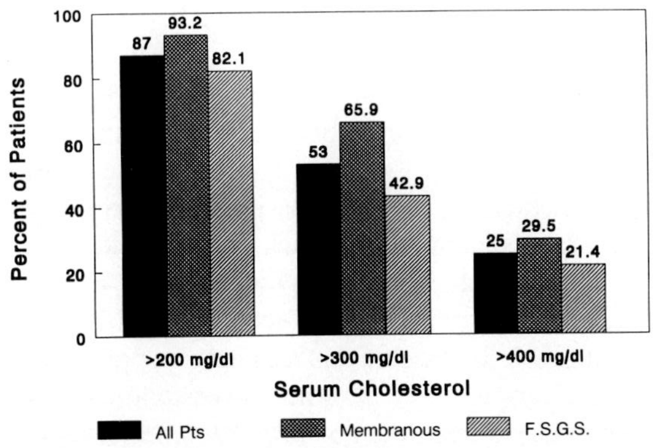

Fig 1. Cardiovascular risk factors in nephrotic patients: total cholesterol levels.

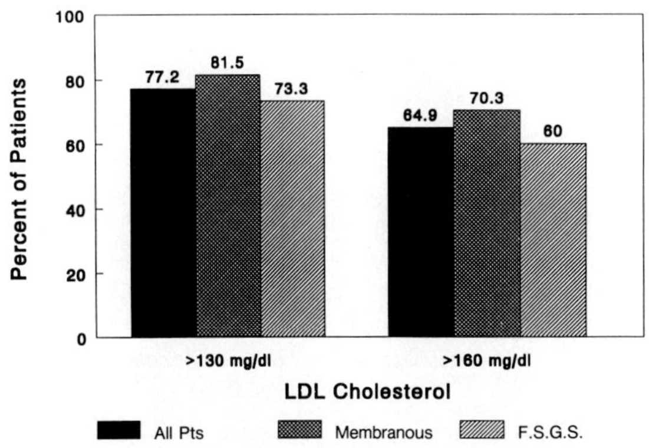

Fig 2. Cardiovascular risk factors in nephrotic patients: LDL cholesterol levels.

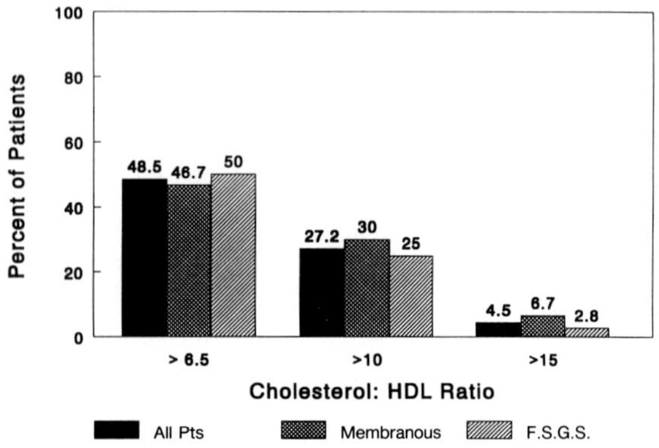

Fig 3. Cardiovascular risk factors in nephrotic patients: cholesterol to HDL ratio.

tion of the cholesterol to HDL cholesterol ratio, the 24-hour proteinuria, or the presence of hypertension with progression to ESRD. Total serum cholesterol, cholesterol to HDL cholesterol ratio, hypertension, and 24-hour proteinuria at baseline evaluation did not predict remission of proteinuria. However, those patients who remitted had a lower serum creatinine at presentation (1.21 mg/dL) than those who did not have a remission of proteinuria (1.64 mg/dL, $P < 0.02$). We could not accurately determine adverse cardiovascular events and evidence for ischemic heart disease and its relationship to the risk factors for cardiovascular disease in this population (vide infra).

DISCUSSION

Hyperlipidemia is an integral part of the full nephrotic syndrome. There is considerable con-

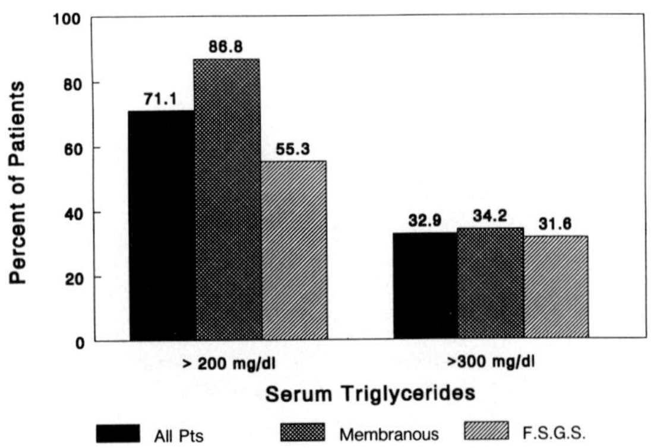

Fig 4. Cardiovascular risk factors in nephrotic patients: triglyceride levels.

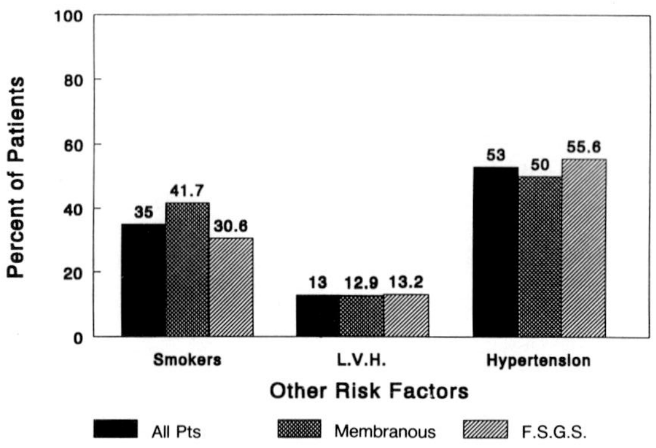

Fig 5. Cardiovascular risk factors in nephrotic patients: other risk factors.

cern that the lipid abnormalities found in patients with the nephrotic syndrome will lead to a more rapid progression to renal failure and an increased risk of atherosclerotic cardiovascular disease. This risk has not been clearly defined despite a number of retrospective studies and a single histologic study of the coronary arteries in the nephrotic population.[24-31] The variable remission rates of patients with different patterns of the nephrotic syndrome, the long duration of follow-up necessary, and the presence of numerous concurrent risk factors makes such analyses difficult. In the general population, the Framingham study and many others have discovered a number of independent risk factors for cardiovascular disease.[10] The presence of multiple risk factors leads to a compounding of the risk for atherosclerotic heart disease. In renal failure and in dialysis populations these factors have been extensively studied.

A number of studies have documented a high risk for atherosclerotic cardiovascular complications in the dialysis population.[13-21,32] It has been debated whether dialysis itself adds to this cardiovascular mortality. Some investigators have documented that the risk of ischemic heart disease in dialysis populations is similar to that of the Framingham study if risk factors such as hypertension, left ventricular hypertrophy, and hyperlipidemia are taken into account.[14,17] Lipid abnormalities in the dialysis and uremic population are common.[4,15,21,33,34] Some investigators have been able to document a correlation between elevated triglycerides and low HDL cholesterol and the presence of coronary heart disease or de-

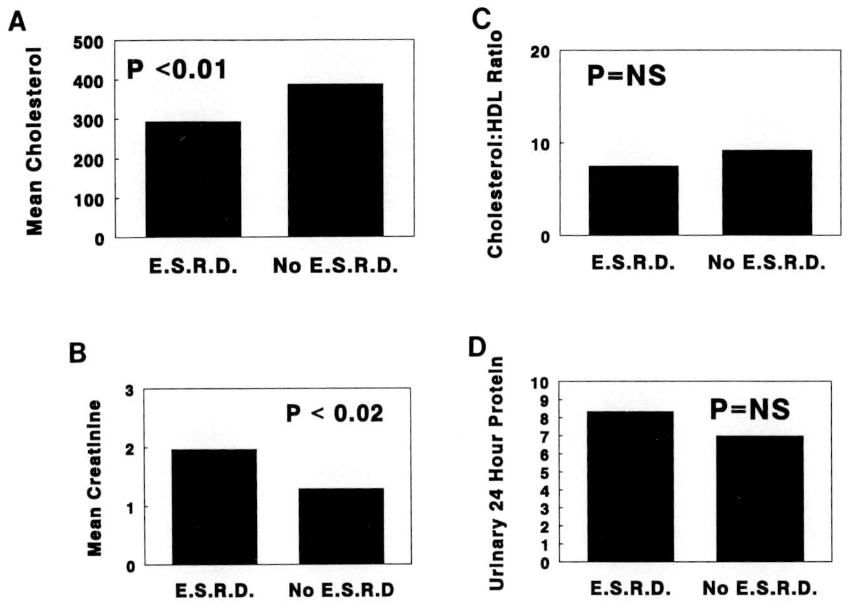

Fig 6. Progression of renal disease. (A) Serum cholesterol, (B) serum creatinine, (C) cholesterol:HDL ratio, (D) urinary 24-hour protein.

creased survival on dialysis.[15,21] In the ESRD population hypertension also has been related to the risk of ischemic heart disease and generalized atherosclerosis.[13,17,18,20,21] Likewise, a number of studies have documented that increased left ventricular mass or left ventricular hypertrophy are common findings in the ESRD population and that survival of patients with left ventricular hypertrophy is lower than in the patients without left ventricular hypertrophy.[35,36] Finally, smoking has been associated with a decreased survival in patients on maintenance dialysis.[21,37] Similar studies have documented these risk factors in patients with hyperlipidemia and other cardiovascular risk factors after renal transplantation.[22,23] Unfortunately, no such studies have been done in the nephrotic population.

In this study we chose to analyze retrospectively the data from 100 patients followed in our center with either focal glomerulosclerosis or membranous nephropathy. These are two of the most common patterns of idiopathic nephrotic syndrome in adults. Unlike minimal change nephrotic syndrome and its variants, such patterns are less likely to have a rapid, spontaneous, or medication-induced remission. Thus, while only a small fraction of the minimal-change nephrotic patients will pose a long-term concern about their hyperlipidemia as a cardiovascular risk factor, clearly a higher percentage of patients we studied will still be at risk from hyperlipidemia at 1, 2, and 5 years after diagnosis. This is true despite recent reports of higher remission rates in membranous and focal sclerosis nephrotic patients treated with more vigorous immunosuppressive regimens.[38-42] Our population was not epidemiologically different from that of other large surveys of patients with these patterns of the nephrotic syndrome.

The lipid analysis of our patients showed that the vast majority had elevated serum cholesterols above the recommended value of 200 mg/dL, and over half had values above 300 mg/dL as well. Low-density lipoprotein cholesterols were significantly elevated in most patients and the total cholesterol to HDL cholesterol ratio was abnormally high in a large number of patients. This confirms our previous work and that of others suggesting that the pattern of hyperlipidemia found in the nephrotic syndrome is typical of that seen in other populations that have been associated with an enhanced risk for atherosclerotic heart disease. We also found that over half this population had hypertension. While this hypertension is probably multifactorial in origin, it nevertheless is a well-documented and potent risk factor for progressive cardiovascular disease and for left ventricular hypertrophy. Left ventricular hypertrophy itself could be documented only in a small percentage of our patients, probably as a result of the insensitive technique we had available in this retrospective study. Echocardiography is a far more reliable and sensitive indicator of left ventricular hypertrophy than is electrocardiography.[19,35,36] It is unclear which factors other than hypertension relate to left ventricular hypertrophy in the nephrotic population. In ESRD patients, hypertension, volume overload, advanced age, anemia, and a number of other factors have been associated with left ventricular hypertrophy.[19,35,36] Finally, one third of our patients had a positive history for cigarette smoking, clearly an additive risk factor for cardiovascular complications. Moreover, two thirds of our patients were either male or of age to be postmenopausal. Thus, many of our patients had a number of cardiovascular risk factors potentially enhancing their risk for adverse cardiovascular events.

In analyzing progression to ESRD, an increased serum creatinine at presentation predicted a poor outcome, as has been shown in many other studies of the nephrotic syndrome.[38-41] It is interesting that the group progressing to ESRD actually had a lower mean serum cholesterol at presentation than that of the patients who did not progress to ESRD. We do not believe this negates the argument that hyperlipidemia may lead to accelerated renal failure. First, both groups, those progressing to ESRD and those that did not, had markedly elevated cholesterol levels (mean cholesterol, 292 and 387 mg/dL, respectively). Second, the effects of treatment cannot be judged from this study. It is possible that patients with more marked hyperlipidemia were more likely to receive vigorous antihyperlipidemic medical therapy. Finally, some subgroups of patients may have higher lipid levels and yet be more likely to experience a remission of their nephrotic syndrome and hence be at less risk of progression to renal failure. Regardless, we could not document an adverse effect of the initial serum lipids on the progression to ESRD in a study of this design.

From this retrospective analysis we cannot yet conclude whether nephrotic patients with these risk factors have increased cardiovascular morbidity and mortality. It is extremely difficult to accurately assess the prevalence of atherosclerotic cardiovascular disease in such a retrospective study. Unlike ESRD, which is a definite end point, anginal episodes and ischemic changes on electrocardiograms are more questionable end points. Including only those patients with documented myocardial infarctions may exclude the majority of patients with ischemic heart disease. Moreover, it is likely that appropriate therapy for some risk factors will influence the patient's ultimate risk of cardiovascular disease. Thus, treatment of hypertension should reduce the risk of this feature and also decrease the incidence of left ventricular hypertrophy. Patients may have been instructed to stop smoking, with a decrease in cardiovascular risk after 5 to 10 years of abstinence. Finally, active dietary and medical intervention has been undertaken in our nephrotic patients with hyperlipidemia for a number of years. Clearly, with the current state of knowledge, designing prospective studies with an untreated control group for most of these risk factors would be unethical. Nevertheless, it is clear from data from other populations that these risk factors are synergistic. We have now documented a high-risk profile in many of our adult nephrotic patients with focal sclerosis and membranous nephropathy. We believe that until further data are available, vigorous treatment should be directed at the combined cardiovascular risk profile in this population. Thus, for example, it can be debated whether the normotensive, nonsmoking young female with membranous nephropathy who has a total serum cholesterol of 250 mg/dL and an LDL cholesterol of 160 mg/dL after dietary counseling warrants vigorous intervention with antihyperlipidemic medication. However, the older male nephrotic patient who presents with the same lipid values but who is hypertensive, has left ventricular hypertrophy, and is a smoker deserves more vigorous treatment of all his risk factors for cardiovascular disease, including his hyperlipidemia.

REFERENCES

1. Cameron JS: The nephrotic syndrome and its complications. Am J Kidney Dis 10:157-171, 1987

2. Appel GB, Valeri A, Appel AS, Blum C: The hyperlipidemia of the nephrotic syndrome. Am J Med 87:5:45N-51N, 1989

3. Appel GB, Blum CB, Chieu S, Kunis CL, Appel AS: The hyperlipidemia of the nephrotic syndrome. N Engl J Med 312:1544-1548, 1985

4. Appel GB: Nephrology forum: Lipid abnormalities in renal disease. Kidney Int 39:169-183, 1991

5. Kaysen GA: Hyperlipidemia of the nephrotic syndrome. Kidney Int 39:S41-48, 1991

6. Appel GB, Moulin P, Tall AR, Cernese-Klein E: In-

crease of plasma cholesteryl transfer ester protein concentration (CETP) in nephrotic syndrome. J Am Soc Nephrol 2:262, 1991 (abstr)

7. Keane WF, Mulcahy WAS, Kasiske BL, Kim Y, O'Donnell MP: Hyperlipidemia and progressive renal disease. Kidney Int 39:S41-48, 1991

8. Rabelink AJ, Hene RJ, Erkelens DW, Joles JA, Koomans HA: Partial remission of the nephrotic syndrome in patients on long-term simvastatin. Lancet 335:1045-1046, 1990

9. Maschio G, Oldrizzi L, Rugiu C, Loschiavo C: Serum lipids in patients with chronic renal failure on long-term protein-restrictive diets. Am J Med 87:51N-54N, 1989

10. Kannel WB: CHD risk factors. A Framingham study update. Hosp Pract 25:119-130, 1990

11. Levy D, Garrison RJ, Savage DD, Kannel WB, Castelli WP: Left ventricular mass predicts coronary disease events independent of standard risk factors. Circulation 76, Pt 2:IV-435, 1987 (abstr)

12. Aronow WS, Koenigsberg M, Schurtz KS: Usefullness of echocardiographic left ventricular hypertrophy in predicting new coronary events and atherembolic brain infarction. Am J Cardiol 61:1130-1132, 1988

13. Ibels LS, Stewart JH, Mahoney JF, Neale FC, Sheil AGR: Occlusive arterial disease in uremic and hemodialysis patients and renal transplant recipients. Q J Med 44:197-214, 1977

14. Rostand SG, Gretes JC, Kirk KA, Rutsky EA, Andreoli TE: Ischemic heart disease in patients with uremia undergoing maintenance hemodialysis. Kidney Int 16:600-611, 1979

15. Hahn R, Oette K, Mondorf H, Finke K, Sieberth HG: Analysis of cardiovascular risk factors in chronic hemodialysis patients with special attention to the hyperlipoproteinemia. Atherosclerosis 48:279-288, 1983

16. Burke JF, Francos GC, Moore LL, Cho SY, Lasker N: Accelerated atherosclerosis in chronic dialysis patients—Another look. Nephron 21:181-185, 1978

17. Rostand SG, Kirk KA, Rutsky EA: Relationship of coronary risk factors to hemodialysis-associated ischemic heart disease. Kidney Int 22:304-308, 1982

18. Vincenti F, Amend WJ, Abele J, Feduska NJ, Salvatierra O, Jr: The role of hypertension in hemodialysis-associated atherosclerosis. Am J Med 68:363-369, 1980

19. Harnett JD, Parfrey PS, Griffiths SM, Gault MH, Gutmann RD: Left ventricular hypertrophy in end stage renal disease. Nephron 48:107-115, 1988

20. Ikran H, Lynn L, Bailey RR, Little PJ: Cardiovascular changes in chronic hemodialysis patients. Kidney Int 24:371-376, 1983

21. Haire HM, Sherrard DJ, Scardapane D, Curtis FK, Brunzell JD: Smoking, hypertension and mortality in a maintenance dialysis population. Cardiovasc Med 3:1163-1168, 1978

22. Vatsala A, Weinberg RB, Schoenberg L, Grevel J, Goldstein RH, Van Buran CT, Lewis RM, Kahan BD: Lipid abnormalities in cyclosporine-prednisone treated renal transplant recipients. Transplantation 48:37-43, 1989

23. Zilleruelo G, Hsia SL, Freundlich M, Gorman KM, Strause J: Persistence of serum lipid abnormalities in children with idiopathic nephrotic syndrome. J Pediatr 104:61-64, 1984

24. Wass VJ, Jarrett RJ, Chilvers C, Cameron JJ: Does the nephrotic syndrome increase the risk of cardiovascular disease? Lancet 2:664-667, 1979

25. Gilboa N: Incidence of coronary heart disease associated with nephrotic syndrome. Med J Aust 1:207-208, 1976

26. Alexander JH, Schapel GJ, Edwards KDG: Increased incidence of coronary heart disease associated with combined elevations of serum triglycerides and cholesterol in the nephrotic syndrome in man. Med J Aust 2:119-122, 1974

27. Hopper J, Ryan P, Lee JC, Rosenman W: Lipid nephrosis in 31 adult patients. Medicine 49:321-341, 1970

28. Vosnides G, Cameron JS: Hyperlipidemia in renal disease. Med J Aust 2:855, 1974

29. Berlyne GM, Mallick NP: Ischemic heart disease as a complication of the nephrotic syndrome. Lancet 2:399-400, 1969

30. Ordonez JD, Hiatt R, Killebrew E, Fireman B: The risk of coronary artery disease among patients with the nephrotic syndrome. Kidney Int 37:243, 1990 (abstr)

31. Curry RC, Roberts WC: Status of the coronary arteries in the nephrotic syndrome. Am J Med 63:183-192, 1977

32. Lindner A, Charra B, Sherrard D, Scribner BM: Accelerated atherosclerosis in prolonged maintenance hemodialysis. N Engl J Med 290:697-701, 1974

33. Attman PO, Alaupovic P: Lipid abnormalities in chronic renal insufficiency. Kidney Int 38:S16-24, 1991

34. Avram MM, Fein PA, Antignani A, Mittman N, Mushnick RA, Lustig AR, Lapuz MH, Goldwasser P: Cholesterol and lipid disturbances in renal disease: The natural history of uremic dyslipidemia and the impact of hemodialysis and CAPD. Am J Med 85:55N-60N, 1989

35. Silberberg JS, Barre PE, Prichard SS, Sniderman AP: Impact of left ventricular hypertrophy on survival in end stage renal disease. Kidney Int 36:286-290, 1989

36. Parfrey PS, Harnett JD, Griffiths SM, Taylor R, Hand J, King A, Barre PE: The clinical course of left ventricular hypertrophy in dialysis patients. Nephron 55:114-120, 1990

37. Rostand SG, Kirk KA, Rutsky EA: Dialysis-associated ischemic heart disease: Insights from coronary angiography. Kidney Int 25:653-659, 1984

38. Ponticelli C, Zucchelli P, Passerini P, Cesana B: Methylprednisolone plus chlorambucil as compared with methylprednisolone alone for the treatment of idiopathic membranous nephropathy. N Engl J Med 327:599-604, 1992

39. Banfi G, Moriggi M, Sabadini E, Fellin G, D'Amico G, Ponticelli C: The impact of prolonged immunosuppression on the outcome of idiopathic focal-segmental glomerulonephritis with nephrotic syndrome in adults. Clin Nephrol 36:53-59, 1991

40. Jindal K, West M, Bear, Goldstein M: Long-term benefits of therapy with cyclophosphomide and prednisone in patients with membranous glomerulonephritis and impaired renal function. Am J Kidney Dis 19:61-67, 1992

41. Bruns FJ, Adler S, Fraley DS, Segel DP: Sustained remission of membranous glomerulonephritis after cyclophosphamide and prednisone. Ann Intern Med 114:725-730, 1991

42. Mendoza SA, Reznik VM, Griswold WR, Krensky AM, Yorgin PD, Tune BM: Treatment of steroid-resistant focal segmental glomerulonephritis with pulse methylprednisolone and alkylating agents. Pediatr Nephrol 4:303-307, 1990

Treatment of Hyperlipidemia in the Nephrotic Syndrome: The Effects of Pravastatin Therapy

Samuel Spitalewitz, MD, Jerome G. Porush, MD, Daniel Cattran, MD, and Noel Wright, MD

● The hyperlipidemia of the nephrotic syndrome is characterized by an elevation of total cholesterol (TC) and low-density lipoprotein cholesterol (LDLC), with a normal or low high-density lipoprotein cholesterol (HDLC), and an increase in triglycerides (TGs) later in the course of the disease. If sustained, this lipid profile probably places these patients at increased risk for cardiovascular disease. Despite extensive trials of diet and drug therapy in patients with primary hyperlipidemias, few such trials exist in patients with the nephrotic syndrome. We conducted a randomized, prospective, double-blind, placebo-controlled trial to investigate the efficacy and safety of pravastatin, the newest cholesterol synthesis inhibitor, in the treatment of the hyperlipidemia of the nephrotic syndrome. After dietary modification was implemented, 13 patients received pravastatin and eight received placebo. All patients were maintained on a low-fat, low-cholesterol diet for the duration of the trial (24 weeks). The dose of pravastatin was increased from the initial 20 mg/d to 40 mg/d at week 10 or 18 if TC remained elevated (>50th percentile). A bile acid sequestrant was added at week 18 if TC remained elevated and if the patient was already receiving the maximal pravastatin dosage. Dietary modification did not significantly change the lipid profile. Pravastatin (20 mg/d) reduced TC by 22% from a baseline of 301 ± 28 mg/dL ($P < 0.05$) and LDLC by 28% from a baseline of 222 ± 28 mg/dL ($P < 0.05$). When used at 40 mg/d (in six patients) no further change in the lipid profile was observed. Pravastatin caused no significant changes in the HDLC fraction (baseline, 44 ± 3 mg/dL) or in TGs (baseline, 221 ± 37 mg/dL). There was, however, a trend for HDLC to increase (8%) and TGs to decrease (19%). Although difficult to evaluate because of poor compliance, bile acid sequestrants (used in six patients) effected no change in the lipid profiles in patients of either group. Placebo baseline TC, LDLC, HDLC and TG values were similar to the pravastatin group and remained unchanged throughout the study. No patient was dropped from the study because of adverse events attributed to the study medication. Renal function and protein excretion were unaffected by pravastatin. Six diabetic patients treated with pravastatin and patients (n = 8) with chronic renal insufficiency (serum creatinine >1.5 mg/dL) had a response to pravastatin similar to that of the other patients. Our results are similar to other studies using 3-hydroxy-3-methylglutaryl-coenzyme A reductase inhibitors and demonstrate the efficacy and safety of pravastatin in the treatment of the hyperlipidemia of the nephrotic syndrome. The lipid profile, however, was not totally normalized even with maximal pravastatin therapy, indicating the need for combination drug therapy. Long-term trials are clearly necessary to determine the long-term safety and efficacy of drug therapy in the treatment of the hyperlipidemia of the nephrotic syndrome and to establish whether the probable risk of atherosclerosis can be reversed and progression of renal insufficiency (suggested to occur in part secondary to the hyperlipdemia per se) slowed.

INDEX WORDS: Hyperlipidemia; nephrotic syndrome; pravastatin.

THE hyperlipidemia of the nephrotic syndrome is characterized by an elevation of total cholesterol (TC) and low density lipoprotein cholesterol (LDLC), with a normal or low high-density lipoprotein cholesterol (HDLC).[1,2] Hypertriglyceridemia may be observed later in the course of the disease.[1] There is little reason to doubt that this lipid profile places patients with prolonged, untreated nephrotic syndrome at higher risk for coronary heart disease, since it clearly does so in the general population.[2-5] In spite of this increased risk and the potential for reversal with treatment,[6-8] there has been a paucity of studies testing the safety and efficacy of both nonpharmacologic and pharmacologic methods of lowering lipids in nephrotic patients.[9] Especially lacking are large, long-term studies of nephrotic diabetic patients who are particularly at risk for accelerated generalized atherosclerosis.[10,11]

Since the introduction of a unique class of cholesterol-lowering drugs, inhibitors of 3-hydroxy-3-methylglutaryl-coenzyme A (HMG-CoA) reductase (the rate-limiting enzyme in the synthesis of cholesterol),[12,13] and because hyperlipidemia per se may contribute to the progression of chronic renal insufficiency,[14-16] there has been renewed interest in treating hyperlipidemia in patients with nephrotic syndrome.[2,9,17] This report describes our experience with the newest HMG-CoA reductase inhibitor, pravastatin,[18-20] in the treatment of hyperlipidemia of nephrotic syndrome due to a variety of renal diseases and summarizes the previous studies of the nonphar-

Supported in part by a grant from Bristol-Myers Squibb Co, Inc.

macologic and pharmacologic therapy of the hyperlipidemia seen in the nephrotic syndrome.

METHODS

Patient Population

Patients between the ages of 18 and 70 years were included in this study if they had nephrotic syndrome (defined for this study as a urinary protein excretion ≥2.0 g/24 hr and a serum albumin of <3.5 g/dL) and the mean of two plasma TC levels (obtained 1 week apart) above the 75th percentile for the US population by age and gender and higher than 220 mg/dL.[21] Excluded from the study were patients with a serum creatinine ≥5.0 mg/dL, poorly controlled diabetes mellitus (fasting glucose >200 mg/dL), taking more than 60 mg of prednisone (or its equivalent) or other immunosuppressive agents, thyroid disease, primary hyperlipidemia, significant liver disease, excessive obesity (>40% above ideal body weight), or excessive ethanol consumption. Patients on thiazide diuretics, beta-adrenergic blockers, and other drugs known to affect blood lipids were included only if the drug and dose had been constant for 8 weeks prior to the study and was expected to be constant throughout the study period.

The protocol was approved by the institutional review boards of the participating institutions and informed consent was obtained from each patient prior to participation.

Study Design

This was a prospective, double-blind, placebo-controlled study with eligible patients randomized 2:1 to receive either pravastatin, administered once daily, or placebo.

All lipid-lowering drugs were withdrawn at least 6 to 12 weeks prior to study. At that time, patients were placed on a low-fat, low-cholesterol diet containing approximately 30% fat and 300 mg/d or less of cholesterol. At 4 weeks prior to randomization, dietary compliance was established by a nutritionist who reviewed a diary kept by the patient that recorded quantities of all foods ingested. Baseline lipids and 24-hour urinary protein excretion and creatinine clearance were determined and repeated at 2- to 4-week intervals throughout the study. Just prior to randomization a history and physical examination were performed as well as a complete blood cell count, Chem-20 (including creatine phosphokinase, to be repeated at 2- to 4-week intervals) thyroid profile, electrocardiogram, chest x-ray, and an ophthalmologic examination (including a slit lamp). Qualifying patients were then randomized to receive either pravastatin 20 mg (one tablet) or placebo, each given once daily. Patients returned at 2- to 4-week intervals for the clinical and laboratory evaluation of the safety and efficacy of therapy. At the 10th week of therapy, a dose change of the study medication was implemented.

If TC at week 8 was higher than the 50th percentile the dose was increased to two tablets per day; if it was between the 25th and 50th percentile there was no dose change; if it was less than the 25th percentile but ≥130 mg/dL there was no dose change, and if it was less than the 25th percentile and less than 130 mg/dL the dose was decreased to half a tablet per day.

At week 18 the regimen was altered again. If the TC at week 16 was higher than the 50th percentile the dose was increased to two tablets or a bile acid-binding resin (20 to 30 g/d) was added if the patient was already taking two tablets per day; if it was between the 25th and 50th percentile there was no dose change; if it was less than the 25th percentile but more than 130 mg/dL there was no dose change, and if it was less than the 25th percentile and ≤130 mg/dL the dose was decreased to half a tablet per day if the patient was taking one tablet.

Liprotein a [Lp(a)] was determined in the first six patients (two on placebo, four on pravastatin) at weeks 2, 8, and 24. Glycosolated hemoglobin ($HgBA_1C$) was determined in the 10 diabetic patients seen at The Brookdale Hospital Medical Center at baseline and at weeks 8, 16, and 24. At completion of the trial, a repeat ophthalmologic examination (including slit lamp) was done, as well as a repeat physical examination and electrocardiogram.

Analytical Methods

Complete blood cell count and blood and urine chemistries were determined by standard autoanalyzer. Total cholesterol and triglycerides (TGs) were determined using standard enzymatic methods. Plasma lipoprotein fractions were measured using Lipid Research Clinics methodology.[22] Lipoprotein (a) was assayed using enzyme-linked immunosorbent assay (Terumo International, Somerset, NJ).

Statistical Analysis

The differences observed after treatment in each group were analyzed with the Wilcoxon signed rank test. The nonparametric Iman-Conover test was used to compare the percentage of changes in the placebo and pravastatin groups.

RESULTS

Patient characteristics are summarized in Tables 1 and 2. Thirteen patients received pravastatin and eight received placebo. Three patients in the pravastatin group did not complete the protocol. One was dropped after week 2 because of poor compliance, one was lost to follow-up after week 12, and another was dropped after week 12 at her own request. Only one patient in the placebo group was dropped (at her own request) after week 16. No patient had to be dropped because of either a clinical or laboratory adverse effect attributed to medication. Four patients reported four separate instances of adverse events (congestive heart failure [CHF], transient ischemic attack [TIA], rash, chest pain) unrelated to the study medication.

The patients ranged in age from 29 to 69 years with a mean age of 55 ± 3 years in the placebo group and 48 ± 4 years in the pravastatin group.

Table 1. Baseline Patient Characteristics: Placebo Group

Patient No.	Age (yr)/Gender	Serum Creatinine (mg/dL)	Creatinine Clearance (mL/min)	Protein Excretion (g/24 hr)	Diagnosis
1.	64/M	3.6	36	2.4	Necrotizing vasculitis
2.	64/M	3.1	34	7.6	Focal glomerulosclerosis
3.	45/F	2.5	—	17.3	Diabetic nephropathy
4.	42/M	1.2	—	2.6	Focal glomerulosclerosis
5.	50/F	5.3	18	11.3	Diabetic nephropathy
6.	57/M	1.3	90	3.4	Diabetic nephropathy
7.	59/M	1.0	140	3.6	Diabetic nephropathy
8.	60/F	0.7	122	3.4	Unknown
Mean ± SEM	55 ± 3	2.3 ± 0.6	73 ± 21	6.5 ± 1.9	

The placebo group was composed of five men and three women; six (75%) were white and two (25%) were black. The pravastatin group comprised seven men and six women; there were six (46%) whites, six (46%) blacks, and one (8%) oriental. There were no renal diagnostic differences between the two treatment groups (Tables 1 and 2). Creatinine clearance was 73 ± 21 mL/min and 62 ± 11 mL/min, the serum creatinine was 2.3 ± 0.6 mg/dL and 1.9 ± 0.2 mg/dL, and the 24-hour protein excretion was 6.5 ± 1.9 g and 5.4 ± 0.6 g in the placebo and pravastatin groups, respectively.

Effect of Therapy on Blood Lipids

Dietary modification had no significant impact on the lipid profile of either group. Figure 1 shows the effect of pravastatin compared with placebo on TC. Through week 24, TC decreased an average of 22% ($P < 0.05$) from a baseline of 301 ± 28 mg/dL compared with no significant change in the placebo group (baseline TC, 281 ± 25 mg/dL). At each time interval, TC was significantly reduced by pravastatin and a significant difference between the two treatment groups was observed (P varied between <0.05 and 0.001). Six of the 13 pravastatin-treated patients required an increase in the dose at 10 weeks to 40 mg/d, which did not reduce TC any further (264 ± 29 mg/dL to 263 ± 37 mg/dL). At week 18, cholestyramine or colestipol (20 to 30 g/d) was added to two of the six patients receiving the maximal pravastatin dose and four of the seven remaining patients on placebo. The addition of

Table 2. Baseline Patient Characteristics: Pravastatin Group

Patient No.	Age (yr)/Gender	Serum Creatinine (mg/dL)	Creatinine Clearance (mL/min)	Protein Excretion (g/24 hr)	Diagnosis
1.	61/F	2.1	23	6.4	Diabetic nephropathy
2.	38/M	0.8	134	8.6	Focal glomerulosclerosis
3.	54/M	0.8	53	4.5	Membranoproliferative glomerulonephritis
4.	30/M	1.9	62	2.7	Diabetic nephropathy
5.	31/M	2.8	—	5.3	IgA nephropathy
6.	45/M	2.1	26	2.8	IgA nephropathy
7.	64/M	2.9	40	4.6	Diabetic nephropathy
8.	59/F	1.9	39	3.9	Diabetic nephropathy
9.	29/F	1.3	67	3.3	Focal glomerulosclerosis
10.	39/F	2.6	42	9.6	Focal glomerulosclerosis
11.	69/F	2.6	30	5.2	Diabetic nephropathy
12.	58/M	1.3	96	5.2	Diabetic nephropathy
13.	51/F	1.4	134	8.6	Focal glomerulosclerosis
Mean ± SEM	48 ± 4	1.9 ± 0.2	62 ± 11	5.4 ± 0.6	

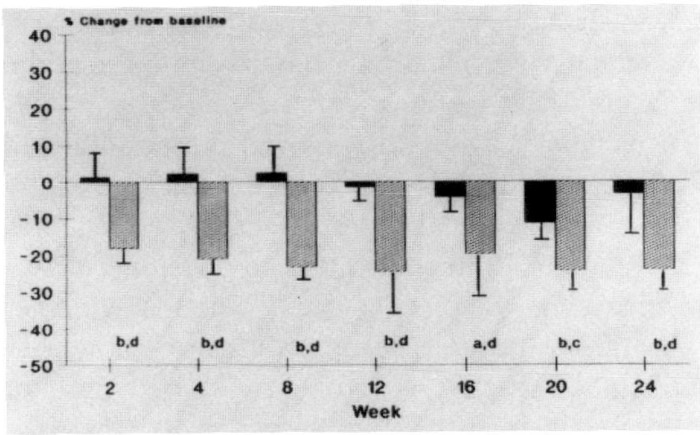

Fig 1. Effects of pravastatin on TC. a, $P < 0.05$ compared with baseline; b, $P < 0.001$ compared with baseline; c, $P < 0.05$ between groups; d, $P < 0.001$ between groups. ■, Control; ▨, pravastatin.

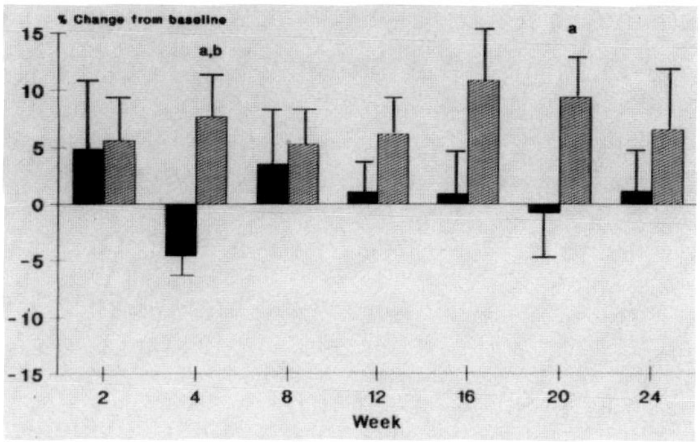

Fig 3. Effects of pravastatin on HDLC. a, $P < 0.05$ compared with baseline; b, $P < 0.001$ between groups. ■, Control; ▨, pravastatin.

the resin did not reduce TC in either group and, as noted, the difference in TC between the two groups was maintained. Since compliance to resin was not specifically checked, the significance of these findings is unclear.

Figure 2 summarizes the effects of pravastatin compared with placebo on LDLC. Through week 24, there was an average decrease in LDLC of 28% ($P < 0.05$) from a baseline of 222 ± 28 mg/dL, while placebo had no significant effect on the baseline LDLC of 208 ± 22 mg/dL. As with TC, the increased dose of pravastatin to 40 mg/d at week 10 did not lower LDLC any further in six patients (179 ± 20 mg/dL to 181 ± 35 mg/dL). The addition of resin did not lower LDLC in either group.

As noted in Fig 3, except for significant increases in HDLC (compared with the baseline of 44 ± 3 mg/dL) in the pravastatin group of 7.7% ± 2.9% at week 4 and 9.4% ± 3.4% at week 20, no other significant changes were noted in this lipid fraction. The baseline HDLC of 43 ± 4 mg/dL in the placebo group remained unchanged. Neither the increased dose of pravastatin nor the addition of resin led to a change in HDLC in either group. Since no consistent change in HDLC was observed while LDLC decreased with pravastatin therapy, the LDLC to HDLC ratio decreased significantly.

The effects of pravastatin and placebo on TG are shown in Fig 4. Baseline TG values were 221 ± 37 mg/dL and 182 ± 31 mg/dL in the pravastatin and placebo groups, respectively. A

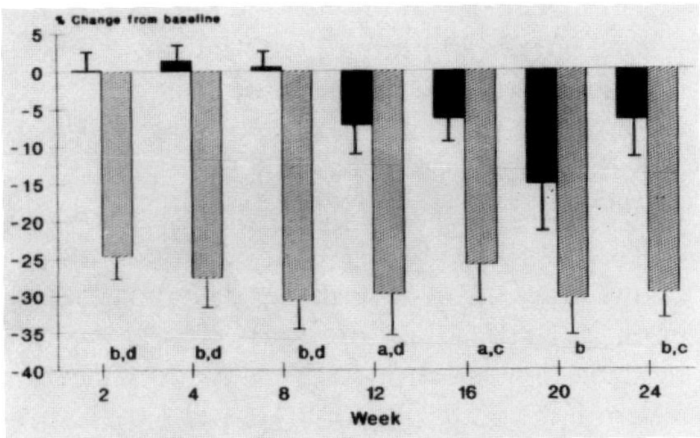

Fig 2. Effects of pravastatin on LDLC. a, $P < 0.05$ compared with baseline; b, $P < 0.001$ compared with baseline; c, $P < 0.05$ between groups; d, $P < 0.001$ between groups. ■, Control; ▨, pravastatin.

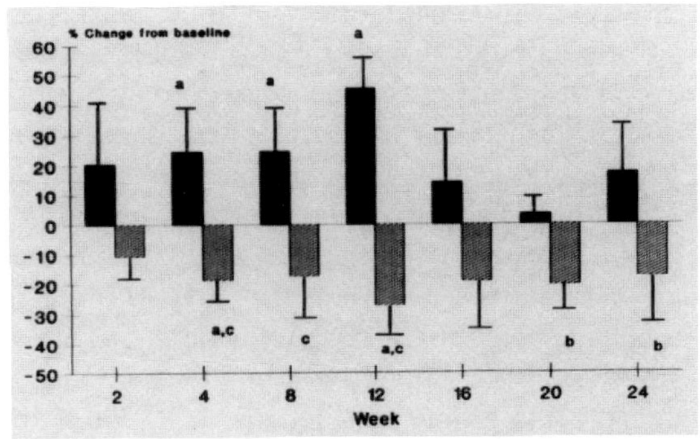

Fig 4. Effect of pravastatin on TGs. a, $P < 0.05$ compared with baseline; b, $P < 0.05$ between groups; c, $P < 0.001$ between groups. ■, Control; ▨, pravastatin.

significant difference was noted between the two groups at all weeks except 2 and 16, with the pravastatin group showing an average reduction of 19%. The addition of resin effected no additional change. As noted in Fig 4, there were significant increases in TG in the control group at weeks 4, 8, and 12.

There was no change in the Lp(a) in the four pravastatin and two placebo patients measured at weeks 2, 8, and 24.

During the 24-week study, serum creatinine, creatinine clearance, and protein excretion did not change significantly in either group, including eight patients in the pravastatin group and four patients in the placebo group with chronic renal insufficiency (serum creatinine, >1.5 mg/dL). Those patients with renal insufficiency responded to pravastatin similarly to those with normal renal function.

When analyzed separately, the response to pravastatin in the six diabetic patients was not different from that of patients with other renal diseases, despite the fact that glucose control, as assessed by fasting blood glucose and $HgbA_1C$, was suboptimal throughout the study (159 ± 12 mg/dL and 8.3% ± 0.3%, respectively). No patient exhibited a significant change in weight, body mass index (kg/m^2), or blood pressure during the study.

DISCUSSION

Although it is well accepted that an increase in TC and its LDL component places patients with primary hyperlipidemia at increased risk for coronary artery disease,[5] some doubt has been expressed whether this lipid profile, characteristic of the nephrotic syndrome, places nephrotic patients at higher risk.[23-25] Others, however, stress the high incidence of coronary artery disease in patients with prolonged, unremitting proteinuria and hyperlipidemia and urge that lipid-lowering therapy be included as part of the treatment.[3,4,26,27] Recent data in experimental animals have suggested that hyperlipidemia may contribute to the development and progression of kidney disease by promoting mesangial damage and glomerulosclerosis.[14-16,28] This process may be reversed with normalization of lipids.[29,30] For these reasons, sustained hyperlipidemia of the nephrotic syndrome should be aggressively treated.

To date, there has only been one study systematically evaluating dietary modification. D'Amico and Gentile[9] demonstrated that a low-fat, vegetarian diet very rich in polyunsaturated fatty acids (unsaturated to saturated ratio, >2) and fiber lowered TC and LDLC by as much as 28% and 33%, respectively, and prompted a 32% decrease in proteinuria in 24 patients with nephrotic syndrome. These investigators, however, concluded that their findings were the result of short-term dietary manipulation (2 months) that necessitated considerable effort and that prolonged compliance might be difficult. Prior to this study, an overall reduction in TC and LDLC of only 6% has been observed with nonsystematic studies of dietary manipulation.[2,31]

The use of bile acid-binding resins recently has been examined by two groups in patients with nephrotic syndrome demonstrating a significant reduction in total cholesterol and in LDLC, with no change in TC or proteinuria in a total of 17 patients studied over 4 to 9 weeks.[32,33] However, there frequently are significant side effects from resins, including constipation, abdominal bloating, and diarrhea, that make compliance difficult and may explain the lack of response to resins in the study described herein.

Nicotinic acid reduces TC, LDLC, and TG and increases HDLC.[17,34,35] There are no reports available on the use of nicotinic acid in the nephrotic syndrome. It may, however, be a poor choice in these patients (particularly in diabetic patients and in patients with renal insufficiency) since it may worsen hyperglycemia and increase serum uric acid.[2,17]

Fibric acids decrease TG and increase HDLC levels, but only minimally inhibit the synthesis of cholesterol.[17,36] Thus, they are of limited usefulness in treating hyperlipidemia in nephrotic patients. Moreover, there is an increase in clofibrate's toxicity in these patients (myopathy), possibly related to an increase in the unbound fraction in serum due to hypoalbuminemia.[37] If used, the dose must be significantly reduced in proportion to the reduction in serum albumin (500 mg of clofibrate per 1.0 g/dL reduction in serum albumin/d). Although gemfibrozil is less toxic than clofibrate it only lowered TC and LDLC minimally in 11 patients studied over 6 weeks.[38]

Table 3. Effects of 3-Hydroxy-3-methylglutaryl-coenzyme A Reductase Inhibitors in Nephrotic Hyperlipidemia

Study	No. of Patients	Drug and Maximum Dose (mg)	Duration (wk)	TC (%)	LDLC (%)	HDLC (%)	TG (%)
Vega and Grundy,[43] 1988	3	Lovastatin (40)	6	−31	−33	+43	−34
Rabelink et al,[33] 1988	10	Simvastatin (40)	6	−36	−39	+21	−39
Golper et al,[44] 1989	10	Lovastatin (80)	18	−33	−45	+1	−25
Kasiske et al,[31] 1990	13	Lovastatin (40)	6	−27	−27	+8	−30
Bazzato et al,[45] 1991	20	Simvastatin (40)	10	−26	−34	+8	−17
Hommel et al,[11] 1992	14	Simvastatin (20)	12	−25	−38	+2	−9
Biesenbach and Zazgornik,[10] 1992	10	Lovastatin (20)	12	−25	−35	+11	−13
Study described herein	13	Pravastatin (40)	24	−22	−28	+7	−19
Prata et al[46]	8	Lovastatin (40)	2 yr	−44	−49		−46
Mean			12	−27	−35	+9	−21

Probucol lowers TC, but also lowers HDLC.[39] This latter unfavorable effect may be offset by probucol-induced inhibition of the oxidation of LDLC, an initial step in the pathogenesis of atherosclerosis.[2,40,41] Two groups of investigators have used probucol to lower cholesterol in 17 nephrotic patients studied over 12 weeks and demonstrated a significant TC-lowering effect.[32,42] Valeri et al[32] noted a 23% reduction in TC and a 24% decrease is LDLC, with HDLC decreasing 12%, but still leading to a decrease in the LDL to HDL ratio. Iida et al[42] showed a similar effect of probucol on TC (30% decrease) and LDLC (25% decrease), but with a more marked decrease in HDLC (25%). Neither group reported any side effects.

HMG-CoA reductase inhibitors are the newest (and most effective) class of lipid-lowering agents that inhibit cholesterol synthesis and enhance the formation of LDL receptors, promoting hepatic clearance of LDL and VLDL.[2,12,13] Their use in patients with hyperlipidemia and the nephrotic syndrome is summarized in Table 3.

Nine studies (including the one described herein) have been carried out.[10,11,31,33,43-46] In most of these studies approximately 10 to 14 patients were given the drug (open label) for 6 to 12 weeks, with the largest study treating 20 patients for 18 weeks.[45] The study we report in this article had a 24-week follow up and is the only one that used a bile-acid resin in combination with an HMG-CoA inhibitor. Our data are consistent with the other investigations; namely, TC and LDLC decreased by an average of 22% and 28%, respectively. Although a trend upward was observed, we did not demonstrate a significant change in HDLC. We included a large proportion of diabetic patients and patients with chronic renal insufficiency in whom the response was similar to other patients. A newer study[46] reports on eight patients with nephrotic syndrome who were administered lovastatin for 2 years. Of the 101 nephrotic patients reported in the literature who received an HMG-CoA inhibitor, therapy was discontinued in only four because of side effects (two had gastrointestinal distress and one had myalgias).[11,31] This class of drug appears to be well tolerated and efficacious in these patients, at least over the short term.

It has been proposed that correction of the hyperlipidemia may decrease proteinuria and/or slow the progression of renal failure.[28,29] The present study, as well as other studies with HMG-CoA reductase inhibitors, did not demonstrate a change in either proteinuria or renal function.

No study has yet demonstrated complete normalization of the lipid profile; therefore, combination therapy needs to be more fully investigated. Groggel et al[38] reported that colestipol added to gemfibrozil further reduced TC from 15% to 41% and TG from 51% to 68%. Long-term tolerance for colestipol and other resins has still not been examined in nephrotic patients. Furthermore, Schapel et al[47] noted that when cholestyramine and clofibrate were used together there was an antagonistic effect, preventing a reduction in TG achieved by either drug alone. Grundy and Vega[2,17] suggest that other combination therapies be tried in nephrotic patients, including bile acid binding resins added to HMG-CoA reductase inhibitors, fibric acids, or nicotinic acid. Probucol can be combined with an HMG-CoA inhibitor, particularly if oxidation of LDLC is a key intermediate step in atherogenesis. The combination of nicotinic acid or a fibric acid with HMG-CoA inhibitor should be avoided because of the risk of severe myopathy.

In summary, we and others have demonstrated the short-term efficacy and safety of HMG-CoA reductase inhibitors in the treatment of nephrotic hyperlipidemia. Additional long-term studies using single and combination drug therapy are needed, however, not only for the demonstration of long-term reversal of the lipid abnormalities in nephrotic syndrome, but also to examine the effects of these agents on proteinuria and renal function. Furthermore, long-term studies are necessary to determine whether the incidence of coronary artery disease is indeed increased in these patients and can be decreased by lowering their serum lipids.

REFERENCES

1. Appel GB, Blum CB, Chien S, Kunis CL, Appel AS: The hyperlipidemia of the nephrotic syndrome: Relation to the plasma albumin concentration, oncotic pressure and viscosity. N Engl J Med 312:1544-1548, 1985

2. Grundy SM: Management of hyperlipidemia of kidney disease. Kidney Int 37:847-853, 1990

3. Mallick NP, Short CD: The nephrotic syndrome and ischemic heart disease. Nephron 27:54-57, 1981

4. Alexander JH, Schapel GJ, Edwards KDG: Increased incidence of coronary heart disease associated with combined elevation of serum triglycerides and cholesterol concentrations in the nephrotic syndrome in man. Med J Aust 2:119-122, 1974

5. The Expert Panel: Report of the National Cholesterol Education Program expert panel on detection, evaluation, and treatment of high blood cholesterol in adults. Arch Intern Med 148:36-69, 1988

6. Blankenhorn DH, Nessim SA, Johnson RL, Sanmarco ME, Azen SP, Cashin-Hemphill LC: Beneficial effects of combined colestipol-niacin therapy on coronary atherosclerosis and coronary venous bypass grafts. JAMA 257:3233-3240, 1987

7. Tyroler HA: Overview of clinical trials of cholesterol lowering in relationship to epidemiologic studies. Am J Med 87:14S-19S, 1989 (suppl 4A)

8. Lipid Research Clinics Program: The lipid research clinics coronary primary prevention trial results. II. The relationship of reduction in incidence of coronary heart disease to cholesterol lowering. JAMA 251:365-374, 1984

9. D'Amico G, Gentile MG: Pharmacological and dietary treatment of lipid abnormalities in nephrotic patients. Kidney Int 39:S65-S69, 1991 (suppl 31)

10. Biesenbach G, Zazgornik J: Lovastatin in the treatment of hypercholesterolemia in nephrotic syndrome due to diabetic nephropathy stage IV-V. Clin Nephrol 37:274-279, 1992

11. Hommel C, Andersen P, Gall MA: Plasma lipoproteins and renal function during simvastatin treatment in diabetic nephropathy. Diabetologia 35:447-451, 1992

12. Mabuchi H, Haba T, Tatami R, Miyamoto S, Sakai Y, Wakasugi T, Watanabe A, Koizumi J, Takeda R: Effects on an inhibitor of 3-hydroxy-3-methylglutaryl coenzyme A reductase on serum lipoproteins and ubiquinone-10 levels in patients with familial hypercholesterolemia. N Engl J Med 305:478-482, 1981

13. Grundy SM: HmG-CoA reductase inhibitors for treatment of hypercholesterolemia. N Engl J Med 319:24-33, 1988

14. Avram MM: Cholesterol and lipids in renal disease. Am J Med 87:1N-2N, 1989 (suppl 5N)

15. Moorhead JF, Wheeler DC, Varghese Z: Glomerular structures and lipids in progressive renal disease. Am J Med 87:12N-20N, 1989 (suppl 5N)

16. Keane WF, Kasiske BL, O'Donnell MP, Schmitz PG: Therapeutic implications of lipid-lowering agents in the progression of renal disease. Am J Med 87:21N-29N, 1989 (suppl 5N)

17. Grundy SM, Vega GL: Rationale and management of hyperlipidemia of the nephrotic syndrome. Am J Med 87:3N-11N, 1989 (suppl 5N)

18. Hunninghake DB, Mellies MJ, Goldberg AC, Kuo PT, Kostis JB, Schrott HO, Insull W Jr, Pan HY: Efficacy and safety of pravastatin in patients with primary hypercholesterolemia. II. Once-daily versus twice-daily dosing. Atherosclerosis 85:219-227, 1990

19. Crepaldi G, Baggio G, Arca M, Avello G, Avogaro P, Bon B, Bompiani GD, Capurso A, Cahin L, D'Alo G, Descovich C, Feruglio FS, Gaddi A, Gnasso A, Liberatore S, Lupatteli G, Mancini M, Miccoli R, Muggeo M, Muntoni S, Navalesi R, Patrizi GF, Pintus F, Quevena M, Resta F, Ricci G, Segato T, Sirtori R, Sirtori M, Ventura A: Pravastatin vs. gemfibrizol in the treatment of primary hypercholesterolemia. The Italian multicenter pravastatin study I. Arch Intern Med 151:146-151, 1991

20. Isley WL: Therapy of hypercholesterolemia with pra-

vastatin: A new HmG-CoA reductase inhibitor. Drugs Today 28:255-279, 1992

21. Heiss G, Tamir I, Davis CE, Tyroler HA, Rifkand BM, Schonfeld G, Jacobs D, Frantz ID, Jr: Lipoprotein-cholesterol distributions in selected North American populations: The lipid research clinics program prevalence study. Circulation 61:302-315, 1980

22. Lipid Research Clinics Manual of Laboratory Operations, vol I. Lipid and Lipoprotein Analysis. Washington DC, Department of Health Education and Welfare, US Government Printing Office, 1974

23. Hopper J, Ryan P, Lee JC, Rosenau W: Lipoid nephrosis in 31 adult patients: Renal biopsy by light, electron and fluorescence microscopy with experience in treatment. Medicine 49:321-341, 1970

24. Wass VJ, Jarrett RJ, Chilvers C, Cameron JS: Does the nephrotic syndrome increase the risk of cardiovascular disease? Lancet 2:664-667, 1979

25. Wass V, Cameron JS: Cardiovascular disease and the nephrotic syndrome: The other side of the coin. Nephron 27:58-61, 1981

26. Berlyne GM, Mallick NP: Ischaemic heart-disease as a complication of nephrotic syndrome. Lancet 2:399-400, 1969

27. Curry RC, Roberts WC: Status of the coronary arteries in the nephrotic syndrome. Am J Med 63:183-192, 1977

28. Moorhead JF: Lipids and progressive kidney disease. Kidney Int 39:S35-S40, 1991 (suppl 31)

29. Harris KP, Purkerson ML, Yates J, Klahr S: Lovastatin ameliorates the development of glomerulosclerosis and uremia in experimental nephrotic syndrome. Am J Kidney Dis 25:16-23, 1990

30. Aurell M, Björck S: Determinants of progressive renal disease in diabetes mellitus. Kidney Int 41:S38-S42, 1992 (suppl 36)

31. Kasiske BL, Velosa JA, Halstenson CE, La Belle P, Langend A, Keane WF: The effects of lovastatin in hyperlipidemic patients with nephrotic syndrome. Am J Kidney Dis 15:8-15, 1990

32. Valeri A, Gelfand J, Blum C, Appel GB: Treatment of the hyperlipidemia of the nephrotic syndrome: A controlled trial. Am J Kidney Dis 8:388-396, 1986

33. Rabelink AJ, Hene RJ, Erkelens DW, Joles JA, Koomans HA: Effects of simvastatin and cholestyramine on lipoprotein profile in hyperlipidemia of nephrotic syndrome. Lancet 2:1335-1338, 1988

34. Canner PL, Berge KG, Wenger NK, Stamler J, Friedman L, Prineas RJ, Friedewald W: Fifteen year mortality in coronary drug project patients: Long term benefit with niacin. J Am Coll Cardiol 8:1245-1255, 1986

35. Grundy SM, Mok HYI, Zech L, Berman M: Influence of nicotinic acid on metabolism of cholesterol and triglycerides in man. J Lipid Res 22:34-36, 1981

36. Grundy SM, Vega GL: Fibric acids: Effects on lipids and lipoprotein metabolism. Am J Med 83:9-20, 1987

37. Bridgman JF, Rosen SM, Thorp JM: Complications during clofibrate treatment of nephrotic syndrome hyperlipoproteinemia. Lancet 2:506-509, 1972

38. Groggel GC, Cheung AK, Ellis-Benigni K, Wilson DE: Treatment of nephrotic hyperlipoproteinemia with gemfibrizol. Kidney Int 36:266-271, 1989

39. Kesaniemi YA, Grundy SM: Influence of probucol on cholesterol and lipoprotein metabolism in man. J Lipid Res 25:780-790, 1984

40. Parthasarathy S, Young SG, Witztum JL, Pittman RC, Steinberg D: Probucol inhibits oxidative modification of low density lipoprotein. J Clin Invest 77:641-644, 1986

41. Steinberg D, Parthasarathy S, Carew TE, Khoo JC, Witztun JL: Beyond cholesterol. Modifications of low-density lipoproteins that increase its atherogenicity. N Engl J Med 320:915-923, 1989

42. Iida H, Izumino K, Asaka M, Fujita M, Nishino A, Sasayama S: Effect of probucol on hyperlipidemia in patients with nephrotic syndrome. Nephron 47:280-283, 1987

43. Vega GL, Grundy SM: Lovastatin therapy in nephrotic hyperlipidemia: Effects on lipoprotein metabolism. Kidney Int 33:1160-1168, 1988

44. Golper TA, Illingworth R, Morris CD, Bennet WM: Lovastatin in the treatment of multifactorial hyperlipidemia associated with proteinuria. Am J Kidney Dis 13:312-320, 1989

45. Bazzato G, Landini S, Fracasso A, Righetto F, Scanferla F, Roncali D, Genchi R, Toffoletto PP: Treatment of nephrotic syndrome hyperlipidemia with simvastatin. Curr Ther Res 50:744-752, 1991

46. Prata MM, Nogueira AC, Pinto JR, Correia AM, Vicente O, Rodrigues MC, Miguel MJP: Long-term effect of lovastatin on lipoprotein profile in patients with primary nephrotic syndrome. Clin Nephrol 41:277-283, 1994

47. Schapel GJ, Edwards KDG, Neale FC: Factorial study of the efficacy of cholestyramine, L-tryptophan and clofibrate in human nephrotic hyperlipidemia. Progr Biochem Pharmacol 9:82-98, 1974

Proteinuria: A Risk Factor for Pregnancy-Related Renal Function Decline in Primary Glomerular Disease?

Marc H. Hemmelder, MD, Dick de Zeeuw, MD, Vaclav Fidler, PhD, and Paul E. de Jong, MD

● Pregnancy may be followed by a postpartum acceleration of renal function loss in patients with renal disease. We retrospectively analyzed the effects of pregnancy on progressive renal function decline, and the risk factors for an acceleration, in a group of 19 renal disease patients with 30 pregnancies and a group of 31 patients who did not become pregnant after onset of glomerular disease. The rate of renal function loss was calculated for each patient by linear regression on reciprocal serum creatinine values over 11 years' follow-up. Multiple regression analysis showed that both pregnancy ($P = 0.03$) and initial proteinuria ($P = 0.005$) were independently related with the rate of renal function loss. Such a relation could not be observed with histologic diagnosis, and initial age, renal function, blood pressure, and serum albumin. Further analysis showed that 10 of 30 pregnancies are followed by a predefined acceleration of renal function loss. These pregnancies were preceded and complicated by a higher proteinuria (4.1 *v* 1.7 g/d, $P < 0.005$; and 3.6 *v* 2.1 g/d, $P < 0.05$, respectively) compared with the other 20 pregnancies that are not followed by such an acceleration. In conclusion, patients with primary glomerular disease complicated by substantial proteinuria are at risk for acceleration of renal function decline after pregnancy.

INDEX WORDS: Pregnancy; proteinuria; primary renal disease; hypertension.

IT IS GENERALLY assumed that pregnancy does not adversely influence the natural course of renal disease in patients with a preserved renal function.[1-8] However, in hypertensive patients with chronic renal failure, pregnancy has more frequently a deleterious effect on renal function outcome.[7,9-11] Therefore, both chronic renal failure and systemic hypertension are considered to be risk factors for an adverse effect of pregnancy on renal function decline in patients with renal disease.

It may well be that other factors play also a role, because a small number of patients have experienced an unexpected postpartum renal function deterioration in the absence of both chronic renal failure and systemic hypertension. Recently, we reported on such a patient with nephrotic range proteinuria, but without chronic renal failure and hypertension, who experienced accelerated renal function loss after each of two successive pregnancies.[12] Because proteinuria has been suggested to have a role in the progressive renal function loss,[13] we questioned whether proteinuria, in addition to renal failure and hypertension, could be involved in a postpartum acceleration of renal function decline in patients with renal disease.

We therefore investigated the effects of pregnancy on the rate of renal function decline in patients with biopsy-proven primary glomerular disease. Because pregnancy indeed was associated with an accelerated renal function decline, we additionally tried to identify the risk factors for this acceleration in our population.

PATIENTS AND METHODS

Patient Population

The records of female patients born between 1940 and 1970 with a biopsy diagnosis of focal segmental glomerulosclerosis, minimal change disease, immunoglobulin (Ig)A glomerulopathy, membranous glomerulopathy, or membranoproliferative glomerulonephritis were collected from the outpatient nephrology division of the State University Hospital Groningen. Patients from this cohort were included in the current analysis only when sufficient data were present to allow a follow-up evaluation on the progression of renal function loss. Patients who became pregnant after onset of glomerular disease had to have at least three serum creatinine values during at least 1 year before and after each pregnancy. Patients who did not became pregnant had to have at least five serum creatinine values available during at least 3 years of follow-up. This resulted in a group of 19 patients who experienced 30 pregnancies after onset of renal disease in the period between 1967 and 1990 and a control group of 31 patients who did not become pregnant after onset of renal disease. Two patients experienced a spontaneous abortion in the first pregnancy trimester, which was therefore not included as a pregnancy in our analysis. All 50 patients were caucasian. The follow-up (median and interquartile range) was 10.8 (6.0 to 13.5) years, whereby the follow-up duration was 12.0 (9.0 to 15.9) years in the group of patients with pregnancies and 7.0 (4.8 to 12.1) years in the control group. The number of serum creatinine values in this period was 28 (21 to 44) in the group of patients with pregnancies and 15 (9 to 31) in the control group.

Data Analysis

We assessed the rate of renal function decline in each of the 50 patients by calculating the slope of linear regression derived from reciprocal serum creatinine values over time.[14] An example of this method is illustrated in Fig 1A. Serum creatinine values obtained during pregnancy were excluded

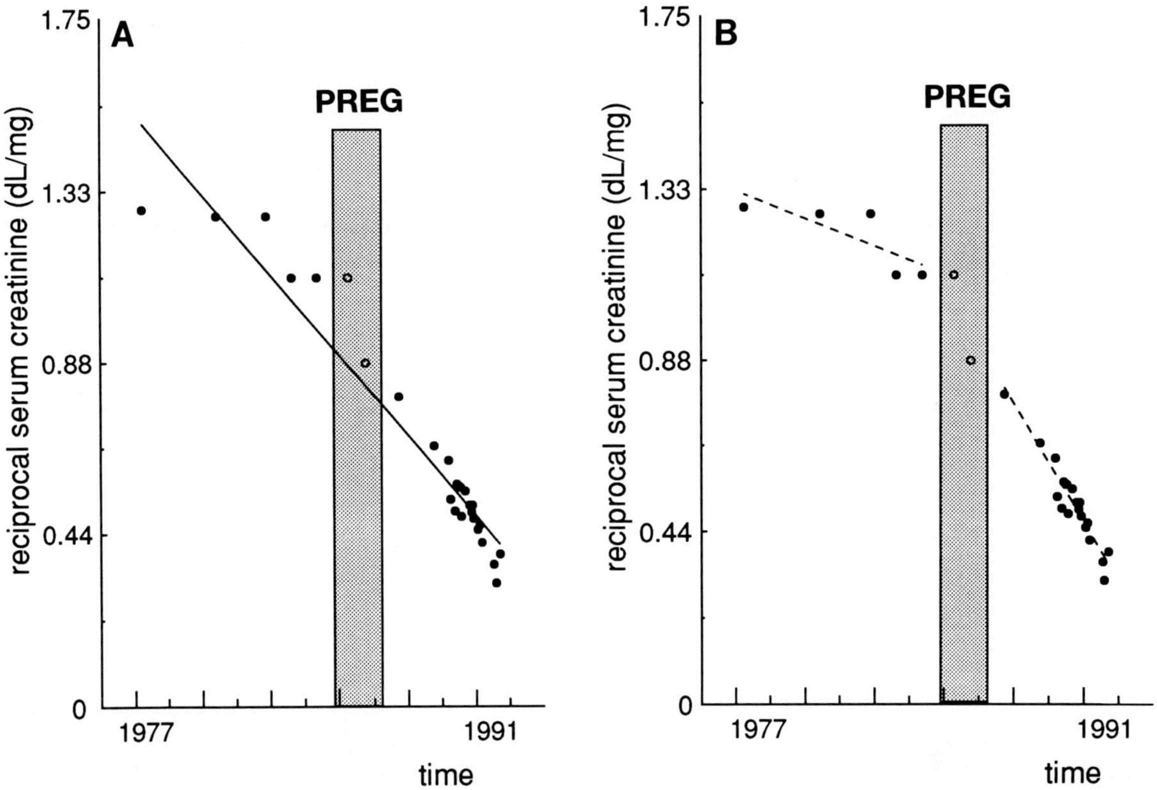

Fig 1. The rate of renal function decline in one patient who became pregnant (PREG) after onset of glomerular disease. (A) The slope of linear regression of reciprocal serum creatinine values (●) during the total follow-up disregarding reciprocal serum creatinine values during pregnancy (○); (B) the breakpoint analysis using the reciprocal serum creatinine slope before and after pregnancy.

from this analysis because these are influenced by functional changes.[1,15] Multiple regression analysis was performed to identify prognostic factors for the rate of renal function decline, taking the following independent variables into account: the presence of pregnancy during follow-up, histologic renal diagnosis, and age, reciprocal serum creatinine, blood pressure, proteinuria, and serum albumin at the onset of glomerular disease. Subsequently, we divided each of the 30 pregnancies in group A of pregnancies followed by postpartum accelerated renal function loss or group B of pregnancies not followed by such an acceleration. Postpartum acceleration of renal function decline was defined by a decreased mean reciprocal serum creatinine value in combination with a steepening of the slope of reciprocal serum creatinines after pregnancy compared with prepregnancy values. An example is shown in Fig 1B. Renal function parameters immediately before and during pregnancies of both groups were compared.

In the current study we defined renal function impairment as a serum creatinine level greater than 1.2 mg/dL, systemic hypertension as a diastolic blood pressure greater than 90 mm Hg (during pregnancy greater than 85 mm Hg) or the need to use antihypertensive treatment, and nephrotic range proteinuria as a proteinuria of more than 3.0 g/day. Data are expressed as median values with their interquartile range. Wilcoxon's rank sum test were used to compare characteristics of patients or pregnancies. Unless otherwise indicated, two-sided tests were used. Significance was assumed at a *P* level of 0.05.

RESULTS

The group of patients with pregnancies was comparable to the control group at the onset of glomerular disease, although patients of the control group were slightly, but significantly, older. Serum creatinine, systolic and diastolic blood pressure, proteinuria, and serum albumin were not different between both groups (Table 1). No difference was present in both groups among the distribution of histologic diagnoses and the incidence of renal function impairment (11% *v* 10%), diastolic hypertension (22% *v* 35%), proteinuria (89% *v* 77%), and nephrotic range proteinuria (42% *v* 48%). Furthermore, the number of patients who needed treatment with nonsteroidal

Table 1. Patient Characteristics at Onset of Glomerular Disease and at the End of Follow-up (Median and Interquartile Range) of the Group of Patients With Pregnancies (n = 19) and the Control Group of Patients Without Pregnancy (n = 31)

	At Onset		At End	
	Pregnant	Control	Pregnant	Control
Age (yr)	22 [19-23]*	26 [18-31]	33 [32-36]	35 [28-42]
Scr (mg/dL)	0.9 [0.8-1.0]	0.9 [0.8-1.0]	1.2 [1.0-2.9]†	0.9 [0.7-1.0]
SBP (mm Hg)	130 [120-150]	130 [120-143]	120 [118-135]	135 [120-143]
DBP (mm Hg)	85 [80-90]	80 [73-95]	80 [75-90]	85 [80-90]
Uprot (g/d)	3.0 [1.3-4.7]	3.0 [0.6-5.4]	1.4 [1.1-2.9]	0.6 [0.0-2.7]
Salb (g/L)	36 [27-43]	36 [30-44]	43 [37-43]	43 [40-47]
MCD	2 (11%)	5 (16%)		
FSGS	8 (41%)	8 (23%)		
IgA-GP	3 (16%)	6 (19%)		
MGP	3 (16%)	7 (23%)		
MPGN	3 (16%)	4 (13%)		
ND	0 (0%)	1 (3%)		

Abbreviations: Scr, serum creatinine; SBP, systolic blood pressure; DBP, diastolic blood pressure; Uprot, urinary protein excretion; Salb, serum albumin; MCD, minimal change disease; FSGS, focal segmental glomerulosclerosis; IgA-GP, IgA glomerulopathy; MGP, membranous glomerulopathy; MPGN, membranoproliferative glomerulonephritis; ND, no histologic diagnosis.

* $P < 0.01$, pregnant *v* control in the comparable period.

† $P < 0.05$, pregnant *v* control in the comparable period.

antiinflammatory drugs (NSAID) or antihypertensive drugs including angiotensin-converting enzyme inhibitors (ACEi) during follow-up were similar in both groups, as was the duration of those treatments. The type and dosage of NSAID and ACEi was similarly distributed over the two groups.

The progression of renal function loss was found to vary considerably in our population of 50 patients when reciprocal serum creatinine values were plotted against time. Multiple regression analysis indicated, after adjustment for age, a significant predictive effect of pregnancy ($P = 0.03$) as well as proteinuria at onset of glomerular disease ($P = 0.005$) on the rate of renal function loss (Table 2). Neither histologic diagnosis, serum creatinine, systolic and diastolic blood pressure, nor serum albumin at the time of the diagnosis of glomerular disease could explain the rate of renal function loss. In accordance with these results, patients with pregnancies had a higher serum creatinine than control patients at the end of follow-up ($P < 0.05$), although serum creatinine immediately before pregnancy was still comparable to that in the control group. During follow-up, 4 of 19 (21%) patients with pregnancies and 4 of 31 (13%) control patients reached end-stage renal failure and needed dialysis. At the end of follow-up, age, systolic and diastolic blood pressure, proteinuria, and serum albumin did again not differ between both groups (Table 1); neither did the incidence of renal function impairment, diastolic hypertension, proteinuria, and nephrotic range proteinuria.

The 30 pregnancies resulted in 32 childbirths, including two pairs of twins, one stillbirth in the 25th gestational week, and three infants who were born between the 30th and the 36th gestational weeks. Ten of those 30 pregnancies were followed by an acceleration of renal function de-

Table 2. Results of the Multiple Regression Analysis With the Rate of Renal Function Loss as Dependent Variable

Variable	Coefficient	SE	*P* Value
Constant	0.64	0.35	
Proteinuria (g/d)	−0.1	0.03	0.005
Pregnancy	−0.4	0.18	0.03
Age (yr)	−0.02	0.01	0.17

NOTE. n = 50, $r^2 = 0.26$ and adjusted $r^2 = 0.24$.

cline because reciprocal serum creatinine decreased from 1.09 dL/mg (0.79 to 1.36) before pregnancy to 0.65 dL/mg (0.46 to 1.11) after pregnancy, and the slope of reciprocal serum creatinine changed by −17.4° (−33.2° to −10.1°). The impact of this decline was such that the time to end-stage renal failure was projected to be 6.2 years (3.2 to 31.0). Renal function decline did not accelerate after the remaining group of 20 pregnancies reflected by a reciprocal serum creatinine of 1.05 dL/mg (0.78 to 1.18) before pregnancy and 1.06 dL/mg (0.80 to 1.23) after pregnancy, whereas the change in slope was −4.9° (−19.1° to +14.3°).

The presence or absence of pregnancy-induced progression could not be predicted for one of multiple pregnancies in one individual. In the nine patients with multiple pregnancies, five had no progression of renal function loss after all their pregnancies, one patient showed accelerated renal function loss after each of two successive pregnancies, and three patients only showed acceleration after their last of multiple pregnancies. Median follow-up duration before pregnancy was 2.7 (1.2 to 6.2) versus 2.2 (1.3 to 4.9) years and after pregnancy 3.6 (2.3 to 9.3) versus 2.0 (1.0 to 4.3) years in groups A and B, respectively. Serum creatinine and systolic and diastolic blood pressure were comparable preceding and during pregnancy in both groups (Table 3). In contrast, proteinuria was higher before and during pregnancy in group A than in group B pregnancies (4.1 *v* 1.7 g/day, $P < 0.005$; and 3.6 *v* 2.1 g/day, $P < 0.05$, respectively). Proteinuria and reciprocal serum creatinine before pregnancies in groups A and B were not different from the values during pregnancy. Only blood pressure was significantly lower during group A pregnancies when compared with the prepregnancy value. We did not find an association between the pregnancy-induced changes in proteinuria, blood pressure, or reciprocal serum creatinine and the pregnancy-related acceleration of renal function loss. The differences in glomerular histology among both groups of pregnancies did not reach statistical significance: 6 focal segmental glomerulonephritis (60%), 2 membranous glomerulopathy (20%), 1 minimal change disease (10%), 1 membranoproliferative glomerulonephritis (10%) in group A, and 8 focal segmental glomerulonephritis (40%), 2 membranous glomerulopathy (10%), 2 minimal change disease (10%), 3 membranoproliferative glomerulonephritis (15%), and 5 IgA-glomerulopathy (25%) in group B. With respect to drug treatment, ACEi was given more often after pregnancy in group A than in group B (7 of 10 pregnancies *v* 3 of 20 pregnancies, $P < 0.05$). The use of NSAID or antihypertensive agents other than ACEi was not different between both groups.

DISCUSSION

In the current study, pregnancy as well as initial proteinuria are associated with a higher rate of renal function decline in patients with primary glomerular disease. In addition, pregnancies followed by an acceleration of renal function decline are especially observed in patients with substantial proteinuria before and during pregnancy.

Previous studies, almost all retrospectively designed, conclude that pregnancy generally does not influence the natural course of renal disease, except for subgroups of patients with renal failure or systemic hypertension.[1-11] This discrepancy with our observations may be found in differences in study design or differences in study population. With respect to study design, we have estimated the rate of renal function loss by using adequate numbers of serum creatinine values at sufficient frequent time intervals.[14,16] In addition, the rate of renal function loss in a group of patients with pregnancies has been compared with that in a control group of patients without pregnancies. In contrast, most previous studies used only cross-sectional serum creatinine measurements at the end of follow-up,[1-5,10,11] or did not include a comparison with a control group consisting of patients who never became pregnant.[1-4,9-11] This makes it impossible to differentiate between an occasional postpartum renal function deterioration, representing the natural course of the renal disease, or a pregnancy-related acceleration of renal function decline in these studies. Although methodologic differences possibly explain the discrepancy, a few studies that did include a control group as well as serial renal function measurements could, however, not show an adverse effect of pregnancy on renal function outcome.[6-8] We therefore believe that differences in study population characteristics may be more important to explain the discrepancy.

Table 3. Patient Characteristics Before and During Group A Pregnancies Followed by Accelerated Renal Function Decline (n = 10) and Group B Pregnancies Not Followed by Such an Acceleration (n = 20)

	Before Pregnancy		During Pregnancy	
	Group A	Group B	Group A	Group B
Scr (mg/dL)	0.9 [0.8-1.1]	1.0 [0.8-1.2]	0.9 [0.7-1.0]	0.9 [0.8-1.2]
SBP (mm Hg)	126 [120-130]	130 [120-145]	128 [118-131]	125 [121-134]
DBP (mm Hg)	90 [85-95]	85 [80-93]	82 [72-83]*	83 [77-86]
Uprot (g/d)	4.1 [2.8-5.3]‡	1.6 [0.0-2.9]	3.6 [2.9-4.7]†	2.1 [0.9-3.4]

NOTE. Values are given as median and interquartile range.

Abbreviations: Scr, serum creatinine; SBP, systolic blood pressure; DBP, diastolic blood pressure; Uprot, urinary protein excretion.

* $P < 0.05$ before pregnancy *v* during pregnancy in the same group.

† $P < 0.05$, group A *v* group B in the comparable period.

‡ $P < 0.005$, group A *v* group B in the comparable period.

In our population, the incidence of proteinuria is much higher compared with that in the other studies. Proteinuria is present over a wide range in 89% of the patients with pregnancy and 77% of the control patients at onset of renal disease. Nine of 19 patients (49%) showed nephrotic range proteinuria just before pregnancy in the current study, while Katz et al[1] report just on 4 of 70 patients (6%), Barcelo et al[5] on 8 of 48 patients (17%), and Rovati et al[8] on 6 of 29 patients (21%). The significant impact of proteinuria on pregnancy-related renal function loss is also suggested by Abe's data[7] on 32 patients with IgA glomerulopathy. In those five patients who had a renal function deterioration after pregnancy, proteinuria was higher before conception (1.0 *v* 0.6 g/day), and more severe lesions were present in their preconceptional renal biopsy specimens. We believe that the high incidence of proteinuria in our population may explain the observed relation between pregnancy and progressive renal function loss. The most outspoken example of this observation is the patient with nephrotic range proteinuria who experienced an acceleration of renal function loss after each of two successive pregnancies.[12] Although it has been suggested that impaired renal function or systemic hypertension are the important determinants for adverse effects of pregnancy on renal function loss,[7,9-11] we could not confirm these findings in the current study. This may well be explained by the absence of patients with renal failure or untreated systemic hypertension in our population.

Lastly, the discrepancy may also be explained by differences in renal histologic diagnosis of included patients. Membranoproliferative glomerulonephritis[2,17] and focal segmental glomerulosclerosis[4,17,18] have been associated with a worse maternal renal function outcome after pregnancy. Reports concerning IgA glomerulopathy show controversial results.[6,7,19] Although we included patients with different renal histologic lesions, a histologic predisposition for the observed adverse effect of pregnancy on renal function decline could not be found in our small number of patients. That the underlying renal disease may still be of importance is suggested by the fact that patients with focal glomerulosclerosis showed accelerated renal function loss after 60% of their pregnancies, whereas renal function remained stable after all pregnancies in patients with IgA nephropathy.

In conclusion, we found that patients with primary glomerular disease, in particular patients with proteinuria, may be at risk for acceleration of renal function decline after pregnancy even in absence of chronic renal failure and systemic hypertension. Because pregnancy outcome in patients with renal disease is rather uncomplicated as a result of more and accurate perinatal care,[20] one may expect more patients with renal disease to become pregnant. To improve antenatal counseling we recommend accurate monitoring of the preceding course of renal function decline, blood pressure, and proteinuria in such patients. In case of accelerated renal function decline after a pregnancy, a subsequent pregnancy may be discouraged. Prospective trials concerning progression of renal function loss before, during, and after pregnancy in patients with renal disease are needed to confirm the current retrospective data.

ACKNOWLEDGMENT

We would like to thank Dr J.G.M. Jordans, Medical Spectrum Twente, and Dr M.P. Leemhuis, Medical Centre Leeuwarden, who allowed the study of patient records from their nephrology units.

REFERENCES

1. Katz AI, Davison JM, Hayslett JP, Singson E, Lindheimer MD: Pregnancy in women with kidney disease. Kidney Int 18:192-206, 1980

2. Surian M, Imbasciatti E, Cosci P, Banfi G, Barbiano di Belgiojoso G, Brancaccio D, Minetti L, Ponticelli C: Glomerular disease and pregnancy. Nephron 36:101-105, 1984

3. Jungers P, Forget MD, Henry-Amar M, Albouze G, Fournier P, Vischer U, Droz D, Noel LH, Grunfeld JP: Chronic kidney disease and pregnancy. Adv Nephrol 15:103-137, 1986

4. Packham DK, North RA, Fairley KF, Kloss M, Whitworth JA, Kincaid-Smith P: Primary glomerulonephritis and pregnancy. Q J Med 266:537-553, 1989

5. Barcelo P, Lopez-Lillo JL, Cabero L, Del Rio G: Successful pregnancy in primary glomerular disease. Kidney Int 30:914-919, 1986

6. Jungers P, Forget D, Houillier P, Henry-Amar M, Grunfeld JP: Pregnancy in IgA nephropathy, reflux nephropathy and focal glomerular sclerosis. Am J Kidney Dis 4:334-338, 1987

7. Abe S: Pregnancy in IgA nephropathy. Kidney Int 40:1098-1102, 1991

8. Rovati C, Perrino ML, Barbiano di Belgiojoso G, Surian M, Radaelli L, Minetti L: Pregnancy and course of primary glomerulonephritis. Contrib Nephrol 37:182-189, 1984

9. Hou SH, Grossman SD, Madias NE: Pregnancy in women with renal disease and moderate renal insufficiency. Am J Med 78:185-194, 1985

10. Imbasciatti E, Pardi G, Capetta P, Ambroso G, Bozetti P, Pagliari B, Ponticelli C: Pregnancy in women with chronic renal failure. Am J Nephrol 6:193-198, 1986

11. Cunningham FG, Cox SM, Harstad TW, Mason RA, Pritchard JA: Chronic renal disease and pregnancy outcome. Am J Obstet Gynecol 163:453-459, 1990

12. Hemmelder MH, de Zeeuw D, de Jong PE: Accelerated progression of renal function loss after 2 pregnancies in a patient with proteinuria [Letter]. Lancet 340:183, 1992

13. Remuzzi G, Bertani T: Is glomerulosclerosis a consequence of altered glomerular permeability to macromolecules? Kidney Int 38:384-394, 1990

14. Mitch WE, Walser M, Buffington GA, Leman J: A simple method of estimating progression of chronic real failure. Lancet 2:1326-1328, 1976

15. Davison JM, Dunlop W: Renal hemodynamics and tubular function in normal human pregnancy. Kidney Int 18:152-161, 1980

16. Walser M, Drew HH, LaFrance ND: Creatinine measurements often yields false estimates of progression of chronic renal disease. Kidney Int 34:412-418, 1988

17. Abe S: An overview of pregnancy in women with underlying renal disease. Am J Kidney Dis 17:112-115, 1991

18. Taylor J, Novak R, Cristiansen R, Sorensen ET: Focal sclerosing glomerulopathy with adverse effects during pregnancy. Arch Intern Med 138:1695-1696, 1978

19. Kincaid-Smith P, Fairley KF: Renal disease in pregnancy: Three controversial areas: Mesangial IgA nephropathy, focal glomerular sclerosis and reflux nephropathy. Am J Kidney Dis 4:328-333, 1987

20. Imbasciatti E, Ponticelli C: Pregnancy and renal disease: Predictors for fetal and maternal outcome. Am J Nephrol 11:353-362, 1991

Effect of Early Hyperlipidemia on Graft and Patient Survival in Cyclosporine-Treated Renal Transplant Patients

Mariana S. Markell, MD, Nabil Sumrani, MD, Annette DiBenedetto, RN, and Eli A. Friedman, MD

● Hyperlipidemia commonly occurs following renal transplantation. As hyperlipidemia has been postulated to contribute to renal dysfunction in animal models, the effect of early hyperlipidemia was studied in a cohort of 43 cyclosporine-treated renal transplant recipients over a 4-year follow-up period. Hypercholesterolemia occurred in 25 patients, with 18 patients remaining normolipidemic during the initial 3 months following transplantation. Prospective follow-up over a 4-year period was available for 16 of the 18 normolipidemic patients and 25 patients who developed hyperlipidemia, as well as 11 other hyperlipidemic patients who were not included in the initial analysis. Graft function was maintained in 11 (69%) of the patients with early normolipidemia and there has been one patient death (7%). Of the hypercholesterolemic group, two patients were lost to follow-up and 23 of the remaining 34 (68%) had persistant graft function. There have been two patient deaths (6%). No deaths from cardiovascular deaths have occurred in either group, all deaths resulting from infection/sepsis. Mean cholesterol values at 4-year follow-up were 202.0 ± 11.2 mg/dL for the patients with early normolipidemia and 282.9 ± 14.3 mg/dL for the patients with early hyperlipidemia ($P < 0.00001$). The most recent cholesterol value was not associated with pretransplant cholesterol value, creatinine, or cyclosporine dose, but was associated with cholesterol value at 3 months both by regression analysis ($P < 0.0001$) and by Pearson R ($r = 0.71$, $P < 0.0001$). Early posttransplant hypercholesterolemia persisted for the 4-year follow-up period despite decreasing doses of immunosuppression and was independent of renal function, weight gain, and cyclosporine dose, but highly correlated with early posttransplant cholesterol value. The relationship of hypercholesterolemia to prednisone dose was complex and did not follow a simple linear correlation. Early posttransplant hypercholesterolemia was not associated with excess patient or graft loss over the 4-year follow-up period. These data suggest that early hypercholesterolemia is not a major determinant of graft loss, although we cannot exclude a role for hypercholesterolemia in accelerating the rate of declining renal dysfunction in patients with chronic rejection or other renal diseases.

INDEX WORDS: Hyperlipidemia; cyclosporine; renal transplant; graft survival.

ATHEROSCLEROTIC cardiovascular disease is the leading cause of death in renal transplant recipients who survive longer than a decade with a functioning renal allograft.[1,2] Cyclosporine-treated renal transplant recipients commonly develop multiple risk factors for cardiovascular disease, including hypertension, obesity, and diabetes, and the majority develop hyperlipidemia posttransplantation.[3-9]

Most surveys of lipid profiles in renal transplant recipients report point prevalence data, either early, within the first 3 to 6 months,[3-5] or later, at 1 year or more posttransplant.[6-9] Recent evidence suggests that early hypercholesterolemia, occurring between 3 and 6 months posttransplant, will persist for years in untreated patients receiving azathioprine and prednisone[6]; whether this effect is true in cyclosporine-treated patients is not known. Neither is it known whether patients who remain normolipidemic at 3 months will develop hyperlipidemia at a later date in the absence of chronic rejection and nephrotic syndrome.

Hypercholesterolemia has been implicated in the progression of renal disease in animal models, including the obese Zucker rat[10] and the cholesterol-fed guinea pig,[11] and treatment of animal models with lipid-lowering therapy has been demonstrated to slow progression of renal disease.[12,13] The contribution of lipid disorders to progression of renal disease has been more difficult to substantiate in humans, although hyperlipidemia has been considered one of the factors that may contribute to the progressive decline in renal function observed in patients with nephrosis[14-16] and chronic rejection.[17] These claims have not been verified empirically, and the influence of prolonged hyperlipidemia on renal allograft survival is not known.

In a previous report,[3] we followed the prospective changes in lipid profile occurring over the first 3 months following transplantation in 43 patients transplanted between May and November 1987. Twenty-five (58%) of these patients developed hypercholesterolemia, defined as a total cholesterol greater than 240 mg/dL. The major determinant of the observed increase in total cholesterol was an increase in the low-density lipoprotein fraction.[3] Follow-up data were obtained from patients who were screened for hyperlipidemia 4 to 5 years earlier, in an attempt to determine whether early lipid abnormalities persist and whether there is a difference in graft and patient survival between patients who develop early hyperlipidemia and those who do not.

METHODS

Of the 43 patients initially screened in 1987, 16 of the 18 patients who remained normolipidemic at 3 months posttransplant and all 25 of the hyperlipidemic patients, as well as 11 additional cyclosporine-treated renal transplant recipients who developed hyperlipidemia by 3 months posttransplant but who were not included in the initial analysis, had follow-up data available. All patients had received their renal transplants between January and December 1987.

Immunosuppression at the time of transplantation was as follows: initial cyclosporine dose 12 to 15 mg/kg/d, tapered to achieve blood levels of 100 to 200 ng/mL by high-performance liquid chromatography. Prednisone was administered in a tapered fashion as well (1 mg/kg/d, tapered to 0.25 mg/kg/d by 6 months posttransplant). Azathioprine was not routinely started at the time of transplantation but was added at 1 to 1.5 mg/kg if the patient had suffered a rejection episode. ALG (Minnesota) or ATGAM (Upjohn) at 15 mg/kg/d or monoclonal antibody OKT3 (Ortho Pharmaceuticals) at 5 to 10 mg/d were used for rejection episodes that did not respond to intravenous methylprednisolone 250 mg/d for 2 to 3 days. None of the patients were treated with antilipemic agents.

Total cholesterol and creatinine values were measured using a Kodak auto-analyzer following a 6- to 8-hour fast. Hypercholesterolemia was defined as total cholesterol ≥ 240 mg/dL on at least two occasions.

Data regarding medication doses and graft and patient survival were obtained through chart review. Graft failure was defined as the necessity for a return to dialysis or retransplantation, regardless of cause. Patient death was counted as graft failure. For statistical comparison, data from patients with graft failure were collected from their last clinic visit prior to restarting dialysis or retransplantation. Statistical significance was evaluated using Student's *t*-test, chi-square analysis, or Pearson correlation as appropriate. A value of $P < 0.05$ was considered significant.

RESULTS

General demographics and patient characteristics are shown in Table 1. Cholesterol values pretransplant did not differ. Cholesterol values at the most recent follow-up reveal persistence of the early lipid abnormality in patients who developed hypercholesterolemia. There was no difference in graft or patient survival between normolipidemic patients and those who developed hyperlipidemia over the 4- to 5-year follow-up period. Graft survival was 69% for normolipidemic patients and 68% for hyperlipidemic patients. Patients who were initially screened included only those whose grafts survived to 3 months with function, eliminating patients with early graft loss from nonfunction or acute rejection, with the result that subsequent graft losses occurred gradually over the ensuing 4 years (Fig 1). There was one patient death in the normolipidemic group and two patient deaths in the hyperlipidemic group. All deaths were from sepsis/infection and there have been no cardiovascular deaths in either group. Two of the hyperlipidemic patients were lost to follow-up. Seven (19%) of the hyperlipidemic patients required treatment for diabetes at last follow-up. Three of these seven patients developed diabetes following transplantation, compared with one patient in the normolipidemic group.

Follow-up data for patients with functioning grafts are shown in Table 2. At the most recent follow-up, there was no difference between the normolipidemic and hyperlipidemic patients with regard to mean weight or weight gain, serum creatinine, prednisone, cyclosporine, or lasix dose, although a larger percentage of patients

Table 1. Demographics and Patient Characteristics for High and Normal Cholesterol Values at 3 Months Posttransplant for All Patients, Including Graft Failures

	"Normal" Cholesterol	High Cholesterol
No. of patients	16	36
No. of diabetic patients	1 (6)	7* (19)
Male/Female	12 (80)/3 (20)	21 (58)/15 (42)
Prednisone dose at 3 mo (mg)	18.6 ± 7.7	16.5 ± 4.9
Most recent prednisone dose (mg)	13.7 ± 4.5†	11.5 ± 6.4†
Pretransplant cholesterol (mg/dL)	181.1 ± 22.1	207.4 ± 56.9
Cholesterol at posttransplant 3 mo (mg/dL)	208.2 ± 22.1	295.7 ± 43.3‡
Most recent cholesterol (mg/dL)	209.8 ± 39.9	282.9 ± 67.7‡
No. of deaths	1 (7)	2 (6)
No. of functioning grafts remaining	11 (69)	23§ (68)

Note. Values are mean ± SEM. The numbers in parentheses are percentages of the total population.

* Three patients developed diabetes posttransplant.

† $P < 0.05$ for 3 months to most recent comparison.

‡ $P < 0.0001$ for between-group comparisons.

§ Two patients were lost to follow-up; the percentage is of 34 patients.

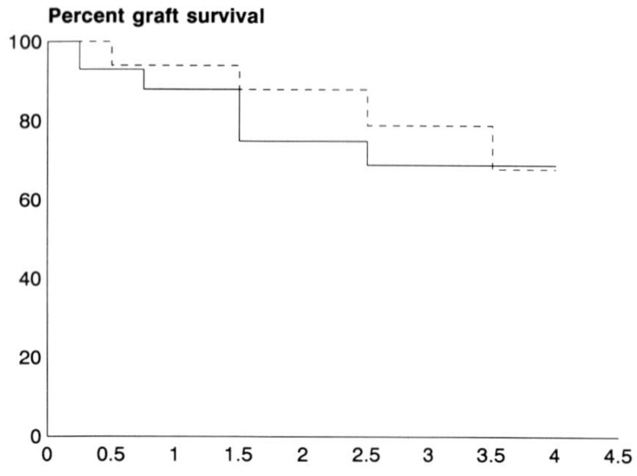

Fig 1. Percentage of graph survival in normolipidemic (solid line) versus hyperlipidemic (broken line) patients followed from 3 months to 4 years posttransplant. There were 16 normolipidemic patients and 36 hyperlipidemic patients.

with hypercholesterolemia were receiving beta-blocking therapy. The prednisone dose did not correlate with the cholesterol value by Pearson R (r = 0.21, P = NS). Only one patient in the group with a functioning transplant and persistent hyperlipidemia had proteinuria.

The data for patients with graft failure are presented in Table 3. There was no significant difference in time to graft failure (''graft survival'') between the two groups and, as would be expected, a high percentage of patients developed significant proteinuria, with 80% of previously normolipidemic patients and 34% of previously hyperlipidemic patients demonstrating greater than 3+ proteinuria on urine dipstick prior to requirement for dialysis or retransplantation.

By multiple regression analysis, the most recent cholesterol value for all patients (with and without a functioning transplant) was not associated with pretransplant cholesterol value, creatinine, or cyclosporine dose. The cholesterol value at 3 months associated highly with most recent value, both by regression analysis ($P < 0.0001$) and by Pearson R ($r = 0.71$, $P < 0.0001$).

Changes in mean cholesterol values over time are show in Fig 2. For patients with functioning transplants, cholesterol values at 3 months remained stable over 4 years of follow-up. For patients who experienced graft failure, there was a marked increase in total mean cholesterol for patients who were initially normolipidemic, although the difference from the 3-month mean value did not achieve significance because of the small number of patients and the large variance.

DISCUSSION

The natural history and significance of posttransplant hyperlipidemia have been unclear. In

Table 2. Laboratory Values and Drug Dosages for Patients With Functioning Grafts at 4 to 5 Years Posttransplant

	"Normal" Cholesterol	High Cholesterol
No. of patients	11	23
Pretransplant weight (kg)	72.8 ± 4.3	68.3 ± 3.0
Weight at 3 mo posttransplant (kg)	73.9 ± 5.1	73.3 ± 3.5
Most recent weight (kg)	79.3 ± 7.0	78.9 ± 4.2*
Change in weight (kg)	6.4 ± 4.3	10.6 ± 1.6
3 mo/most recent furosemide dose (mg)	64 ± 13.6/66 ± 29.5	54.8 ± 9.4/61.7 ± 11.3
No. of patients receiving beta-blockers (3 mo/most recent)	4 (36)/4 (36)	16 (69)/17 (74)
Pretransplant cholesterol (mg/dL)	158.7 ± 18.6	208.2 ± 11.2†
Cholesterol at 3 mo posttransplant (mg/dL)	203.1 ± 5.0	296.8 ± 8.9‡
Most recent cholesterol (mg/dL)	202.0 ± 11.2	282.9 ± 14.3‡
Most recent creatinine (mg/dL)	2.4 ± 0.39	2.2 ± 0.19
>3 + dipstick proteinuria	0 (0)	1 (4)
Most recent prednisone dose (mg)	12.9 ± 1.1	10.9 ± 1.4
Most recent cyclosporine dose (mg/kg)	3.5 ± 0.42	3.6 ± 0.3

Note. The data are presented as means ± SEM. Differences not noted otherwise are not significant. The numbers in parentheses are the percentages of the total population.

* $P < 0.05$ for comparison with pretransplant weight.

† $P < 0.05$.

‡ $P < 0.0001$ for between-group comparisons.

Table 3. Cholesterol Values and Time to Graft Failure for Patients With Failed Transplants (Including Death With Functioning Transplant)

	"Normal" Cholesterol	High Cholesterol
No. of patients	5 (31)	11 (32)
Pretransplant cholesterol (mg/dL)	195.8 ± 5.8	203.2 ± 20.5
Cholesterol at 3 mo posttransplant (mg/dL)	205.9 ± 15.5	292.6 ± 15.1*
Last recorded cholesterol (mg/dL)	239.2 ± 24.0	270.9 ± 17.8
>3 + dipstick proteinuria	4 (80)	4 (34)
Graft survival (mo)	17 ± 4.2	25.5 ± 3.8

Note. The data are presented as means ± SEM. Differences not noted otherwise are not significant. The numbers in parentheses are the percentages of total population.

* $P < 0.005$ for between-group comparisons.

this study, patients with early posttransplant hypercholesterolemia continued to remain hypercholesterolemic as long as 4 years posttransplant and patients who were normolipidemic at 3 months posttransplant maintained normolipidemia, unless they developed graft dysfunction.

Multiple factors have been implicated as contributing to posttransplant hyperlipidemia.[3-10, 18-23] The use of corticosteroids, including predni-sone and methylprednisolone, is associated with insulin resistance[24] and alteration of postheparin lipolytic activity,[25] resulting in hypertriglyceridemia and hypercholesterolemia.[26,27] In the patients we studied, the relationship between cholesterol and prednisone dose was complex and did not follow a simple linear correlation. In fact, prednisone dose was higher in normolipidemic patients at the most recent follow-up and, although the mean prednisone dose was lower for both hyperlipidemic and normolipidemic patients at the most recent follow-up than at 3 months posttransplant, lipid values did not decrease appreciably over the follow-up period.

Although prednisone use did not appear to be a major co-factor in the maintenance of posttransplant hyperlipidemia, the number of patients with diabetes, half of whom developed diabetes following transplantation, was higher in the hyperlipidemic group, suggesting that glucose intolerance per se may have played a contributory role. We have previously reported a high incidence of subclinical glucose intolerance in hypercholesterolemic renal transplant recipients,[18] which might reflect an effect of corticosteroids in a genetically primed subpopulation.

Cyclosporine use also has been implicated as contributing both to glucose intolerance[28-30] and to hyperlipidemia.[3-6] Several mechanisms have been postulated by which cyclosporine could contribute to hyperlipidemia in addition to exacerbation of glucose intolerance. Cyclosporine has been associated with alteration of post heparin lipolytic activity,[31] which could lead to hyperlipidemia through alteration of very low-density lipoprotein synthesis. It is a highly lipophilic compound, which travels in the plasma bound to lipoproteins[32,33] and could theoretically alter cholesterol feedback through interference with the low-density lipoprotein receptor.[7,34] In addition, in vitro work suggests that cyclosporine alters hepatic bile acid synthesis.[35] In our patients, there was no discernable difference in cyclosporine dose between hyperlipidemic and normolipidemic patients, although it has been suggested that because of its lipophilicity, cyclosporine kinetics are altered by hyperlipidemia, resulting in higher blood levels for a given dose.[5]

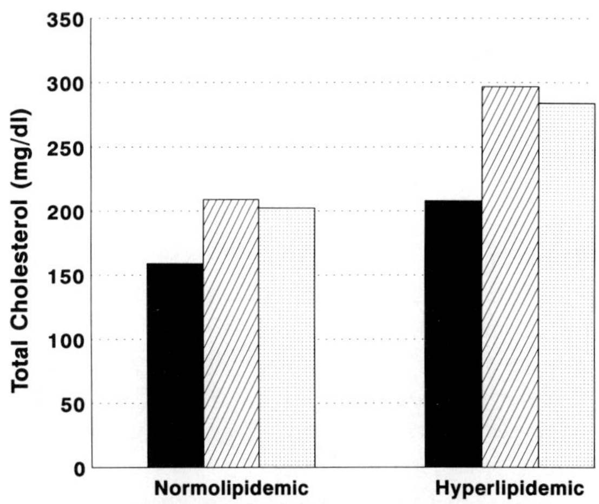

Fig 2. Change in mean cholesterol value over time. There were 16 patients who were normolipidemic at 3 months posttransplant and 36 patients who were hyperlipidemic. $P < 0.0001$ for 3-month and 4-year cholesterol values in hyperlipidemic patients compared with pretransplant value and values in normolipidemic patients at the same time period. All other values are not significant. ■, Pretransplant; ▨, 3 months posttransplant; ▤, 4 years posttransplant.

The use of antihypertensive agents, particularly drugs of the beta-blocker class, and diuretic agents has been associated with hyperlipidemia in the nonrenal transplant population.[36] This effect is felt to be mediated in part through promotion of insulin resistance or alteration in insulin secretion[37] secondary to the development of hypokalemia or beta-blockade. Although there was no difference in actual furosemide dose taken by hyperlipidemic and normolipidemic patients, a higher percentage of patients with hyperlipidemia were receiving beta-blocking drugs. Poor dietary habits and weight gain have been associated with hyperlipidemia in the renal transplant population.[7,37,38] In our population, the majority of patients gained weight following transplantation, and there was no difference in the mean amount of weight gained between patients who remained normolipidemic and those who remained hyperlipidemic, suggesting that this was not a major factor, although, again, weight gain may have contributed to hyperlipidemia in patients with underlying genetic susceptibility to hyperinsulinemia, which is exacerbated by being overweight.[39]

The development of nephrosis appeared to play an exacerbating role in the development of hyperlipidemia only in the normolipidemic patients whose grafts lost function and in whom elevation in cholesterol from baseline was associated with an 80% incidence of significant proteinuria (Table 3). Patients with persistent hyperlipidemia and good renal function, however, had a very low incidence of significant proteinuria, as measured grossly by urine dipstick. The mean creatinine value for hyperlipidemic patients was similar to that of patients who remained normolipidemic, suggesting that renal insufficiency was not responsible for the persistence of their lipid abnormality; however, subtle differences in glomerular filtration rate may have been present that were not obvious from using serum creatinine as a measure of renal function.

Although pretransplant cholesterol values did not correlate with later values, patients who developed hyperlipidemia had a higher mean total cholesterol prior to transplantation. Late posttransplant cholesterol values correlated highly with early posttransplant values, suggesting that as early as 3 months posttransplant, a subpopulation of "at risk" patients can be identified and that hyperlipidemia does not remit over time. In our population, hypercholesterolemia did not result in excess patient mortality over the 4-year follow-up period. Maintenance of normolipidemia did not appear to offer protection against graft loss during the follow-up period; conversely, hypercholesterolemia did not appear to increase the risk of graft loss. However, although this finding suggests that hypercholesterolemia per se is not a major factor in graft loss, it does not rule out the possibility that hypercholesterolemia could play a role in ongoing renal injury, once injury has been established through acute rejection or ischemia. In addition, more complex relationships between graft loss and cholesterol subfractions such as low- and high-density lipoprotein may exist, which would not be possible to discern from examination of total cholesterol values. It remains possible that intervention with lipid-lowering therapy early in the course of renal insufficiency with nephrosis will decrease the rate of progression to renal failure in patients with chronic rejection and that lipids are playing an intermediary role in renal injury.[15,40]

Thus, it appears that in the majority of patients genetic factors may be the most important determinants in the development of post-renal transplant hypercholesterolemia when the patient is exposed to exacerbating factors, including immunosuppression, a high-fat diet, weight gain, antihypertensive medications, and diuretics. Hypercholesterolemia does not spontaneously remit over time, despite reduction in steroid and cyclosporine doses and the presence of stable renal function. Whether persistent hyperlipidemia contributes to the high mortality from coronary disease that is observed in the late posttransplant period is not known at present, although several studies have suggested that transplant patients who suffer cardiovascular events have a high incidence of hyperlipidemia.[41,42] Large, long-term population studies will be required to establish risk factor profile analyses for cardiovascular disease in renal transplant recipients, with follow-up intervention studies as have been carried out in the nontransplant population.

REFERENCES

1. Fassbinder W, Challah S, Brynger H: Long term results of renal transplantation in Europe. Transplant Proc 19:3754-3757, 1987

2. Mahoney JF, Caterson RJ, Pollock CA, Jones M, Waugh DA, Sheil AGR: Coronary artery disease is the major late complication of successful cadaveric renal transplantation. Clin Transplant 4:129-132, 1990

3. Markell MS, Brown CD, Friedman EA, Butt KMH: Prospective evaluation of changes in lipid profiles in cyclosporine treated renal transplant patients. Transplant Proc 21:1497-1499, 1987

4. Raine AEG, Carter R, Mann JI, Chapman JR, Morris PJ: Increased plasma LDL cholesterol after renal transplantation associated with cyclosporine immunosuppression. Transplant Proc 19:1820-1821, 1987

5. Kasiske BL, Tortorice KL, Heim-Duthoy KL, Awni WM, Rao KV: The adverse impact of cyclosporine on serum lipids in renal transplant recipients. Am J Kidney Dis 17:700-707, 1991

6. Vathsala A, Weinberg RB, Schoenberg L, Grevel J, Goldstein RA, VanBuren CT, Lewis RM, Kahan BD: Lipid abnormalities in cyclosporine-prednisone treated renal transplant recipients. Transplantation 48:37-43, 1989

7. Markell MS, Friedman EA: Hyperlipidemia after organ transplantation. Am J Med 87:5-61N-5-67N, 1989

8. Kasiske BL, Uman AJ: Persistent hyperlipidemia in renal transplant patients. Medicine 66:309-316, 1987

9. Cassader M, Ruiu G, Gambino R, Alemanno N, Triolo G, Pagano G: Lipoprotein-apolipoprotein changes in renal transplant recipients: A 2-year follow-up. Metabolism 40:922-925, 1991

10. Divaker D, Bailey RR, Frampton CM, Geoprge PM, Walmsley TA, Murphy J: Hyperlipidemia in stable renal transplant recipients. Nephron 59:423-428, 1991

11. Al-Shebab T, Frolich J, Magil AB: Glomerular disease in hypercholesterolemic guinea pigs. Kidney Int 33:498-507, 1988

12. Kasiske BL, ODonnell MP, Keane WF: The Zucker rat model of obesity, insulin resistance, hyperlipidemia and renal injury. Hypertension 19:I110-115, 1992 (suppl)

13. Kasiske BL, ODonnell MP, Cleary MP, Keane WF: Treatment of hyperlipdiemia reduces glomerular injury in obese Zucker rats. Kidney Int 33:667-672, 1988

14. Harris KPG, Purkerson ML, Yates J, Klahr S: Lovastatin ameliorates the development of glomerulosclerosis and uremia in experimental nephrotic syndrome. Am J Kidney Dis 15:16-23, 1990

15. Moorehead JF: Lipids and progressive kidney disease. Kidney Int 39:S35-S40, 1991 (suppl 31)

16. Keane WF, Mulcahy WS, Kasiske BL, Kim Y, ODonnell MP: Hyperlipidemia and progressive renal disease. Kidney Int 39:S41-S48, 1991 (suppl 31)

17. Paul LC, Fellstrom B: Chronic vascular rejection of the heart and the kidney—Have rational treatment options emerged? Transplantation 53:1169-1179, 1992

18. Markell MS, Zara CP, Brown CD, Sumrani N, Hong JH, Friedman EA: Hyperinsulinemia and glucose intolerance in hypercholesterolemic cyclosporine treated renal transplant recipients. J Am Soc Nephrol 1:764, 1990 (abstr)

19. Nyberg G, Fager G, Mjornstedt L, Olausson M: Metabolic risk factors for cardiovascular disease in pancreas and kidney transplant recipients. Diabetologia 34:S44-S46, 1991 (suppl 1)

20. Ballantyne CM, Podet EJ, Patsch WP, Harati Y, Appel V, Gotto AM, Jr, Young JB: Effects of cyclosporine therapy on plasma lipoprotein levels. JAMA 262:53-56, 1989

21. Cattran DC, Steiner G, Wilson DR, Fenton SSA: Hyperlipidimia after renal transplantation: Natural history and pathophysiology. Ann Intern Med 91:554-559, 1979

22. Chan MK, Varghese Z, Persaud JW, Fernando ON, Moorehead JF: The role of multiple pharmacotherapy in the pathogenesis of hyperlipidemia after renal transplantation. Clin Nephrol 15:309-313, 1981

23. Arnadottir M, Thysell H, Nilsson-Ehle P: Lipoprotein levels and post-heparin lipase activities in kidney transplant recipients: Ciclosporine- versus non–ciclosporine-treated patients. Am J Nephrol 11:391-396, 1991

24. Grill V, Pigon SG, Hartling C, Binder C, Efendici S: Effects of dexamethasone on glucose-induced insulin and proinsulin release in low and high insulin responders. Metabolism 39:251-258, 1990

25. Ettinger WH, Jr, Hazzard WR: Prednisone increases very low density lipoprotein and high density lipoprotein in healthy men. Metabolism 37:1055-1058, 1988

26. Zimmerman J, Fainaru M, Eisenberg S: The effects of prednisone therapy on plasma lipoproteins and apolipoproteins. Metabolism 33:521-522, 1984

27. Ettinger WH, Hazzard WR: Prednisone increases very low density lipoprotein and high density lipoprotein in healthy men. Metabolism 37:1055-1058, 1986

28. Dresner LS, Anderson DK, Khang KU, Munshi IA, Wait RB: Effects of cyclosporine on glucose metabolism. Surgery 106:163-169, 1989

29. Baumgartner D, Schlumpf R, Largiader F: Cyclosporine A interferes with postoperative blood glucose control after clinical pancreas transplantation. Transplant Proc 19:4009-4010, 1987

30. Ost L, Tyden G, Fehrman I: Inpaired glucose tolerance in cyclosporine treated renal graft recipients. Transplantation 46:370-372, 1988

31. Derfler K, Hayde M, Heinz G, Hirschl MM, Steger G, Hauser AC, Baucke P, Widhauser K: Decreased post-heparin lipolytic activity in renal transplant recipients with cyclosporine A. Kidney Int 40:720-727, 1991

32. Sgoutas D, Macmahon W, Love A, Jerkunica I: Interaction of cyclosporine A with human lipoproteins. J Pharm Pharmacol 38:583-588, 1986

33. Lemaire M, Tillement P: Role of lipoproteins and erythrocytes in the in vitro binding and distribution of cyclosporine A in the blood. J Pharm Pharmacol 34:715-718, 1982

34. DeGroen P: Cyclosporine, low-density lipoprotein, and cholesterol. Mayo Clin Proc 63:1012-1021, 1988

35. Princen HMG, Meijer P, Hofstee B, Havekes LM, Kuipers F, Vonk RJ: Effects of cyclosporine A on LDL receptor activity and bile acid synthesis in hepatocyte monolayer cultures and in vivo in the rat. Hepatology 7:1109, 1987 (abstr)

36. Perez-Stable E, Caralis PV: Thiazide-induced disturbances in carbohydrate, lipid and potassium metabolism. Am Heart J 106:245-251, 1983

37. Divaker D, Bailey RR, Price M, Frampton C, George PM: Effect of diet on post-transplant hyperlipidemia. N Z Med J 105:79-80, 1992

38. Gonyea JE, Anderson CF: Weight change and serum

lipoproteins in recipients of renal allografts. Mayo Clin Proc 67:653-657, 1992

39. Winocour PH, Kaluvya S, Ramaiya K, Brown L, Millar JP, Farrer M, Neil HA, Laker MF, Alberti KG: Relationship between insulinemia, body mass index and lipoprotein composition in healthy, nondiabetic men and women. Arterioscler Thromb 12:393-402, 1992

40. Moorehead JF, Chan MK, El-Nahas M, Varghese Z: Lipid nephrotoxicity in chronic progressive glomerular and tubulo-interstitial disease. Lancet 2:1309-1312, 1982

41. Kasiske BL: Risk factors for accelerated atherosclerosis in renal transplant recipients. Am J Med 84:458-463, 1988

42. Abdulmassih Z, Chevalier A, Bader C, Druecke TB, Kreis H, Lacour B: Role of lipid disturbances in the atherosclerosis of renal transplant patients. Clin Transplant 6:106-113, 1992

Progressive Renal Insufficiency Following Cardiac Transplantation: Cyclosporine, Lipids, and Hypertension

Vinita Sehgal, MD, Jai Radhakrishnan, MD, MRCP, Gerald B. Appel, MD, Anthony Valeri, MD, and David J. Cohen, MD

● The increasing success of cardiac transplantation has been attributed to the availability of potent immunosuppressive agents, including cyclosporine. With improved graft and patient survival, the incidence of chronic renal insufficiency has increased. We reviewed the medical records of patients who had undergone orthotopic cardiac transplantation and had been followed for at least 3 years posttransplantation to determine the risk factors at initial evaluation and in the early posttransplantation period for subsequent renal insufficiency. We followed 80 adult patients over a mean period of 4.7 years: 39 patients had a serum creatinine ≥2.4 mg/dL at last follow-up (renal insufficiency or RI group); 41 patients had a serum creatinine ≤1.7 mg/dL at last follow-up (controls). RI patients tended to be older and had a lower mean glomerular filtration rate (GFR) at initial evaluation. There were no differences in race, gender, or previous history of hypertension between the two groups. Although both groups experienced an improvement in GFR at transplantation and a subsequent decline in GFR by 6 months posttransplantation, the RI group achieved a lower peak GFR at transplantation and a far lower mean GFR at the 6-month analysis. Only the RI group showed a continued decline in GFR. The RI group had more severe hypertension and required a significantly greater number of antihypertensive medications. The RI group had a higher mean total cholesterol at 6 months, but this difference was not sustained. They also had higher triglyceride levels and lower high-density lipoprotein (HDL) levels; there was no difference in low-density lipoprotein (LDL) levels. There was no difference in initial, maximum, or mean doses of cyclosporine at 6 months, or of cyclosporine levels at any time. We conclude that older patients with greater prior renal insufficiency and those whose 6-month GFR is more markedly depressed are at a higher risk for progressive renal failure. This group should be targeted for newer interventions to avoid renal failure.

INDEX WORDS: Cardiac transplantation; renal insufficiency; risk factors; lipids; cyclosporine.

THERE have been over 15,000 orthotopic cardiac transplantations performed, over 90% since 1985.[1] Patient survival after cardiac transplantation has progressively increased and is now greater than 75% at 5 years.[1] There is little doubt that the use of the potent immunosuppressive agent cyclosporine has contributed to the prolonged allograft and patient survival rates. As patient survival has increased, concerns about long-term problems such as progressive renal insufficiency have grown. Although progressive renal insufficiency was generally attributed to the very high nephrotoxic doses of cyclosporine originally used in cardiac transplantation, the use of lower doses in recent years does not appear to have eliminated this problem. Most cyclosporine-treated cardiac transplant patients develop some degree of renal insufficiency in the first 6 months after transplantation.[2,3] Many then appear to have stable renal function over the subsequent 3 to 4 years of follow-up. Only a few develop renal failure and require dialysis during this period.[2,3] However, there is clinical, morphologic, and physiologic evidence indicating that at least a subset of this population suffers a progressive decline in renal function at longer follow-up. In some programs, an increased incidence of severe renal insufficiency has been noted 7 to 8 years after transplantation.[4,5] On renal biopsy, Myers et al[6-8] documented evidence of arteriolopathy, interstitial scarring, and glomerulosclerosis, even when renal function appeared stable. Physiologic studies showed increased renal vascular resistance and decreased glomerular filtration rate (GFR) and renal plasma flow, which remained abnormal despite progressive lowering of the dose of cyclosporine over time.[6,8-12] In the renal transplant population the long-term influence of cyclosporine on renal function is clouded by the effects of rejection on graft morphology and function.[13,14] In nontransplant populations receiving cyclosporine for autoimmune disease, a number of factors have been correlated with biopsy-proven cyclosporine nephrotoxicity, including patient age, cyclosporine dose, and maximum percentage increase in the serum creatinine.[15] After a reduction in cyclosporine dose, these patients had only a partial improvement in renal function. None developed progressive renal failure in the relatively

Dr Sehgal is supported in part by a clinical fellowship grant from the National Kidney Foundation of New York/New Jersey.

short 2-year follow-up period. In another study of patients with autoimmune disease, even low-dose cyclosporine (<4 mg/kg/day) for prolonged periods was associated with morphologic evidence of progressive renal damage on repeat biopsies.[16] In cardiac transplant patients little is known about other risk factors for developing renal insufficiency. Some investigators reported that episodes of acute renal insufficiency secondary to hemodynamically mediated dose-related cyclosporine nephrotoxicity did not correlate with long-term renal insufficiency, whereas others did find a correlation.[17,18] Hypertension has been an extremely common finding in cyclosporine-treated patients and may also contribute to renal insufficiency in the cardiac transplant population.[19] Studies of the effects of various antihypertensives on blood pressure and renal function have been inconclusive.[10,20-24] Cyclosporine has also been reported to increase serum cholesterol levels in allograft recipients, which may be a factor in the accelerated atherosclerosis observed in the transplant population.[25-28] The influence of dyslipidemia on the progression of renal disease has been documented in animal models.[29] It is unclear if dyslipidemia contributes to the renal insufficiency of cardiac transplant patients.

At Columbia Presbyterian Medical Center a preliminary analysis of cardiac transplant patients showed renal insufficiency to be a significant problem. Over 15% of cardiac transplant patients followed over 1 year had serum creatinine values over 2.5 mg/dL. At least 10 patients have developed end-stage renal disease (ESRD) related to cardiac transplant. To identify the risk factors associated with the development of progressive renal insufficiency in cardiac transplant patients, we analyzed data from a cohort of cardiac transplant patients with severe renal insufficiency (serum creatinine ≥ 2.4 mg/dL) and compared them with cardiac transplant patients without evidence of severe renal dysfunction at last follow-up (serum creatinine ≤ 1.7 mg/dL).

PATIENTS AND METHODS

Of a total of 334 patients undergoing cardiac transplantation at Columbia Presbyterian Medical Center from 1988 to 1991, 257 were adults. We considered only those patients surviving at least 3 years for our analysis. There were 39 adult patients who had survived at least 3 years and had a serum creatinine at last follow-up that was ≥2.4 mg/dL (renal insufficiency or RI group). There were 41 patients with a serum creatinine at last follow-up ≤1.7 mg/dL and an equal survival time, who served as controls. Patients with serum creatinine levels between 1.7 mg/dL and 2.3 mg/dL were excluded from analysis because it was unclear whether they would develop progressive renal insufficiency.

Oliguric patients and patients with baseline renal dysfunction at the time of transplantation (serum creatinine > 2.0 mg/dL) were treated initially with OKT3 induction. Cyclosporine therapy was started between days 0 to 4 posttransplantation, and was given initially at a dose of 6 mg/kg/day and titrated up to a trough level of approximately 250 ng/mL. The maintenance dose of cyclosporine was 4 to 6 mg/kg/day, with the dose titrated to maintain trough serum levels during the first year at 250 ng/mL. After the first year of therapy cyclosporine levels were adjusted downward to a level above 100 ng/mL. Trough cyclosporine levels were measured using a nonspecific, serum polyclonal radioimmunoassay (normal therapeutic range for renal transplant, 100 to 250 ng/mL). During the initial 2 years of the study, patients received cyclosporine plus prednisone maintenance therapy, and they received triple therapy including azathioprine during the later years of the study.

Information obtained from medical records and computer-based files included patient age, gender, race, history of hypertension, diabetes, and presence of underlying renal disease. Cyclosporine doses in mg/kg/day were recorded and analyzed as follows: initial dose, maximum dose, mean dose for the first 6 months posttransplantation, and dose at yearly intervals thereafter. Severity of hypertension was graded on a scale of zero to three, based on the mean of at least two blood pressure readings obtained by patients, visiting nurses at home, or during routine office visits. The following blood pressure ranges were assigned grades of 0, 1, 2, and 3, respectively: ≤140/90 mm Hg, 140 to 159/90 to 99 mm Hg, 160 to 179/100 to 109 mm Hg, and ≥180/110 mm Hg. The number of antihypertensive medications used for treatment were recorded at patient listing for cardiac transplantation, at time of transplant, at 6 months posttransplantation, and at yearly intervals thereafter. The use of potentially nephrotoxic medications, medications that might interfere with cyclosporine metabolism, and antihyperlipidemic agents was also recorded at similar intervals. All available serum creatinine levels, cyclosporine levels, and lipid profiles were reviewed from the time of listing for cardiac transplantation. The maximum percent increase in serum creatinine above the nadir posttransplantation value at 1 month, 6 months, and 12 months after transplantation was recorded. GFRs were calculated for each interval based on the formula of Cockcroft and Gault.[30] The parameters used to assess cyclosporine toxicity were the number of months during which toxic levels (>250 ng/mL) were obtained and the number of episodes of reversible azotemia associated with toxic cyclosporine levels.

Statistical analysis was performed using the SAS software system. Wilcoxon rank sum analyses were used to compare age, severity of hypertension, and episodes of cyclosporine toxicity. The natural logarithms of the data were used to obtain normalized distributions, and *t*-tests were used to compare cyclosporine doses, lipid data, and maximum percent increase in creatinine. Patients who were using medications that interfere with cyclosporine metabolism were excluded from the analysis of cyclosporine dosing. Spearman's rho tests were used to test correlations between cholesterol and episodes of cyclosporine toxicity. Two-tailed Fisher's exact tests were used to compare demographic data.

RESULTS

The patients were followed for a mean of 4.7 years (range, 3 to 6 years). There was no difference in length of follow-up between the study group and controls. Three of the patients with renal insufficiency had a known history of renal disease (nephrolithiasis, contrast nephropathy, uninephrectomy), compared with one of the controls (nephrolithiasis). Four of the RI patients had a history of diabetes mellitus before transplant, compared with two control patients. After transplantation, three patients in the control group and four in the RI group were exposed to nephrotoxic drugs (amphotericin, gancyclovir, high-dose nonsteroidal antiinflammatory agents). Three patients in the RI group developed illnesses that may have contributed to chronic renal insufficiency (two had abdominal aortic aneurysms and one had prostate cancer with ureteral obstruction), but none progressed to ESRD. There were two deaths in the control group and three in the RI group. Six of the 39 study patients progressed to ESRD in a mean time of 4.7 years after transplantation (range, 3 to 6 years). None had a history of renal disease or any subsequent complications that may have contributed to their renal disease. No patient in the control group progressed to ESRD.

Patients in the RI group were significantly older than controls ($P < 0.01$). There were no differences in race or gender between the RI group and controls. Demographic data are shown in Table 1.

Patients who developed renal insufficiency had lower mean GFR at evaluation, at time of transplantation, and at every interval after transplantation ($P < 0.001$). Both groups experienced an improvement in GFR at the time of transplantation and similar absolute declines in renal function within 6 months of transplantation, but only the RI group experienced a continued decline thereafter. At last follow-up, the RI group had a mean GFR of 28.5 ± 3.7 mL/min, compared with 84.1 ± 8.5 mL/min in the control group (Fig 1). The maximum percent increase in serum creatinine was greater in the RI group between 1 and 6 months after transplantation (218% ± 20% *v* 158% ± 21%, $P < 0.005$), but not within 1 month of transplantation (109% ± 11% *v* 125% ± 16%, P = NS), or between 6 and 12 months afterwards (203% ± 17% *v* 147% ± 10%, $P = 0.05$).

Table 1. Demographic and Clinical Data at the Time of Evaluation for Cardiac Transplantation in 80 Patients

At Time of Transplantation	RI (n = 39)	Controls (n = 41)	*P* Value
Age (yrs)	53.4 + 1.5	45.8 + 2.0	<0.01
Male:female	32:7	32:9	NS
White race	35	32	NS
History of hypertension	27	31	NS
History of diabetes	4	2	NS
History of renal disease	3	1	NS

Abbreviation: RI, renal insufficiency at last follow-up.

Twenty-seven of the RI patients had a known history of hypertension, compared with 31 controls (P = NS). After transplantation, 36 RI patients and 28 controls developed hypertension (P = NS). Patients with RI had more severe hypertension than controls. From years 1 to 4 after transplantation, their blood pressures were higher than the control group (Fig 2). They required a significantly greater number of antihypertensive medications within 2 years after transplantation (mean number of medications, 1.87 *v* 1.09, $P < 0.05$). The RI group had a higher mean total cholesterol level at 6 months after transplantation (262 ± 13 mg/dL *v* 220 ± 11 mg/dL, $P < 0.05$), but this difference was not sustained (Fig 3). They also had a higher mean triglyceride level (298 ± 42 mg/dL *v* 181 ± 18 mg/dL, $P < 0.01$) and lower high-density lipoprotein (HDL) (44 ± 3 mg/dL *v* 51 ± 3 mg/dL, $P < 0.05$). There was no difference in the low-density lipoprotein (LDL) (162 ± 10 mg/dL *v* 185 ± 14 mg/dL, P = NS). There was no correlation between serum cholesterol and creatinine or serum cholesterol and episodes of cyclosporine toxicity. Fourteen controls and 10 RI patients were treated for hyperlipidemia.

There were no differences in initial (7.79 ± 0.64 *v* 7.38 ± 0.55 mg/kg/day), maximum (13.8 ± 0.92 *v* 14.7 ± 1.76 mg/kg/day), or mean

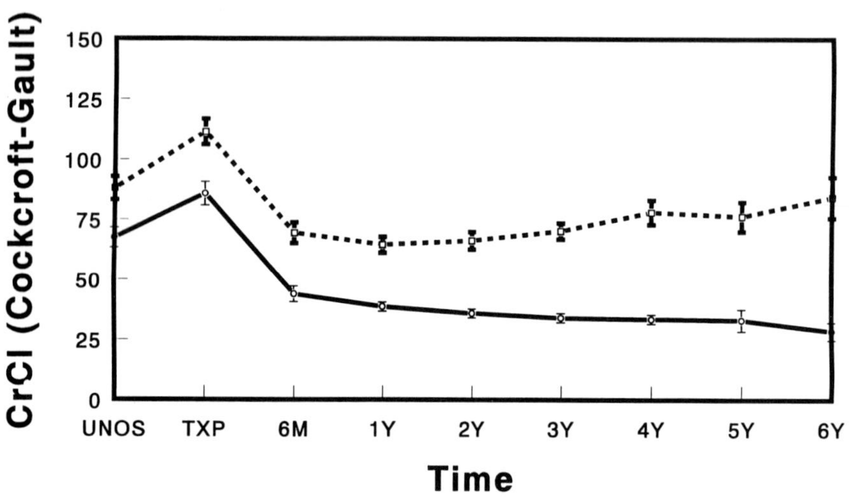

Fig 1. Graph showing the course of creatinine clearance before transplantation and over 6 years of follow-up in patients with renal insufficiency (RI) (— ○ —) and controls (- - □ - -).

6-month (9.71 ± 0.43 *v* 9.91 ± 0.60 mg/kg/day) cyclosporine doses, mean cyclosporine levels at any interval, or episodes of cyclosporine toxicity associated with reversible azotemia between the two groups. The control group had a significantly greater number of months during which toxic cyclosporine levels were recorded at 2 years after transplantation ($P < 0.05$).

DISCUSSION

With improved graft and patient survival through the use of cyclosporine A, the prospect of long-term nephrotoxicity and renal insufficiency has become a significant concern for patients with organ transplants. In renal transplant recipients, a number of studies have shown that, despite initially higher levels of plasma creatinine and reduced GFRs in patients receiving cyclosporine, renal survival is improved when compared with patients receiving non–cyclosporine-based immunosuppressive regimens. A recent multicenter study of more than 1,500 cyclosporine-treated renal transplant recipients reported a 78% graft survival at 36 months after the transplantation.[31] Despite an initial decline in renal function, serum creatinine remained stable in this population at over 4.5 years. Only 22% of the patients were followed at least 4 years posttransplantation, making conclusions on the safety of long-term cyclosporine use difficult. One study of 347 cyclosporine-treated renal transplant recipients who had renal function for 55 months showed that subsequent graft loss was attributable to death, chronic rejection, noncompliance, or recurrence of the primary disease.[32] There was no change in the mean serum creatinine in 100 patients followed for 7 years and in seven patients followed for 10 years after transplantation, and the authors concluded that there was no evidence of progressive deterioration in renal allograft function attributable to cyclosporine nephrotoxicity. However, study of cyclosporine nephrotoxicity and the progression of renal damage in the renal allograft is complicated by the residua of episodes of acute and chronic rejection. The cardiac transplant population with presumably normal native kidneys should provide an excellent group in which to study chronic cyclosporine nephrotoxicity and the factors associated with progressive renal

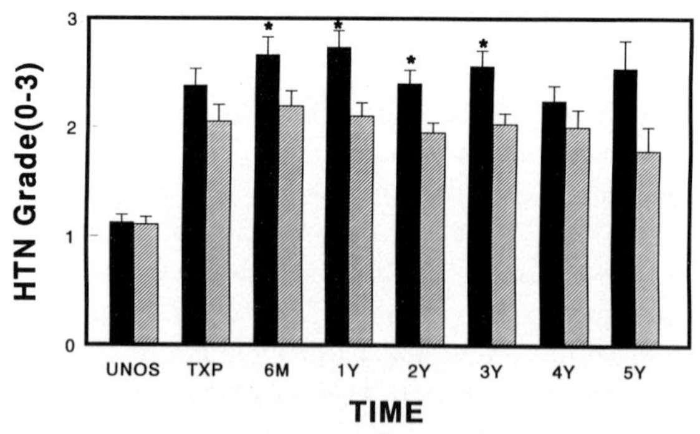

Fig 2. Severity of hypertension over the period of follow-up (grades of blood pressure 0, 1, 2, and 3, respectively: ≤140/90 mm hg, 140-159/90-99 mm hg, 160-179/100-109 mm hg, and ≥180/110 mm hg). *$P < 0.05$. (■) RI; (▨) controls.

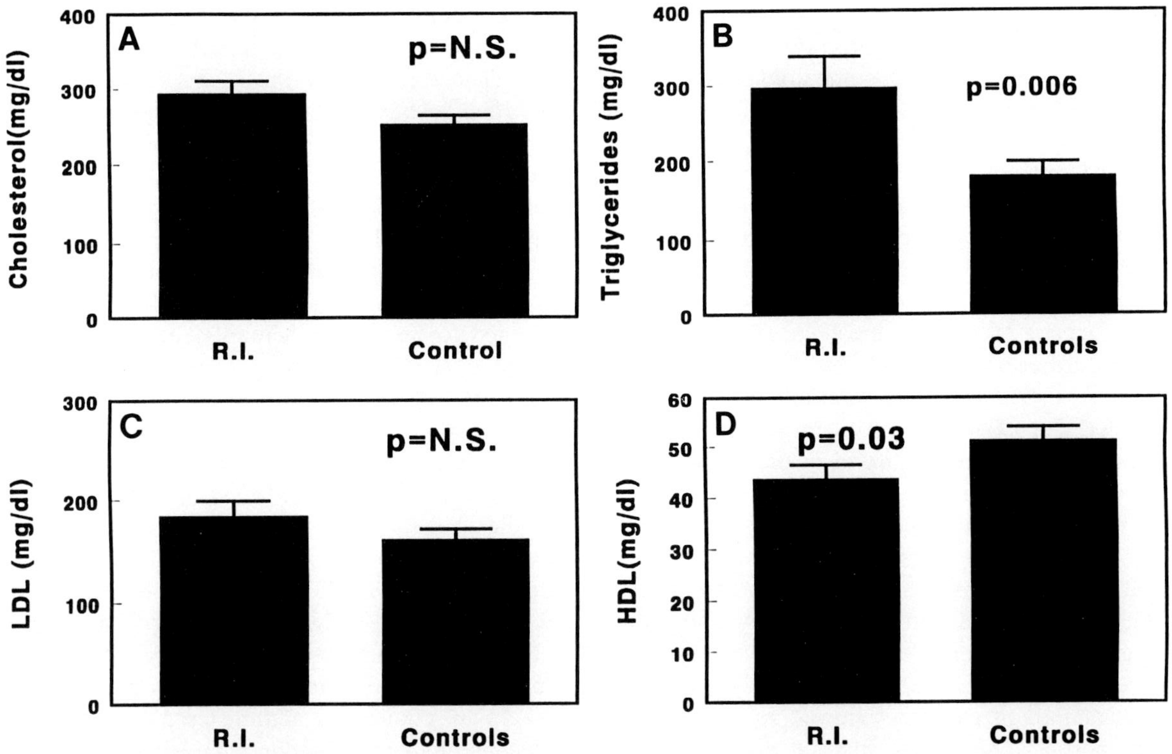

Fig 3. **Mean lipid profiles for total cholesterol (A), triglycerides (B), LDL cholesterol (C), and HDL cholesterol 2 to 5 years after transplantation.**

damage. In a preliminary analysis at Columbia Presbyterian Medical Center we found that, of approximately 500 current cardiac transplantation patients, 15% have a serum creatinine over 2.5 mg/dL. As in other heart transplantation populations we have documented cases progressing to ESRD with biopsy changes compatible with cyclosporine nephrotoxicity.

Myers and the group at Stanford first called attention to this problem a decade ago.[7] They evaluated the GFR in 17 heart transplantation patients treated with cyclosporine and compared them with 15 heart transplantation patients treated with azathioprine. Despite equivalent cardiac outputs, the GFR was markedly depressed in the cyclosporine-treated patients. This was associated with decreased renal function as well as a trend toward restricted transport of neutral dextrans, suggesting loss of ultrafiltration capacity by glomerular capillaries. Histologic examination of the kidneys of five patients showed degrees of tubulointerstitial nephritis and focal glomerular sclerosis. A follow-up study by the Stanford group showed a larger population of cyclosporine-treated patients who developed a similar decreased GFR when compared with azathioprine-treated patients.[6] The cyclosporine-treated patients had elevated renal vascular resistance, proteinuria, and hypertension, as well as an obliterative arteriolopathy and tubulointerstitial damage. Although cyclosporine dose was decreased over 48 months in this population, the reduction in GFR and the other hemodynamic changes persisted. Repeat renal biopsies showed progressive renal damage in some patients, and three patients developed ESRD. Similar histologic and physiologic findings have been documented by others in cardiac transplantation populations.[8,10]

Many other groups have found that after an initial decline from preoperative levels the GFR remains stable over 4 to 6 years of follow-up.[3,10,11,12] Even with biologic induction therapy (OKT3, antilymphocyte globulin, antithrombocyte globulin) and low-dose cyclosporine the initial decrease in GFR still occurs. Although it has been suggested that this stable renal function after the initial decline predicts better preserved renal function over time, some argue that hyperfiltration of remaining nephrons and increased tubular secretion of creatinine are compensating for the reduced renal function, and that, based on both morphologic and physiologic measurements, progressive, irreversible nephron damage is being produced by cyclosporine.[6,8] It is hypothesized that when the fraction of impaired nephrons exceeds a certain threshold, GFR will decline further and lead to ESRD.[5]

Few studies have longer periods of follow-up. A study of 10 heart transplant patients whose renal function was evaluated in detail by inulin and para-aminohippurate clearance at 2 to 3 and 6 years posttransplantation showed stabilized renal function at long-term follow-up, after an initial decline in GFR.[12] The number of patients studied was small in this analysis, and they started with normal renal function as a group. Greenberg et al[4] reported their findings on heart transplantation patients followed for 7 years at Pittsburgh.[4] They found that the plasma creatinine rose from a mean of 1.2 mg/dL at transplantation to 2.0 mg/dL at 2 to 4 years to 3.3 mg/dL at 7 years posttransplantation.[4] There was a biphasic decline in the renal function with a rapid decline initially (despite the use of lower cyclosporine dose regimens), and then a slower decline. Of 385 cardiac transplants followed at Stanford, approximately 10% progressed to ESRD over 8 years of follow-up.[5] The cumulative incidence rose sharply after 7 years of follow-up. This was true despite the use of reduced doses of cyclosporine (with 8 mg/kg daily as initial and 4 mg/kg daily as maintenance therapy). Similar data have been reported from Stanford on heart-lung transplantation patients.[5] Although cyclosporine has been incriminated as a major factor related to this decline in renal function, other potential factors such as hyperlipidemia and hypertension have not been examined as extensively.

To assess what factors might be related to renal dysfunction in the cardiac transplant population, we culled from a group of 257 adult heart transplant patients transplanted from 1988 to 1991 at Columbia Presbyterian Medical Center a subset of patients with depressed renal function (serum creatinine $\geq$ 2.4 mg/dL at last follow-up) and a control population with preserved renal function (serum creatinine $\leq$ 1.7 mg/dL at last follow-up). The selection of these cut-off values was justified because 6 of the 39 RI patients reached ESRD as opposed to none of the control patients during the same mean follow-up time. The difference in GFR between the two groups was highly significant at all times (GFR 28.5 $\pm$ 3.7 mL/min *v* 84.1 $\pm$ 8.5 mL/min in RI *v* controls at last follow-up). Records and computer files were examined for features potentially relating to renal damage at various times during the mean 4.7 years of follow-up after transplantation. Neither the initial, maximal, or 6-month mean cyclosporine dose, nor the blood cyclosporine levels at any interval, predicted renal insufficiency. In studies of nontransplant patients receiving cyclosporine for autoimmune disease, the daily dose in mg/kg/day of cyclosporine has correlated with histologic evidence of toxicity.[15] In transplant patients the drug dose is frequently adjusted, and medications interfering with blood levels are commonly administered (eg, calcium channel blockers, antiepileptic medications) with appropriate correction of the drug dose. In addition, when renal insufficiency develops, cyclosporine doses are often reduced. Despite these adjustments in dose, blood levels might be expected to correlate with renal damage, but they did not in our study. Indeed, the control population actually had a greater number of months with toxic levels recorded. In other transplant populations the correlation of chronic nephrotoxicity with blood levels of cyclosporine has also proven difficult.

Other factors such as race, gender, and age of the patient may affect the progression of certain forms of renal disease. For example, focal sclerosis is often a more aggressive disease in blacks, and certain glomerulopathies are more severe in men.[33] In our heart transplantation population neither race nor gender were associated with renal dysfunction. Increased age has been found to be a factor related to renal dysfunction in autoimmune populations treated with cyclosporine[15] and in some cardiac transplant patients.[4,17] In our study the group with renal insufficiency was significantly older at time of transplantation. Older patients may have reduced renal reserve with more severe effects of hyperfiltration on fewer remaining nephrons, alterations in vascular tone, and alterations in cyclosporine metabolism, or alterations in other factors such as diminished prostaglandin formation or increased growth factors promoting sclerosis and interstitial fibrosis. Clearly, as heart transplantation becomes more successful, older patients will be increasingly accepted into transplantation programs, and the risks of renal damage in this population will become a more important problem.

In populations of patients with autoimmune disease treated with cyclosporine, a known risk factor has been the initial rise in the serum creatinine level.[15] Those patients with a greater than 50% increase from their baseline serum creatinine were more likely to suffer chronic renal damage than those without such increase, regardless of dose administered or other risk factors. In our study, although the absolute magnitude of the decline in creatinine clearance was equal in both groups, the maximum percent decline in renal function from baseline was far greater in the group that had eventual worse renal function and was associated with progressively declining renal function subsequently. The group without eventual renal dysfunction had reduced function at 6 months, which remained stable over time. In both populations the initial posttransplantation GFR may represent a balance between improvement of prerenal azotemia, with the new heart improving renal perfusion, and the acute vasoconstriction of cyclosporine leading to a decrease in GFR. The fact that patients who did not manifest long-term renal dysfunction had greater absolute values for the GFR at transplantation may reflect either better intrinsic renal function once prerenal factors have been corrected or less of a vascular hemodynamic effect from the cyclosporine. Akin to patients with autoimmune disease, the larger increase in serum creatinine and decrease in GFR at 6 months did predict ultimate renal dysfunction.[15]

Although some studies have reported that episodes of perioperative acute renal insufficiency are associated with subsequent renal dysfunction,[18,19] others have not found such an association.[4] Neither of these studies reported the long-term renal outcomes of these patients. In our patients, acute renal dysfunction during the month after transplantation, as measured by the maximum percent increase in creatinine, was not associated with a poor renal outcome a mean of 4.7 years after transplantation.

Hyperlipidemia has long been known to be a clinical finding in many patients with renal insufficiency.[25,27,34-36] A survey of over 500 renal transplantation patients documented a 38% incidence of severe hypercholesterolemia (>300 mg/dL) within 6 months of transplantation, which decreased to 13% by 3 years.[26] Hyperlipidemia has been proposed as a factor in both accelerated atherosclerosis and in late renal allograft loss.[28] Renal transplantation patients with higher total cholesterol, triglyceride, and apolipoprotein-B levels have been shown to have a higher incidence of cardiovascular disease.[27] A number of factors have been related to the hyperlipidemia in both azathioprine- and cyclosporine-treated patients.[28] In the latter population renal dysfunction, pretransplantation lipid values, dose of corticosteroids, and doses and levels of cyclosporine have all been related to the hypercholesterolemia noted.[28] Conversion of patients from cyclosporine to azathioprine immunosuppression has resulted in lowering of serum cholesterol and triglyceride level, but without alteration in HDL cholesterol levels.[37]

Analysis of the lipids in our heart transplant population showed a trend toward hypercholesterolemia in the group that progressed to renal insufficiency. This was statistically significant only at 6 months posttransplantation. Triglycerides, however, were significantly elevated in the renal insufficiency group at the 2- to 5-year period posttransplantation. There was no significant difference in LDL cholesterol between the groups, but HDL cholesterol was lower in the group with renal insufficiency. It is possible that the elevated triglycerides and low HDL cholesterol reflect merely worsening renal function because this is the pattern noted in chronic renal failure and uremic populations.[25] It is also possible that the lipid abnormalities lead to accelerated atherosclerosis. Whether the elevated cholesterol levels in some patients contribute to the progression of renal dysfunction in this population is unknown.[29] It is of interest that seven of the nine patients with long-term cholesterol levels greater than 300 mg/dL were in the renal insufficiency group.

Hypertension is a well-documented factor in the progression of many renal diseases. In the cardiac transplantation population, hypertension occurs in 44% to 90% of patients 2 years after transplant.[6,18] In most studies, the majority of cyclosporine-treated patients have been hypertensive. Cyclosporine use can contribute to hypertension in a number of ways. It increases vascular smooth muscle tone, the response of the vascular smooth muscle to vasoconstrictors, and the production of endothelin, while inhibiting the production of vasodilators such as prostaglandins.[22] Hypertension has been present in patients treated with both low-dose and high-dose cyclosporine.[20] There is considerable debate as to which antihypertensive regimen is most beneficial in this population.[10,19,21-24] Some studies have found renal dysfunction to correlate with the presence of hypertension.[19] In our population the incidence of hypertension at transplantation was not significantly greater in the renal insufficiency group. However, the patients who developed renal insufficiency had more severe hypertension in spite of treatment with a greater number of medications. Presumably this hypertension may have contributed to the progression of renal insufficiency in this population.

As cardiac and other solid organ transplantation become more successful, physicians will focus not only on short-term survival, but on the long-term complications of transplantation as well. The cardiac transplantation population with intrinsically normal native kidney function provides a good group to analyze factors leading to renal dysfunction. The potent immunosuppressive cyclosporine has made long-term survival after cardiac transplantation more commonplace. It is also associated with renal dysfunction, hyperlipidemia, and hypertension. In this study we have compared a group of long-term survivors after heart transplantation with renal dysfunction with a group with preserved renal function. Increased age, the severity of hypertension of the patient, lower initial and subsequent GFR at transplant, and certain posttransplantation lipid abnormalities correlate with poor function at last follow-up. It remains to be clarified in what manner such factors are related to the renal dysfunction, whether they can be modified, or whether different immunosuppressive regimens can preserve renal function in this segment of the heart transplantation population.

ACKNOWLEDGMENT

The authors thank Dr Beverly Diamond, The Irving Center for Clinical Research (National Institutes of Health, Bethesda, MD, grant no. RR00645), for help with statistical methods.

REFERENCES

1. Kaye MP: The long-term effects of cyclosporine in heart transplant patients. Transplant Proc 22:12-14, 1990 (Suppl 1)

2. Lewis RM, Van Buren CT, Radovancevic B, Frazier OH, Janney RP, Powers PL, Golden DL, Giannakis JG, Macris MP, Kerman RH, Kahan BD: Impact of long-term cyclosporine immunosuppressive therapy on native kidneys versus renal allografts: Serial renal function in heart and kidney transplant recipients. J Heart Lung Transplant 10:63-70, 1991

3. Gonwa TA, Mai ML, Pilcher J, Johnson C, Pierson S, Capehart JE, Alivizatos PA: Stability of long-term renal function in heart transplant patients treated with induction therapy and low-dose cyclosporine. J Heart Lung Transplant 11:926-928, 1992

4. Greenberg A, Thompson ME, Griffith BJ, Hardesty RL, Kormos RL, El-Shahawy MA, Janosky JE, Puschett JB: Cyclosporine nephrotoxicity in cardiac allograft patients: A seven-year follow-up. Transplantation 50:589-593, 1990

5. Myers BD, Newton L, Oyer P: The case against the indefinite use of cyclosporine. Transplant Proc 23:41-42, 1991

6. Myers BD, Sibley R, Newton L, Tomlanoivich SJ, Boshkos C, Stinson E, Luetscher JA, Whitney DJ, Krasny D, Coplon NS, Perlroth MG: The long-term course of cyclosporine-associated chronic nephropathy. Kidney Int 33:590-600, 1988

7. Myers BD, Ross J, Newton L, Luetscher J, Perlroth M: Cyclosporine-associated chronic nephropathy. N Engl J Med 311:699-705, 1984

8. Bertani T, Ferrazzi P, Schieppati A, Ruggenenti P, Gamba A, Parenzan L, Mecca G, Perico N, Imberti O, Remuzzi A, Remuzzi G: Nature and extent of glomerular injury induced by cyclosporine in heart transplant patients. Kidney Int 40:243-250, 1991

9. Myers BD, Newton L, Boshkos C, Macoviak JA, Frist WH, Derby GC, Perlroth MG, Sibley RK: Chronic injury of human renal microvessels with low-dose cyclosporine therapy. Transplantation 46:694-703, 1988

10. Bantle JP, Paller MS, Boudreau RJ, Olivari MT, Ferris TF: Long-term effects of cyclosporine on renal function in organ transplant recipients. J Lab Clin Med 115:233-240, 1990

11. Waser M, Maggiorini M, Binswanger U, Keusch G, Carrel T, von Segesser L, Gallino A, Turina M: Irreversibility of cyclosporine-induced renal function impairment in heart transplant recipients. J Heart Lung Transplant 12:846-850, 1993

12. Ruggenenti P, Perico N, Amuchastegui S, Ferrazzi P, Mamprin F, Remuzzi G: Following an initial decline, glomerular filtration rate stabilizes in heart transplant patients on chronic cyclosporine. Am J Kidney Dis 24:549-553, 1994

13. Luke RG: New issues in therapy after renal transplantation. N Engl J Med 331:393-394, 1994

14. Myers BD: Nephrology Forum: Cyclosporine nephrotoxicity. Kidney Int 30:964-974, 1986

15. Feutren G, Mihatsch MJ: Risk factors for cyclosporine-induced nephropathy in patients with autoimmune diseases. N Engl J Med 326:1654-1660, 1992

16. Young EW, Ellis CN, Messana JM, Johynson KJ, Leichtman AB, Mihatsch MJ, Hamilton TA, Groisser DS, Fradin MS, Voorhees JJ: A prospective study of renal structure and function in psoriasis patients treated with cyclosporine. Kidney Int 45:1216-1222, 1994

17. Greenberg A, Egel JW, Thompson ME, Hardesty RL, Griffith BP, Bahnson HT, Bernstein RL, Hastillo A, Hess ML, Puschett JB: Early and late forms of cyclosporine nephrotoxicity: Studies in cardiac transplant patients. Am J Kidney Dis 9:12-22, 1987

18. Miller LW, Pennington DG, McBride LR: Long-term effects of cyclosporine in cardiac transplantation. Transplant Proc 22:15-20, 1990 (Suppl 1)

19. Miller LW, O'Connell JB: Long-term use of cyclosporine in cardiac transplantation. Transplant Proc 22:1, 1990 (Suppl 1)

20. Moore CK, Renlund LG, Rasmussen LG, O'Connell JB: Long-term morbidity of cyclosporine with corticosteroid-free maintenance immunosuppression in cardiac transplantation. Transplant Proc 22:25-29, 1990 (Suppl 1)

21. Schecter D, Ziady GM, Lee A, Armitage JM, Kormos RL, Griffith BP, Hardesty RL: Efficacy of antihypertensive medication in orthotopic heart transplant recipients and its effect on renal function. Angiology 43:585-589, 1992

22. Bunke M, Ganzel B: Effect of calcium channel antagonists on renal function in hypertensive heart transplant recipients. J Heart Lung Transplant 11:1194-1199, 1992

23. Elliott WJ, Murphy MB, Karp R: Long-term preservation of renal function in hypertensive heart transplant recipients treated with enalapril and a diuretic. J Heart Lung Transplant 10:373-379, 1991

24. Ruggenenti P, Perico N, Mosconi L, Gaspari F, Benigni A, Amuchastegui CS, Bruzzi I, Remuzzi G: Calcium channel blockers protect transplant patients from cyclosporine-induced daily renal hypoperfusion. Kidney Int 43:706-711, 1993

25. Appel GB: Nephrology Forum: Lipid abnormalities in renal disease. Kidney Int 39:169-183, 1991

26. Vathsala A, Weinberg RB, Schoenberg L, Grevel J, Dunn J, Goldstein RA, Van Buren CT, Lewis RM, Kahan BD: Lipid abnormalities in cyclosporine-prednisone-treated renal transplant recipients. Transplantation 48:37-43, 1989

27. Drueke TB, Abdulmassih Z, Lacour B, Bader C, Chevalier A, Kreis H: Atherosclerosis and lipid disorders after renal transplantation. Kidney Int 39:S24-S28, 1991 (Suppl 31)

28. Markell MS, Friedman EA: Hyperlipidemia after organ transplantation. Am J Med 87:5-61N-5-67N, 1989

29. Keane WF, Mulcahy WS, Kasiske BL, Kim Y, O'Donnell MP: Hyperlipidemia and progressive renal disease. Kidney Int 39:S41-S48, 1991 (Suppl 31)

30. Cockroft DW, Gault MH: Prediction of creatinine clearance from serum creatinine. Nephron 16:31-41, 1976

31. Burke JF, Pirsch JD, Ramos EL, Salomon DR, Stablein DM, Van Buren DH, West JC: Long-term efficacy and safety of cyclosporine in renal-transplant recipients. N Engl J Med 331:358-363, 1994

32. Almond PS, Gillingham KJ, Sibley R, Moss A, Melin M, Leventhal J, Manivel C, Kyriakides P, Payne WD, Dunn DL, Sutherland DER, Gores PF, Najarian JS, Matas AJ: Renal transplant function after ten years of cyclosporine. Transplantation 53:316-323, 1992

33. Ingulli E, Tejani A: Racial differences in the incidence and renal outcome of idiopathic focal segmental glomerulosclerosis in children. Pediatr Nephrol 5:393-397, 1991

34. Ibels LS, Simons LA, King JO, Williams PF, Neale FC, Stewart JH: Studies on the nature and causes of hyperlipidaemia in uraemia, maintenance dialysis, and renal transplantation. Q J Med XLIV:601-614, 1975

35. Ponticelli C, Barbi GL, Cantaluppi A, DeVecchi A, Annoni G, Donati C, Cecchettin M: Lipid disorders in renal transplant recipients. Nephron 20:189-195, 1978

36. Cattran DC, Steiner G, Wilson DR, Fenton SA: Hyperlipidemia after renal transplantation: Natural history and pathophysiology. Ann Intern Med 91:554-559, 1979

37. Harris KPG, Russell GI, Parvin SD, Veitch PS, Walls J: Alterations in lipid and carbohydrate metabolism attributable to cyclosporin A in renal transplant recipients. BMJ 292:16, 1986

UREMIA AND RENAL REPLACEMENT THERAPY

Introduction

A host of metabolic and nutritional disorders develop in the course of progressive renal failure. These include changes in water and electrolyte metabolism, carbohydrate intolerance, alterations in lipid and protein metabolism, endocrine disorders, and musculoskeletal and neurological abnormalities. Renal replacement therapy (dialysis, transplantation) may ameliorate or aggravate some of the manifestations due to chronic renal insufficiency. Malnutrition is a major cause of morbidity and mortality in patients with end-stage renal disease on replacement therapy.

Levine and Gordon review the data available on measurement of lipoprotein(a) [LP(a)], a genetically determined risk factor for atherosclerosis and vascular disease, in patients receiving renal replacement therapy. They describe the difficulties in accurate measurement of LP(a), the way it functions as an acute phase reactant, and the marked ethnic variation in LP(a) levels. Although variability in results was seen, Lp(a) levels are elevated in dialysis patients. Renal transplantation partially reverses this effect. It is tempting to speculate on the role of elevated levels in the vascular complications observed in dialysis patients.

Goldwasser et al expand on their studies and on those of others that identified low serum cholesterol and albumin as important markers in dialysis patients. In a 14-month study of hemodialysis patients, the authors examined the prognostic value of LP(a) as an independent correlate of coronary risk and other vascular disease in the general population and of serum prealbumin as a sensitive indicator of nutritional status. They found that reduced serum prealbumin, independent of the levels of other visceral and somatic protein markers, was an important predictor of mortality in hemodialysis patients and that increased serum LP(a) predicted vascular access thrombosis and stenosis.

Thillet et al confirm (1) a significant elevation of LP(a) concentration in patients treated by continuous ambulatory peritoneal dialysis (CAPD) versus healthy controls and (2) no correlation of LP(a) concentration with any other lipid-lipoprotein parameter investigated or with the patients' age, previous clinical history, and duration of CAPD treatment. The study does not highlight any specific value of LP(a) concentration as an independent risk factor for cardiovascular complications in uremic patients treated with CAPD.

Brown et al report a clinical study of pharmacologic treatment of hyperlipidemia associated with the nephrotic syndrome using lovostatin. After 8 weeks of treatment, total cholesterol and LDL cholesterol levels decreased significantly. Interestingly, plasma Lp(a) levels were decreased, but only in patients with elevated baseline levels.

Avram et al report a 7-year prospective study of predictors for mortality risk in hemodialysis and CAPD patients, noting that age, diabetic status, and single enrollment levels of serum albumin and creatinine are independent predictors of long-term survival. Prealbumin was an important risk predictor, as well, and was more highly correlated with other nutritional markers than was albumin. These findings suggest that biochemical measures associated with visceral and somatic protein depletion are predominant long-term mortality risk factors in patients on renal replacement therapy.

Lowrie et al retrospectively analyzed variables associated with 1-year survival in a large, multicenter dialysis population, and found strikingly similar correlates associated with peritoneal dialysis and hemodialysis. The important variables were similar among patients receiving peritoneal dialysis or hemodialysis and were related to nutrition, acid-base status (which is related to nutrition), and age.

Bergström provides a review of the multiple causes of protein-calorie malnutrition in maintenance dialysis patients, some related to comorbidity factors but many related to the toxic and metabolic effects of renal failure and its dialytic replacement. Low intake of protein and energy as well as catabolic effects of acidosis, energy depletion, loss of nutrients, and inflammatory responses to dialysis are involved to varying degrees.

Metabolic acidosis is common in patients with renal failure and is associated with increased mortality risk. Reaich et al report that metabolic acidosis stimulates both amino acid oxidation and protein degradation in muscle and, therefore, could overcome adaptive responses to limited dietary protein intake. This may explain the common occurrence of somatic protein wasting in uremia, which has been associated with excessive morbidity and mortality.

Kopple et al find decreased insulin-like growth factor-1 (IGF-1) receptor activity in the skeletal muscle of uremic rats, which may explain resistance to IGF-1 and, therefore, skeletal muscle atrophy, altered physiology, and dysfunction in chronic renal failure.

Ikizler et al document prospectively a progressive decrease in dietary protein intake in patients with progressive renal failure and review the measures that can be taken to improve the nutritional status of long-term dialysis patients, including early institution of dialysis, increasing dialysis doses, and use of biocompatible membranes or dialysis solutions and intensive nutritional interventions. Results with intradialytic parenteral nutrition in hemodialysis and amino acid dialysate solutions are inconclusive, but the use of pronutritional agents, such as recombinant human growth hormone and IGF-1 appears to be promising.

Lipoprotein(a) Levels in Patients Receiving Renal Replacement Therapy: Methodologic Issues and Clinical Implications

Daniel M. Levine, PhD, and Bruce R. Gordon, MD

● Lipoprotein(a) [Lp(a)] is a genetically determined risk factor for vascular disease and a potential link between coagulation, lipoproteins, and the development of atherosclerosis. Its role in the vascular complications of patients with chronic renal disease is unclear. We review methodologic issues involved in measuring Lp(a), particularly as they relate to studies of patients with chronic renal disease. The accurate measurement of Lp(a) is difficult because all the commercially available assays are sensitive to apolipoprotein(a) isoform size, Lp(a) behaves like an acute phase reactant, and levels vary markedly among ethnic groups. The results of 12 studies that included data on median Lp(a) levels in controls and patients receiving renal replacement therapy were analyzed. Although there was variation among studies, most found elevated levels of Lp(a) in patients receiving hemodialysis (range of medians, 9.0 to 38.4 mg/dL) compared with controls (range of medians, 4.7 to 19.7 mg/dL). With the exception of one study, Lp(a) levels also were elevated in patients receiving continuous ambulatory peritoneal dialysis compared with controls and patients receiving hemodialysis. In one study, an elevated Lp(a) level in patients receiving hemodialysis correlated with subsequent development of vascular events. A separate study associated the occurrence of vascular access occlusion with Lp(a) level. Following renal transplantation, Lp(a) levels decreased in all four studies, which included data before and after transplantation. Although variability in results were seen, Lp(a) levels appear to be elevated in patients receiving renal replacement therapy. Renal transplantation at least partially reverses this effect. The variability in results is probably related to methodologic difficulties in measuring Lp(a) and failure to segregate ethnic groups in study design and analysis. Therefore, current and prior studies of Lp(a) should be interpreted cautiously.

INDEX WORDS: Lipoprotein(a); dialysis; renal transplant.

LIPOPROTEIN(a) [Lp(a)] holds a special fascination for clinicians and researchers with an interest in lipid disorders because it represents a potential link between coagulation, lipoproteins, and the development of atherosclerosis. The importance of Lp(a) in patients with renal disease is just now beginning to be appreciated.

Kare Berg discovered Lp(a) in 1963,[1,2] at which time it was considered to be a variant of low-density lipoprotein. By the mid-1980s it was recognized as a genetically determined risk factor for vascular disease.[3,4] Lipoprotein(a) is a heterogeneous family of carbohydrate-rich particles consisting of an apolipoprotein(a) [apo(a)] molecule joined by a disulfide linkage to apolipoprotein B-100 as part of low-density lipoprotein. In addition to this common form, Lp(a) also may circulate in a triglyceride-rich particle or in small amounts as a lipid-free complex.[5] In 1987, the gene for the apo(a) portion of Lp(a) was cloned and the protein sequence was deduced and found to have a striking homology to the sequence for plasminogen.[6,7] The structure of plasminogen includes an active serine protease domain and a single copy of kringles types 1 to 5. Apolipoprotein(a) contains an inactive serine protease domain, a variable number of copies of the kringle 4 domain, and one copy of kringle 5.[8] (The term "kringle" refers to a pretzel-shaped structure that is stabilized by three disulfide bonds.)

Although the association of Lp(a) with increased risk for atherosclerosis is apparent, the mechanism for this effect is unclear. Determination of mechanisms is made more difficult by the lack of understanding of Lp(a)'s normal biologic function. The similarity of components of Lp(a) to both low-density lipoprotein and plasminogen has led to the suggestion that Lp(a) may represent a bridge between the fields of atherosclerosis and thrombosis.[9] Possible mechanisms for a pro-atherogenic effect of Lp(a) include inhibition of fibrinolysis,[10-15] increase in plasminogen activator inhibitor,[16] inhibition of transforming growth factor-β, which can cause an increase in smooth muscle cell proliferation,[17,18] and incorporation of apo(a), Lp(a), and Lp(a) cholesterol into plaque.[19-26]

MEASUREMENT OF LIPOPROTEIN(a)

There are a number of potential difficulties in accurately measuring Lp(a) (for review, see Marcovina et al[27]). Apolipoprotein(a) is one of the most polymorphic proteins in blood. There are 10 different types of kringle 4 in apo(a); type 1 and types 3 to 10 are found singly. The number of copies of kringle 4 type 2 has been demon-

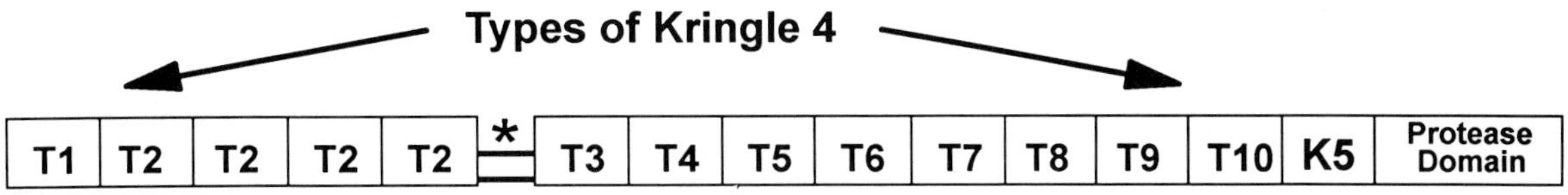

Fig 1. Apolipoprotein(a) is composed of 10 types (T1 to T10) of kringle 4, one copy of kringle 5 (K5), and an inactive protease domain. Kringle 4 type 2 may be repeated up to 40 times.

strated to vary between 3 and 40, and it is the number of these repeats that determines the size of apo(a) and, consequently, the size of Lp(a), and gives origin to the 34 isoforms that have been identified to date (Fig 1).[28-30] Most individuals have two different isoforms of Lp(a), which are genetically determined and can differ in size and structure. Lipoprotein(a) levels and isoforms vary greatly between ethnic groups.[8,31-33]

Cross-reactivity with apolipoprotein B or plasminogen was a potential difficulty for early assays, but most antibodies in use today have been immunopurified against these interferents. Polyclonal and monoclonal antibodies to apo(a) will be reactive primarily to kringle 4 type 2 repeats, since these are the most common epitopes and the ones most likely to be antigenic in the host animal. The immunoreactivity of antibodies directed to kringle 4 type 2 repeats will vary depending on the size of apo(a). Because of the high degree of polymorphism, it is impossible to match the isoform of the assay calibrator with that of the unknown samples. Some of the unknown samples will have isoforms smaller than those present in the calibrator, while others will be larger. Marcovina et al[34] recently demonstrated that the consequence of immunoreactivity to kringle 4 type 2 repeats is that apo(a) levels in samples with apo(a) isoforms smaller than those in the calibrator are underestimated, while those with larger isoforms are overestimated. In an attempt to determine the incidence of misclassification of patients by an assay sensitive to isoform size, Marcovina et al chose the 80th percentile as an arbitrary cutoff point for an elevated Lp(a). Comparison of Lp(a) levels measured in a population of 723 individuals with single banded apo(a) isoforms with an enzyme-linked immunosorbent assay (ELISA) sensitive to isoform size compared with one that is not demonstrated that 5.1% of the population was misclassified above the 80th percentile as false positive and 11% were misclassified as false negative.[34]

We recently reported that the INCSTAR Lp(a) assay (INCSTAR Corporation, Stillwater, MN) was not affected by apo(a) isoform size. This conclusion was based on a study of 13 individuals with apo(a) isoforms ranging in molecular weight from 419 to 838 kd.[35,36] Because we felt that 13 patients did not adequately represent the possible combinations of apo(a) isoforms in the general population, we conducted a collaborative study with Dr Marcovina at the Northwest Lipid Research Laboratories, Seattle, WA. Lipoprotein(a) levels in 172 patient samples with single- and double-banded apo(a) isoforms ranging from isoform 4 to 26[30] were measured using the INCSTAR method and the ELISA method using an antibody that is not sensitive to apo(a) isoform size. Figure 2 shows bias plots comparing results obtained by both methods plotted by isoform. Double-banded samples were graphed by plotting the major isoform. The isoforms are numbered in decreasing order, with number 1 indicating the largest apo(a) size isoform. Isoforms larger in size than isoform 15 were overestimated, while those smaller in size were underestimated. These results highlight the importance of designing studies of Lp(a) with sample sizes large enough to adequately represent the range and frequency of apo(a) isoforms present in the general population. Studies conducted on small numbers of samples may yield misleading results.

A common misconception is that the use of apo B detection in the ELISA format will result in measurement of Lp(a) level independent of isoform size. In fact, if the value to the assay calibrator is assigned in terms of total lipoprotein or protein mass of Lp(a), the values in the sample will vary as a function of the size of apo(a) in the samples with respect to the size of apo(a) in the calibrator.[37] Only if the value to the assay calibrator is assigned in terms of moles of Lp(a) proteins [apo(a) plus apo B][34] or in terms of mass of apo B in Lp(a), will the values generated by

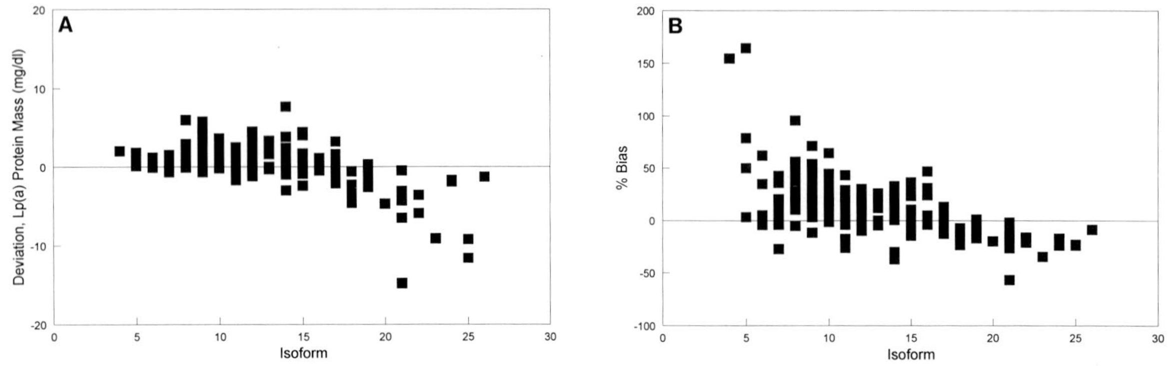

Fig 2. Bias plots comparing the INCSTAR Lp(a) assay, which is sensitive to kringle 4 type 2 repeats and is therefore sensitive to apo(a) isoform size, with an ELISA assay that is not sensitive to isoform size. In panel A, the bias is expressed in terms of protein mass and panel B shows the percent bias plotted as a function of apo(a) isoform size. The isoforms are numbered in decreasing order, with number 1 indicating the largest apo(a) size isoform. The effect illustrated in panel B is magnified by the fact that Lp(a) levels for large isoforms (small numbers) are low.

the apo B detection ELISA be independent of the apo(a) size polymorphism. Therefore, considering that all the assays commercially available, including one ELISA using apo B detection,[38] are calibrated in terms of total lipoprotein or total protein mass of Lp(a), there are no Lp(a) test kits that are unaffected by apo(a) isoform size.

An additional problem for measuring and interpreting Lp(a) levels in clinical studies is that Lp(a) has been shown to be an acute-phase reactant with levels increasing after a myocardial infarction,[39] stroke,[40] or coronary artery bypass graft surgery.[41] Lipoprotein(a) should not be measured less than 1 month after an acute clinical event.[42] It also has been suggested that Lp(a) may play a role in inflammation.[15,43] Clearly, the clinical state of the patient is an important consideration for determining the timing of Lp(a) measurements in clinical studies. Unless the patient is clinically stable it is difficult to interpret the Lp(a) data.

Finally, there is no standardization for the measurement of Lp(a). Despite the fact that suggestions for standardization have been published,[27,44] no international standardization program has been established for Lp(a) measurement. A program modeled after the successful International Federation of Clinical Chemistry study for the standardization of apo A-I and B[45,46] involving manufacturers and academics is needed for Lp(a). However, Lp(a) standardization constitutes a greater challenge than did apo A-I and B, and therefore the structural peculiarities of Lp(a) should be taken into consideration in designing a rigorous multistep project. Additionally, before any project can be implemented, it requires the development of a reference or "designated comparison method" with proven independence from apo(a) size polymorphism to be used for value assignment to calibrators and reference material and to evaluate the performance of the various Lp(a) methods.

LIPOPROTEIN(a) LEVELS IN PATIENTS RECEIVING RENAL REPLACEMENT THERAPY

Thirteen studies[47-59] that reported Lp(a) levels in controls and patients receiving renal replacement therapy were analyzed; the median Lp(a) levels for 12 of these studies are shown in Fig 3. One study that reported mean values instead of median values was excluded (Irish et al[50]), since the distribution of Lp(a) levels in most ethnic groups is not normally distributed and mean values can be misleading. Methods for measuring Lp(a) varied. Four studies[50,54,57,59] used a sandwich ELISA (Tint-Elize; Biopool AB, Umea, Sweden), two studies[49,52] used a radioimmunoassay (Pharmacia, Uppsala, Sweden), one study[48] used a turbidimetric assay (INCSTAR), and five studies used assays that were developed in house (radioimmunoassay,[47,58] latex immunoadsorption,[55] and ELISA[53,56]). Calibrators for these assays varied widely and included plasma from single donors to pooled plasma. Lipoprotein(a)

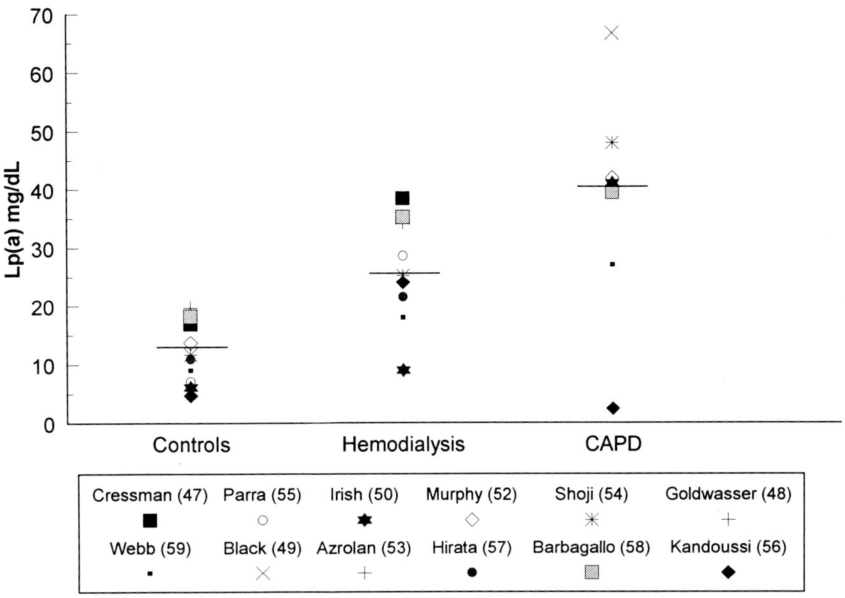

Fig 3. Median Lp(a) levels for controls and patients receiving hemodialysis or continuous ambulatory peritoneal dialysis. Data were obtained from 12 studies that reported median Lp(a) levels in controls and patients undergoing renal replacement therapy. References are indicated in parentheses.

values in all cases were expressed in terms of total Lp(a) lipoprotein mass or total apo(a) apolipoprotein mass.

There was extensive variability in Lp(a) levels in controls and patients receiving renal replacement therapy. Study median Lp(a) levels in controls ranged between 4.7 and 19.7 mg/dL. There was even greater variability in the Lp(a) levels in patients receiving hemodialysis (median range, 9 to 38.4 mg/dL). However, all studies demonstrated higher Lp(a) levels in patients receiving hemodialysis than in healthy controls. Lipoprotein(a) levels were considerably higher in patients receiving continuous ambulatory peritoneal dialysis than in patients receiving hemodialysis, with the exception of one study.[56]

Another possible etiology for the variation in Lp(a) levels are ethnic differences. The large differences in Lp(a) levels within ethnic groups make this an important variable to control for in analyzing data. Only three of the 13 studies[47,48,53] included data analysis by race or matched patients with controls by race. The necessity of segregating ethnic groups for data analysis makes it even more difficult to obtain adequate sample sizes to represent the isoform distributions characteristic of these groups.

The elevated levels of Lp(a) observed in dialysis patients may be due to an inflammatory response since Lp(a) has been shown to behave like an acute phase protein.[39,40,41] Release of tumor necrosis factor-α, interleukin-1, interleukin-6,[60] and C-reactive protein[61] has been reported in hemodialysis patients, and is possibly a result of chronic exposure to dialysis membranes.[62] Interleukin-6 is a potent activator of the synthesis of acute-phase proteins by hepatocytes[63,64] and also may play a role in inflammation.[42,43] Similar cytokine production has been reported in continuous ambulatory peritoneal dialysis patients.[65] These findings may explain why Lp(a) concentrations are elevated in patients undergoing chronic dialysis treatment.

EFFECT OF RENAL TRANSPLANTATION ON LIPOPROTEIN(a) LEVELS

Nine studies[49,50,51,53,58,66-69] reported Lp(a) levels in patients who had a renal transplant. Four of these studies[49,53,67,68] also reported Lp(a) levels when patients were receiving dialytic therapy, thereby permitting analysis of the effects of renal transplantation on Lp(a) levels (Fig 4). All four of these studies demonstrated that Lp(a) levels decreased as a result of renal transplantation. These changes in Lp(a) levels are in contrast to the increase in low-density lipoprotein cholesterol levels following renal transplantation.

Since elevated Lp(a) levels respond poorly to low-fat diet and drug therapy,[70,71] it is of great interest to determine why Lp(a) levels sometimes decrease following renal transplantation. Various studies have examined the effect of cyclosporine

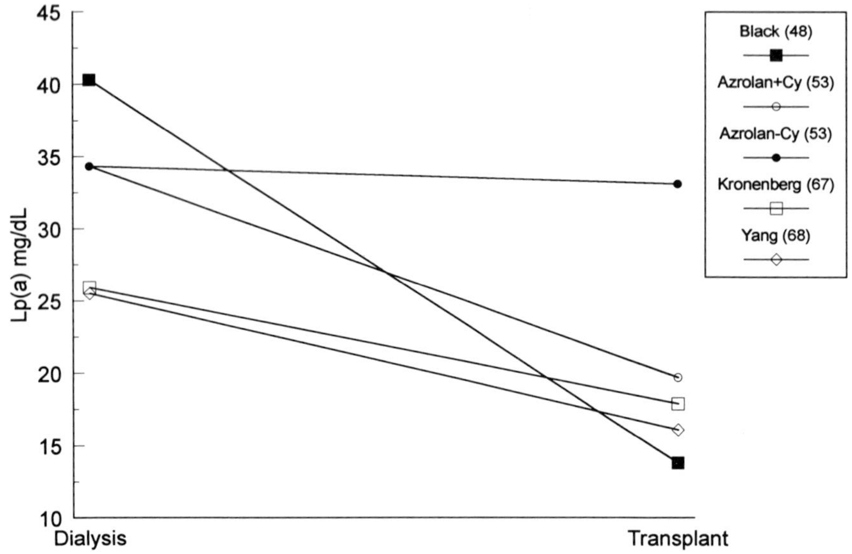

Fig 4. Change in Lp(a) level as a result of renal transplantation in four studies that reported Lp(a) levels prior to and at least 3 weeks after renal transplantation. References are indicated in parentheses. +cy, patients received cyclosporine; -cy, patients did not receive cyclosporine.

on Lp(a) levels with conflicting results. Azrolan et al[53] suggest that the Lp(a) lowering effect of renal transplantation may be related to the administration of cyclosporine. In individuals who received cyclosporine for immunosuppression, Lp(a) levels decreased from 34.3 mg/dL to 19.7 mg/dL (Fig 4). Patients receiving immunosuppressive therapy other than cyclosporine had little change in their Lp(a) levels. In contrast, Webb et al[69] demonstrated higher Lp(a) levels in patients receiving cyclosporine as part of their immunosuppressive regimen compared with patients not receiving cyclosporine. This study, however, did not observe patients prior to transplantation. Kronenberg et al[67] demonstrated no correlation between cyclosporine use and reduction in Lp(a) level following renal transplantation. These investigators demonstrated a statistically significant Lp(a)-lowering effect of transplantation only in those patients who had large apo(a) isoforms.

CLINICAL SIGNIFICANCE OF ELEVATED LIPOPROTEIN(a) LEVELS IN PATIENTS RECEIVING RENAL REPLACEMENT THERAPY

Although Lp(a) may be a risk factor for atherosclerosis in patients without renal disease, it is necessary to prove that elevated Lp(a) levels observed in patients receiving renal replacement therapy are associated with an increased risk for vascular disease. One study reported a correlation between Lp(a) level and the development of vascular events in patients receiving dialytic therapy.[47] In this study, 129 patients on hemodialysis were followed for 48 months. In those patients who developed atherosclerotic-related events, the Lp(a) level was approximately twice that of individuals without events. Of interest, the baseline Lp(a) level did not correlate with prior vascular events, suggesting that the increased Lp(a) level was of more recent origin.

In a study by Goldwasser et al,[48] Lp(a) levels did not correlate with atherosclerotic events in patients receiving dialysis therapy. The follow-up period of 14 months may have been too short to reveal any trends. Elevated Lp(a) levels, however, were associated with an enhanced risk for either thrombosis or occlusion of the vascular access. This correlation was observed when the data were analyzed for all patients or for white and Hispanic patients. No correlation between Lp(a) level and vascular access problems was observed for African-American patients. These observations highlight the heterogeneity of Lp(a) levels between different patient populations.

SUMMARY AND CONCLUSION

Lipoprotein(a) has been found to be a risk factor for atherosclerosis in patients without renal disease. It has been found to be elevated in most studies of patients receiving hemodialysis or continuous ambulatory peritoneal dialysis, and a risk factor for clinical atherosclerotic events in one study of patients receiving hemodialysis therapy.

It generally decreases following renal transplantation, possibly because of the effect of cyclosporine. Due to the difficulties in measuring Lp(a) and lack of standardization, current and prior studies should be interpreted cautiously.

REFERENCES

1. Berg K: A new serum type system in man: The Lp system. Acta Pathol Microbiol Scand 59:362-382, 1963
2. Berg K: The Lp system. Ser Haemotol 1:111-136, 1968 (review)
3. Koltringer P, Jurgens G: A dominant role of lipoprotein(a) in the investigation and evaluation of parameters indicating development of cervical atherosclerosis. Atherosclerosis 58:187-198, 1985
4. Dahlen GH, Guyton JR, Mohammad A, Farmer JA, Kautz JA, Gotto AM: Association of levels of lipoprotein Lp(a), plasma lipids, and other lipoproteins with coronary artery disease documented by angiography. Circulation 74:758-765, 1986
5. Scanu AM: Lipoprotein(a): A genetically determined cardiovascular pathogen in search of a function. J Lab Clin Med 116:142-146, 1990
6. Eaton D, Fless G, Kohr W, McClean J, Xu Q, Miller C, Lawn R, Scanu A: Partial amino acid sequence of apolipoprotein(a) shows that it is homologous to plasminogen. Proc Natl Acad Sci U S A 84:3224-3228, 1987
7. McClean JW, Tomlinson JE, Kuang WJ, Eaton DL, Chen EY, Fless GM, Scanu AM, Lawn RM: cDNA sequence of human apolipoprotein(a) is homologous to plasminogen. Nature 330:132-137, 1987
8. Utermann G: The mysteries of lipoprotein(a). Science 246:904-910, 1989
9. Scanu AM: Lipoprotein(a): A potential bridge between the fields of atherosclerosis and thrombosis. Arch Pathol Lab Med 112:1045-1047, 1988
10. Harpel PC, Gordon BR, Parker TS: Plasmin catalyzes binding of lipoprotein(a) to immobilized fibrinogen and fibrin. Proc Natl Acad Sci U S A 86:3847-3851, 1989
11. Gonzalez-Gronow M, Edelberg JM, Pizzo SV: Further characterization of the cellular plasminogen binding site: Evidence that plasminogen 2 and lipoprotein(a) compete for the same site. Biochemistry 28:2374-2377, 1989
12. Loscalzo J, Weinfeld M, Fless GM, Scanu AM: Lipoprotein(a), fibrin binding, and plasminogen activation. Arteriosclerosis 10:240-245, 1990
13. Rouy D, Grailhe P, Nigon F, Chapman J, Angles-Cano E: Lipoprotein(a) impairs generation of plasmin by fibrin-bound tissue-type plasminogen activator. In vitro studies in a plasma milieu. Arterioscler Thromb 11:629-638, 1991
14. Miles LA, Fless GM, Levin EG, Scanu AM, Plow E: A potential basis for the thrombotic risks associated with lipoprotein(a). Nature 339:301-303, 1989
15. Hajjar KA, Gavish D, Breslow JL, Nachman RL: Lipoprotein(a) modulation of endothelial cell surface fibrinolysis and its potential role in atherosclerosis. Nature 339:303-305, 1989
16. Etingin OR, Hajjar DP, Hajjar KA, Harpel PC, Nachman RL: Lipoprotein(a) regulates plasminogen activator inhibitor-1 expression in endothelial cells. A potential mechanism in thrombogenesis. J Biol Chem 266:2459-2465, 1991
17. Kojima S, Harpel PC, Rifkin DB: Lipoprotein(a) inhibits the generation of transforming growth factor beta: An endogenous inhibitor of smooth muscle cell migration. J Cell Biol 113:1439-1445, 1991
18. Grainger DJ, Kemp PR, Liu AC, Lawn RM, Metcalfe JC: Activation of transforming growth factor-β is inhibited in transgenic apolipoprotein(a) mice. Nature 370:460-462, 1994
19. Walton KW, Hitchens J, Magnani HN, Kahn M: A study of methods of identification and estimation of Lp(a) lipoprotein and of its significance in health, hyperlipidaemia and atherosclerosis. Atherosclerosis 20:323-346, 1974
20. Cushing GL, Gaubatz JW, Nava ML, Burdick BJ, Bocan TM, Guyton JR, Weilbaecher D, DeBakey ME, Lawrie GM, Morrisett JD: Quantitation and localization of apolipoproteins(a) and B in coronary artery bypass vein grafts at reoperation. Arteriosclerosis 9:593-603, 1989
21. Rath M, Niendorf A, Reblin T, Dietel M, Krebber HJ, Beisiegel U: Detection and quantification of lipoprotein(a) in the arterial wall of 107 coronary artery bypass patients. Arteriosclerosis 9:579-592, 1989
22. Niendorf A, Rath M, Wolf K, Peters S, Arps H, Beisiegel U, Dietel M: Morphological detection and quantification of lipoprotein(a) deposition in atheromatous lesions of human aorta and coronary arteries. Virchows Arch A Pathol Anat Histopathol 417:105-111, 1990
23. Beisiegel U, Niendorf A, Wolf K, Reblin T, Rath M: Lipoprotein(a) in the arterial wall. Eur Heart J 11:174-83, 1990 (suppl E)
24. Hoff HF, O'Neil J, Yashiro A: Partial characterization of lipoproteins containing apo(a) in human atherosclerotic lesions. J Lipid Res 34:789-798, 1993
25. Wolf K, Rath M, Niendorf A, Beisiegel U, Dietel M: Morphological co-localization of apoprotein(a) and fibrin(ogen) in human coronary atheromas. Circulation 80:II-522, 1989 (abstr)
26. Smith EB, Cochran S: Factors influencing the accumulation in fibrous plaques of lipid derived from low density lipoprotein. II. Preferential immobilization of lipoprotein(a) (Lp(a)). Atherosclerosis 84:173-181, 1990
27. Marcovina SM, Levine DM, Lippi G: Lipoprotein(a): Structure, measurement, and clinical significance, in Rifai N, Warnick GR (eds): Laboratory Measurement of Lipids, Lipoproteins and Apolipoproteins. Washington, DC, AACC Press, 1994, pp 235-264
28. Lackner C, Cohen JC, Hobbs HH: Molecular definition of the extreme size polymorphism in apolipoprotein(a). Hum Mol Genet 2:933-940, 1993
29. van der Hoek YY, Wittekoek ME, Beisiegel U, Kastelein JJ, Koschinsky ML: The apolipoprotein(a) kringle IV repeats which differs from the major repeat kringle are present in variably-sized isoforms. Hum Mol Genet 2:361-366, 1993
30. Marcovina SM, Zhang ZH, Gaur VP, Albers JJ: Identification of 34 apolipoprotein(a) isoforms: Differential expression of apolipoprotein(a) alleles between American blacks and whites. Biochem Biophys Res Commun 191:1192-1196, 1993
31. Guyton JR, Dahlen GH, Patsch W, Kautz JA, Gotto

AM Jr: Relationship of plasma lipoprotein Lp(a) levels to race and to apolipoprotein B, Arteriosclerosis 5:265-272, 1985

32. Helmhold M, Bigge J, Muche R, Mainoo J, Thiery J, Seidel D, Armstrong VW: Contribution of the apo(a) phenotype to plasma Lp(a) concentration shows considerable ethnic variation. J Lipid Res 32:1919-1928, 1991

33. Sandholzer C, Saha N, Kark JD, Rees A, Jaross W, Dieplinger H, Hoppichler F, Boerwinkle E, Utermann G: Apo(a) isoforms predict risk for coronary heart disease. A study in six populations. Arterioscler Thromb 12:1214-1226, 1992

34. Marcovina SM, Albers JJ, Gabel B, Kochinsky ML, Gaur VP: Effect of the number of apolipoprotein(a) kringle 4 domains on the immunochemical measurements of lipoprotein(a). Clin Chem 41:246-255, 1995

35. Levine DM, Sloan B-J, Parker TS, Donner JE, Heinzerling RH: Equivalent recovery of Lp(a) polymorphs by an automated assay: Analysis by a model of dilution parallelism. Clin Chem 39:1125, 1993 (abstr)

36. Levine DM, Parker TS, Sloan B-J, Heinzerling RH, Lorenz JD: Lipid risk factors as predictors of coronary disease. Clin Chem 39:1755-1756, 1993 (letter)

37. Albers JJ, Marcovina SM: Standardization of Lp(a) measurement. Chem Phys Lipids 67/68:257-263, 1994

38. Taddei-Peters WC, Butman BT, Jones GR, Venetta TM, Macomber PF, Ransom H: Quantification of lipoprotein(a) particles containing various apolipoprotein(a) isoforms by a monoclonal anti-apo(a) capture antibody and a polyclonal anti-apolipoprotein B detection antibody sandwich enzyme immunoassay. Clin Chem 39:1382-1389, 1993

39. Slunga L, Johnson O, Dahlen GH, Eriksson S: Lipoprotein(a) and acute-phase proteins in acute myocardial infarction. Scand J Clin Lab Invest 52:95-101, 1992

40. Woo J, Lam CWK, Kay R, Wong HY, Teoh R, Nicholls MG: Acute and long-term changes in serum lipids after acute stroke. Stroke 21:1407-1411, 1990

41. Cobbaert C, Sergeant P, Meyns B, Szecsi J, Kesteloot H: Time course of serum Lp(a) in men after coronary artery bypass grafting. Acta Cardiol 47:529-542, 1992

42. Maeda S, Abe A, Seishima M, Makino K, Noma A, Kawade M: Transient changes of serum lipoprotein(a) as an acute phase protein. Atherosclerosis 78:145-150, 1989

43. Rantapaa-Dahlqvist S, Wallberg-Jonsson S, Dahlen G: Lipoprotein(a), lipids, and lipoproteins in patients with rheumatoid arthritis. Ann Rheum Dis 50:366-368, 1991

44. Albers JJ, Marcovina SM, Lodge MS: The unique lipoprotein(a): Properties and immunochemical measurement. Clin Chem 36:2019-2026, 1990

45. Albers JJ, Marcovina SM, Kennedy H: International Federation of Clinical Chemistry standardization project for measurements of apolipoproteins A-I and B. II. Evaluation and selection of candidate reference materials. Clin Chem 38:658-662, 1992

46. Marcovina SM, Albers JJ, Henderson LO, Hannon WH: International Federation of Clinical Chemistry standardization project for measurements of apolipoproteins A-I and B. III. Comparability of apolipoprotein A-I values by use of international reference material. Clin Chem 39:773-781, 1993

47. Cressman MD, Heyka RJ, Paganini EP, O'Neil J, Skibinski CI, Hoff HF: Lipoprotein(a) is an independent risk factor for cardiovascular disease in hemodialysis patients. Circulation 86:475-482, 1992

48. Goldwasser P, Michel MA, Collier J, Mittman N, Fein PA, Gusik SA, Avram MM: Prealbumin and lipoprotein(a) in hemodialysis: Relationships with patient and vascular access survival. Am J Kidney Dis 22:215-225, 1993

49. Black IW, Wilcken DEL: Decreases in apolipoprotein(a) after renal transplantation: Implications for lipoprotein(a) metabolism. Clin Chem 38:353-357, 1992

50. Irish AB, Simons LA, Savdie E, Hayes JM, Simons J: Lipoprotein(a) levels in chronic renal disease states, dialysis and transplantation. Aust N Z J Med 22:243-248, 1992

51. Heimann P, Josephson MA, Fellner SK, Thistlethwaite JR Jr, Stuart FP, Dasgupta A: Elevated lipoprotein(a) levels in renal transplantation and hemodialysis patients. Am J Nephrol 11:470-474, 1991

52. Murphy BG, McNamee P, Duly E, Henry W, Archbold P, Trinick T: Increased serum apolipoprotein(a) in patients with chronic renal failure treated with continuous ambulatory peritoneal dialysis. Atherosclerosis 93:53-57, 1992

53. Azrolan N, Brown CD, Thomas L, Hayek T, Zhao ZH, Roberts KG, Scheiner C, Friedman EA: Cyclosporin A has divergent effects on plasma LDL cholesterol (LDL-C) and lipoprotein(a) [Lp(a)] levels in renal transplant recipients. Evidence for renal involvement in the maintenance of LDL-C and the evaluation of Lp(a) concentrations in hemodialysis patients. Arterioscler Thromb 14:1393-1398, 1994

54. Shoji T, Nishizawa Y, Nishitani H, Yamakawa M, Morii H: High serum lipoprotein(a) concentrations in uremic patients treated with continuous ambulatory peritoneal dialysis. Clin Nephrol 38:271-276, 1992

55. Parra HJ, Mezdour H, Cachera C, Dracon M, Tacquet A, Fruchart JC: Lp(a) lipoprotein in patients with chronic renal failure treated by hemodialysis. Clin Chem 33:721, 1987

56. Kandoussi A, Cachera C, Pagniez D, Dracon M, Fruchart JC, Tacquet A: Plasma level of lipoprotein Lp(a) is high in predialysis or hemodialysis, but not in CAPD. Kidney Int 42:424-425, 1992

57. Hirata K, Kikuchi S, Saku K, Jimi S, Zhang B, Naito S, Hamaguchi H, Arakawa K: Apolipoprotein(a) phenotypes and serum lipoprotein(a) levels in maintenance hemodialysis patients with/without diabetes mellitus. Kidney Int 44:1062-1070, 1993

58. Barbagallo CM, Averna MR, Sparacino V, Galione A, Caputo F, Scafidi V, Amato S, Mancino C, Cefalù AB, Notarbartolo A: Lipoprotein(a) levels in end-stage renal failure and renal transplantation. Nephron 64:560-564, 1993

59. Webb AT, Reaveley DA, O'Donnell M, O'Connor B, Seed M, Brown EA: Lipoprotein(a) in patients on maintenance haemodialysis and continuous ambulatory peritoneal dialysis. Nephrol Dial Transplant 8:609-613, 1993

60. Cavaillon JM, Poignet JL, Fitting C, Delons S: Serum interleukin-6 in long-term hemodialyzed patients. Nephron 60:307-313, 1992

61. Docci D, Bilancioni R, Buscaroli A, Baldrati L, Capponcini C, Mengozzi S, Turci F, Feletti C: Elevated serum levels of C-reactive protein in hemodialysis patients. Nephron 56:364-367, 1990

62. Mege JL, Olmer M, Purgus R, Bertocchio P, Farnarier C, Kaplanski S, Capo C, Bongrand P: Haemodialysis mem-

branes modulate chronically the production of TNF alpha, IL1beta and IL6. Nephrol Dial Transplant 6:868-875, 1991

63. Le JM, Vilcek J: Interleukin-6: A multifunctional cytokine regulating immune reactions and the acute phase protein response. Lab Invest 61:588-602, 1989

64. Kishimoto T: The biology of interleukin-6. Blood 74:1-10, 1989

65. Steinhauer HB, Brugger U, Atmanspacher R, Lubrich-Birkner I, Schollmeyer P: Effect of CAPD dialysate on the release of eicosanoids and cytokines from human peritoneal macrophages. Adv Perit Dial 8:47-52, 1992

66. Webb AT, Plant M, Reaveley DA, O'Donnell M, Luck VA, O'Connor B, Seed M, Brown EA: Lipid and lipoprotein(a) concentrations in renal transplant patients. Nephrol Dial Transplant 7:636-641, 1992

67. Kronenberg F, König P, Lhotta K, Ofner D, Sandholzer C, Margreiter R, Dosch E, Utermann G, Dieplinger H: Apolipoprotein(a) phenotype-associated decrease in lipoprotein(a) plasma concentrations after renal transplantation. Arterioscler Thromb 14:1399-1404, 1994

68. Yang CW, Kim YS, Kim SY, Chang YS, Yoon YS, Bang BK: Serum levels of lipoprotein(a) after renal transplantation: Short-term follow-up. Nephron 67:364, 1994

69. Webb AT, Reaveley DA, O'Donnell M, O'Connor B, Seed M, Brown EA: Does cyclosporin increase lipoprotein(a) concentrations in renal transplant recipients? Lancet 341:268-270, 1993

70. Kostner G, Gavish D, Leopold B, Bolzano K, Weintraub MS, Breslow JL: HMG-CoA reductase inhibitors lower LDL cholesterol without reducing Lp(a) levels. Circulation 80:1313-1319, 1989

71. Brewer HB: Effectiveness of diet and drugs in the treatment of patients with elevated Lp(a) levels, in Scanu AM (ed): Lipoprotein(a). New York, NY, Academic, 1990, pp 211-220

Prealbumin and Lipoprotein(a) in Hemodialysis: Relationships With Patient and Vascular Access Survival

Philip Goldwasser, MD, Marie-Alex Michel, MD, James Collier, MD, Neal Mittman, MD, Paul A. Fein, MD, Sara-Ann Gusik, MS, and M.M. Avram, MD

● The high morbidity and mortality of hemodialysis patients has led to a search for early markers of risk. Because cardiovascular and nutritional risk are prevalent in this population, we examined the prognostic value of the serum levels of two markers of risk in the general population: (1) lipoprotein(a) [Lp(a)], a low-density lipoprotein-like particle linked to myocardial infarction and coronary bypass stenosis, and (2) prealbumin, a marker of visceral protein status, with a shorter half-life than that of serum albumin. Baseline demographics, clinical information, dialysis prescription, and serum biochemistry measurements of 125 hemodialysis patients followed for up to 14 months were recorded on enrollment. Vascular access events and deaths were recorded prospectively. The hypotheses tested were that increased serum Lp(a) levels would predict cardiovascular mortality and vascular access stenosis and thrombosis, and that reduced serum prealbumin levels would predict mortality risk independently of established risk predictors. Cross-sectional analysis of serum Lp(a) demonstrated a skewed distribution with a median value of 38.3 mg/dL (upper tertile, ≥57 mg/dL). Lipoprotein(a) was significantly higher in black patients ($P < 0.001$) and was significantly correlated ($P < 0.005$) with total cholesterol and apoprotein B (apoB), but not with a history of prior coronary disease. Serum prealbumin was strongly correlated with serum albumin ($r = 0.49$, $P < 0.001$). However, prealbumin correlated ($P < 0.001$) more strongly with other serum nutrition markers (total cholesterol, apoB, creatinine, urea) than did serum albumin. Fourteen-month cumulative survival was 80%. Age, diabetes, and serum levels of albumin, prealbumin, creatinine, total cholesterol and apoB, but not Lp(a), were correlated with survival in univariate analysis. Using the Cox proportional hazards model, independent predictors of mortality risk were prealbumin less than 15 mg/dL versus higher values (relative risk [RR] = 4.48, $P < 0.01$), apoB (RR = 0.97 per 1 mg/dL increase, $P < 0.02$), creatinine less than 10 mg/dL versus higher values (RR = 3.51, $P = 0.04$), and age (RR = 1.04 per year, $P = 0.10$). Thirty-eight patients experienced at least one vascular access thrombosis (n = 33) or stenosis (n = 5) during the study. Patients with Lp(a) ≥57 mg/dL had decreased vascular access event-free survival compared with patients with Lp(a) less than 57 mg/dL (56% *v* 73%, $P < 0.06$). This trend was increased in magnitude and statistically significant for white and Hispanic patients (31% *v* 79%, $P < 0.01$). Lipoprotein(a) ≥57 mg/dL was not associated with reduced access event-free survival in black patients (64% *v* 64%, P = NS). In summary, two serum risk markers, Lp(a) and prealbumin, were evaluated prospectively in 125 hemodialysis patients. Increased serum Lp(a) was found to be a new predictor of vascular access occlusion in white and Hispanic patients. Reduced serum levels of prealbumin, apoB, and creatinine were found to be important independent predictors of mortality risk in hemodialysis patients.

INDEX WORDS: Lipoprotein(a); prealbumin; hemodialysis; mortality; dialysis vascular access.

DESPITE improvements in technology over the past decade, hemodialysis patients continue to have a high mortality, especially from cardiovascular disease.[1-5] Early reports suggested that atherosclerosis is accelerated by end-stage renal disease (ESRD),[6,7] prompting research into potentially treatable proatherogenic disturbances. The lipid disturbances seen in uremia were believed to be particularly atherogenic.[8-12] Hemodialysis patients have impaired reverse cholesterol transport, decreased serum levels of high-density lipoprotein cholesterol (HDLC), and increased levels of potentially atherogenic intermediate particles.[13-15] We and others reported that in ESRD the total cholesterol to HDLC ratio (TC/HDLC) is abnormally high and the ratio of apoprotein A-I (apoAI) to apoprotein B (apoB) is in the low-normal range, and that the TC/HDLC ratio is significantly higher in patients treated with continuous ambulatory peritoneal dialysis than in patients on hemodialysis.[16-18] However, recent studies have failed to support the early viewpoint that atherosclerosis is accelerated by uremia; pre-existing disease is generally felt to be responsible.[9-11,19-21] Comparisons of the lipids and apoproteins in patients with renal failure with and without vascular disease have revealed inconsistent differences or none at all.[21-24] In several studies, coronary disease itself has not been found to be a significant mortality predictor.[25-27]

Ironically, although uremia tends to induce an atherogenic lipid profile, 1-year mortality risk in dialysis patients is inversely related to serum cholesterol, as well as to serum albumin and creatinine.[28-33] We established that single measure-

Supported in part by grants from The National Kidney Foundation of New York/New Jersey and the Nephrology Foundation of Brooklyn.

ments of serum albumin and cholesterol are independent predictors of survival for at least 2 years in both recently diagnosed and longstanding dialysis patients, and these markers remain predictive even in patients receiving adequate dialysis.[34] Since serum cholesterol and albumin are visceral protein markers and serum creatinine reflects somatic protein stores, the evidence suggests that protein malnutrition is a more important mortality risk factor in the dialysis population than is atherosclerosis.[17,35] However, low serum albumin and cholesterol are not considered early markers of malnutrition.[36,37] Therefore, a more sensitive serum marker may improve our ability to identify patients at risk. One such marker has been found to be prealbumin.[38] Because of its rapid turnover, the concentration of serum prealbumin can change more rapidly than that of serum albumin in response to changes in nutritional status.[39,40] Cano et al reported that low serum levels of creatinine and prealbumin, but not albumin, were associated with increased 1-year mortality in hemodialysis patients.[32] However, they did not determine whether the prognostic information of prealbumin concentration was independent from that of other biochemical risk factors, demographic factors (such as age or sex), or comorbidity (such as diabetes).

Our ability to detect dialysis patients at cardiovascular risk would be improved by identifying a serum risk marker that, unlike serum cholesterol, is not confounded by nutritional status.[17] Serum lipoprotein(a) [Lp(a)] has been found to be an independent predictor of coronary risk and coronary bypass stenosis in white and Asian populations.[41-45] Values in the upper third of the population are associated with increased risk.[41,42] End-stage renal disease is associated with a threefold increase in the median level of this lipoprotein.[46] Increased Lp(a) in hemodialysis patients was found to be associated with an increased rate of cardiovascular events in a recent cohort study,[47] but the relationship of Lp(a) to vascular access occlusion in these patients has not been reported.

To study the prognostic value of serum levels of Lp(a) and prealbumin, cross-sectional and longitudinal analyses were performed in 125 hemodialysis patients followed for up to 14 months. We tested whether increased Lp(a) correlated with baseline coronary status. Using Cox's proportional hazards model, we tested the hypothesis that low prealbumin and increased Lp(a) concentrations are important mortality predictors, independent of previously established predictors and, in a cohort design, we tested the hypothesis that increased Lp(a) levels predict vascular access occlusion.

METHODS

Patients

A group of 125 hemodialysis outpatients at The Long Island College Hospital was enrolled in February 1991 and followed for up to 14 months. On enrollment, clinical and laboratory data were collected. Follow-up was censored on transplantation, transfer to continuous ambulatory peritoneal dialysis treatment, or transfer to another dialysis center. Average follow-up was 12 months and median follow-up was 14 months.

Clinical Data

The clinical data included age, race, gender, etiology of ESRD and total months on dialysis, estimated dry weight, treatment time, access type (endogenous fistula *v* polytetrafluoroethylene graft), heparin dose, dialyzer membrane, mean predialysis blood pressure (of three consecutive treatments), diabetic status prior to uremia, and coronary status. The causes of ESRD were hypertensive nephrosclerosis (34.9% of patients), diabetes mellitus (34.9%), chronic glomerulonephritis (9.5%), polycystic kidney disease (8.7%), obstruction (4.8%), miscellaneous (4.8%), and unknown (2.4%). For the purpose of this study, coronary disease (CAD) was considered to be present if there was a proven myocardial infarction by history or electrocardiogram, or positive angiography or thallium stress testing. Angina alone was considered to be present in patients who had anginal symptoms and were being treated with antianginal medications but who had no proof of CAD. The remaining patients were classified as having no CAD.

Description of Dialysis Prescription

All patients were on thrice weekly hemodialysis with bicarbonate bath using Cobe Centrysystem 3 dialysis machines (Cobe, Lakewood, CO). Dialyzer membranes were cellulose acetate (55% of patients), saponified cellulose ester (32%), polysulfone (6%), hemophane (3%), cuprophane (3%), and cuprammonium rayon (1%). Blood flows ranged from 300 to 500 mL/min. Dialysis prescription was guided in part by a goal of achieving a value of ≥ 2.5 for the ratio of pretreatment serum urea nitrogen (BUN) to 5 minute posttreatment BUN.[48-50] The posttreatment BUN was drawn 5 minutes after treatment to minimize the problem of spurious low post-BUN values that results from graft recirculation and from disequilibrium. The mean BUN ratio was 2.73 ± 0.54 SD (range, 1.37 to 4.60). The mean treatment time was 3.01 ± 0.36 hours (range, 2 to 4 hours). At enrollment, 105 patients were receiving heparin with each dialysis treatment and 70 patients were receiving erythropoietin therapy at the conclusion of each dialysis session.

Elevated venous pressure on dialysis or abnormally low or high monthly BUN ratio values were used by clinicians as indications for investigation of the vascular access with recirculation studies and/or angiography.

Biochemical Data

On enrollment, nonfasting baseline blood was drawn immediately prior to the first treatment of the week from the arteriovenous access. A multiphasic biochemistry screen was obtained for each patient using the SMAC autoanalyzer (Technicon, Tarrytown, NY). Total cholesterol was measured by the SMAC autoanalyzer (120 to 200 mg/dL). High-density lipoprotein cholesterol was measured on the DuPont ACA, (Wilmington, DE) using an assay from EM Diagnostic Systems, (Gibbstown, NJ) (reference range, 32 to 96 mg/dL). Hematocrit was measured using the Technicon H1 analyzer (Technicon).

Prealbumin (reference range, 17 to 42 mg/dL in a normal healthy population; linear range, 7 to 50 mg/dL), apoAI (reference range, 96 to 176 mg/dL in normal males, 109 to 203 mg/dL in normal females; linear range, 25 to 225 mg/dL), and apoB (reference range, 43.0 to 128 mg/dL in normal males, 42.0 to 112 mg/dL in normal females; linear range, 30 to 200 mg/dL) were determined by rate nephelometry on a Beckman Array Protein System (Beckman Instruments Inc, Brea, CA). Appropriate blanks were used to correct for turbidity in samples.

Lipoprotein(a) was determined by Dr Daniel Levine of The Rogosin Institute, The New York Hospital-Cornell Medical Center (New York, NY). Lipoprotein(a) (reference range, 0 to 24 mg/dL; linear range, 5 to 105 mg/dL) was measured by immunoturbidometric analysis (SPQ II kits, INCSTAR Corp, Stillwater, MN) on the Roche COBAS FARA II clinical chemistry analyzer. The Lp(a) assay has been standardized to the double monoclonal enzyme-linked immunosorbent assay used at the Northwest Lipid Research Laboratory, University of Washington School of Medicine, Harborview Medical Center, Seattle, WA.[51] The antibodies used to measure Lp(a) do not cross-react with plasminogen up to 230 mg/dL and do not cross-react with apoB up to 436 mg/dL. There is no interference in the Lp(a) assay from triglycerides up to 4 g/L. Renal patients often have elevated triglyceride levels; therefore, patient samples with levels above 4 g/L were diluted prior to analysis.

Study Design and Data Analysis

In the cross-sectional analyses, comparisons of continuous variables and proportions were made using ANOVA and the Chi-square test, respectively. Continuous variables are reported as the mean ± SD. For selected comparisons, nonparametric methods were used, as indicated in the text. Correlations are reported as either the Pearson correlation coefficient (r) or the Spearman rank correlation coefficient (r_s). Multiple logistic regression was used to construct models that predicted baseline coronary classification. The upper third of the population by Lp(a) values was hypothesized to be at increased risk of CAD for this analysis.

Patient survival for up to 14 months was analyzed with the Cox proportional hazards model[52,53] using baseline age, race, gender, diabetes, coronary status, duration of ESRD, BUN, creatinine, albumin, cholesterol, HDLC, apoAI, apoB, Lp(a), prealbumin, treatment time, and BUN ratio as independent variables. The variables chosen reflected our previous experience as well as reports in the literature. Variables were selected for the final models with a backward stepwise approach. The proportional hazard assumption was tested by plotting baseline hazards across strata. If the hazards were parallel among the strata, the variable was modeled as a covariate; otherwise, the analysis was stratified. The fit of the models were assessed by comparing predicted survival to that of the observed probabilities of survival for selected subgroups of patients. Observed survival was computed by the Kaplan-Meier method.[54] Data presented include the regression coefficients, the relative risk ratios and their 95% confidence intervals, and the actual probability values for the odds ratios. The risk ratios reflect the level of risk associated with a variable assuming other factors are held constant. Certain serum measurements were transformed into categoric variables with clinically relevant break points. Kaplan-Meier estimates of survival across these categories were compared by the log rank test.[55]

Angioaccess survival to first thrombosis or stenosis was analyzed by the Kaplan-Meier method. The upper third of the population by Lp(a) was hypothesized to be at increased risk for thrombosis or stenosis. A one-tailed probability value is reported for the test of the primary hypothesis. Two-tailed probability values are reported for subgroup analysis. For analysis of vascular access survival, outcome was censored on death, transplantation, or transfer to peritoneal dialysis or to another institution. One patient who was receiving coumadin (for mitral valve replacement) was excluded from this analysis. No patients were receiving aspirin.

Calculations were performed using SPSS for Windows 5.0.2. (SPSS Inc, Chicago, IL) and Egret (SERC, Seattle, WA) statistical software.

RESULTS

Cross-sectional Analysis

The mean age of the population was 60 ± 15 (SD) years and the mean duration of ESRD was 56 ± 52 months. Forty percent of the population was diabetic and 52% were female. The diabetic patients were significantly older than the nondiabetic patients (66 ± 12 years *v* 56 ± 16 years, $P < 0.001$) and the female patients were significantly older than the male patients (63 ± 13 years *v* 56 ± 17 years, $P < 0.01$). The population was 52% black, 32% white, and 16% Hispanic. The coronary status distribution was 18% with evidence of CAD, 26% with angina alone, and 56% with no clinical disease.

The distribution of serum Lp(a) in the population was skewed (Fig 1). The median value of Lp(a) was 38.3 mg/dL. Seventeen percent of cases had values below 5 mg/dL. One third of the cases had values of 57 mg/dL or above. Age

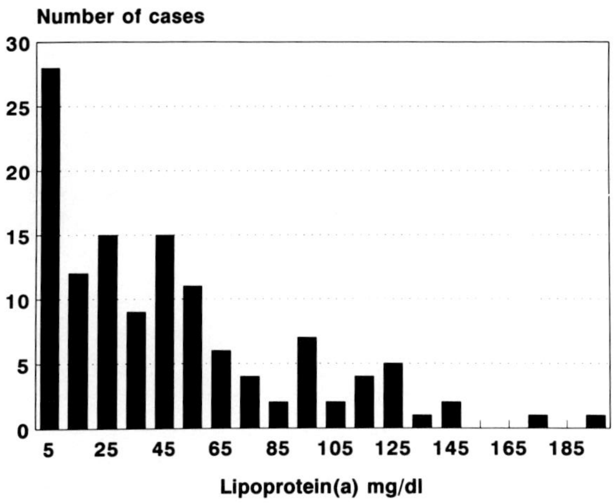

Fig 1. Distribution of serum Lp(a) values in 125 hemodialysis patients. The range of each bar is ±5 mg/dL.

and duration of ESRD did not correlate with Lp(a). Mean Lp(a) level was higher in black patients than in white or Hispanic patients (57.9 ± 39.9 mg/dL *v* 38.0 ± 41.8 mg/dL *v* 32.1 ± 38.9 mg/dL, respectively, P = 0.0004 by Kruskal-Wallis test). Women had higher values than men (53.4 ± 40.0 mg/dL *v* 40.9 ± 42.6 mg/dL, $P < 0.02$ by Mann-Whitney test). Lipoprotein(a) was similar in diabetic and nondiabetic patients (48.8 ± 39.7 mg/dL *v* 46.5 ± 43.0 mg/dL, $P = 0.59$ by Mann-Whitney test). Lipoprotein(a) correlated significantly with serum cholesterol, apoB, and HDLC, but not with apoAI, prealbumin, or albumin (Table 1). The trends observed were similar for black patients and for white and Hispanic patients analyzed separately.

Demographic and biochemical comparison of the patients grouped by coronary status is shown in Tables 2 and 3. Patients with CAD or angina alone were older and more likely to be diabetic

Table 1. Correlations of Serum Lipoprotein (a)

	r_s	Probability Value
ApoA	0.14	0.110
ApoB	0.25	0.004
TC	0.28	0.002
HDLC	0.20	0.029
Prealbumin	0.13	0.136
Albumin	0.001	0.995
Creatinine	−0.07	0.433

Table 2. Demographic Comparison of Coronary Groups

	No CAD (n = 70)	Angina Without Proven CAD (n = 32)	CAD (n = 23)	Probability Value
Age (yr)	56 ± 17	64 ± 12	66 ± 12	<0.005
Male (%)	51	34	57	0.185
Race (%)				0.619
White	34	22	39	
Black	51	56	48	
Hispanic	14	22	13	
Diabetes (%)	29	56	52	0.013

than patients classified as having no CAD (Table 2). The mean value of the TC/HDLC ratio was significantly higher in patients with CAD compared with patients with angina alone or with no disease (Table 3). The occurrence of Lp(a) values of 57 mg/dL or higher was more frequent in CAD than angina (39% *v* 16%, $P = 0.05$). Although mean TC/HDLC ratio was lower in non-CAD patients than in patients with CAD, mean Lp(a) values were similar in the two groups (Table 3). The pattern of differences among the three coronary groups persisted when the analysis was performed separately for black patients and for white and Hispanic patients. Independent predictors of baseline coronary class were derived using multiple logistic regression with age, diabetes, gender, TC/HDLC ratio, and Lp(a) ≥ 57 mg/dL as independent variables. The strongest independent discriminators of CAD (*v* angina) were TC/HDLC ratio (mean odds ratio [OR] = 1.22, $P = 0.10$) and Lp(a) ≥ 57 mg/dL (OR = 3.17, $P = 0.06$, by one-tailed P). Thus, an Lp(a) value of 57 mg/dL or greater tripled the likelihood of being classified as having CAD rather than angina. Similarly, each unit increase in the TC/HDLC ratio independently increased the likelihood of being classified as having CAD rather than angina by 22%. The strongest independent discriminators of CAD (*v* no disease) were age (OR = 1.05, $P < 0.05$), diabetes (OR = 2.66, $P = 0.05$), and TC/HDLC (OR = 1.21, $P = 0.06$).

Mean serum prealbumin level was 26.5 ± 6.4 mg/dL. The mean value was lower in diabetic patients than nondiabetic patients (24.2 ± 6.9

Table 3. Biochemical Comparison of Coronary Groups

	No CAD (n = 70)	Angina Without Proven CAD (n = 32)	CAD (n = 23)	Probability Value
TC (mmol/L)	169.5 ± 46.2	167.4 ± 47.8	188.5 ± 47.6*	0.20
HDLC (mmol/L)	39.0 ± 14.1†	37.6 ± 12.0	35.7 ± 14.1*	0.60
TC/HDLC	4.9 ± 2.1†	4.9 ± 2.2‡	6.5 ± 3.5§	0.02
Lp(a) (mg/dL)	51.1 ± 44.5	35.3 ± 29.3‡	53.1 ± 45.1	0.29‖
Lp(a) ≥ 57 mg/dL (%)	39	16	39	<0.06
Apo AI (mg/L)	99.0 ± 22.0	98.6 ± 20.9	95.0 ± 18.4	0.72
Apo B (mg/L)	64.1 ± 22.5	62.5 ± 21.1	75.6 ± 23.5	<0.07
Apo AI/Apo B	1.75 ± 0.75	1.79 ± 0.79	1.38 ± 0.55	<0.08

*n = 22.
†n = 69.
‡n = 31.
§n = 21.
‖Comparison by Kruskal-Wallis test.

mg/dL v 28.1 ± 5.6 mg/dL, $P < 0.001$) and in females compared with males (25.3 ± 6.9 mg/dL v 27.9 ± 5.6 mg/dL, $P = 0.02$). These differences remained significant after adjusting for age by ANOVA with covariance. Serum prealbumin was correlated strongly with serum albumin ($r = 0.49$, $P < 0.001$). Serum prealbumin was more strongly correlated with other nutritional markers (total cholesterol, apoB, creatinine, BUN) than was serum albumin (Table 4). Serum total cholesterol and apoB were highly correlated with each other ($r = 0.87$, $P < 10^{-4}$), but neither correlated with serum creatinine.

Prospective Study of Survival

Twenty-three patients died during the study. Cumulative survival was 80% (by the Kaplan-Meier method). Lipoprotein(a) less than 57 mg/dL was associated with a survival of 78% compared with 83.7% for Lp(a) ≥ 57 mg/dL ($P = 0.23$ by log-rank test). When survival was stratified by race and Lp(a) (<57 mg/dL v ≥57 mg/dL), the results were similar for black patients (77% v 84%, $P = 0.22$) and for white and Hispanic patients (78% v 80%, $P = 0.80$). Serum albumin (Table 5), prealbumin (Table 6), creatinine, cholesterol, apoB, diabetes, and age were significantly correlated with survival in univariate analysis. Independent predictors of mortality risk were derived using the Cox proportional hazards model with stepwise removal of variables. The final model is shown in Table 7. The significant predictors were prealbumin, apoB, and creatinine. Adjusting for the other variables in the model, serum prealbumin below 15 mg/dL increased risk fourfold to fivefold ($P < 0.01$). Each 1 mg/dL increase in apoB lowered mortality risk by 3% ($P < 0.02$). A serum creatinine below 10 mg/dL increased risk threefold to fourfold (P

Table 4. Correlations of Serum Albumin and Prealbumin

	Pearson Correlation Coefficient	
	Albumin	Prealbumin
Creatinine	0.38*	0.48*
TC	0.21†	0.44*
ApoB	0.18†	0.46*
BUN	0.15‡	0.32*
Age	−0.15‡	−0.15‡
BUN ratio	0.04	−0.03

*$P < 0.001$.
†$P < 0.05$.
‡$P \leq 0.10$.

Table 5. Cumulative Survival by Serum Albumin Level

Range	N	Survival Rate*
≤3.0 g/dL	5	60%
3.1-3.4 g/dL	14	59%
3.5-3.9 g/dL	63	88%
≥4.0 g/dL	42	76%

*$P < 0.04$ by log rank test.

Table 6. Cumulative Survival by Serum Prealbumin Level

Range	N	Survival Rate*
<15.0 mg/dL	7	0%
15.0-17.9 mg/dL	12	83%
18.0-26.9 mg/dL	39	76%
≥27.0 mg/dL	67	89%

* $P < 10^{-4}$ by log rank test.

< 0.04). Age was not quite significant; relative risk was increased by 4% for each additional year of age at study entry (P = 0.10).

Prospective Study of Vascular Access Events

The relationship of vascular access occlusion events to serum Lp(a) was compared in cohorts defined by Lp(a) level. The cohorts were well-matched for all characteristics except race (Table 8). Thirty-eight patients developed at least one vascular access thrombosis (n = 33) or stenosis (n = 5). Using the Kaplan-Meier method, the cumulative survival without a vascular access occlusion event was lower for Lp(a) ≥ 57 mg/dL compared with Lp(a) less than 57 mg/dL (56% *v* 73%, $P < 0.06$ by one-tailed log rank test) (Fig 2). Because Lp(a) levels were significantly higher in the black patients, access event-free survival was examined separately in black patients and in white and Hispanic patients. There were no statistically significant differences in the baseline characteristics of the two Lp(a) cohorts for black patients alone. However, for white and Hispanic patients, the high Lp(a) cohort had a greater proportion of diabetic patients (82% *v* 35%, $P < 0.01$). Lipoprotein(a) ≥ 57 mg/dL was associated with significantly decreased access event-free survival in white and Hispanic patients (31% *v* 79%, $P < 0.01$ by two-tailed log rank test) (Fig 3). The influence of Lp(a) ≥ 57 mg/dL (*v* Lp(a) < 57 mg/dL) on first occlusion rate was similar in both diabetic patients (0.63 *v* 0.27 events/person-year) and nondiabetic patients (0.63 *v* 0.15 events/person year). However, in black patients Lp(a) ≥ 57 mg/dL did not predict access events (64% *v* 64%, $P > 0.90$) (Fig 4).

DISCUSSION

The high morbidity and mortality of dialysis patients has led to a search for early markers of risk. Because cardiovascular and nutritional risk are prevalent in hemodialysis,[4-7,33,35,56] we examined the prognostic value of serum levels of Lp(a) and prealbumin, markers of cardiovascular risk and nutritional risk, respectively. Despite the disturbances of lipid metabolism in uremia, the traditional serum markers of cardiovascular mortality risk have not been useful in dialysis patients.[21-24] High levels of serum Lp(a) have been found to be independent predictors of coronary risk (including coronary bypass stenosis) in white and Asian populations with normal renal function.[41-45] Serum Lp(a) is markedly increased in dialysis patients.[46,47] Consequently, we tested whether high Lp(a) is correlated cross-sectionally with coronary disease and prospectively with mortality risk and angioaccess occlusion in a 14-month study of 125 hemodialysis patients. Low serum albumin, cholesterol, and creatinine have been found to be predictive of mortality in dialysis.[28,29,32-34] Since these markers reflect visceral and somatic nutritional status, we also tested whether a more sensitive nutritional marker, serum prealbumin, would add prognostic information to these established risk predictors.

In cross-sectional analysis, elevated mean Lp(a) levels were found in black patients, compatible with other studies of dialysis patients and the general population.[47,57] Women had higher

Table 7. Predictors of Mortality Over 14 Months

Predictor	Regression Coefficient	Relative Risk (95% CI)	Probability Value
Prealbumin < 15 mg/dL (*v* ≥ 15 mg/dL)	1.500	4.48 (1.57-13.79)	0.009
ApoB (per mg/dL)	−0.030	0.97 (0.95-0.99)	0.016
Creatinine < 10 mg/dL (*v* ≥ 10 mg/dL)	1.256	3.51 (1.09-11.31)	0.035
Age (per year)	0.034	1.04 (0.99-1.08)	0.100

Abbreviation: CI, confidence interval.

Table 8. Comparison of Lipoprotein (a) Cohorts

	Lp(a) < 57 mg/dL (n = 84)	Lp(a) ≥ 57 mg/dL (n = 40)	Probability Value
Lp(a) (mg/dL)*	23.5 ± 16.8	96.3 ± 33.8	$<10^{-4}$ †
Age (yr)	60 ± 16	61 ± 13	0.61
Race (%)			<0.02
White	38%	19%	
Black	43%	71%	
Hispanic	19%	10%	
Male (%)	52%	39%	0.22
Diabetes (%)	38%	44%	0.67
PTFE access (%)	70%	73%	0.90
Systolic BP (mm Hg)	133 ± 25	139 ± 19	0.20
Diastolic BP (mm Hg)	76 ± 12	78 ± 8.1	0.51
Hematocrit (%)	27.6 ± 5.3	27.4 ± 5.1	0.90
Erythropoietin (U/wk)	3,940 ± 3,678	3,425 ± 3,448	0.50†
Heparin (U/treatment)	1,469 ± 899	1,524 ± 987	0.90†
Treatment time (hr)	2.98 ± 0.35	3.06 ± 0.37	0.25
BUN ratio	2.72 ± 0.49	2.75 ± 0.66	0.84

Abbreviations: PTFE, polytetrafluoroethylene; BP, blood pressure.
* Median values were 21.6 mg/dL and 94.3 mg/dL (for Lp(a) cohorts <57 mg/dL and ≥57 mg/dL), respectively.
† Comparison by Mann-Whitney U-test.

Lp(a) levels than men. Since the women were older, their higher mean Lp(a) may reflect the postmenopausal state that was associated with higher Lp(a) in several studies.[58] The correlations observed for Lp(a) with total cholesterol and apoB probably reflect the cholesterol and apoB content of Lp(a). The strength of the observed correlation with total cholesterol was comparable to that found in other populations, although the correlation observed with apoB was somewhat stronger.[41,44,57,59,60] In this study, serum Lp(a) and the TC/HDLC ratio appeared to be independent correlates of baseline coronary status and were particularly useful in distinguishing patients with CAD from those with clinical angina. However, due to the small sample size, the correlations were only of borderline significance. Moreover, owing to biases inherent in the study of prevalent groups and imprecision in the baseline classification of cases in this study (eg, false-positive and false-negative stress testing), the correlation of Lp(a) and coronary status needs to be confirmed in other dialysis populations. Cressman et al did not find any correlation between Lp(a) and atherosclerosis in their cross-sectional study of a group of hemodialysis patients.[47]

In prospective analysis, Lp(a) did not predict mortality risk over 14 months. This is in agreement with the 48-month cohort study of Cressman et al.[47] In that study, the high Lp(a) cohort did not show an increase in cardiovascular morbidity or mortality at 18 months; at 48 months, however, they had significantly increased cardiovascular morbidity and mortality. In our 14-month study, there were too few cardiovascular events for meaningful analysis. Importantly, high Lp(a)

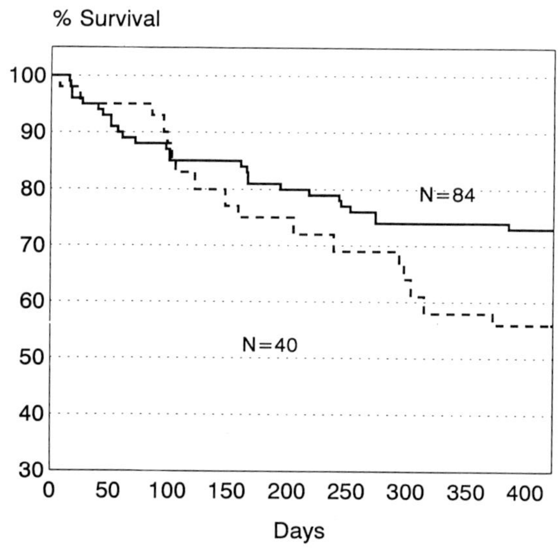

Fig 2. Vascular access event-free survival over 14 months in 84 patients with serum Lp(a) < 57 mg/dL (——) and 40 patients with serum Lp(a) ≥ 57 mg/dL (- - -) (*P* < 0.06).

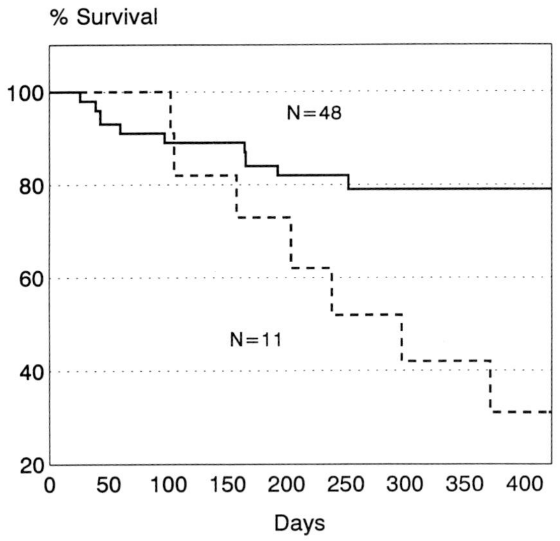

Fig 3. Vascular access event-free survival over 14 months in 59 white or Hispanic patients stratified by serum Lp(a) $<$ 57 mg/dL (——) (n = 48) versus $\geq$57 mg/dL (---) (n = 11) (P $<$ 0.01).

was associated with an increased risk of vascular access occlusion. This trend was of borderline significance when all patients were analyzed, but increased in magnitude and was statistically significant for white and Hispanic patients. Although there was potential confounding of high Lp(a) by diabetes in the white and Hispanic group, the relationship of Lp(a) to access occlusion was consistent for both diabetic and nondiabetic patients. The apparent lack of influence of Lp(a) on vascular access occlusion in black patients is compatible with the speculation that Lp(a) may be less thrombogenic and atherogenic in black patients.[43,57,61] In the study of Cressman et al, the cohorts were not stratified by race.[47] If Lp(a) is a new risk predictor for vascular access events, Lp(a)-lowering therapy may be of benefit. At present, only nicotinic acid, its derivatives, and apheresis methods have been reported to lower Lp(a) in dialysis patients.[62,63]

Cross-sectional analysis of serum prealbumin demonstrated significant correlations with the other serum nutritional markers. The correlations of serum albumin with the same markers were somewhat weaker. In the proportional hazards analysis, the independent predictors of mortality risk were low concentrations of prealbumin, apoB, and creatinine and increased age. Serum albumin and total cholesterol were not independent predictors of mortality in the final model. Despite being more strongly correlated with and hence confounded by creatinine and apoB, prealbumin was actually a stronger independent correlate of mortality risk than albumin concentration (Tables 4 to 7). This implies that prealbumin concentration may be more reflective of a distinctive aspect of mortality risk than albumin or, conversely, that albumin concentration may be more influenced by factors unrelated to mortality risk. The increased predictive power of serum prealbumin compared with albumin may be due to the short half-life of serum prealbumin, which permits rapid changes in its concentration in response to undernutrition or catabolism.[38-40] Similarly, it is noteworthy that apoB, although highly correlated with total cholesterol cross-sectionally, was a significantly stronger correlate of mortality in univariate analysis (data not shown) and in the multivariate model (Table 7). In any event, circulating visceral and somatic protein markers, prealbumin, apoB, and creatinine all appear to contribute independent information to risk assessment. The BUN ratio measured on enrollment was not a significant risk predictor in the final model. The BUN ratio is a measurement of the delivered dialysis dose normalized to the urea space. Although other preliminary studies have found increased mortality risk associated with lower dialysis doses,[64] the design of this

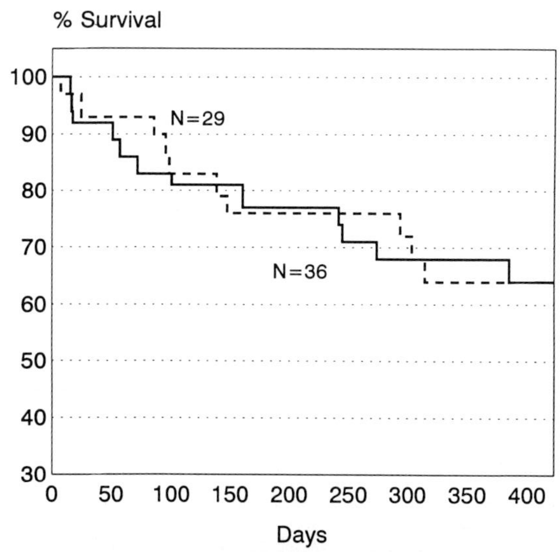

Fig 4. Vascular access event-free survival over 14 months in 65 black patients stratified by serum Lp(a) $<$ 57 mg/dL (——) (n = 36) versus $\geq$57 mg/dL (---) (n = 29) (P $>$ 0.90).

study may have minimized both the apparent risk associated with low initial BUN ratio values and the apparent benefit associated with higher initial values. For example, selective physician interventions tend to increase the dialysis doses of the patients with the lowest initial values. Additionally, patients who were losing weight owing to a co-morbid condition may have drifted up to higher BUN ratio values prior to study enrollment as their weight (and urea distribution volume) fell. The upward drift of these cases would result in less apparent benefit with the higher BUN ratios. Similarly, since dialysis dose was not randomly allocated, physicians may have empirically prescribed higher dialysis doses for patients who were not "doing well" because of unsuspected co-morbid illness.

In summary, two serum risk markers, Lp(a) and prealbumin, were evaluated prospectively in hemodialysis patients and found to contribute important prognostic information. Increased serum Lp(a) concentration correlated with vascular access occlusion in white and Hispanic patients. Reduced serum levels of prealbumin, together with reduced levels of apoB and creatinine, were found to be important, independent predictors of mortality risk. These markers will enable clinicians to identify patients at high risk and investigators to improve stratification of patient risk in future observational and interventional studies.

ACKNOWLEDGMENT

The authors thank Dr Joseph Feldman for his assistance in the statistical analysis, Dr Daniel Levine of The Rogosin Institute, New York Hospital-Cornell Medical Center, to whom we are much indebted for the Lp(a) determinations, INCSTAR Corp for their donation of Lp(a) assay kits, Antoinette Antignani for her expert technical assistance, and Marilyn Collins for her assistance in preparing this manuscript.

REFERENCES

1. End-Stage Renal Disease Program Facility Survey Tables 1982 through 1988. Baltimore, MD, ESRD Information Analysis Branch, Division of Information Analysis, Health Care Financing Administration, 1989

2. Hull AR, Parker TF III: Proceedings from the Morbidity, Mortality and Prescription of Dialysis Symposium, Dallas, TX, September 15-17, 1989. Am J Kidney Dis 15:375-383, 1990

3. United States Renal Data System, USRDS 1989 Annual Report. Bethesda, MD, National Institutes of Health, National Institute of Diabetes, and Digestive and Kidney Diseases, August 1989

4. Broyer M, Brunner FP, Brynger H, Fassbinder W, Guillou PJ, Oules R, Rizzoni G, Selwood NH, Wing AJ, Challah S, Dykes SR: Demography of dialysis and transplantation in Europe, 1984. Nephrol Dial Transplant 1:1-8, 1986

5. Port FK, Garcia JR, Whelton P, Fitzsimmons SC, Moulton LH: Changes in causes of death among ESRD patients in the U.S. US Renal Data System, Washington, DC. Kidney Int 37:283, 1990 (abstr)

6. Lindner A, Charra B, Sherrard DJ, Scribner BH: Accelerated atherosclerosis in prolonged maintenance hemodialysis. N Engl J Med 290:697-701, 1974

7. Lowrie ED, Lazarus JM, Mocelin AJ, Bailey GL, Hampers CL, Wilson RE, Merrill JP: Survival of patients undergoing chronic hemodialysis and renal transplantation. N Engl J Med 288:863-867, 1973

8. Green D, Stone NJ, Krumlovsky FA: Putative atherogenic factors in patients with chronic renal failure. Prog Cardiovasc Dis 26:133-144, 1983

9. Rostand SG, Gretes JC, Kirk KA, Rutsky EA, Andreoli TE: Ischemic heart disease in patients with uremia undergoing maintenance hemodialysis. Kidney Int 16:600-611, 1979

10. Rostand SG, Kirk KA, Rutsky EA: Relationship of coronary risk factors to hemodialysis-associated ischemic heart disease. Kidney Int 22:304-308, 1982

11. Rostand SG, Kirk KA, Rutsky EA: Dialysis-associated ischemic heart disease: Insights from coronary angiography. Kidney Int 25:653-659, 1984

12. Goldberg AP, Harter HR, Patsch W, Schectman KB, Province M, Weerts C, Kuisk I, McCrate MM, Schonfeld G: Racial differences in plasma high-density lipoproteins in patients receiving hemodialysis. N Engl J Med 308:1245-1252, 1983

13. Dieplinger H, Schoenfeld PY, Fielding CJ: Plasma cholesterol metabolism in end-stage renal disease—difference between treatment by hemodialysis or peritoneal dialysis. J Clin Inv 77:1071-1083, 1986

14. Bagdade JD, Albers JJ: Plasma high-density lipoprotein concentrations in chronic hemodialysis and renal-transplant patients. N Engl J Med 296:1436-1439, 1977

15. Chan MK, Persaud J, Varghese Z, Moorhead JF: Pathogenic roles of post-heparin lipases in lipid abnormalities in hemodialysis patients. Kidney Int 25:812-818, 1984

16. Avram MM, Fein PA, Antignani A, Mittman N, Mushnick RA, Lustig AR, Lapuz MH, Goldwasser P: Cholesterol and lipid disturbances in renal disease: The natural history of the uremic dyslipidemia and continuous ambulatory peritoneal dialysis. Am J Med 87:55N-60N, 1989

17. Avram MM, Goldwasser P, Burrell DE, Antignani A, Fein PA, Mittman N: The uremic dyslipidemia: A cross-sectional and longitudinal study. Am J Kidney Dis 20:324-335, 1992

18. Lacour B, Roullet JB, Beyne P, Kreis H, Thevenin M, Drüeke T: Comparison of several atherogenicity indices by the analysis of serum lipoprotein composition in patients with chronic renal failure with or without hemodialysis, and in renal transplant patients. J Clin Chem Biochem 23:805-810, 1985

19. Burke JF, Francos GC, Moore LL, Cho SY, Lasker N: Accelerated atherosclerosis in chronic dialysis patients—Another look. Nephron 21:181-185, 1978

20. Ritz E, Querfeld U: Atherogenesis—Is it accelerated in uremia? Semin Dialysis 2:246-252, 1989

21. Bergesio F, Ciuti R, Salvadori M, Galli GA, Monzani G, Bestoni E, Salerno A, Frizzi V: Are lipid abnormalities reliable cardiovascular risk factors in dialysis patients? Int J Artif Organs 12:677-682, 1989

22. Attman PO, Alaupovic P, Gustafson A: Serum apolipoprotein profile of patients with chronic renal failure. Kidney Int 32:368-375, 1987

23. Manske CL: Low HDL cholesterol is not associated with coronary artery disease in azotemic diabetics. Kidney Int 37:280, 1990 (abstr)

24. Parsy D, Dracon M, Cachera C, Parra H-J, Vanhouette G, Tacquet A, Fruchart J-C: Lipoprotein abnormalities in chronic hemodialysis patients. Dialysis Transplant 3:51-56, 1988

25. Hutchinson TA, Thomas DC, MacGibbon B: Predicting survival in adults with end-stage renal disease: An age equivalence index. Ann Intern Med 96:417-423, 1982

26. Maiorca R, Vonesh E, Cancarini GC, Cantaluppi A, Manili L, Brunori MG, Camerini C, Feller P, Strada A: A six-year comparison of patient and technique survivals in CAPD and HD. Kidney Int 34:518-524, 1988

27. Silberberg JS, Barre PE, Prichard SS, Sniderman AD: Impact of left ventricular hypertrophy on survival in end-stage renal disease. Kidney Int 36:268-290, 1989

28. Collier JT, Erroa M, Goldwasser P, Antignani A, Mittman N, Avram MM: Prospective study of one-year survival on hemodialysis. Am J Kidney Dis 19:A3, 1992 (abstr)

29. Erroa M, Goldwasser P, Mittman N, Fein PA, Avram MM: Predictors of one-year survival in CAPD. Perit Dial Int 12:116, 1992 (abstr)

30. Avram MM, Slater PA, Gan A, Iancu M, Pahilan AN, Okanya D, Rajpal K, Paik SK, Zouabi M, Fein PA: Predialysis BUN and creatinine do not predict adequate dialysis, clinical rehabilitation, or longevity. Kidney Int 28:S100-S104, 1985

31. Shapiro JI, Argy WB, Rakowski TA, Chester A, Siemsen AS, Schreiner GA: The unsuitability of BUN as a criterion for prescription dialysis. ASAIO Trans 29:129-132, 1983

32. Cano N, Fernandez JP, Lacombe P, Lankester M, Pascal S, DeFayolle M, Labastie J, Saingra S: Statistical selection of nutritional parameters in hemodialyzed patients. Kidney Int 32:S178-S180, 1987 (suppl 22)

33. Lowrie EG, Lew NL: Death risk in hemodialysis patients: The predictive value of commonly measured variables and an evaluation of the death rate differences between facilities. Am J Kidney Dis 15:458-482, 1990

34. Goldwasser P, Mittman N, Antignani A, Burrell D, Michel M-A, Collier JC, Avram MM: Predictors of mortality in hemodialysis patients. J Am Soc Nephrol 3:1613-1622, 1993

35. Acchiardo SR, Moore LW, Latour PA: Malnutrition as the main factor in morbidity and mortality of dialysis patients. Kidney Int 24:S199-S203, 1983 (suppl 16)

36. Blumenkrantz MJ, Kopple JD, Gutman RA, Chan YK, Barbour GL, Roberts C, Shen FH, Gandhi VC, Tucker T, Curtis FK, Coburn JW: Methods for assessing nutritional status of patients with renal failure. Am J Clin Nutr 33:1567-1585, 1980

37. Torún B, Viteri FE: Protein-energy malnutrition, in Shils ME, Young VR (eds): Modern Nutrition in Health and Disease (ed 7). Philadelphia, PA, Lea & Feibiger, 1988, pp 746-773

38. Tuten MB, Wogt S, Dasse F, Lieder Z: Utilization of prealbumin as a nutritional parameter. J Parenter Enteral Nutr 9:709-711, 1985

39. Robbins J, Cheng SY, Gershengorn MC, Glinoer D, Cahnmann J, Edelnoch H: Thyroxine transport proteins of plasma: Molecular properties and biosynthesis. Recent Prog Horm Res 34:477-519, 1979

40. Ingenbleek Y, DeVisscher M, DeNayer P: Measurement of prealbumin as index of protein-calorie malnutrition. Lancet 2:106-108, 1972

41. Murai A, Miyahara T, Fujimoto N, Matusada M, Kameyama M: Lp(a) lipoprotein as a risk factor for coronary heart disease and cerebral infarction. Atherosclerosis 59:199-204, 1986

42. Dahlén GH, Guyton JR, Attar M, Farmer JA, Kautz JA, Gotto M: Association of levels of lipoprotein Lp(a), plasma lipids and other lipoproteins with coronary disease documented by angiography. Circulation 74:758-765, 1986

43. Scanu A: Lipoprotein(a): A genetic risk factor for premature coronary disease. JAMA 267:3326-3329, 1992

44. Rosengren A, Wilhelmsen L, Eriksson E, Risberg B, Wedel H: Lipoprotein(a) and coronary heart disease: A prospective case control study in a general population sample of middle aged men. Br Med J 301:1248-1251, 1990

45. Hoff HF, Beck GJ, Skibinski CI, Jürgens G, O'Neil J, Kramer J, Lytle B: Serum Lp(a) level as a predictor of vein graft stenosis after coronary bypass surgery in patients. Circulation 77:1238-1244, 1988

46. Parra HJ, Mezdour H, Cachera C, Dracon M, Jacquet A, Fruchart JC: Lipoprotein(a) in patients with chronic renal failure treated by hemodialysis. Clin Chem 33:721, 1987

47. Cressman MD, Heyka RJ, Paganini EP, O'Neil J, Skibinski CI, Hoff HF: Lipoprotein(a) is an independent risk factor for cardiovascular disease in hemodialysis patients. Circulation 86:475-482, 1992

48. Daugirdas JT, Dumler F, Zasuwa GA, Levin NW: Chronic hemodialysis prescription, in Daugirdas JT, Ing TS (eds): Handbook of Dialysis (ed 1): Boston, MA, Little, Brown, 1988, pp 72-86

49. Keshaviah PR, Hanson GL, Berkseth RO, Collins AJ: A simplified approach to monitoring in vivo therapy prescription. Trans Am Soc Artif Intern Organs 34:620-622, 1988

50. Soundararajan R, Soundararajan P: A simple and practical method for assessing the adequacy of dialysis. ASAIO Trans 37:M393-M394, 1991

51. Levine DM, Sloan BJ, Lorenz JD, Donner JE, Heinzcoling RH: Automated measurement of lipoprotein(a) by immunoturbidimetric analysis. Int J Clin Lab Res 22:173-178, 1992

52. Cox DR: Regression models and life tables (with discussion). J R Stat Soc Series B 34:187-220, 1992

53. Kelbfleisch J, Prentice R: The Statistical Analysis of Failure Time Data. New York, NY, Wiley, 1980

54. Kaplan EL, Meier P: Nonparametric estimation from incomplete observations. J Am Stat Assoc 53:457-481, 1958

55. Nouřsis MJ: SPSS for Windows Advanced Statistics Release 5.0.2. Chicago, IL, SPSS Inc, 1992, pp 259-274

56. Steinman TI, Mitch WE: Nutrition in dialysis patients, in Maher JF (ed): Replacement of Renal Function by Dialysis. Dordrecht, Holland, Kluwer Academic, 1988, pp 1088-1106

57. Guyton JR, Dahlen GH, Ratsch W, Kautz JA, Gotto

AM: Relationship of plasma lipoprotein Lp(a) levels to race and to apolipoprotein B. Arteriosclerosis 5:265-272, 1985

58. Rader DJ, Brewer HB, Jr: Lipoprotein(a): Clinical approach to a unique atherogenic lipoprotein. JAMA 267:1109-1112, 1992

59. Berg K: Genetics of atherogenic lipoprotein(a) and its relation to other atherosclerotic risk factors, in Scanu AM, moderator: Lipoprotein(a) and Atherosclerosis. Ann Intern Med 115:209-218, 1991

60. Irish AB, Hayes JM, Simons LA, Simons J, Sardie E: Lipoprotein(a) levels in chronic disease states, dialysis and transplantation. Aust N Z J Med 22:243-248, 1992

61. Srinivasan SR, Dahlen GH, Jarpa RA, Webber LS, Berenson GS: Racial (black-white) differences in serum lipoprotein(a) distribution and its relation to parental myocardial infarction in children. Circulation 84:160-167, 1991

62. Bosch T, Thiery J, Samtleben W, Seidel D: Combined simultaneous LDL-apheresis and hemodialysis in hypercholesterolemic ESRD patients: A new mode of therapy. J Am Soc Nephrol 2:233, 1991 (abstr)

63. Nakahama H, Miyazaki M, Imai N, Yokokawa T, Okada M, Kubori S, Okamural K, Tanaka Y, Shirai D: Reduction of plasma lipoprotein(a) levels by niceritrol in patients on maintenance hemodialysis. J Am Soc Nephrol 2:340, 1991 (abstr)

64. Hakim RM, Depner TA, Parker TF: Adequacy of hemodialysis. Am J Kidney Dis 20:107-123, 1992

Lipoprotein(a) in Patients Treated by Continuous Ambulatory Peritoneal Dialysis

Joëlle Thillet, PhD, Claire Faucher, MD, Belkacem Issad, MD, Mahmoud Allouache, MD, John Chapman, PhD, and Claude Jacobs, MD, FRCP

● **Lipoprotein(a) [Lp(a)] has been identified as an independent, inherited risk factor for atherosclerotic vascular disease. An elevation of Lp(a) plasma levels has been documented in several series of uremic patients submitted to maintenance dialysis treatment methods or after renal transplantation. We have measured the plasma levels of Lp(a) using an enzyme-linked immunosorbent enzyme method in 19 patients treated with continuous ambulatory peritoneal dialysis (CAPD). Mean (±SD) concentration of Lp(a) was significantly higher in the patients than in the 19 healthy controls (51 ± 48 mg/dL *v* 16 ± 15 mg/dL, *P* < 0.005). No significant differences in Lp(a) levels were found between diabetic patients (n = 5) and nondiabetic patients (n = 14) or between patients who had (n = 6) or had not (n = 13) suffered a previous major cardiovascular complication. No correlation was evident between Lp(a) levels and the patients' ages, period of time on CAPD treatment, or any other lipid-lipoprotein investigated parameter. The mechanisms accounting for the elevation of Lp(a) levels in CAPD patients as well as the specific value of increased Lp(a) concentration as a cardiovascular risk predictor in uremic patients remain thus far speculative. Additional experimental and clinical studies are warranted before the administration of drugs to attempt to lower Lp(a) levels in CAPD patients can be recommended.**

INDEX WORDS: Lipoprotein(a); dyslipidemia; end-stage renal failure; continuous ambulatory peritoneal dialysis.

ATHEROSCLEROTIC vascular disease is widely recognized as a leading cause of morbidity and mortality in terminally uremic patients undergoing any mode of renal replacement therapy, extracorporeal dialysis, peritoneal dialysis, or renal transplantation.[1-3] Whether these patients actually show a truly accelerated atherosclerosis profile has remained a matter of ongoing debate for more than 15 years.[4-6] The extent to which disturbances of lipid and lipoprotein metabolism may contribute specifically among many other atherogenic risk factors to the vascular complications afflicting the uremic patients is also diversely appreciated.[7-10]

The dyslipidemic profiles encountered in terminally uremic patients treated with continuous ambulatory peritoneal dialysis (CAPD) have been extensively documented in several studies published in the literature during the past 10 years.[11-16] These investigations revealed certain features that are distinct from those recorded in patients treated by maintenance hemodialysis or renal transplantation.[17-21] Indeed, the most common profile documented in CAPD patients includes a near-normal or moderately elevated level of total cholesterol (TC), a reduced level of high-density lipoprotein cholesterol (HDLC) and apolipoprotein A (apoA), and an often marked elevation of low-density lipoprotein cholesterol (LDLC), triglycerides, and apolipoprotein B (apoB), the latter being considered as the prevalent dyslipoproteinemia recorded in CAPD-treated patients.[15,21] The mechanisms involved in the genesis and development of these abnormalities remain uncompletely elucidated; however, for several investigators these include to a variable extent the continuous absorption of glucose from the peritoneal dialysate, the reduced activity of lipoprotein lipase and hepatic lipase causing delayed clearance of triglyceride-rich lipoproteins and a greater loss in the dialysis fluid of apoA over that of apoB, the resulting elevation of plasma concentration of apoB exposing the patients to a greater risk of atherosclerotic vascular disease.[14,16,22]

In recent years, lipoprotein(a) [Lp(a)], discovered in 1963 by Kâre Berg, has been clearly identified as a further independent, inherited risk factor for atherosclerotic cardiovascular disease.[23-26] The atherogenicity and thrombogenicity of Lp(a) are deemed to be related to its structure, consisting of an LDL-like particle with a molecule of apoB-100 linked by a disulphide bridge to a large glycosylated apoprotein (apoA), which is structurally homogenous to plasminogen.[27] Lipoprotein(a) competes with plasminogen for binding sites on endothelial cells and fibrin. Binding of Lp(a) to fibrin may thus accelerate the formation of atherosclerotic plaques at sites of endothelial injury by inhibiting the generation of plasmin on fibrin clots, blocking fibrinolysis,

Supported by a research grant from AURA (Paris).

Table 1. Continuous Ambulatory Peritoneal Dialysis Patients: Clinical Data

No. of Patients	19
Sex (M/F)	12/7
Age (yr)	65 ± 14 (range, 31-86)
Etiology of renal disease	
Glomerulonephritis	8
Diabetic nephropathy	5
Interstitial nephritis	1
Renal vascular disease	1
Polycystic kidney disease	1
Undetermined	3
Time on CAPD (months)	21 ± 24 (range, 5-113)

and promoting thrombosis. These properties have prompted numerous studies on Lp(a) levels in populations of patients particularly prone to atherosclerotic cardiovascular complications, such as diabetic patients,[28,29] patients with proteinuria or nephrotic syndrome,[30,31] and terminally uremic patients treated with maintenance hemodialysis,[32-39] peritoneal dialysis,[36-43] or renal transplantation.[33,41,44,45] We report in this study the results of Lp(a) determination in 19 patients submitted to CAPD for the treatment of end-stage renal failure.

PATIENTS AND METHODS

Plasma Lp(a) concentration was determined together with other lipid-apolipoprotein parameters in 19 patients submitted to CAPD treatment for end-stage renal failure. The clinical characteristics of the patients and the etiology of their underlying renal disease are described in Table 1. Four of the five diabetic patients were insulin dependent/treated and four patients had suffered a myocardial infarction prior to initiation of renal replacement therapy. Continuous ambulatory peritoneal dialysis was composed of four daily exchanges of 2-L bags of dialysate, of which three contained 1.36% glucose and one contained 3.86% glucose. The dietary recommendations included a caloric intake of 35 to 40 kcal/kg body weight with 1 to 1.20 g protein/kg body weight, no specific limitation in lipid intake, and carbohydrate intake restricted to approximately 220 g/d for the diabetic patients. Four patients were taking lipid-lowering drugs at the time of the study.

For measurement of Lp(a), venous blood was drawn after a normal overnight fast and without interruption of CAPD. Blood was collected in tubes containing EDTA (final concentration, 0.1%). Plasma was immediately separated by low-speed centrifugation at 4°C and was stored at −20°C prior to assays.

Lipoprotein(a) was quantified using a noncompetitive enzyme-linked immunosorbent assay developed in our laboratory with two polyclonal antibodies. An anti-human apo(A) antibody prepared in sheep was used as the "capture" antibody and a peroxidase-conjugate anti-human apoB100 antibody as the detecting antibody. Both antibodies were purified by caprylic acid precipitation and then concentrated by ammonium sulfate precipitation (40%). Polystyrene microtiter plates (96-well immunoplates; Costar, Cambridge, UK) were coated overnight at 4°C with 100 μL of a 10 μg/mL dilution of antiapo(A) antibody in phosphate-buffered saline (PBS), pH 7.4. After washing to remove unbound antibodies (washing buffer, PBS containing 0.05% Tween), the wells were blocked by incubation with 3% bovine serum albumin in PBS at room temperature for 1 hour. After a further wash, 100 μL of appropriately diluted Lp(a) samples in PBS containing 0.05% Tween and 1% bovine serum albumin, pH 7.4, were added to the wells. The plates were incubated for 2 hours at 37°C; they were then washed and a peroxidase-labeled, anti-apoB100 antibody (1:800 in PBS/Tween/bovine serum albumin) was added. After an additional 1.5-hour incubation at 37°C, the plates were washed and the substrate (1 mg/mL O-phenylenediamine dihydrochloride [OPD Sigma, St Louis, MO] in 0.05 mol/L citrate buffer at pH 5.5 containing 0.01% H_2O_2) was added. The reaction was then allowed to proceed in the dark for 20 minutes and was stopped with HCl 3N. Absorbance was then read at 492 nm using a Titertek multiscan microplate reader. Each plate contained eight dilutions (4 ng to 500 ng total Lp(a)/well) of a reference standard (Immuno-France). Periodically, purified Lp(a) was compared with the reference standard for calibration purposes. For the present enzyme-linked immunosorbent assay, the working concentration range was 40 ng to 5 μg/mL Lp(a) lipoprotein mass. Intracoefficient and intercoefficient of variation for the enzyme-linked immunosorbent assay used in the study were 1.0% (n = 32) and 2.6% (n = 18), respectively.

The plasma samples were stored at −20°C. Previous examination demonstrated the absence of any effect on Lp(a) assays from freezing the samples over a 3-month period. Two determinations of plasma Lp(a) concentration were performed in the 19 patients at an interval of 1 month, yielding similar average results (51 ± 48 mg/dL and 51 ± 51 mg/dL, respectively, P = NS). Correlations between Lp(a) plasma concentrations and other lipid-apolipoprotein parameters were therefore made against the first assay. Plasma Lp(a) concentration was furthermore determined in 19 healthy subjects aged 50 ± 17 years (range, 33 to 93 years) who served as controls. Plasma total cholesterol and triglycerides were determined enzymatically with Boehringer-Mannheim reagents (Mannheim, Germany); total protein and albumin were assessed with standard laboratory methods. The quantification of apoAI and apoB in whole plasma was performed by nephelometry using commercial antibodies (Behring, Marburg, Germany). Plasma HDLC was estimated enzymatically (Boehringer-Mannheim), apoB lipoprotein being initially precipitated with phosphotungstate/$MgCl_2$. Low-density lipoprotein cholesterol was calculated according to the formula of Friedewald: LDLC = total cholesterol − (HDLC + triglycerides/5). The results are expressed as mean ± SD. Statistical analyses were performed with the Statview TMII computer program (Abacus Concepts Inc, Berkeley, CA) using Student's t-test for paired or unpaired data as appropriate, and single linear regression with a statistical level of significance set at 5%.

RESULTS

The mean plasma concentrations of Lp(a) in the 19 CAPD patients measured twice at an inter-

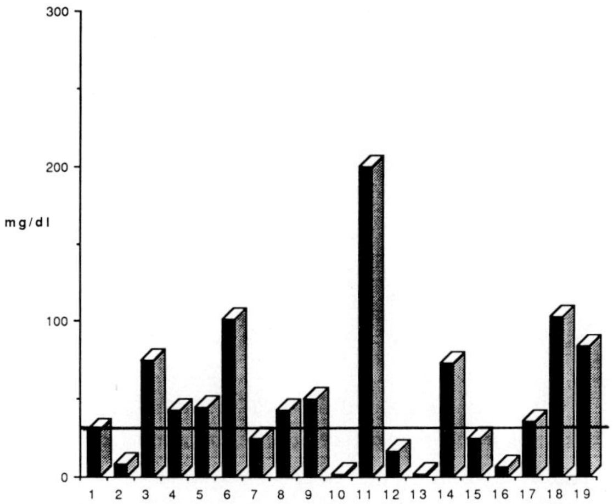

Fig 1. Serum Lp(a) concentrations in 19 patients treated by CAPD (mean ± SD, 51 ± 48 mg/dL; range, 2 to 201 mg/dL). The horizontal line at 30 mg/dL represents the level above which elevation of Lp(a) is considered to be an increased risk factor for coronary heart disease.

val of 1 month were 51 ± 48 mg/dL and 51 ± 51 mg/dL, respectively ($P = 0.98$ [NS]). The individual values that were observed at the first determination are shown in Fig 1. The mean values recorded in the CAPD patients are very significantly higher than those found in the 19 healthy control subjects: 16 mg/dL ± 15 ($P < 0.005$, Fig 2). The plasma concentrations of lipid-lipoprotein parameters, total protein, and albumin determined in the CAPD patients are described in Table 2; total cholesterol, HDLC, LDLC, and triglyceride levels being not considered for the four patients who were taking a lipid-lowering drug. No correlation could be detected between the plasma concentration of Lp(a) and the following parameters: age, ($P = 0.98$), duration of CAPD treatment ($P = 0.27$), and any of the other biologic parameters investigated (Table 3). No statistical difference in plasma Lp(a) levels was found between the diabetic and nondiabetic patients (unpaired *t*-test: 0.24; $P = 0.98$ [NS]) and between those who had or had not suffered a myocardial infarction (*t*-test: 1.0; $P = 0.32$ [NS]).

DISCUSSION

The overall lipid profile observed in this group of patients treated with CAPD is well in accordance with the results reported by several other

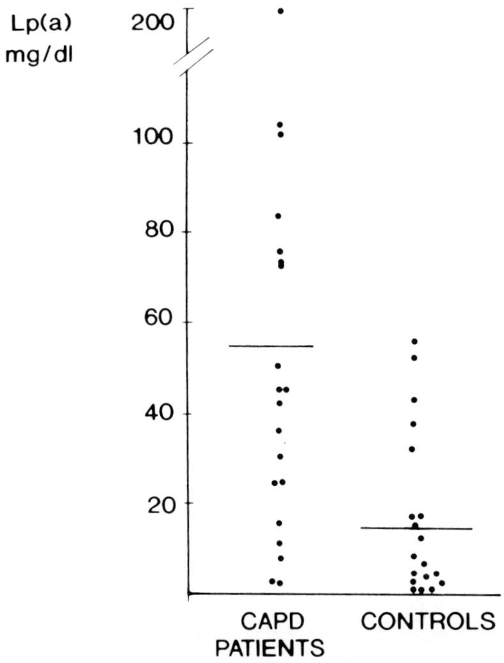

Fig 2. Serum Lp(a) concentrations in 19 patients treated with CAPD (51 ± 48 mg/dL) and in 19 healthy control subjects (16 ± 15 mg/dL) ($P < 0.005$).

investigators in patients submitted to this mode of renal replacement therapy.[11,12,14] The mean levels of total cholesterol, HDLC, LDLC, and apoA1 are within the normal reference values of the laboratory, with, on the other hand, an elevation of triglycerides and apoB concentrations. Atherogenic risk ratios (total cholesterol/HDLC

Table 2. Plasma Lipids, Lipoproteins, Total Protein, and Albumin Concentrations in Continuous Ambulatory Peritoneal Dialysis Patients

	CAPD Patients	No. of Patients	Reference Values
Total cholesterol (mg/dL)	241 ± 60	15	147-251
HDLC (mg/dL)	48 ± 18	15	39-67
Total cholesterol/HDLC	5.7 ± 2.5	15	<4
LDLC (mg/dL)	157 ± 75	15	170
Triglycerides (mg/dL)	152 ± 47	15	35-144
Lp(a) (mg/dL)	51 ± 48	19	1-53
ApoA1 (mg/dL)	146 ± 40	19	113-185
ApoB (mg/dL)	144 ± 26	19	63-134
ApoA1/ApoB	1.01 ± 1.6	19	1.4-1.8
Total protein (g/dL)	6.1 ± 0.4	19	6.5-7.8
Albumin (g/dL)	3.5 ± 0.4	19	3.7-4.6

Table 3. Correlations Between Lipoprotein(a) Levels and Biologic Parameters in Continous Ambulatory Peritoneal Dialysis Patients

	No. of Patients	*r*	Probability Value
Total cholesterol	15	0.26	0.34
HDLC	15	0.37	0.17
LDLC	15	0.35	0.19
Total cholesterol/HDLC	15	0.17	0.54
Triglycerides	15	0.28	0.31
ApoA1	19	0.04	0.85
ApoB	19	0.11	0.64
ApoA/ApoB	19	0.07	0.77
Total plasma protein	19	0.26	0.27
Plasma albumin	19	0.01	0.97

and apoA1/apoB) are both in the ''higher-risk'' range. The mean Lp(a) level in the CAPD patients is more than threefold higher that of the healthy controls. In keeping with the results reported in several other studies involving uremic nondialyzed, dialyzed, or transplanted patients, no statistically significant correlation could be detected in the CAPD patients either with clinical characteristics (age, sex, duration of renal replacement therapy) or any other lipid-profile parameter investigated,[31,33,34] whereas a significant correlation between Lp(a) concentrations and apoB levels has been reported in a recent work by Shoji et al.[40] There were no significant differences in Lp(a) levels between our CAPD diabetic and nondiabetic patients or between those who had or had not experienced an overt clinical cardiovascular complication during the course of their renal disease. The lack of correlation between Lp(a) concentrations and cardiovascular events recorded in these series of patients, however, may be related to the small sample size of the population included in the study.

A marked increased risk for coronary heart disease has been documented in patients with a Lp(a) concentration greater than 30 mg/dL.[24] Cardiovascular risk is considered as enhanced by a concomittant elevation of LDLC levels.[23] Eleven of our 19 patients had a Lp(a) level higher than 30 mg/dL; four of the 15 patients not taking a lipid-lowering medication displayed an LDLC level above the upper normal range. Lipoprotein(a) and LDLC levels were both elevated in only two of these 15 patients, one of whom had by far the highest Lp(a) concentration (201 mg/dL) and the second highest LDLC level (246 mg/dL). This patient was a 76-year-old man with primary glomerulonephritis who had been treated by CAPD for 35 months at the time of the study and had not suffered a major atherosclerotic cardiovascular complication during his past history.

An increase in plasma Lp(a) concentration has been documented in several recent studies performed in limited groups of uremic patients, either prior to initiation of renal replacement therapy,[36,39,46] during maintenance hemodialysis,[33-38] or after successful renal transplantation.[34,41,44] However, Cressman et al[32] found normal levels of Lp(a) in their transplanted patients with good renal function, in contrast to elevated levels in hemodialysis and CAPD patients; this finding led these investigators to hypothesize that renal dysfunction is implicated in the elevation of Lp(a) levels in uremic patients. Increased Lp(a) levels have been described in all published studies performed in patients treated by CAPD except in that by Kandoussi et al, who reported Lp(a) concentrations to be within the normal range in 24 CAPD patients in contrast to elevated levels evidenced in 24 uremic nondialyzed patients and in 18 patients treated by maintenance hemodialysis.[36] No clear explanation is apparent for this rather surprising discrepancy.

The underlying mechanisms that may account for the elevation of Lp(a) levels in uremic patients, and more specifically in those submitted to maintenance dialysis methods, remain thus far obscure. According to Boerwinckle et al, genetic factors account for more than 90% of the variation of plasma Lp(a) concentration in normal subjects.[47] The differences in plasma levels are considered to be related more to the variation of hepatic synthesis of Lp(a) than to its catabolism, whose pathway(s) remains to date largely unknown. It has not been established whether the elevation of Lp(a) in uremic patients results from an overproduction by the liver, impaired catabolism, or both.[31,33] Impairment of renal function could interfere with the catabolism of Lp(a) and induce an elevation of its plasma concentration.[32] This hypothesis, however, is not supported by the results reported by Thomas, et al, who found no correlation between plasma Lp(a) concentrations and plasma creatinine or creatinine clearance in a population of patients whose plasma creatinine ranged from 71 to 510 μmol/L.[31] A similar finding was reported by Webb et al in a group of transplanted patients who had a plasma creatinine ranging from 140 to 680 μmol/L.[48] Alternatively, it has been suggested that high levels of Lp(a) may be related to hypertriglyceridemia,[33] but we, like other investigators, failed to detect a correlation between Lp(a) and triglyceride levels in our population of CAPD patients. As mentioned previously, plasma Lp(a) levels are found in some (but not all) studies to be significantly higher in CAPD patients than in a control group of hemodialysis patients; the possible contribution of the continuous absorption of glucose from the peritoneal cavity to an increased synthesis of Lp(a) by the liver is therefore suggested, but thus far unproven.[36]

Whether plasma Lp(a) levels may be useful and reliable predictors for atherosclerotic cardiovascular complications in uremic patients, particularly in those submitted to maintenance dialysis therapies, remains to be demonstrated by further carefully conducted clinical studies. In a recently published study conducted prospectively in a population of 129 hemodialysis patients with a 48-month follow-up, Cressman et al[49] showed by a stepwise multiple regression analysis that Lp(a) concentration and the presence of a previous clinical event of presumed atherosclerotic etiology were the only independent contributors to the risk of a clinical atherosclerotic event during the period of follow-up, whereas age, gender, race, duration of hemodialysis, baseline total cholesterol, triglyceride, HDLC, and LDLC were unrelated to this type of risk. It is probably too early to recommend routine measurements of Lp(a) levels in patients who are not included in research protocols oriented in this field. Among controversial reports,[50-53] a few studies have shown some beneficial effect of lipid-lowering medications, such as bezafibrate,[54] gemfibrozil,[43] or nicotinic acid precursors,[34] on Lp(a) levels of hemodialysis/CAPD patients or of an HMG-CoA reductase inhibitor (lovastatin) in transplanted patients.[45] However, at the present stage of knowledge, it seems prudent to await the results of additional experimental and clinical studies before extending the prescription of lipid-lowering drugs to patients with elevated Lp(a) levels who would not present at the same time with significant disturbances of lipid parameters that are also well recognized as vascular risk factors, such as elevation of LDLC and ApoB.[15,21,23]

ACKNOWLEDGMENT

The authors thank Mrs J. Barbereau for preparing the manuscript.

REFERENCES

1. Churchill DN, Taylor W, Cook RJ, Laplante P, Barre P, Cartier P, Fay WP, Goldstein MB, Jindal K, Mandin H, MacKenzie JK, Muirhead N, Parfray PS, Posen GA, Slaughter D, Ulan RA, Werb R: Canadian hemodialysis morbidity study. Am J Kidney Dis 19:214-234, 1992

2. Raine AEG, and The EDTA Registry Committee: Combined report on regular dialysis and transplantation in Europe, XXII, 1991 Nephrol Dial Transplant 2:7-35, 1992

3. US Renal Data System (USRDS) 1991, Annual Data Report. Survival probabilities and causes of death. Bethesda, MD NIH, NIDDK, 1991, pp 31-40

4. Lindner A, Charra B, Sherrard D, Scribner BH: Accelerated atherosclerosis in prolonged maintenance hemodialysis. N Engl J Med 290:697-701, 1974

5. Burke JF, Francos GC, Moore LL, CHO SY, Lasker N: Accelerated atherosclerosis in chronic dialysis patients. Another look. Nephron 21:181-185, 1978

6. Nicholls AJ, Catto GRD, Engeset EN, MacLeod M: Accelerated atherosclerosis in long-term dialysis and renal transplant patients: Fact or fiction? Lancet 1:276-278, 1980

7. Hahn R, Oette K, Mondorf M, Finke K, Sieberth HG: Analysis of cardiovascular risk factors in chronic hemodialysis patients with special attention to hyperlipoproteinemias. Atherosclerosis 48:279-288, 1983

8. Ma KW, Greene EL, Raij L: Cardiovascular risk factors in chronic renal failure and hemodialysis populations. Am J Kidney Dis 19:505-513, 1992

9. Wheeler DC, Sweny P, Varghese Z, Moorhead JF: Hyperlipidemia and atherosclerosis in chronic dialysis patients, in Maher JF (ed): Replacement of Renal Function by Dialysis (ed 3). Dordrecht, Germany, Kluwer, 1989, pp 798-808

10. Burrell D, Antignani A, Fein PA, Goldwasser PH, Mittman N, Avram MM: Longitudinal survey of apolipoproteins and atherogenic risk in hemodialysis and continuous ambulatory peritoneal dialysis patients. ASAIO Trans 36:M331-M335, 1990

11. Lindholm B, Norbeck HE: Serum lipids and lipoproteins during continuous ambulatory peritoneal dialysis. Acta Med Scand 220:143-151, 1986

12. Tan D, Fein PA, Antignani A, Mittman N, Avram MM: The impact of CAPD treatment on lipid metabolism and cardiovascular risk. Perit Dial Bull 10:233-237, 1990

13. Lameire N, Matthys D, Matthys E, Beheydt R: Effect of long-term CAPD on carbohydrate and lipid metabolism. Clin Nephrol 30:553-558, 1988 (suppl 1)

14. Steele J, Billington T, Janus E, Moran J: Lipids, lipoproteins and apolipoproteins A-I and B and apolipoprotein losses in continuous ambulatory peritoneal dialysis. Atherosclerosis 79:47-50, 1989

15. Sniderman A, Cianflone K, Kwiterovich PO, Jr, Hutchinson T, Barre P, Prichard S: Hyperapobetalipoproteinemia: The major dyslipoproteinemia in patients with chronic renal failure treated with chronic ambulatory peritoneal dialysis. Atherosclerosis 65:257-264, 1987

16. Saku K, Sasaku J, Naito S, Arakawa K: Lipoprotein

and apolipoprotein losses during continuous ambulatory peritoneal dialysis. Nephron 51:220-224, 1989

17. Appel G: Lipid abnormalities in renal disease. Nephrology forum. Kidney Int 39:169-183, 1991

18. Avram MM, Fein PA, Antignani A, Mittman N, Muschnick RA, Lustig AR, Lapuz MG, Goldwasser P: Cholesterol and lipid disturbances in renal disease. The natural history of uremic dyslipidemia and the impact of hemodialysis and continuous ambulatory peritoneal dialysis. Am J Med 87:55-61, 1989

19. Senti M, Romero R, Pedro-Botet J, Pelegri A, Nogues X, Rubies-Prat J: Lipoprotein abnormalities in hyperlipidemic and normolipidemic men on hemodialysis with chronic renal failure. Kidney Int 41:1394-1399, 1992

20. Avram MM, Antignani A, Goldwasser Ph, Lustig A, Fein PA, Muschnick R, Quinones E, Rao Y, Mittman N: Lipids in diabetic and non diabetic hemodialysis and CAPD patients. ASAIO Trans 34:314-316, 1988

21. Gault MM, Longerich L, Prabhakaran V, Purchase L: Ischemic heart disease, serum cholesterol and apolipoproteins in CAPD. ASAIO Trans 37:M513-514, 1991

22. Fein PA, Fletcher D, Antignani A, Lustig A, Goldwasser Ph, Mittman A, Avram MM: Variability of peritoneal clearances for apolipoprotein and its relationship to susceptibility for atherosclerotic changes in CAPD, in Khanna R, Nolph KD (eds): Advances in Peritoneal Dialysis. Toronto, Canada, University of Toronto. Press, 1989, pp 185-190

23. Armstrong VW, Cremer P, Eberle E: The association between Lp(a) concentrations and angiographically assessed coronary atherosclerosis: Dependence on serum LDL levels. Atherosclerosis 62:249-257, 1986

24. Kostner GM, Avogaro P, Cazzolato G, Marth E, Bittolo-Bon G, Quinili GB: Lipoprotein (a) and the risk for myocardial infarction. Atherosclerosis 38:51-61, 1981

25. Rhoads GG, Dahlen G, Berg K, Morton NE, Dannenberg AL: Lp(a) lipoprotein as a risk factor for myocardial infarction. JAMA 256:2540-2544, 1986

26. Scanu AM, Lawn RM, Berg K: lipoprotein(a) and atherosclerosis. Ann Intern Med 115:209-218, 1991

27. MacLean JW, Tomlinson JE, Kuang WJ, Eaton DL, Chien Ey, Fless GM, Scanu AM, Lawn RM: cDNA sequence of human apolipoprotein(a) is homologous to plasminogen. Nature 330:132-137, 1987

28. Takegoshi T, Haba T, Hirai JI, Kitoh C, Saga T, Yamazaki Y: Alterations of lipoprotein(a) in patients with diabetic nephropathy. Atherosclerosis 83:99-100, 1990

29. Kapelrud H, Bangstad HJ, Dahl-Jorgensen K, Berg K, Manssen KF: Serum Lp(a) lipoprotein concentrations in insulin dependent diabetic patients with microalbuminuria. Br Med J 303:675-678, 1991

30. Karadi I, Romica L, Palos G, Doman J, Kaszas I, Hesz A: Lp(a) lipoprotein concentration in serum of patients with heavy proteinuria of different origin. Clin Chem 35:21-23, 1989

31. Thomas ME, Freestone A, Varghese Z, Persaud JW, Moorhead JF: Lipoprotein(a) in patients with proteinuria. Nephrol Dial Transplant 7:597-601, 1992

32. Cressman MD, Hoff HF, Nally JV, Jr, Schreiber M, Jr, Van Lante F: Lipoprotein(a) and the cardiovascular risk of end stage renal disease: J Am Soc Nephrol 2:234, 1992 (abstr)

33. Heimann P, Josephson MA, Fellner SK, Thistlethwaite RJ, Jr, Stuart FP, Dasgupta A: Elevated lipoprotein(a) levels in renal transplantation and hemodialysis patients. Am J Nephrol 11:470-474, 1991

34. Nakahama H, Miyazaki M, Imai M, Yokokawa T, Odaka M, Kubiri S, Okamura K, Tanaka Y, Shirai D, et al: Reduction of plasma lipoprotein(a) levels by niceritrol in patients on maintenance hemodialysis. J Am Soc Nephrol 2:340, 1992 (abstr)

35. Parra MJ, Mezdour H, Cachera C, Dracon M, Tacquet A, Fruchart JC: Lp(a) lipoprotein in patients with chronic renal failure treated by hemodialysis. Clin Chem 33:721-724, 1987

36. Kandoussi A, Cachera C, Pagniez D, Dracon M, Fruchart JC, Tacquet A: Plasma level of lipoprotein Lp(a) is high in predialysis or hemodialysis, but not in CAPD. Kidney Int 42:424-425, 1992

37. Modi KS, MA JZ, Kasiske BL, Collins AJ, Keane WF: Lipoprotein(a) in hemodialysis patients. J Am Soc Nephrol 3:380, 1992 (abstr)

38. Barbagallo CM, Averna MR, Scafidi V, Galione A, Notarbartolo A: Increased lipoprotein(a) levels in subjects with chronic renal failure on hemodialysis. Nephron 62:44-72, 1992

39. Massy ZA, Lacour B, Chauveau Ph, Zingraff J, Lambrey G, Drueke T, Bader CA, Jungers P: Serum lipoprotein(a) in patients with different degrees of chronic renal failure and after initiation of dialysis therapy. J Am Soc Nephrol 3:378, 1992 (abstr)

40. Shoji T, Nishizawa Y, Nishitani H, Yamakawa M, Morii H: High serum lipoprotein(a) concentrations in uremic patients treated with continuous ambulatory peritoneal dialysis. Clin Nephrol 38:271-276, 1992

41. Short CD, Anwar N, Durrington PN, Khan A, Bhatnagar D, Bewu AM, Mallick NP, Gokal R: Serum lipoprotein(a) levels in nephrotic syndrome, CAPD patients and renal transplant recipients. J Am Soc Nephrol 2:244, 1991 (abstr)

42. Ross EA, Shah GM, Gupta AK, Kashyap ML: Elevated lipoprotein(a) in peritoneal dialysis patients. J Am Soc Nephrol 3:418, 1992 (abstr)

43. Henriquez MA, Esquivel J, Bemis JA: Effect of gemfibrozil on lipid abnormalities in CAPD patients. J Am Soc Nephrol 3:412, 1992 (abstr)

44. Brown JH, Anwar N, Short CD, Bhatnagur D, Durrington PN, Mallick NP: Lipoprotein(a) levels in renal allograft recipients maintained on cyclosporin monotherapy. 29th Congress of the EDTA-ERA, Book of Abstracts, Paris, France, 1992, p 224 (abstr)

45. Traindl O, Reading S, Frans M, Watschinger B, Klauser R, Pidlich H, Widhalm K, Pohanka E, Kovarik J: Treatment of hyperlipidemic kidney graft recipients with lovastatin: Effect on LDL cholesterol and lipoprotein(a). Nephron 62:394-398, 1992

46. Grüber KK, Haffner St M, Tuttle RR: Increased Lp(a) concentrations in chronic renal failure. J Am Soc Neprol 3:333, 1992 (abstr)

47. Boerwinckle E, Leffert CC, Lin J, Lackner C, Chiesa G, Hobbs HH: Apolipoprotein(a) Gene accounts for greater than 90% of the variation in plasma lipoprotein(a) concentrations. J Clin Invest 90:52-60, 1992

48. Webb AT, Plant M, Reaveley DA, O'Donnell M, Luck

VA, O'Connor B, Seed M, Brown EA: Lipid and lipoprotein(a) concentrations in renal transplant patients. Nephrol Dial Transpl 7:636-641, 1992

49. Cressman MD, Heyka RJ, Paganini EP, O'Neil J, Skibinski CI, Hoff HE: Lipoprotein(a) is an independent risk factor for cardiovascular disease in hemodialysis patients. Circulation 86:475-482, 1992

50. Matthys E, Schurgers M, Lamberigts G, Lameire N, Vandecasteele N, Labeur C, Beisigel U, Rosseneu M: Effects of simvastatin treatment on the dyslipoproteinemia in CAPD patients. Atherosclerosis 86:183-192, 1991

51. Crook D, Sidhu M, Bruce R: Simvastatin and lipoprotein(a). Lancet 339:313-314, 1992 (letter)

52. Kostner GM, Gavish D, Leopold B, Bolzano K, Weintraub MS, Breslow JL: HMGCoA reductase inhibitors lower LDL cholesterol without reducing Lp(a) levels. Circulation 80:313-319, 1989

53. Wanner C, Lubrich-Birkner I, Summ O, Wieland M, Schollmeyer P: Effect of simvastatin on qualitative and quantitative changes of lipoprotein metabolism in CAPD patients. Nephron 62:40-46, 1992

54. Pelegri A, Romero R, Senti M, Nogues X, Pedro-Botet J, Rubies-Piat J: Effects of bezafibrate on lipoprotein(a) and triglyceride rich lipoproteins, including intermediate density lipoproteins, in patients with chronic renal failure receiving hemodialysis. Nephrol Dial Transplant 7:623-626, 1992

Reduction of Lipoprotein(a) Following Treatment With Lovastatin in Patients With Unremitting Nephrotic Syndrome

Clinton D. Brown, MD, Neal Azrolan, PhD, Lorraine Thomas, AA, Kathleen G. Roberts, BA, Andrew Bostom, MD, Zhong H. Zhao, MD, and E.A. Friedman, MD

● Pharmocologic treatment of the hyperlipidemia associated with the nephrotic syndrome with lovastatin has been previously shown to be safe and effective. However, there is no information on the effect of lovastatin treatment on plasma lipoprotein(a) [Lp(a)] levels in patients with the nephrotic syndrome. We administered lovastatin (40 to 80 mg/day) to 20 adult patients with unremitting nephrotic syndrome for 8 weeks to assess its effect on plasma Lp(a) and other plasma lipid concentrations. Apoprotein(a) (apo(a)) phenotype was determined in all patients. Patients were grouped according to their plasma Lp(a) levels. Those with elevated plasma Lp(a) (≥30 mg/dL) were placed in group I and those with normal Lp(a) levels (<30 mg/dL) were placed in group II. Mean total cholesterol and LDL cholesterol were similarly and significantly reduced in groups I and II (−35.9% and −43.3%, *P* < 0.0005, *P* < 0.0005 group I, and −31.0% and −42.0%, *P* < 0.02, *P* < 0.03 group II, respectively). The median reduction in plasma Lp(a) was −32% (*P* < 0.003) in nephrotic patients in group I, whereas the median decline in plasma Lp(a) levels in nephrotic patients in group II was only −8.0% (*P* = 0.052). The overall frequency of the high molecular weight (M_r) apo(a) phenotype S_4 was 70% in nephrotic patients. There was no correlation between plasma Lp(a) and apo(a) phenotype. Treatment with lovastatin results in a favorable response in terms of total and low-density lipoprotein cholesterol lowering in patients with the nephrotic syndrome; however, plasma Lp(a) levels are uniformly and significantly reduced only in nephrotic patients with elevated baseline plasma Lp(a) concentrations. There was no correlation between plasma Lp(a) concentration and other lipid and biochemical parameters.

INDEX WORDS: Lipoprotein(a); low-density lipoprotein-cholesterol; nephrotic syndrome; lovastatin; Apo(a) phenotype.

HYPERCHOLESTEROLEMIA is a common feature of the nephrotic syndrome.[1,2] Recently it has been shown that plasma levels of lipoprotein(a) [Lp(a)] are elevated in the nephrotic syndrome, presumably related to heavy proteinuria.[3-5] In normal populations, plasma Lp(a) concentration is heritable and inversely related to the molecular weight (M_r) of apoprotein(a) (apo(a)),[6-8] although complete elucidation of the mechanisms regulating plasma levels of Lp(a) are not known.

In patients with unremitting nephrotic syndrome, persistent hyperlipidemia may increase the risk for premature atherosclerotic cardiovascular disease.[9-11] This risk may be compounded by the concurrence of elevated plasma concentration of Lp(a), a potent independent risk factor for coronary artery and cerebral vascular disease.[12,13]

Treatment of the hypercholesterolemia associated with the nephrotic syndrome has been safely and effectively achieved with 3-hydroxy-3-methylglutaryl coenzyme A (HMG-CoA) reductase inhibitors.[14,15] However, there are no reports on the effect of treatment on elevated plasma Lp(a) that is associated with the nephrotic syndrome. Reports on the treatment of patients with primary elevation in plasma Lp(a) concentration with HMG-CoA reductase inhibitors have been disappointing and indicate an ineffectiveness of this class of drug on lowering plasma Lp(a) levels.[16,17] The current study was carried out to investigate the effect of the HMG-CoA reductase inhibitor lovastatin on plasma Lp(a) concentration in patients with unremitting nephrotic syndrome.

STATISTICS

Student's *t*-test was used for comparison of paired and unpaired data. Correlations between plasma Lp(a) concentration and clinical and lipid parameters were assessed by Spearman rank-order test. Comparison of plasma Lp(a) concentration at baseline and after treatment with lovastatin was assessed with the Wilcoxon signed rank test. Differences between group I and group II nephrotic patients were assessed with the Mann-Whitney rank sum test. Data on plasma Lp(a) are expressed as median and range other data are expressed as mean and standard deviation. A *P* value of <0.05 was considered to be statistically significant.

Funded in part by a grant from Merck Research Laboratories, West Point, PA.

PATIENTS AND METHODS

Patients

This study was designed as an open-label trial with lovastatin. Twenty adult patients with unremitting nephrotic syndrome defined as persistent for 6 months or longer were recruited from the renal clinic of University Hospital at Brooklyn and the medical service of Kings County Hospital Center. All patients met the following criteria of: proteinuria ≥ 3.5 g/day, low-density lipoprotein (LDL)-cholesterol > the 75th percentile of normal population values.[18] All patients, with one exception, had biopsy-proven glomerular disease. Patient 1 refused renal biopsy but had no evidence of diabetic retinopathy, a normal glucose tolerance test, a normal thyroid function test, and a negative antinuclear antibody titer. Immunosuppressive therapy was discontinued in all patients, not less than 2 months before study participation. No patient had diabetes mellitus or received angiotensin converting enzyme inhibitors or estrogen therapy. For the purpose of intragroup and intergroup analyses and comparisons, nephrotic patients were grouped according to their baseline plasma Lp(a) concentrations. Patients in group I had plasma Lp(a) concentration at or above the atherosclerosis threshold (≥30 mg/dL),[13] and patients in group II had plasma Lp(a) concentration of <30 mg/dL. Patient demographics and clinical characteristics are summarized in Table 1. On average group I patients tended to be older than patients in group II; however, the difference was marginally significant ($P = 0.053$). There were no significant differences in group mean creatinine clearance, serum albumin concentration, proteinuria, and plasma total and LDL cholesterol. Mean high-density lipoprotein (HDL) cholesterol concentration in group II was significantly greater in comparison with group I (40.8 ± 9.6 *v* 56.8 ± 18.6 mg/dL, $P < 0.05$). Mean triglyceride concentration was much higher in group I (compared with group II), but the difference did not reach statistical significance because of high patient-to-patient variability ($P = 0.11$). The median Lp(a) plasma concentration in group I was more than fivefold higher than in group II ($P < 0.0005$). Ten of 12 (83.3%) patients in group I and eight of eight (100%) patients in group II were found to have at least one S_4 Lp(a) isoform.

All patients followed a cholesterol-lowering diet for at least 2 to 3 months before receiving lovastatin. Patients received lovastatin according to their plasma LDL-cholesterol concentration (20 mg twice daily was given to patients with plasma LDL-cholesterol < 190 mg/dL; 40 mg twice daily was given for plasma LDL-cholesterol ≥ 190 mg/dL). The intent in selecting this drug regimen was to achieve a plasma LDL-cholesterol concentration of <130 mg/dL.

Patients were seen at 4-week intervals, at which time 24-hour urine collections for protein excretion and creatinine clearance, routine blood chemistries (including liver function tests and muscle enzymes), and complete blood count were repeated. Venous blood samples for plasma lipid and lipoprotein determination were obtained after a 12-hour overnight fast at baseline and repeated after 8 full weeks of lovastatin administration. All patients tolerated lovastatin treatment without complication. Plasma for Lp(a) concentration and apo(a) phenotype determination were frozen at −80°C.

Lipid and Lipoprotein Analysis

Plasma triglyceride, total and HDL cholesterol levels were measured enzymatically on fresh plasma (Kodak, Rochester, NY), with HDL cholesterol determined after dextran-sulfate-magnesium precipitation of lipoproteins, and LDL-cholesterol was calculated by the Friedewald equation.[19]

In one patient plasma triglyceride exceeded 400 mg/dL. In the latter case HDL- and LDL-cholesterol were measured in the infranatant after a 2-hour spin in an airfuge (Beckman, Brea, CA) to float the very-low-density lipoprotein (VLDL) fraction. HDL-cholesterol was measured after precipitation of the whole plasma with dextran-sulfate-magnesium, and LDL-cholesterol was calculated by difference. LDL-cholesterol was corrected by accounting for the cholesterol contained in the Lp(a) fraction[20]; therefore, LDL-cholesterol concentration reported herein was derived by subtracting 0.3 × Lp(a) mass from the calculated LDL-cholesterol. A sandwich enzyme-linked immunosorbent assay (ELISA) was used to quantify plasma Lp(a) levels as previously described.[21] The coefficient of variation of the measurement was less than 3%.

Apo(a) Phenotyping

Apo(a) phenotyping was determined by a previously described method.[22] Apo(a) size was calculated using apo B-100 (550 kd), thyroglobulin (330 kd), alpha-2 macroglobullin (180 kd), and apo(a) standards of 760, 680, 536, and 419 kd.[20]

RESULTS

After Treatment With Lovastatin

The effect of treatment with lovastatin is shown in Table 2. In group II patients (plasma Lp(a) < 30 mg/dL) the median reduction in plasma Lp(a) concentration was relatively small (−8.0%; range, 14.3 to −47.3%, borderline significance, $P = 0.052$) with six of eight patients responding favorably. In contrast, in group I patients (plasma Lp(a) ≥ 30 mg/dL), there was a substantial and highly significant median reduction in plasma Lp(a) concentration of −32% (range, −5.6 to −60.2%; $P < 0.003$). All patients in group I experienced a reduction in plasma Lp(a) concentration (Fig 1). In groups I and II there were similar and highly significant reductions in mean total plasma cholesterol (−35.5 and −31.0%; P 0.0005 and $P < 0.03$, respectively) and in mean plasma LDL-cholesterol concentration (−43.3 and −42.0%; $P < 0.0005$ and $P < 0.03$, respectively). Nephrotic patients in group I tended to be hypertriglyceridemic at baseline and responded to lovastatin treatment with a significant reduction in mean plasma triglyceride concentration of −51.6% ($P < 0.05$) and an 18.6% increase in mean plasma HDL cholesterol concentration ($P < 0.05$). Conversely, in group II (which had normal mean plasma triglyc-

Table 1. Clinical Features of Patients With the Nephrotic Syndrome

Patient No.	Age (yr)	Race/ Sex	Histology	Creatinine Clearance (mL/min)	Serum Albumin (g/dL)	Proteinuria (g/day)	Total Cholesterol (mg/dL)	Triglyceride (mg/dL)	LDL Cholesterol (mg/dL)	HDL Cholesterol (mg/dL)	Lp(a)* (mg/dL)	Apo(a) Phenotype
Group I												
1	58	C/W	NB	11	4.1	4.3	324	268	173	36	204	S4
2	37	C/M	MEM	134	3.0	5.0	319	201	224	33	72	S4
3	38	C/W	MEM	98	2.0	16.5	345	227	222	46	104	S2
4	44	B/W	FS	22	2.1	5.5	435	334	295	62	36	S4
5	25	B/M	MEM	63	2.8	3.6	314	242	201	35	99	S4
6	45	B/M	FS	64	2.5	9.1	626	1191	391	28	35	S4
7	59	B/M	FS	49	2.5	10.4	346	263	203	45	150	S4
8	61	B/W	MEM	64	2.1	11.1	351	227	232	38	117	S3/S4
9	70	B/W	MEM	31	2.4	8.1	336	232	207	32	170	S3/S4
10	31	B/M	MEM	150	2.0	5.8	434	367	299	48	44	S2
11	50	B/M	MEM	82	2.3	18.0	425	353	290	37	93	S4
12	60	B/W	MEM	72	2.8	4.8	305	200	161	50	180	S1/S4
Mean	48.2			70.0	2.5	8.5	380	343	241	40.8	101.5†	
(SD)	(13.8)			(41.9)	(0.6)	(4.8)	(90)	(273)	(66)	(9.6)	[36-204]	
Group II												
13	20	B/M	IgM	52	2.3	6.1	328	65	235	78	7	S4
14	22	C/M	FS	67	2.0	7.1	357	264	242	56	21	S4
15	29	B/M	FS	99	2.9	14.0	529	124	418	79	25	S4
16	48	B/W	MEM	84	2.7	6.2	282	324	177	30	21	S2/S4
17	43	B/W	MEM	106	2.7	4.8	325	174	210	72	27	S4
18	38	B/W	PGN	50	3.2	11.6	289	190	195	52	12.5	S4
19	35	B/W	MEM	71	3.9	4.0	260	138	173	52	24	S4
20	56	B/M	MPGN	90	3.0	4.9	216	103	152	35	28	S4
Mean	35.8			77.4	2.8	7.3	323	173	225	56.8‡	22.5	
(SD)	(11.9)			(20.8)	(0.6)	(3.6)	(90)	(86)	(84)	(18.6)	[7-28]	

NOTE. Unmarked parameters were not significantly different.

Abbreviations: C, caucasian; B, black; W, woman; M, man; NB, no biopsy; MEM, membranous glomerulonephritis; FS, focal sclerosis; IgM, IgM nephropathy; PGN, proliferative glomerulonephritis; MPGN, membranoproliferative glomerulonephritis.

* Lp(a) data are expressed as median and [range].

† $P < 0.0005$ compared with group II.

‡ $P < 0.05$ compared with group I.

eride and HDL-cholesterol concentrations at baseline), there was no significant change in either of these parameters. There was a modest but significant decline in mean creatinine clearance in group I from 70.0 to 60.4 mL/min ($P = 0.01$); however, proteinuria and serum albumin concentration did not change significantly. There was no significant change in mean creatinine clearance, serum albumin, or proteinuria in group II nephrotic patients.

Lp(a) Concentration and Apo(a) Phenotype

A comparison between the frequency distribution of apo(a) phenotypes and median plasma Lp(a) concentrations of nephrotic patients is shown in Table 3. In both groups, the S_4 apo(a) phenotype, is by far the most predominate (58.3, group I and 87.5%, group II). The overall prevalence of S_4 phenotype in nephrotic patients (n = 20) was 70%. However, within the S_4 apo(a) phenotype class the median plasma Lp(a) concentration in group I was nearly fivefold greater than in group II ($P < 0.002$) despite intergroup similarity in factors that might influence Lp(a) concentration, ie, creatinine clearance[23,24] ($P = 0.39$), 24-hour protein excretion[4] ($P = 0.87$), serum albumin concentration[3] ($P = 0.77$), and race[25,26] (five of seven patients in group I and six of seven in group II with the S_4 apo(a) phenotype were black).

DISCUSSION

Elevated plasma total and LDL-cholesterol[27,28] and in almost all instances elevated plasma Lp(a) concentrations[29-32] have been shown to be closely linked with the development of premature atherosclerosis. Although the association between atherosclerosis and the nephrotic syndrome has been

Table 2. Mean (SD) of Parameters at Baseline and After Treatment With Lovastatin

		Creatinine Clearance (mL/min)	Serum Albumin (g/dL)	Proteinuria (g/day)	Total Cholesterol (mg/dL)	Triglyceride (mg/dL)	LDL Cholesterol (mg/dL)	HDL Cholesterol (mg/dL)	Lp(a)* (mg/dL)
Group I (n = 12)	Baseline	70.0 (41.9)	2.5 (0.6)	8.5 (4.8)	380.0 (90.0)	342.0 (273.0)	242.0 (66.0)	40.8 (9.6)	101.5 [36-204]
	After	60.4† (39.8)	2.8 (0.5)	6.9 (4.2)	243.3‡ (39.6)	166.1§ (72.5)	138.7‡ (36.5)	48.8§ (12.9)	74.0‖¶ [16-180]
Group II (n = 8)	Baseline	77.4 (20.8)	2.8 (0.6)	7.3 (3.6)	323.0 (90.0)	173.0 (86.0)	225.0 (84.0)	56.8 (18.6)	22.5 [7-28]
	After	75.3 (22.7)	2.7 (0.6)	7.1 (5.4)	223.4§ (28.3)	161.8 (96.4)	132.0§ (29.3)	56.4 (17.4)	21.0 [8.0-23]

NOTE. Unmarked parameters were not statistically significant.
* Plasma Lp(a) data are expressed as median and [range].
† $P < 0.02$ compared with baseline mean.
‡ $P < 0.005$ compared with baseline mean.
§ $P < 0.05$ compared with baseline mean.
‖ $P < 0.003$ compared with baseline Lp(a) data, Wilcoxon signed rank test.
¶ $P < 0.001$ compared with group II plasma Lp(a) data, Mann-Whitney rank sum test.

disputed,[33] there is mounting evidence suggesting that patients with unremitting nephrotic syndrome are at increased risk of atherosclerotic cardiovascular disease.[9-13] Therefore, correction of the lipid abnormalities in these patients may be of clinical importance. Previous reports are consistent with our finding that plasma Lp(a) concentration is elevated in most (60%) patients with the nephrotic syndrome.[5] However, our study is the first to show that treatment with the HMG-CoA reductase inhibitor lovastatin lowers plasma Lp(a) concentration significantly by −32.2% in nephrotic patients with elevated plasma Lp(a) levels. In comparison, nephrotic patients with plasma Lp(a) concentration of less than 30 mg/dL responded inconsistently to lovastatin treatment with a relatively small median reduction in plasma Lp(a) concentration.

In agreement with previous reports,[15,34-36] both groups of nephrotic patients treated with lovastatin responded favorably with significant reductions in mean total and LDL-cholesterol. Also, treatment with lovastatin had further beneficial effects on group I nephrotic patients who were hypertriglyceridemic at baseline by significantly lowering mean plasma triglyceride concentration ($P < 0.05$) and raising plasma HDL-cholesterol ($P < 0.05$). Reduction in plasma triglyceride concentration during treatment with lovastatin and pravastatin in patients with the nephrotic syndrome has been previously reported[34,36] and was shown to be secondary to a drug-induced increase in the hepatic removal of triglyceride rich VLDL remnants.[34] Whether the favorable change in mean plasma HDL-cholesterol found in group I nephrotic patients is a direct or indirect effect of lovastatin treatment is not known.

Nevertheless, during lovastatin treatment there was marked improvement in the mean LDL/HDL ratio in the two groups of nephrotic patients (from 6.3 ± 2.8 to 2.8 ± 0.8, $P = 0.001$, group I; and from 4.1 ± 1.1 to 2.6 ± 1.1, $P = 0.01$, group II) (data not shown).

There is no consensus on the mechanism underlying the high plasma LDL content in the nephrotic syndrome. Vega and Grundy[34] used isotope kinetic turnover studies in a small group of nephrotic patients and showed that elevated plasma LDL concentration is not due to impaired receptor-mediated catabolism of this lipoprotein but to increased LDL production. They also showed that LDL production in the nephrotic syndrome is inhibited by lovastatin, which significantly reduced plasma total and LDL-cholesterol. Also, Joven et al[37] reported normal fractional catabolic rate (FCR) and elevated production rate of LDL in patients with the ne-

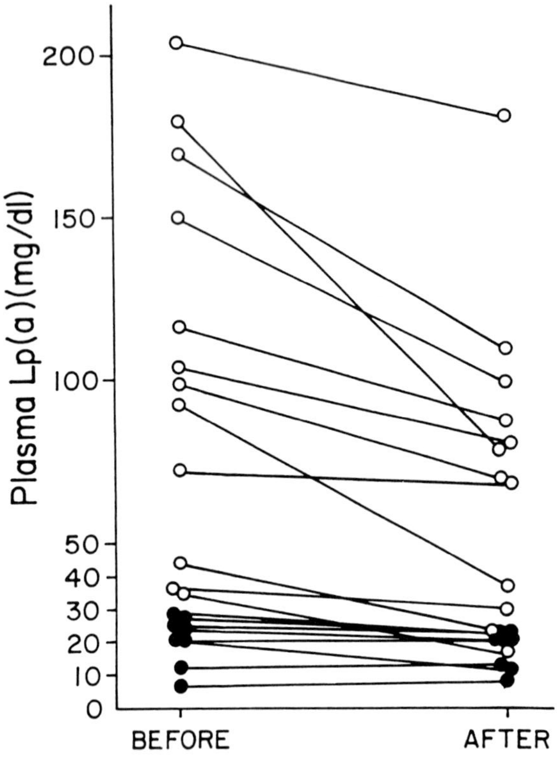

Fig 1. Plasma Lp(a) concentration in patients with the nephrotic syndrome at baseline and after 8 weeks of treatment with lovastatin. Open circles represent patients with elevated plasma Lp(a) concentration at baseline (group I); closed circles represent patients with normal plasma Lp(a) concentration at baseline (group II).

phrotic syndrome. In contrast, Warwick et al[35] showed a low FCR of LDL in a group of nephrotic patients. There are no kinetic turnover studies, however, that would explain the changes in Lp(a) metabolism observed in humans with the nephrotic syndrome.

The mechanism by which lovastatin lowers plasma Lp(a) in the nephrotic syndrome is not known. Studies have shown that HMG-CoA reductase inhibitors are not effective in lowering plasma Lp(a) concentration in normal subjects or in patients with primary hypercholesterolemia.[16,17,38] The major effect of HMG-CoA reductase inhibitors in nonnephrotic patients is to enhance receptor-mediated catabolism of LDL.[39,40] Lp(a) is a poor ligand for the LDL receptor,[41] and several studies have shown that plasma Lp(a) levels are mainly determined by hepatic synthesis and are correlated with apo(a) mRNA abundance.[22,42-44] Therefore, increased receptor-mediated catabolism (induced by treatment with HMG-CoA reductase inhibitors) would not appear to affect plasma Lp(a) concentrations significantly.[16,17] Because receptor-mediated catabolism plays either no or, at most, a minor role in determining plasma Lp(a) concentration,[42,43] it is probable that Lp(a) production may be increased over a wide range in nephrotic patients (see below). The mechanism of Lp(a) assembly involves the association of apo(a) with the apo B moiety of an LDL particle. Current data suggest that the linkage of apo(a) to apo B occurs outside of the hepatocyte.[44] We postulate that lovastatin may lower plasma Lp(a) levels in nephrotic patients (with increased Lp(a) production) by an effect on hepatic LDL production (as suggested by Vega and Grundy[34]), which would reduce LDL availability for Lp(a) assembly. Conversely, the plasma concentration of Lp(a) in nephrotic patients with Lp(a) production at the lower end of the spectrum may not be affected significantly by a lovastatin-induced reduction in hepatic LDL production. This hypothesis may, in part, explain the different effects on plasma Lp(a) lowering in response to lovastatin therapy that was exhibited by group I and group II nephrotic patients.

Another possible explanation for the reduction in plasma Lp(a) demonstrated in group I nephrotic patients (elevated plasma Lp(a) and triglyceride levels at baseline) may be related to triglyceride metabolism. In the fasting state both triglyceride rich and cholesterol ester rich lipoprotein apo(a)-apo(B) particles are measured together as total Lp(a).[45] The affiliation of apo(a)-apo(B) with triglyceride-rich lipoproteins in individuals with primary hypertriglyceridemia is quite variable, accounting for 1.3% to 50% of total plasma Lp(a).[46] It is possible that apo(a)-apo(B) may be linked to endogenous hepatic triglyceride production in hypertriglyceridemic patients with the nephrotic syndrome. Previous work suggests that lovastatin increases catabolism of triglyceride-rich lipoproteins in hypertriglyceridemic nephrotic patients.[34] Therefore the concurrent decline in plasma triglyceride and Lp(a) levels in group I nephrotic patients may be due to a lovastatin-induced increased receptor-mediated removal of triglyceride-rich lipoproteins including triglyceride-rich apo(a)-apo(B)

Table 3. Frequency of Apo(a) Phenotypes (%) in Nephrotic Patients With Elevated (Group I) and Normal (Group II) Plasma Lp(a) Concentration

Apo(a) Phenotype	Group I (n = 12) No. of Patients	Group I %	Group I Lp(a) (mg/dL)	Group II (n = 8) No. of Patients	Group II %	Group II Lp(a) (mg/dL)	Overall Frequency (n = 20) (%)
S2	2	16.7	44,102	—	—	—	10.0
S4	7	58.3	93.0* (35-204)	7	87.5	24.0 (7-28)	70.0
S1/S4	1	8.3	72.0	—	—	—	5.0
S2/S4	—	—	—	1	12.5	21.0	5.0
S3/S4	2	16.7	117,170	—	—	—	10.0

NOTE. Plasma Lp(a) data are expressed as median (range).
* $P = 0.002$, group I compared with group II.

particles. This action would result in a reduction in total plasma Lp(a) concentration. In contrast, less than 5% of apo(a)-apo(B) associates with triglyceride-rich lipoproteins in hypercholesterolemic subjects who have normal plasma triglycerides.[46] If this situation pertains to nephrotic patients who have normal or near normal triglyceride levels (ie, group II), then failure of lovastatin to significantly lower plasma triglycerides would not alter total plasma Lp(a) concentration. Presumably, plasma Lp(a) concentration in group II nephrotic patients is determined mainly by hepatic production, which we speculate is low in these individuals.

Wanner et al[5] suggest that individual heterogeneity of genetic factors within the nephrotic population may be responsible for the variability in plasma Lp(a) concentrations. We determined apo(a) phenotypes in nephrotic patients with normal and elevated plasma Lp(a) concentration and found in each group an extremely high frequency of high Mr apo(a) isoforms (75.0%, group I and 87.5%, group II, respectively) (Table 3). However, intergroup comparison of median plasma Lp(a) concentration within the same (and most prevalent) apo(a) phenotype class (S_4) showed a fourfold increase in plasma Lp(a) concentration (group I *v* group II) despite intergroup similarity in renal function, proteinuria, serum albumin concentration, and race (Table 1). In their study of normal volunteers, Rader et al[42] have shown that wide variability in plasma Lp(a) concentration among subjects with the same apo(a) phenotype is caused by differences in Lp(a) production rate. It is not known whether the same reasoning pertains to the nephrotic syndrome, although we speculate that the conclusion reported by Rader et al[42] may apply to our study. Plasma Lp(a) concentration has been reported to be elevated in patients with renal insufficiency.[23,24] Both groups of nephrotic patients had a similar magnitude of renal insufficiency at baseline ($P = 0.34$) and after treatment with lovastatin ($P = 0.35$). Group I nephrotic patients had a mild and significant decline in renal function (from 70.0 to 60.4 mL/min, $P < 0.01$), suggesting that these patients had less stable renal function during the study course compared with group II patients. On very rare occasion, lovastatin has been implicated in the causation of myopathy and acute renal failure.[47] In the current study, there was no biochemical or clinical evidence suggesting that lovastatin caused a decline in renal function in patients assigned to group I.

There was no significant correlation between plasma Lp(a) concentration and creatinine clearance ($P = 0.35$, baseline; $P = 0.18$, during treatment). Therefore, we conclude that the difference in plasma Lp(a) concentration between the two groups of nephrotic patients cannot be explained on the basis of renal function.

In in vitro experiments, homocysteine (in mmol concentration) has been shown to reduce the immunoreactivity of Lp(a) and thereby impair detection of this lipoprotein by enzyme-linked immunosorbent assay.[48] Plasma homocysteine levels are known to be elevated in patients with reduced creatinine clearance.[49] However, the levels of homocysteine reported in patients with reduced creatinine clearance are far less (by one order of magnitude[48] than the concentration of homocysteine that was shown to be minimally effective in impairing Lp(a) detection by enzyme-linked immunosorbent assay.[46] Therefore we do not think that homocysteine played a role in confounding our results pertaining to the effect of lovastatin on plasma Lp(a) levels.

Our results support our conclusion that lovastatin lowers plasma Lp(a) concentration safely, effectively, and consistently in nephrotic patients with elevated plasma Lp(a) concentration. The mechanism(s) by which lovastatin lowers plasma Lp(a) in nephrotic patients with elevated levels of this lipoprotein is not clear. Also, our data support the contention that apo(a) phenotype does not influence plasma Lp(a) concentration in the nephrotic syndrome.

There is considerable need for future studies to further explore the mysteries surrounding lipoprotein and especially Lp(a) metabolism in the nephrotic syndrome; with information in hand, treatment of hyperlipidemia can be optimized to reduce the risk for atherosclerosis in those patients in whom the nephrotic syndrome is persistent.

REFERENCES

1. Kaysen GA: Hyperlipidemia of the nephrotic syndrome. Kidney Int 39:S8-S15, 1991 (Suppl 31)

2. Newmark SR, Anderson CF, Donadio FV, Ellefson RD: Lipoprotein profiles in adult nephrotics. Mayo Clinic Proc 50:359-365, 1975

3. Stenvinkel P, Berglund L, Heimburger O, Pettersson E, Alvestrand A: Lipoprotein(a) in nephrotic syndrome. Kidney Int 44:1116-1123, 1993

4. Karadi I, Romics L, Palos G, Doman J, Kaszas I, Hesz A, Kostner GM: Lp(a) lipoprotein concentration in serum of patients with heavy proteinuria of different origin. Clin Chem 35(10):2121-2123, 1989

5. Wanner C, Rader D, Bartens W, Kramer J, Brewer HB, Schollmyer P, Wieland H: Elevated plasma lipoprotein(a) in patients with the nephrotic syndrome. Ann Intern Med 119:263-269, 1993

6. Utermann G, Kraft HG, Menzel HJ, Hopferwieser T, Seitz C: Genetics of the quantitative Lp(a) lipoprotein trait. Hum Genet 78:41-46, 1988

7. Utermann G, Duba C, Menzel HJ: Genetics of the quantitative Lp(a) lipoprotein trait. Hum Genet 78:47-50, 1988

8. Utermann G: Mysteries of Lp(a). Science 246:904-910, 1989

9. Berlyne GM, Mallick NP: Ischaemic heart disease as a complication of nephrotic syndrome. Lancet 2:399-400, 1969

10. Curry RC, Roberts WC: Status of the coronary arteries in the nephrotic syndrome. Am J Med 63:183-192, 1977

11. Ordonez JD, Hiatt RA, Killebrew EJ, Fireman BH: The increased risk of coronary heart disease associated with nephrotic syndrome. Kidney Int 44:638-642, 1993

12. Rhoads GG, Dahlen G, Berg K, Morton NE, Dannenberg AL: Lp(a) lipoprotein as a risk factor for myocardial infarction. JAMA 256:2540-2544, 1986

13. Kostner GM, Avogaro P, Cazzolato G, Marth E, Bittolo-Bon G, Qunici GB: Lipoprotein Lp(a) and the risk for myocardial infarction. Atherosclerosis 38:51-61, 1981

14. Thomas ME, Harris KPG, Ramaswamy C, Hattersley JM, Wheeler DC, Varghese Z, Williams JD, Walls J, Moorhead JF: Simvastatin therapy for hypercholesterolemic patients with nephrotic syndrome or significant proteinuria. Kidney Int 44:1124-1129, 1993

15. Kasiske BL, Velosa JA, Halstenson CE, La Belle P, Langendorfer A, Keane WF: The effects of lovastatin in hyperlipidemic patients with the nephrotic syndrome. Am J Kidney Dis 15:8-15, 1990

16. Hunninghake DB, Stein EA, Dujovne CA, Harris WS, Fedman EB, Miller VT, Tobert JA, Laskarzewski PM, Quiter E, Held J, Taylor AM, Hopper S, Leonard SB, Brewer BK: The efficacy of intensive dietary therapy alone or combined with lovastatin in outpatients with hypercholesterolemia. N Engl J Med 328:1213-1219, 1993

17. Kostner GM, Gavish D, Leopold B, Bolzano K, Weintraub MS, Breslow JL: HMG CoA reductase inhibitors lower LDL cholesterol without reducing Lp(a) levels. Circulation 80:1313-1319, 1989

18. Heiss G, Tamir I, Davis CE, Tyroler HA, Rifkind BM, Schonfeld G, Jacobs D, Frantz ID, Jr: Lipoprotein-cholesterol distributions in selected North American populations: The lipid research clinics program prevalence study. Circulation 61:302-315, 1980

19. Friedewald WT, Levy RI, Fredrickson DS: Estimation of the concentration of low-density lipoprotein cholesterol in plasma, without use of the preparative ultracentrifuge. Clin Chem 18:499-502, 1972

20. Gaubatz JW, Heideman C, Gotto AM, Morrisett JD, Dahlen GH: Human plasma lipoprotein(a): Structural properties. J Biol Chem 258:4582-4589, 1983

21. Gavish D, Azrolan N, Breslow JL: Plasma Lp(a) concentration is inversely correlated with the ratio of kringle IV/kringle V encoding domains in the apo(a) gene. J Clin Invest 84:2021-2027, 1989

22. Azrolan N, Gavish D, Breslow JL: Plasma lipoprotein(a) concentration is controlled by apolipoprotein(a) (apo(a)) protein size and the abundance of hepatic apo(a) mRNA in a cynomolgus monkey model. J Biol Chem 266:13866-13872, 1991

23. Para HJ, Mezdour H, Cachera C, Dracon M, Tacquet A, Fruchart JC: Lp(a) lipoprotein in patients with chronic renal failure treated by hemodialysis. Clin Chem 33:721, 1987

24. Irish AB, Simons LA, Savdie E, Hayes JM, Simons J: Lipoprotein(a) levels in chronic renal disease states, dialysis and transplantation. Aust N Z J Med 22:243-248, 1992

25. Para H-J, Luyeye I, Bouramoue C, Demarquilly C, Fruchart J-C: Black-white differences in serum Lp(a) lipoprotein levels. Clin Chim Acta 167:27-31, 1987

26. Sandholzer C, Hallman DM, Saha N, Sigurdsson G, Lackner C, Csaszar A, Boerwinkle E, Utermann G: Effects of the apolipoprotein(a) size polymorphism on the lipoprotein(a) concentration in 7 ethnic groups. Hum Genet 86:607-614, 1991

27. Castelli WP, Garrison RJ, Wilson PWF, Abbott RD, Kalousdian S, Kannel WB: Incidence of coronary heart disease and lipoprotein cholesterol levels: The Framingham Heart Study. JAMA 256:2835-2838, 1986

28. Kannel WB, Castelli WP, Gordon T: Lipoprotein cholesterol in th prediction of atherosclerotic disease: New perspectives based on the Framingham Heart Study. Ann Intern Med 90:85-91, 1979

29. Hoefler G, Harnoncourt F, Paschke E, Mirtl W, Pfeiffer KH, Kostner GM: Lipoprotein Lp(a): A risk factor for myocardial infarction. Arteriosclerosis 8:398-401, 1988

30. Seed M, Hoppichler F, Reaveley D, McCarthy S, Thompson GR, Boerwinkle E, Utermann G: Relation of serum lipoprotein(a) phenotype to coronary heart disease in patients with familial hypercholesterolemia. N Engl J Med 322:1494-1499, 1990

31. Sandholzer CH, Boerwinkle E, Saha N, Tong MC, Utermann G: Apolipoprotein(a) phenotypes, Lp(a) concentration and plasma lipid levels in relation to coronary heart disease in a chinese population: Evidence for the role of the apo(a) gene in coronary heart disease. J Clin Invest 89:1040-1046, 1992

32. Ridker PM, Hennekens CH, Stampfer MJ: A prospective study of lipoprotein(a) and the risk of myocardial infarction. JAMA 270:2195-2199, 1993

33. Wass VJ, Jarrett RJ, Chilvers C, Cameron JS: Does the nephrotic syndrome increase the risk of cardiovascular disease? Lancet 2:664-667, 1979

34. Vega GL, Grundy SM: Lovastatin therapy in nephrotic hyperlipidemia: Effects on lipoprotein metabolism. Kidney Int 33:1160-1168, 1988

35. Warwick GL, Packard CJ, Murray L, Grierson D, Stewart JP, Shepherd J, Bolten-Jones M: Effect of simvastatin on plasma lipid and lipoprotein concentrations and low-density lipoprotein metabolism in the nephrotic syndrome. Clin Sci 82:701-708, 1992

36. Spitalewitz S, Porush JG, Cattran D, Wright N: Treatment of hyperlipidemia in the nephrotic syndrome: The effects of pravastatin therapy. Am J Kidney Dis 22:143-150, 1993

37. Joven J, Villabona C, Vilella E, Masana L, Alberti R, Valles M: Abnormalities of lipoprotein metabolism in patients with the nephrotic syndrome. N Engl J Med 323:579-584, 1990

38. Malmendier CL, Lontie JF, Delcroix C, Magot T: Effect of simvastatin on receptor-dependent low density lipoprotein catabolism in normocholesterolemic human volunteers. Atherosclerosis 80:101-109, 1989

39. Raveh D, Israeli A, Aron R, Eisenberg S: Effects of lovastatin therapy on LDL receptor activity in circulation monocytes and on structure and composition of plasma lipoproteins. Atherosclerosis 82:19-26, 1990

40. Slunga L, Johnson O, Dahlen GH: Changes in Lp(a) lipoprotein levels during the treatment of hypercholesterolemia with simvastatin. Eur J Clin Pharm 43:369-373, 1992

41. Armstrong VW, Walli AK, Seided D: Isolation, characterization and uptake in human fibroblasts of an apo(a)-free lipoprotein obtained on reduction of lipoprotein(a). J Lipids Res 26:1314-1323, 1985

42. Rader DJ, Cain W, Zech LA, Usher D, Brewer HB, Jr: Variation in lipoprotein(a) concentrations among individuals with the same apolipoprotein(a) isoform is determined by the rate of lipoprotein(a) production. J Clin Invest 91:443-447, 1993

43. Krempler F, Kostner GM, Bolzano K: Turnover of lipoprotein(a) in man. J Clin Invest 65:1483-1490, 1980

44. Koschinsky ML, Cote GP, Gabel B, van der Hoek YY: Identification of the cysteine residue in apolipoprotein(a) that mediates extracellular coupling with apolipoprotein B-100. J Biol Chem 268:19819-19825, 1993

45. Scanu AM, Edelstein C, Fless GM, Eisenbart J, Sitrin M, Kasawa B, Hinman J: Postprandial lipoprotein(a) response to a single meal containing either saturated or *w*-3 polyunstaturated fatty acids in subjects with hypoalphalipoproteinemia. Metabolism 41:1361-1366, 1992

46. Selinger E, Sallongeville J, Davignon J: Apolipoprotein(a) is present in the triglyceride-rich fraction type IV hypertriglyceridemia. Clin Biochem 26:59-64, 1993

47. Manoukian AA, Bhagavan NV, Hayashi T, Nestor TA, Rios C, Scottolini AG: Rhabdomyolysis secondary to lovastatin therapy. Clin Chem 36:2145-2147, 1990

48. Scanu AM, Pfaffinger D, Fless GM, Makino K, Eisenbart J, Hinman J: Attenuation of immunologic reactivity of lipoprotein(a) by thiols and cystein-containing compounds: Structural implications. Arterioscler Thromb 12:424-429, 1992

49. Soria C, Chadefaux B, Coude M, Gaillard O, Kamoun P: Concentrations of total homocysteine in plasma in chronic renal failure. Clin Chem 36:2137-2138, 1990

Markers for Survival in Dialysis: A Seven-Year Prospective Study

M.M. Avram, MD, Neal Mittman, MD, Luigi Bonomini, MD, PhD, Jyoti Chattopadhyay, PhD, and Paul Fein, MD

● Serum biochemical markers suggestive of undernutrition are directly correlated with mortality in hemodialysis and peritoneal dialysis patients. In particular, serum albumin is the most powerful predictor of survival. We have prospectively examined the relationship of single baseline measurements of serum albumin, cholesterol, creatinine, apoproteins, and prealbumin in 250 hemodialysis patients and 140 patients maintained on continuous ambulatory peritoneal dialysis (CAPD) monitored up to 7 years (1987 to 1994). Other variables studied included age, race, gender, diabetes, and number of months on dialysis. Observed survival was computed by the Kaplan-Meier method. Cox's proportional hazards model was used to determine independent predictors of mortality risk. Age, diabetes, prior months on dialysis, and low levels of serum albumin, creatinine, and cholesterol were important and independent predictors of mortality risk in hemodialysis patients. For peritoneal dialysis patients, the independent predictors of mortality risk were age, diabetes, and low serum albumin and serum creatinine. Prealbumin, a serum protein with rapid turnover and relatively small pool, was an important and independent risk predictor in both hemodialysis and CAPD patients. In addition, prealbumin was more highly correlated with other nutritional markers than was albumin. In summary, these findings suggest that biochemical measures associated with visceral and somatic protein depletion are predominant long-term mortality risk factors in patients maintained on hemodialysis and CAPD.

INDEX WORDS: Hemodialysis; continuous ambulatory peritoneal dialysis; mortality; malnutrition; serum albumin; serum prealbumin.

CARDIOVASCULAR disease is the most important cause of mortality in end-stage renal disease (ESRD). Although both dyslipidemia and accelerated atherosclerosis are common in this population[1,2] autopsy studies have failed to provide a strong link between the two.[3,4] Moreover, several studies have failed to show an increased occurrence of new atherosclerosis in ESRD.[5,6] We reported a survey of atherogenicity indicators in a cross-sectional survey of patients with renal insufficiency (non-ESRD), and patients with ESRD on different treatment modalities.[7] Patients with renal insufficiency had marked dyslipidemia well described in this population[8] but were at a disadvantage relative to patients undergoing dialysis (ie, they had a more "atherogenic" profile). Lipid levels were inversely correlated to months on dialysis.[7] When we followed dialysis patients longitudinally over 3 years, we found that the profile of nonsurvivors was less atherogenic, characterized by lower total cholesterol and apoprotein B, and higher apoprotein A-1/B ratio.[9] Given the direct correlation of serum albumin with total cholesterol and apoprotein B, and the inverse relationship between albumin and apoprotein A-1/B, the most likely interpretation is that patients with preserved visceral protein stores have reduced mortality risk, although potentially increased atherogenic risk.

We later reported a 4-year prospective study of the influence of biochemical risk factors on survival in patients on hemodialysis using a proportional hazards model.[10] Low serum albumin and low serum cholesterol were independent predictors of mortality risk for up to 2 years in both new (in their first 12 months of dialysis) and long-standing dialysis patients. These findings extended and confirmed the observations of Lowrie and Lew's cross-sectional study of 1-year survival.[11] We recently reported the increased predictive value of prealbumin over albumin in 14-month survival in patients on hemodialysis[12] and in 20-month survival in patients on continuous ambulatory peritoneal dialysis (CAPD).[13] Cano et al[14] found that serum prealbumin, but not serum albumin or anthropometrics, correlated with 1-year mortality risk in hemodialysis patients.

We now extend our findings with an analysis of the survival of 250 hemodialysis patients and 140 peritoneal dialysis patients monitored up to 7 years (1987 to 1994) to determine the independent relationship to mortality risk of a spectrum of demographic, clinical, and biochemical variables.

PATIENTS AND METHODS

Patients

Hemodialysis and CAPD patients treated at the Long Island College Hospital were enrolled into the study beginning in April 1987 through June 1994.

Supported in part by grants from the National Kidney Foundation of New York/New Jersey and the Nephrology Foundation of Brooklyn.

On enrollment and once per year, clinical and laboratory data were collected. Survival was recorded up to September 1994. Two hundred fifty hemodialysis and 140 peritoneal dialysis patients were enrolled over a 7-year period.

Demographic and Clinical Data

Demographic data included age, gender, and race. Clinical data included cause of ESRD, total months on dialysis, estimated dry weight, diabetic status before uremia, and medications. For hemodialysis patients, length of dialysis treatment, dialyzer membrane, dialysate, total heparin dose, mean predialysis blood pressure (of three consecutive treatments), and ratio of pretreatment blood urea nitrogen (BUN) to 5-minute posttreatment BUN were recorded. For peritoneal dialysis patients, mean blood pressure at three consecutive visits were recorded.

Hemodialysis patients. On enrollment, mean age was 60.0 + 15.5 (SD) years (range, 19 to 93 years) and mean prior months on dialysis was 31.7 + 41.0 (SD) (range, 0 to 230 months). There were 55.6% women. The racial composition was black (55.8%), white (28.1%), and hispanic (16.1%). Forty percent were diabetic. The causes of ESRD were diabetes (34.6%), hypertension (35.0%), chronic glomerulonephritis (7.1%), polycystic disease (6.3%), obstructive uropathy (3.5%), human immunodeficiency virus–associated (2.0%), miscellaneous (7.5%), and unknown (3.9%).

Hemodialysis prescription was evolving during the 7-year study period. In 1987, they were treated with acetate (85%) or bicarbonate (15%) dialysate on conventional membranes with Cobe Centry 2 or Centry 2x machines (Cobe, Lakewood, CO). In 1988, a small number of patients were being treated with shorter, high-efficiency or high-flux prescriptions, and 62% of the population received bicarbonate dialysis. Beginning in 1989, all treatments were performed on Cobe Centry-system 3 machines with bicarbonate bath and volumetric ultrafiltration control. Dialysis prescription was guided, in part, by the goal of achieving a value of >2.5 for pretreatment BUN to 5-minute posttreatment BUN.[15-17] The posttreatment BUN was drawn 5 minutes after treatment to minimize the potential problem of spuriously low posttreatment BUN values from the disequilibrium between intracellular and extracellular fluid spaces, as well as cardiopulmonary and access recirculation.

Peritoneal dialysis patients. The mean age of patients maintained with peritoneal dialysis was 52.0 + 15.4 (SD) years (range, 22 to 82 years), and mean months on dialysis at enrollment was 13.5 + 19.4 (SD) months (range, 0 to 127 months). There were 50.4% women. The racial composition was black (61.8%), white (17.6%), and hispanic (16.9%). Thirty-three percent were diabetic. The causes of ESRD were diabetes (30.1%), hypertension (30.9%), chronic glomerulonephritis (13.2%), polycystic disease (3.7%), obstructive uropathy (2.9%), human immunodeficiency virus–associated (5.9%), miscellaneous (10.3%), and unknown (2.9%).

CAPD prescription was four 2-L exchanges per day in most patients. Dextrose concentration varied with the need for ultrafiltration. Frequency and volume were adjusted appropriately based on patient size, peritoneal equilibration testing, and clinical impression throughout the study. Weekly creatinine clearance was estimated by extrapolating the 4-hour peritoneal equilibration test,[18] and adjustments were made to keep the creatinine clearance above 40 L/wk/1.7 m^2. Equilibration characteristics were monitored routinely semiannually with the peritoneal equilibration test, and more often if clinically warranted.

Biochemical Data

On enrollment, nonfasting baseline blood was drawn immediately before the first treatment of the week from the arteriovenous access for hemodialysis patients, or from a peripheral vein in CAPD patients during a routine monthly visit. A multiphasic biochemistry screen was obtained for each patient using the SMAC autoanalyzer (Technicon, Tarrytown, NY). High-density lipoprotein cholesterol was measured on the DuPont ACA (Wilmington, DE) using an assay from EM Diagnostic Systems (Gibbstown, NJ). Prealbumin (added to the profile in 1991), and apoproteins A-I and B (added to the profile in 1988) were measured by rate nephelometry on a Beckman Array Protein System (Beckman Instruments Inc, Brea, CA). Appropriate blanks were used to correct for turbidity in samples. Parathyroid hormone was measured with the Allegro intact PTH assay (Nichols Institute Diagnostics, San Juan Capistrano, CA).

Study Design

We examined patient survival using a proportional hazards model based on the data recorded on initial enrollment. Patients were classified as ''new'' cases if their time on dialysis before initial enrollment was 12 months or less. Patients who were maintained on dialysis for more than 12 months were considered to be ''long-standing'' cases. Hemodialysis patients were prospectively followed for a mean 33 months, range of 2 months to 7 years. CAPD patients were followed for a mean of 24 months, range of 2 months to 6 years. To adjust for survivor bias in patient selection, survival data for the ''new'' and ''long-standing'' groups were analyzed separately. Follow-up was censored on transplantation, transfer between dialysis modalities, or transfer to another dialysis center.

In a separate analysis, to highlight differences between patients with good versus poor survival, we selected two extreme groups of patients: Long-term or ''good'' survival were those patients surviving at least 4 years after enrollment, whereas those dying within the first year after enrollment were categorized as having ''poor'' survival.

Data Analysis

Survival was analyzed using Cox's proportional hazards model[19,20] with baseline age, race, gender, diabetes, duration of ESRD, BUN, creatinine, albumin, cholesterol, high-density lipoprotein cholesterol, apoproteins A-I and B, prealbumin, and parathyroid hormone as independent variables. The variables chosen reflected our previous experience as well as reports in the literature. Variables were selected for the final models by a backward stepwise approach. In general, Cox's model assumes that the risk associated with independent factors is multiplicative and consistent (ie, proportional) during the study period. The proportional hazards assumption was tested by plotting baseline hazards across strata. If the hazards were parallel among the strata, the variable was modeled as a covariate; otherwise, the analysis was stratified. The fit of

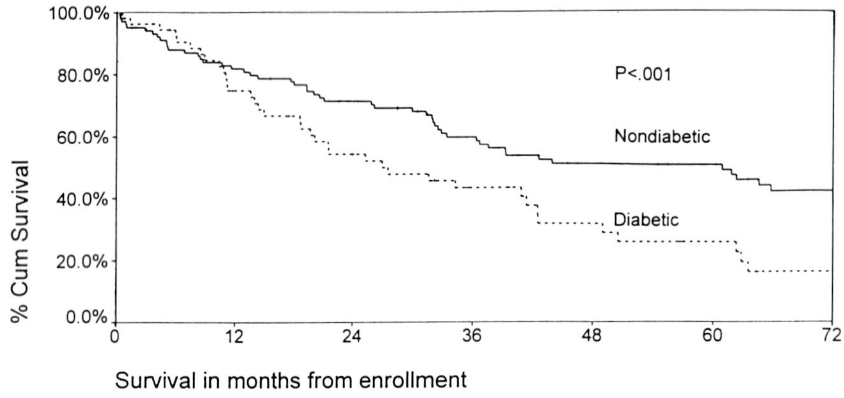

Fig 1. Survival by diabetic status in 157 long-standing HD patients. Long-standing cases were on HD for more than 12 months at the time of study enrollment.

the models was assessed by comparing predicted survival with that of the observed probabilities of survival for selected subgroups of patients. Observed survival was computed by the Kaplan-Meier method.[21] The number of patients represented in Figs 1 through 5 varies because the number with missing data varied for each of the biochemical markers. Data presented include the regression coefficients, the relative risk ratios and their 95% confidence intervals (CI), and the actual *P* values for the risk ratios. The relative risk reflects the risk associated with a variable, assuming other factors are held constant. Variables were analyzed as catagorical, with clinically relevant breakpoints, or as continuous variables.

In cross-sectional analyses, comparisons of continuous variables and proportions were made using ANOVA and the chi-squared test, respectively, unless otherwise stated. Continuous variables are reported as the mean + SD. Simple correlations are reported as the Pearson correlation coefficient or the Spearman rank correlation coefficient (*r*).

RESULTS

Hemodialysis

Long-standing cases. Figures 1 to 4 show observed survival stratified by diabetic status, baseline serum albumin, creatinine, and cholesterol computed by the Kaplan-Meier method for long-standing patients (on dialysis greater than 12 months at enrollment). Significant differences in observed survival over 72 months were seen with each stratification. The independent predictors of patient survival for up to 72 months were determined using Cox's proportional hazards model. The final model is shown in Table 1. Diabetes, age, baseline serum albumin, and serum cholesterol were independent predictors of mortality risk. Adjusting for the other variables in the model, diabetes was associated with almost 1.5-fold increase in mortality risk compared with nondiabetic patients. Each additional year of age imparted a 2% increase in mortality risk. Patients with a serum albumin less than 3.5 g/dL at baseline had greater than twofold mortality risk relative to those with serum albumin 4.0 g/dL or greater. Patients with the lowest cholesterol had almost 2.5-fold mortality risk relative to those with the highest stratification.

New cases. Observed Kaplan-Meier survival curves stratified by diabetic status and baseline serum albumin, creatinine, and cholesterol were

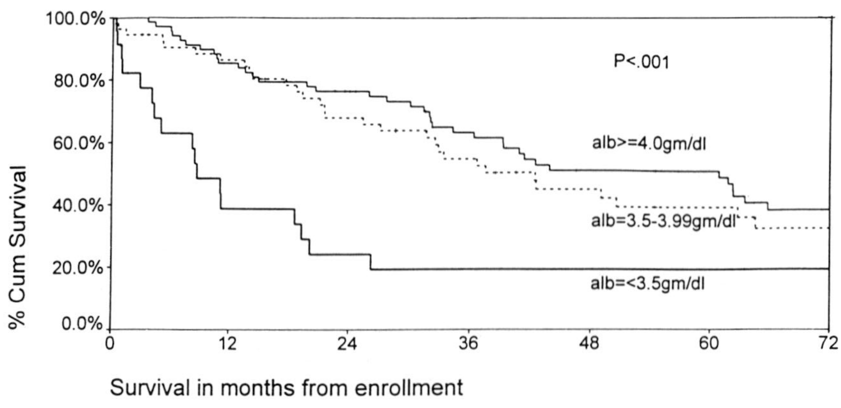

Fig 2. Survival by baseline albumin level in 145 long-standing HD patients. Long-standing cases were on HD for more than 12 months at the time of study enrollment.

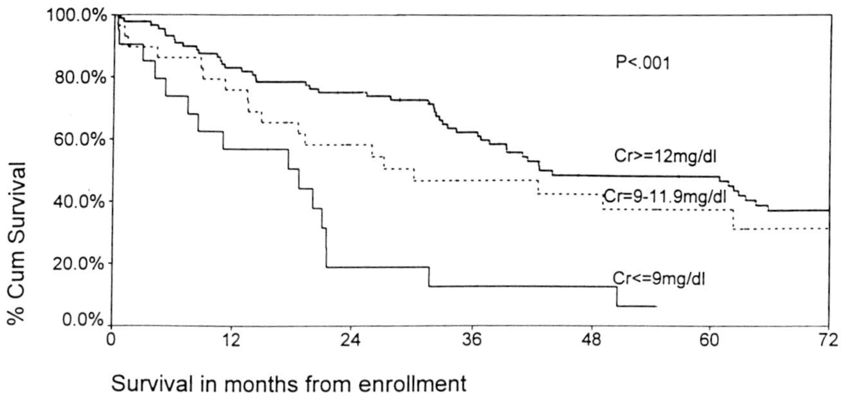

Fig 3. Survival by baseline creatinine level in 141 long-standing HD patients. Long-standing cases were on HD for more than 12 months at the time of study enrollment.

similar to those seen in long-standing cases (not shown). Diabetics had poorer survival than nondiabetics ($P < 0.05$). Significant differences were seen in patient survival at 72 months by differences in baseline measurement of serum albumin ($P < 0.001$ for albumin <3.5 g/dL *v* albumin >3.5 g/dL), and serum creatinine ($P < 0.001$ for creatinine < 9 mg/dL *v* creatinine > 12 mg/dL). Significant differences noted at 36 months by baseline serum cholesterol were not seen at 72 months. The independent predictors of patient survival by Cox's model is seen in Table 2. Adjusting for the other variables in the model, diabetic status, age, race, and baseline serum albumin were important predictors of mortality risk over 72 months. Diabetics had nearly twice the mortality risk as nondiabetics. Each year of life imparted a 4% increase in mortality risk. White hemodialysis patients had greater than fourfold increased mortality risk compared with Hispanics and more than threefold increased risk compared with blacks. Patients with baseline serum albumin below 3.5 g/dL were at 2.5-fold increased mortality risk relative to patients with baseline serum albumin >4.0 g/dL over 72 months of follow-up.

New and long-standing patients. Because the relationship between risk factors and survival was consistent for the most part between long-standing and new cases, we combined both groups in the following analysis. Table 3 shows the independent and multiplicative baseline predictors of mortality risk for the entire group of hemodialysis patients followed up to 72 months. Diabetics had 1.5-fold increased mortality risk compared with nondiabetics. Patients older than 75 years were almost three and one-half times as likely to die as those less than 50 years old at enrollment, and those between 50 and 75 years of age had intermediate risk. Long-standing patients had twice the mortality risk as new patients (for those on hemodialysis between 1 and 3 years as well as those dialyzed more than 3 years at enrollment). Low baseline serum levels of albumin, creatinine, and cholesterol imparted a twofold mortality risk compared with the highest

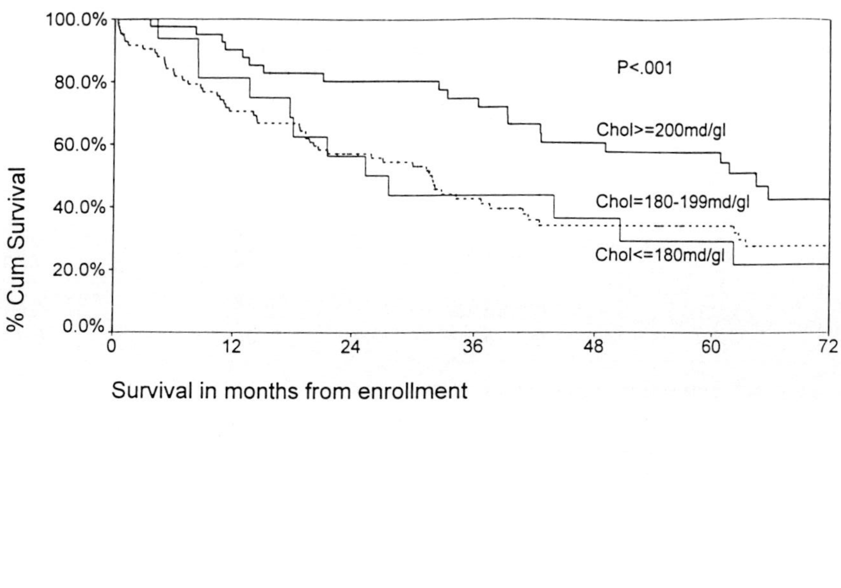

Fig 4. Survival by baseline cholesterol level in 144 long-standing HD patients. Long-standing cases were on HD for more than 12 months at the time of study enrollment.

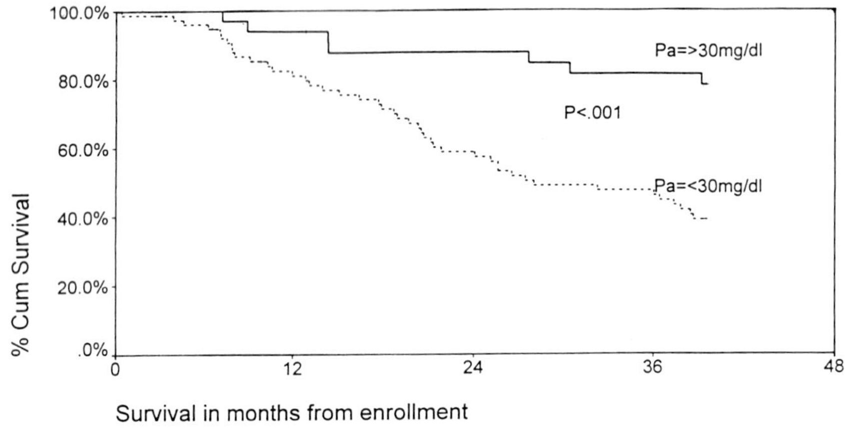

Fig 5. Survival by baseline prealbumin level in 112 HD patients.

range in each categorical variable. Serum albumin was less than 3.5 g/dL in approximately 21% of cases, whereas 42% had serum albumin above 4.0 g/dL. Approximately 25% of cases had serum creatinine less than 9 mg/dL, compared with 49% above 12 mg/dL. Seventy percent of the patients had baseline serum cholesterol below 200 mg/dL.

Figure 5 shows observed survival stratified by baseline serum prealbumin level, computed by the Kaplan-Meier method, for 112 hemodialysis patients followed up to 40 months. Patients with serum prealbumin level of 30 mg/dL or above (n = 77 or 69% of patients) had significantly better survival, above 80% at 40 months ($P < 0.001$), versus patients with baseline values lower than 30 mg/dL, who had only 40% survival. Table 4 shows Cox's proportional hazards models for a subset of patients enrolled between 1991 and 1994 for diabetes and several biochemical markers; prealbumin, apoprotein B, and creatinine. When combined with diabetes alone, or with diabetes and apoprotein B, prealbumin was an independent predictor of mortality risk. When creatinine was added to the model, prealbumin was no longer a significant risk predictor. Note also that diabetes, which is a mortality risk predictor, loses discrimination after biochemical markers are considered. Table 5 shows the Spearman rank correlation coefficients for selected biochemical markers. Baseline serum prealbumin was highly correlated ($P < 0.001$) with all of the biochemical markers; albumin, creatinine, apoprotein B, and cholesterol, but not with baseline BUN ratio (Kt/V) or dialysis hours.

Good versus poor survival. Figure 6 compares baseline demographic and biochemical characteristics of patients who ultimately survived more than 4 years compared with patients who died within 12 months of enrollment. Hemodialysis patients with good survival were younger (55.0 ± 15.1 years *v* 65.3 ± 12.1, $P < 0.001$), and had higher baseline values of serum albumin (4.0 ± 0.4 g/dL *v* 3.5 ± 0.5, $P < 0.001$), serum

Table 1. Proportional Hazard Analysis of 142 Long-Standing Hemodialysis Patients

Predictor	Relative Risk	95% CI	Partial Correlation *R*	*P*
Diabetes (Y *v* N)	1.4	0.90-2.18	0.015	0.14
Age (per year)	1.02	1.01-1.04	0.085	0.01
Serum albumin (g/dL)				
3.5 *v* ≥4.0	2.2	1.15-4.10	0.070	0.02
3.5-3.9 *v* ≥4.0	1.0	0.60-1.56	0.001	0.88
Serum cholesterol (mg/dL)				
<180 *v* ≥200	2.43	1.43-4.13	0.107	0.01
180-199 *v* ≥200	1.84	0.87-3.88	0.028	0.11

NOTE. Long-standing cases were on HD >12 months at the time of study enrollment.

Table 2. Proportional Hazard Analysis of 105 New Hemodialysis Patients

Predictor	Relative Risk	95% CI	Partial Correlation *R*	*P*
Diabetes (Y *v* N)	1.8	0.94-3.42	0.061	0.08
Age (per year)	1.04	1.01-1.07	0.124	0.01
Serum albumin (g/dL)				
<3.5 *v* ≥4.0	2.5	1.12-5.79	0.098	0.03
3.5-3.9 *v* ≥4.0	0.7	0.33-1.68	0.001	0.48
Race				
Blacks *v* whites	0.32	0.15-0.67	−0.199	0.01
Hispanics *v* whites	0.24	0.09-0.69	−0.127	0.01

NOTE. New cases were on HD <12 months at the time of study enrollment.

creatinine (14.7 ± 4.5 mg/dL *v* 10.9 ± 4.3, $P < 0.001$), total serum cholesterol (193.3 ± 46.7 mg/dL *v* 167.9 ± 49.0, $P < 0.02$), and apoprotein B (72.9 ± 27.7 mg/dL *v* 53.2 ± 11.7, $P < 0.001$). Baseline estimated dry weights were similar ($P < 0.96$).

Peritoneal Dialysis

Baseline biochemical values. Peritoneal dialysis patients had lower baseline serum albumin and higher baseline serum cholesterol than hemodialysis patients. Approximately 35% had serum albumin less than 3.2 g/dL, 35% were 3.2 to 3.7 g/dL, and only 30% had values above 3.7 g/dL. Fifty-eight percent had baseline total serum cholesterol above 200 mg/dL. At enrollment, they were on peritoneal dialysis for a mean of 10.6 + 18.2 months. Sixty-seven percent were new cases (on peritoneal dialysis fewer than 12 months at enrollment). Approximately 10% of patients were on peritoneal dialysis more than 3 years at enrollment.

Correlates of mortality. The independent predictors of mortality risk for 140 patients followed on peritoneal dialysis are summarized in Table 6. Diabetes, age, baseline serum albumin, and baseline serum creatinine were important and independent predictors of mortality risk. Adjusting for other predictors, diabetes was associated with 1.5-fold increase in mortality risk compared with nondiabetics. Age older than 65 years imparted greater than three times, and age between 40 and 65 more than twice the mortality risk compared with those younger than age 40.

Figure 7 shows observed survival stratified by baseline serum prealbumin level, computed by

Table 3. Proportional Hazard Analysis of 247 New and Long-Standing Hemodialysis Patients

Predictor	Relative Risk	95% CI	Partial Correlation *R*	*P*
Age				
50-74 *v* <50	1.8	1.07-3.12	0.048	0.03
>75 *v* <50	3.4	1.74-6.66	0.094	0.01
Diabetes (yes *v* no)	1.5	1.01-2.31	0.040	0.05
Months on HD				
12-36 *v* <12	2.0	1.22-3.14	0.080	0.01
>36 *v* <12	2.1	1.35-3.35	0.068	0.01
Serum albumin (g/dL)				
<3.5 *v* ≥4.0	2.22	1.31-3.74	0.074	0.01
3.5-3.9 *v* ≥4.0	0.9	0.56-1.37	0.001	0.57
Serum creatinine (mg/dL)				
<9 *v* >12	1.9	1.03-3.75	0.042	0.04
9-12 *v* >12	0.9	0.53-1.50	0.001	0.67
Serum cholesterol (mg/dL)				
<180 *v* >200	2.0	1.29-3.10	0.078	0.01
180-200 *v* >200	1.4	0.77-2.57	0.001	0.27

Table 4. Proportional Hazard Models for Prealbumin, Creatinine, Apo B, and Diabetes for Hemodialysis Patients 1991 to 1994

	Relative Risk	95% CI	Partial Correlation Coefficient *R*	*P*
I				
Diabetes	1.64	1.33-3.54	−0.09	0.015
Prealbumin	0.91	0.87-0.95	−0.19	0.001
II				
Diabetes	2.22	1.15-3.64	−0.09	0.01
Apo B	0.98	0.97-1.00	−0.06	0.07
Prealbumin	0.93	0.88-0.98	−0.11	0.001
III				
Diabetes	1.62	0.87-3.03	−0.03	0.13
Apo B	0.98	0.96-0.99	−0.11	0.009
Creatinine	0.86	0.78-0.96	−0.12	0.005
Prealbumin	0.99	0.92-1.05	0.01	0.654

the Kaplan-Meier method, for 33 peritoneal dialysis patients followed up to 40 months. Patients with prealbumin level of 30 mg/dL or above had significantly better survival. Table 7 shows the Spearman rank correlation coefficients for selected biochemical markers in peritoneal dialysis patients (n = 79). As with hemodialysis patients, serum prealbumin correlated strongly ($P < 0.01$) with other baseline biochemical markers: albumin, creatinine, and total cholesterol.

DISCUSSION

This report confirms our findings that baseline serum biochemical measurements are independent predictors of long-term mortality risk in patients maintained by hemodialysis and peritoneal dialysis. In hemodialysis patients, using Cox's proportional hazards model to study survival up to 72 months, we found that low baseline level of serum albumin is an independent predictor of long-term mortality risk in both new and long-standing patients. Low baseline serum albumin was also an independent predictor of mortality risk in CAPD using the Cox model. Lower values were seen for serum albumin in CAPD for the entire population, as reported previously.[22] The combination of large effluent protein losses and large carbohydrate load associated with CAPD predisposes those patients to protein depletion.[23] For the entire hemodialysis population, low baseline serum albumin, creatinine, and cholesterol each imparted twofold increases in risk compared with patients with higher values. Low serum creatinine was also an independent predictor of mortality for CAPD patients in the Cox model.

Low level of serum prealbumin was an important and independent predictor of mortality risk for hemodialysis and peritoneal dialysis patients followed up to 40 months. Using the pro-

Table 5. Spearman's Rank Correlation Coefficient for Selected Nutritional Markers in Hemodialysis Patients

	PA	ALB	CR	Apo B	TC	BUN	HRS
PA	—	—	—	—	—	—	—
ALB	0.43*	—	—	—	—	—	—
CR	0.51*	0.38*	—	—	—	—	—
Apo B	0.47*	0.17	0.06	—	—	—	—
TC	0.44*	0.18	0.06	0.85*	—	—	—
BUN	−0.04	0.06	−0.07	0.11	0.15	—	—
HRS	−0.14	−0.11	−0.12	−0.03	−0.05	0.03	—

Abbreviations: PA, prealbumin; ALB, albumin; CR, creatinine; TC, total cholesterol; BUN, blood urea nitrogen ratio; HRS, dialysis hours.

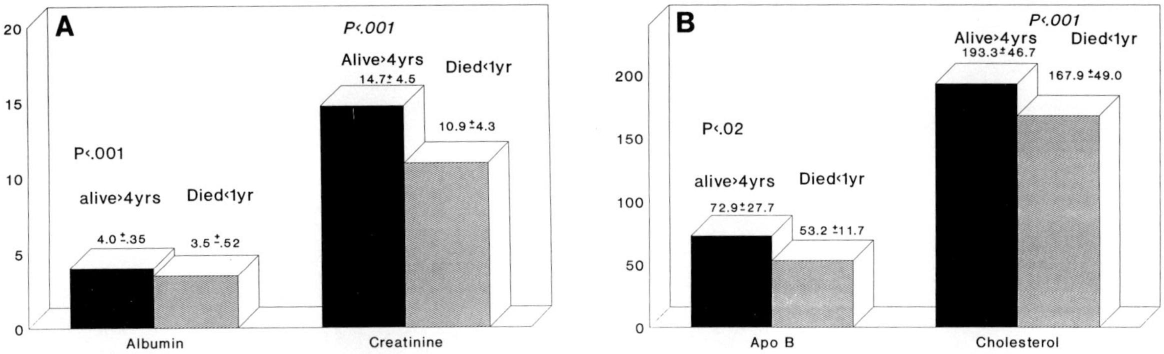

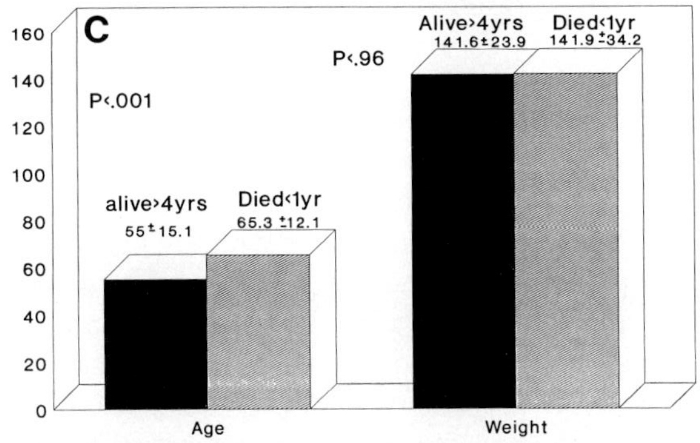

Fig 6. **(A) Difference in baseline albumin and creatinine between short- and long-term survivors. (B) Difference in baseline cholesterol and apo-B between short- and long-term survivors. (C) Difference in baseline age and weight between short- and long-term survivors.**

portional hazards model for hemodialysis patients, prealbumin ceased to be an independent predictor when added to apoprotein B and creatinine. This is likely explained by the strong correlation seen between prealbumin and the other biochemical markers, ie, it loses discrimination because it is measuring the same factors.

The serum levels of secretory proteins, such as albumin and lipoproteins (hence cholesterol), reflect the size and function of the visceral protein pool.[24,25] Serum creatinine is a marker of somatic protein content.[26,27] The finding that visceral and somatic protein depletion are important risk predictors is compatible with the view expressed by Acchiardo et al[28] that malnutrition is the most important cause of mortality in dialysis patients. However, low serum albumin and cholesterol are not considered early markers of malnutrition.[29,30] Therefore, a more sensitive marker may improve our ability to identify patients at risk. Prealbumin, a serum protein with rapid turnover and relatively small pool, has been found to be a practical and sensitive nutrition marker in the general population.[31,32] The serum level of

Table 6. Proportional Hazard Analysis of 140 New and Long-Standing Peritoneal Dialysis Patients

Predictor	Relative Risk	95% CI	Partial Correlation *R*	*P*
Diabetes (yes *v* no)	1.5	0.86-2.62	0.001	0.16
Age				
40-64 yrs *v* <40 yrs	2.3	1.01-5.10	0.063	0.05
≥65 *v* <40 yrs	3.2	1.29-7.80	0.096	0.01
Serum albumin (g/dL)				
<3.2 *v* >3.7	2.3	1.08-4.82	0.075	0.03
3.2-3.7 *v* >3.7	1.8	0.79-4.06	0.001	0.17
Serum creatinine (mg/dL)				
<9 *v* >12	2.4	1.18-4.85	0.090	0.02
9-12 *v* >12	1.3	0.65-2.73	0.001	0.44

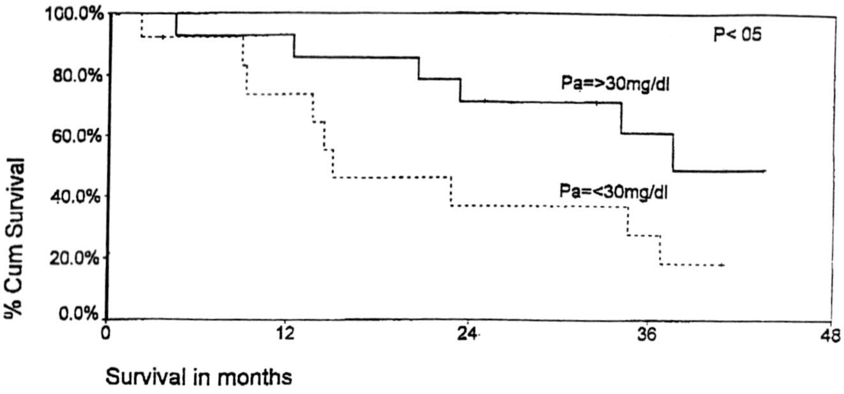

Fig 7. Survival by baseline prealbumin level (N = 33 PD patients; n = 14 < 30 mg/dL; n = 19 > 30 mg/dL).

prealbumin can change more rapidly than that of serum albumin in response to changes in nutritional status.[33] Cano et al[14] reported that low serum levels of creatinine and prealbumin, but not albumin, were associated with increased 1-year mortality in hemodialysis patients. We found that serum prealbumin correlated more highly with other nutritional markers than albumin for hemodialysis and peritoneal dialysis patients.

In addition to biochemical risk predictors, demographic parameters were important predictors of long-term mortality risk. Not surprisingly, age at enrollment was an independent predictor of mortality risk for both new and long-standing hemodialysis patients and for patients maintained on CAPD. Race was found to be important mortality risk predictor in new hemodialysis patients, that is, those enrolled within their first 12 months on dialysis. White patients were at greater mortality risk, similar to findings reported by others.[34,35] Lowrie et al[34] linked this finding to genetic differences in serum creatinine, creatinine generation rate, and somatic protein content,

Table 7. Spearman's Rank Correlation Coefficients for Selected Nutritional Markers in Peritoneal Dialysis Patients

	PA	ALB	CR	TC
PA	—	—	—	—
ALB	0.42*	—	—	—
CR	0.44*	0.28*	—	—
TC	0.57*	0.18	−0.15	—

Abbreviations: PA, prealbumin; ALB, albumin; CR, creatinine; TC, total cholesterol.

*$P < 0.01$.

which might affect ability to respond to nutritional changes. In addition, there is a selection bias in that transplantation rates for whites exceed those for blacks, thereby removing a subgroup disproportionately from whites who would be expected to have a better prognosis. Diabetes was an important and independent risk factor for long-term survival for hemodialysis and CAPD patients. Interestingly, similar to the findings of Lowrie and Lew,[11,34] diabetes loses discrimination in hemodialysis patients when biochemical markers are considered. This suggests that biochemical markers reflect an aspect of mortality risk that is characteristic of diabetes, eg, reduced somatic protein. Excess mortality among diabetic patients with ESRD has been associated with differences in nutrition and the intensity of dialysis.[34,36] Inadequate dialysis is believed to be a dominant factor in excess mortality in the entire United States ESRD population relative to other major industrialized nations.[37,38] We have noted a relationship between BUN ratio (Kt/V) and mortality risk in a 2-year period.[10] The design of the current study did not permit any meaningful analysis of the effect of treatment dose or time on long-term mortality risk. There was no relation between baseline BUN ratio or treatment time and any of the baseline biochemical markers. Recent studies have shown that prospective increases in Kt/V can impact morbidity and mortality favorably.[38,39] However, although speculated, there are no prospective studies demonstrating nutritional improvement through increased dialysis dose or time. In fact, Owen et al,[36] in a retrospective analysis, found no difference in interval serum albumin change between two subgroups of hemodialysis patients, one with urea reduction ratio that increased during the study period, and one group with decreased interval urea reduction ratio; both groups experienced similar decreases in serum albumin.

In summary, we examined mortality risk in 250 hemodialysis and 140 peritoneal dialysis patients followed up to 7 years using a proportional hazards model. Biochemical markers suggestive of visceral and somatic protein malnutrition, as well as diabetes and age, were independent predictors of mortality risk. Protein-calorie malnutrition is highly prevalent in ESRD (reviewed in depth in references 40 and 41) and is a dominant cause of mortality in this population. The use of risk profiles that permit early identification of high-risk patients may allow for early intervention in these individuals. Prospective trials to improve dietary intake, increase dialysis dose, lessen catabolism, and correct acidosis are sorely needed to assess their ability to improve nutriture and ultimately, patient survival. Embryonal reports of successful intervention using intradialytic parenteral nutrition and pronutritional agents such as growth hormone must be confirmed.

ACKNOWLEDGMENT

The authors thank Dr Joseph Feldman for his assistance in the statistical analysis.

REFERENCES

1. Lindner A, Charra B, Sherrard DJ, Scribner BH: Accelerated atherosclerosis on prolonged maintenance hemodialysis. N Engl J Med 290:697-701, 1974

2. Gurland HJ, Brunner FP, Dehn H von: Combined report on regular dialysis and transplantation in Europe. Proc Eur Dial Transplant Assoc 10:XVII-LVII, 1978

3. Green D, Stone NJ, Krumlovsky FA: Putative atherogenic factors in patients with chronic renal failure. Prog Cardiovasc Dis 26:1133-1144, 1983

4. Ibels LS, Alfrey AC, Huffer WE, Craswell PW, Anderson JJ, Weil R: Arterial calcification and pathology in uremic patients undergoing dialysis. Am J Med 66:790-796, 1979

5. Burke JF, Francos GC, Moore LL, Cho SY, Lasker N: Accelerated atherosclerosis in chronic-dialysis patients: Another look. Nephron 21:181-185, 1978

6. Nicholls AJ, Edward N, Catto GRD, Engeset J, Macleod M: Accelerated atherosclerosis in long-term dialysis and renal transplantation: Fact or fiction? Lancet 1:276-278, 1980

7. Avram MM, Fein PA, Antignani A, Mittman N, Mushnick RA, Lustig AR, Lapuz MH, Goldwasser P: Cholesterol and lipid disturbances in renal disease: The natural history of uremic dyslipidemia and the impact of hemodialysis and continuous ambulatory peritoneal dialysis. Am J Med 87:55N-60N, 1989

8. Grutzmacher P, Marz W, Peschke B, Gross W, Schoeppe W: Ischemic heart disease in patients with uremia undergoing maintenance hemodialysis. Kidney Int 126:600-611, 1979

9. Avram MM, Goldwasser P, Burrell DE, Antignani A, Fein PA, Mittman N: The uremic dyslipidemia: A cross-sectional and longitudinal study. Am J Kidney Dis 20:325-335, 1992

10. Goldwasser P, Mittman N, Antignani A, Burrell D, Michel MA, Collier J, Avram MM: Predictors of mortality in hemodialysis patients. J Am Soc Nephrol 3:1613-1622, 1993

11. Lowrie EG, Lew NL: Death risk in hemodialysis patients: The predictive value of commonly measured variables and an evaluation of the death rate differences between facilities. Am J Kidney Dis 15:458-482, 1990

12. Goldwasser P, Michel M-A, Collier J, Mittman N, Fein PA, Gusik SA, Avram MM: Prealbumin and lipoprotein(a) in hemodialysis: Relationships with patient and vacular access survival. Am J Kidney Dis 22:215-225, 1993

13. Avram MM, Goldwasser P, Erroa M, Fein PA: Predictors of survival in continuous ambulatory peritoneal dialysis: The importance of prealbumin and other nutritional and metabolic markers. Am J Kidney Dis 23:91-98, 1994

14. Cano N, Fernandez JP, Lacombe P, Lankester M, Pascal S, DeFayolle M, Labastie J, Saingra S: Statistical selection of nutritional parameters in hemodialyzed patients. Kidney Int 32:S178-S180, 1987

15. Daugirdas TJ, Dumler F, Zasuwa GA, Levin NW: Chronic hemodialysis prescription, in Daugirdas TJ, Ing TS (eds): Handbook of Dialysis (ed 1). Boston, MA, Little Brown, 1988, pp 72-86

16. Keshaviah PR, Hanson GL, Berkseth RO, Collins AJ: A simplified approach to monitoring in vivo therapy prescription. Trans Am Soc Artif Intern Organs 34:620-622, 1988

17. Soundararajan R, Soundararajan P: A simple and practical method for assessing the adequacy of dialysis. Trans Am Soc Artif Intern Organs 37:M393-M394, 1991

18. Twardowski Z: Clinical value of standardized equilibrium tests in CAPD patients. Blood Purif 7:95-108, 1989

19. Cox DR: Regression models and life tables (with discussion): J R Stat Soc (Series B) 43:187-220, 1972

20. Kelbfleisch J: The Statistical Analysis of Failure Time Data. New York, NY, John Wiley & Sons, 1980

21. Kaplan EL, Meier P: Nonparametric estimation from incomplete observations. J Am Stat Assoc 53:457-481, 1958

22. Fine A, Cox D: Modest reduction of serum albumin in continuous ambulatory peritoneal dialysis patients is common and of no apparent clinical consequence. Am J Kidney Dis 20:50-54, 1992

23. Kaysen GA, Schoenfeld P: Albumin homeostasis in patients undergoing continuous ambulatory peritoneal dialysis. Kidney Int 25:107-114, 1984

24. Young GA, Hill GL: Assessment of protein-calorie malnutrition in surgical patients from plasma proteins and anthropometric measurements. Am J Clin Nutr 31:429-435, 1978

25. Carpentier YA, Barthel J, Bruyns J: Plasma protein concentration in nutritional assessment. Proc Nutr Soc 41:405-417, 1982

26. Heymsfield SB, Arteaga C, McManus C, Smith J,

Moffitt S: Measurement of muscle mass in humans: Validity of the 24-hour urinary creatinine method. Am J Clin Nutr 37:478-494, 1983

27. Bleiler RE, Schedl HP: Creatinine excretion: Variability and relationships to diet and body size. J Lab Clin Med 59:945-955, 1962

28. Acchiardo SR, Moore LW, Latour PA: Malnutrition as the main factor in morbidity and mortality of hemodialysis patients. Kidney Int 24:199-203, 1983 (Suppl 16)

29. Blumenkrantz MJ, Kopple J, Gutman RA, Chan YK, Barbour GL, Roberts C, Shen FH, Grandhi VC, Tucker T, Curtis FK, Coburn JW: Methods for assessing nutritional status of patients with renal failure. Am J Clin Nutr 33:1567-1585, 1980

30. Torun B, Viteri FE: Protein-energy malnutrition, in Shils ME, Young VR (eds): Modern Nutrition in Health and Disease, Philadelphia, PA, Lea & Feiberger, 1988, pp 746-773

31. Shetty PS, Watrasiewicz KE, Jung RT, James WP: Rapid turnover transplant patients: An index of sublinical protein-energy malnutrition. Lancet 2:230-232, 1979

32. Tuten MB, Wogt S, Dasse F, Lieder Z: Utilization of prealbumin as a nutritional parameter. J Parenter Enteral Nutr 9:709-711, 1985

33. Ingenbleek Y, DeVisscher M, Denayer P: Measurement of prealbumin as an index of protein-calorie malnutrition. Lancet 2:106-108, 1972

34. Lowrie EG, Lew NL, Huang WH: Race and diabetes as death risk predictors in hemodialysis patients. Kidney Int 42:S22-S31, 1992 (Suppl 38)

35. Eggers PW: Mortality rates among dialysis patients in Medicare's end-stage renal disease program. Am J Kidney Dis 25:414-421, 1990

36. Owen WF, Lew NL, Liu Y, Lowrie EG, Lazarus JM: The urea reduction ratio and serum albumin concentration as predictors of mortality in patients undergoing hemodialysis. N Engl J Med 329:1001-1006, 1993

37. Parker TF, Husni L, Huang W, Lew N, Lowrie EG, Dallas Nephrology Associates: Survival of hemodialysis patients in the United States is improved with a greater quantity of dialysis. Am J Kidney Dis 23:670-680, 1994

38. Hakim RM, Depner TA, Parker TF: Adequacy of hemodialysis. Am J Kidney Dis 20:107-123, 1992

39. Hakim RM, Breyer J, Ismail N, Schulman G: Effects of dose of dialysis on morbidity and mortality. Am J Kidney Dis 23:661-669, 1994

40. Hakim RM, Levin N: Malnutrition in hemodialysis patients. Am J Kidney Dis 21:125-137, 1993

41. Avram MM, Mittman N: Malnutrition in uremia. Semin Nephrol 14:238-244, 1994

Death Risk Predictors Among Peritoneal Dialysis and Hemodialysis Patients: A Preliminary Comparison

Edmund G. Lowrie, MD, Wei H. Huang, MS, and Nancy L. Lew, SM

● Variables associated with survival among 1,522 peritoneal dialysis patients and 16,404 hemodialysis patients who received treatment during 1992 were evaluated. Analysis was performed separately for the treatment types and for the combined patient group. In general, the associates of survival appear similar among patients receiving peritoneal or hemodialysis. Important variables appear related to nutrition, acid-base status (which is related to nutrition), and age.

INDEX WORDS: Hemodialysis; peritoneal dialysis; survival.

NATIONAL Medical Care, Inc. (NMC) maintains a clinical database, the Patient Statistical Profile System (PSP), that supports ongoing quality enhancement activities. Data are summarized statistically each calendar quarter and are distributed to affiliated dialysis centers for their use in quality enhancement activities. The data are also used to evaluate timely topics of clinical interest. We posit that better understanding of associations between the outcomes and processes of care, combined with monitoring by centers of both outcomes and processes, will lead to improved care outcome systemwide.[1]

Much recent effort has been devoted to evaluating the relationship between various care processes and the outcome, survival (reflected by the odds of death), among hemodialysis patients.[2-6] We chose survival because it is a highly relevant outcome of care.[1] We focused on hemodialysis patients because most patients with end-stage kidney failure are treated by hemodialysis. The statistical studies described below represent a first attempt to retrospectively explore the relationship between survival and the processes of care among peritoneal dialysis patients and to compare them with patients receiving hemodialysis.

PATIENTS AND METHODS

Patients receiving three times weekly hemodialysis or peritoneal dialysis (continuous ambulatory peritoneal dialysis [CAPD] and automated peritoneal dialysis [APD]) on January 1, 1992 and those starting dialysis during 1992 were chosen for the initial sample. Precautions were taken to assure that patients were properly assigned to a single therapy. Patients who switched dialysis types during the year were censored at the time of therapy change and were not reclassified into the new treatment. All patients treated by intermittent peritoneal dialysis were eliminated form the sample.

Working files were constructed from the PSP database as previously described[6] and included demographic, laboratory, and outcome data. Only patients with complete clinical and laboratory data were included in the final sample. Laboratory data from up to 3 months before and during the observation period were included in these files. This violates the general practice of including only those data measured before start of the observation period but allowed inclusion of patients starting peritoneal dialysis during the year. Sample size was therefore increased, permitting categorized analysis of measurements such as serum albumin concentration. Compared with most analysis using Cox techniques, these observation times are short—1 year or less—making significant biasing unlikely. Further, separate analysis including only subsamples of hemodialysis and peritoneal dialysis patients with laboratory data obtained before start of the observation period identified the same primary risk factors as found with the complete sample analyses and in the analysis combining all patients. All analyses (five of them, three reported herein) extracted remarkably similar risk coefficients.

The final data set included 1,522 peritoneal dialysis patients and 16,404 hemodialysis patients. Factors contributing to survival time, from the later of January 1, 1992 or the date of first dialysis to December 31, 1992, were evaluated by Cox proportional hazards modeling processes.[7,8] The analytic logic has been described previously.[1-3,5] Differences between means were evaluated by Student's *t*-test.[9] Frequency differences of categorical counts between groups were evaluated by chi-square tests.[9]

RESULTS

Table 1 compares respectively the demographic and laboratory data from peritoneal and hemodialysis patients. The median age of patients receiving peritoneal dialysis was more than 9 years younger than patients on hemodialysis. Peritoneal dialysis patients were more likely to be white and less likely to be diabetic.

Mean serum albumin concentration was significantly lower among peritoneal than hemodialysis patients and so was iron-binding capacity. Triglyceride and cholesterol concentrations, however, were higher among peritoneal than hemodialysis patients. Lactate dehydrogenase and serum glutamic-pyruvic transaminase were somewhat higher, but bilirubin was slightly lower among peritoneal than hemodialysis patients. Hematocrit, serum iron, and ferritin con-

Table 1. Descriptive Statistics: Hemodialysis and Peritoneal Dialysis Patients

	Peritoneal Dialysis	Hemodialysis	*P*
Case mix predictors			
Number	1,522	16,404	
Age (yrs)			
Median	52.57	61.70	
Mean	52.52	58.91	<0.001
Race (%)			
White	61.50	49.34	<0.001
Black	31.73	41.25	—
Asian	1.18	1.50	—
Native American	0.92	0.59	—
Other	4.66	7.32	—
Sex (%)			
Female	49.01	48.65	NS
Diabetes (%)	37.19	40.14	0.025
Primary renal diagnosis (%)			
Diabetes mellitus	31.08	30.95	—
Essential hypertension	19.91	22.42	—
Nephrosclerosis	7.36	9.85	—
Chronic glomerulonephritis	10.58	9.83	—
Interstitial nephritis	3.29	2.58	—
Cystic kidney disease	3.48	2.89	—
Other	17.74	21.48	—
Laboratory predictors (mean)			
Albumin (g/dL)	3.44	3.68	<0.001
Creatinine (mg/dL)	10.98	10.76	0.053
Anion gap (mEq/L)	21.10	23.50	<0.001
Chloride (mEq/L)	98.93	99.68	<0.001
Iron (μg/dL)	60.38	53.95	<0.001
LDH (μ/L)	226.16	207.92	<0.001
Ferritin (ng/mL)	357.08	309.06	0.006
WBC (1,000/μL)	7.66	7.06	<0.001
Bilirubin (mg/dL)	0.47	0.51	<0.001
Cholesterol (mg/dL)	201.31	171.94	<0.001
Protein (g/dL)	6.50	6.82	<0.001
SGPT (U/L)	18.15	16.50	<0.001
HCT (%)	31.53	30.43	<0.001
Platelet (1,000/μL)	282.05	242.78	<0.001
Uric acid (mg/dL)	6.62	6.90	<0.001
BUN (mg/dL)	63.34	71.16	<0.001
PO_4 (mg/dL)	5.64	5.96	<0.001
Alkaline Phosphatase (U/L)	121.75	140.51	<0.001
Ca (mg/dL)	9.07	8.96	<0.001
CO_2 (mEq/L)	21.98	18.55	<0.001
K (mEq/L)	4.49	4.99	<0.001
Na (mEq/L)	137.53	136.74	<0.001
SGOT (U/L)	19.24	18.14	0.002
TIBC (μg/dL)	241.53	247.51	<0.001
Triglycerides (mg/dL)	216.57	175.45	<0.001

Abbreviations: —, not done; NS, not significant; LDH, lactate dehydrogenase; WBC, white blood cells; SGPT, serum glutamic-pyruvic transaminase; HCT, hematocrit; BUN, blood urea nitrogen; Ca, calcium; SGOT, serum glutamic oxaloacetic transaminase; TIBC, total iron-binding capacity.

Table 2. Case Mix and Laboratory Death Risk Predictors Among Peritoneal Dialysis Patients

Predictors	Risk Ratio	χ^2	*P*
Case mix			
Age (yrs)	1.047	40.9	0.0001
Sex (Ref = male)	0.417	23.8	0.0001
Diagnosis			
Collagen vascular disease	11.094	10.5	0.0012
Essential hypertension	1.634	5.3	0.0213
Laboratory			
Albumin (g/dL)	0.164	71.6	0.0001
Anion gap (mEq/L)	1.159	32.1	0.0001
Creatinine (mg/dL)	0.841	28.2	0.0001
LDH (U/L)	1.004	9.8	0.0018
Protein (g/dL)	1.489	9.5	0.0021
Chloride (mEq/dL)	0.943	8.4	0.0037
Bilirubin (mg/dL)	1.837	5.6	0.0183
Alkaline phosphatase (U/L)	1.001	4.7	0.0302
Automated peritoneal dialysis (Ref = CAPD)	0.986	0.0	NS

NOTE. N = 1,522; Cox Model.

Abbreviations: *P*, associated probability for accepting the null hypothesis; NS, not significant; Ref, reference.

centration were all higher among peritoneal dialysis patients.

Serum creatinine, blood urea nitrogen, CO_2 concentrations, and anion gap may not be comparable, strictly speaking, between the therapy types because blood samples are collected before hemodialysis but are more likely to be time-averaged values among peritoneal dialysis patients. Nonetheless, anion gap was greater and CO_2 lower among hemodialysis than peritoneal dialysis patients. The values of serum creatinine were comparable. Blood urea nitrogen was higher among hemodialysis than peritoneal dialysis patients.

Peritoneal Dialysis

Table 2 describes the risk ratios for those variables shown in Table 1 that were found significantly associated with the risk of death. The type of peritoneal dialysis was forced into the statistical model and was not associated with survival time. Serum albumin concentration was the variable most closely associated with death risk, followed by age, anion gap, and serum creatinine concentration. Higher values of both albumin and creatinine were associated with lower risk. Higher values of both age and anion gap were associated with greater risk. Both diabetes and

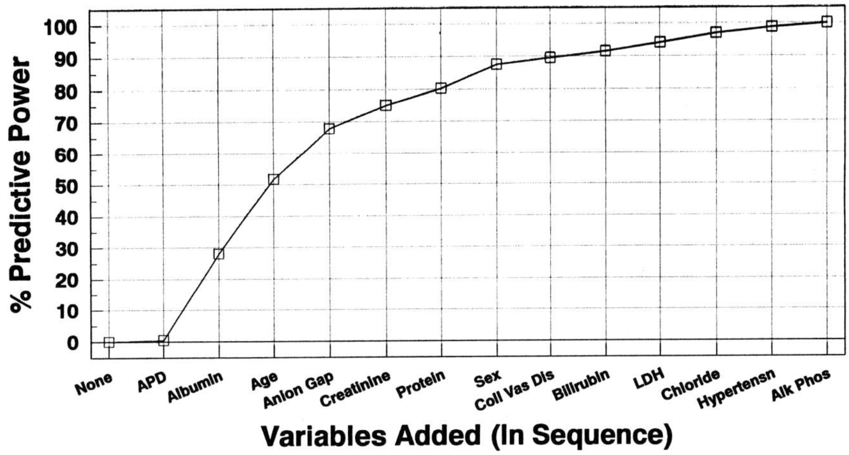

Fig 1. The fraction of final predictive power of a Cox model is shown as variables are added sequentially to it.

race were significant predictors before the addition of laboratory variables to the statistical model (analysis not shown). Neither was significant after laboratory variables were added. The finding has been observed among hemodialysis patients as well.[4]

Figure 1 shows the evolution of the statistical model described by Table 2. The type of peritoneal dialysis did not contribute to the predictive power of the final model. The combination of albumin, age, anion gap, and creatinine contribute approximately 75% of its final predictive power. Hence, those four variables, out of approximately 30 evaluated, are most closely associated with explainable death risk differences among peritoneal dialysis patients.

These findings are remarkably similar to those reported for the hemodialysis population.[1,2] They suggest that the combination of nutrition-related markers (albumin and creatinine), age, and anion gap are closely associated with risk among dialysis patients in general.

Figure 2 shows the risk profile for serum albumin concentration. Two analyses are shown. The first adjusts only for the case mix predictors. The second adjusts for both those and the other laboratory variables in the statistical model. Patients with values >4.0 g/dL were chosen for the reference group. The risk ratio was approximately 1.7 among patients with albumin >3.5 g/dL but ≤4.0 g/dL (P = NS). When albumin was ≤3.5 g/dL, death risk exceeded 3.5 to 4 times that of persons with albumin >4.0 g/dL.

Figure 3 is a similar profile for serum creatinine concentration. In general, risk increased as creatinine decreased, particularly after adjustment for laboratory values, most notably serum albumin concentration.

Figure 4 shows the risk profile for anion gap. Patients with values <20 mEq/L were chosen for the reference group. Risk increases as anion gap increases but only after adjustment for other laboratory values such as albumin and creatinine. The observation has been reported previously among hemodialysis patients.[1,2] We are unable to explain lower risk at an anion gap of 26 to 28 mEq/L. The relatively small number of patients in that group—only 81—may contribute to the disparate finding.

Hemodialysis

We do not discuss this analysis in detail because its findings are similar to earlier analyses already published.[1,2] Table 3 shows the risk ratios

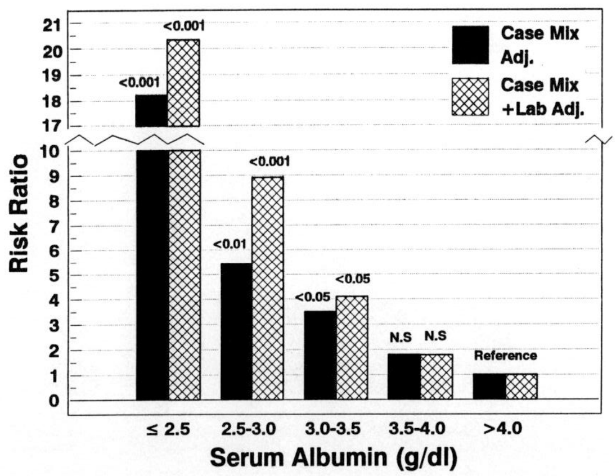

Fig 2. Risk profile for serum albumin concentration among peritoneal dialysis patients.

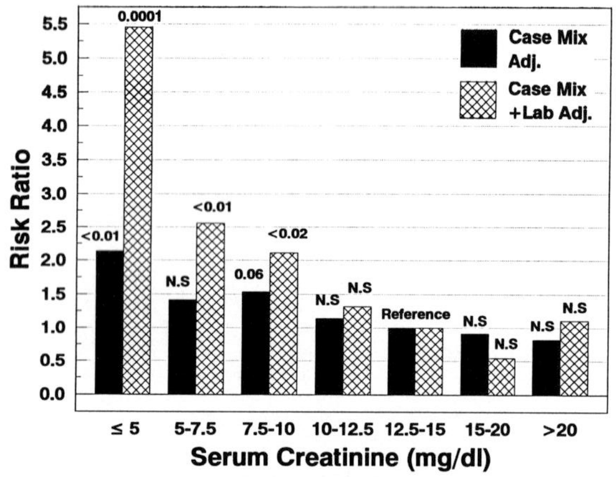

Fig 3. Risk profile for serum creatinine concentration among peritoneal dialysis patients.

associated with the case mix and laboratory predictors significantly associated with survival time.

The risk ratio (RR) associated with age was 1.024, suggesting increasing risk with advancing age. The earlier analysis,[2] which used logistic modeling (rather than Cox analysis) to evaluate data gathered during 1991 (rather than 1992) suggested an odds ratio for death (OR) of 1.029. Females experienced less risk than males in both analyses (RR = 0.680 in 1992; OR = 0.745 in 1991). Albumin, creatinine, and anion gap were the three laboratory variables most closely associated with death risk in both (RR = 0.241, 0.865, and 1.114, respectively; and OR = 0.396, 0.841, and 1.072). Cholesterol (RR = .996; OR = .998) was also a significant factor in both,

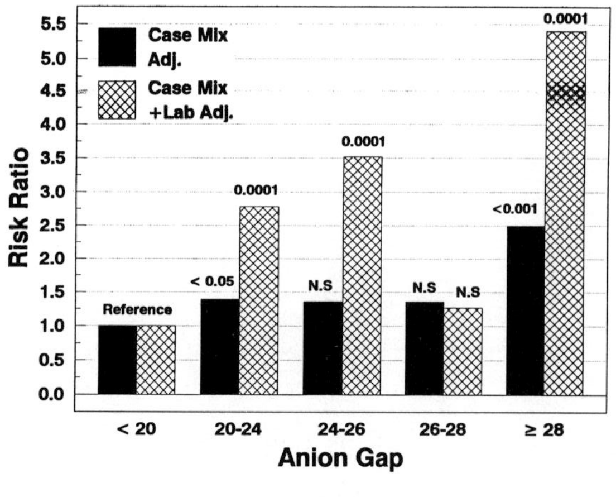

Fig 4. Risk profile for anion gap among peritoneal dialysis patients.

Table 3. Case Mix and Laboratory Death Risk Predictors Among Hemodialysis Patients

Predictors	Risk Ratio	χ^2	*P*
Case mix			
Age (yrs)	1.024	148.6	0.0001
Sex (Ref = male)	0.680	60.2	0.0001
Diagnosis			
Collagen vascular disease	2.386	6.7	0.0094
Multiple myeloma	1.627	4.4	0.0368
Laboratory			
Albumin (g/dL)	0.241	359.4	0.0001
Creatinine (mg/dL)	0.865	172.2	0.0001
Anion gap (mEq/L)	1.114	141.6	0.0001
Iron (μg/dL)	0.990	61.8	0.0001
Chloride (mEq/dL)	0.951	60.6	0.0001
LDH (U/L)	1.001	44.9	0.0001
Ferritin (ng/mL)	1.000*	41.1	0.0001
WBC (1,000/μL)	1.059	37.8	0.0001
Bilirubin (mg/dL)	1.181	32.0	0.0001
Cholesterol (mg/dL)	0.996	29.7	0.0001
SGPT (U/L)	1.004	23.6	0.0001
Hct (%)	0.970	17.3	0.0001
Protein (g/dL)	1.150	13.1	0.0003
Platelet (1,000/μL)	0.999	10.4	0.0012
Phosphorus (mg/dL)	0.965	4.3	0.0388

NOTE. n = 16,404; Cox Model.

Abbreviations: *P*, associated probability for accepting the Null hypothesis; Ref, reference.

* 1.000171.

as was lactate dehydrogenase (RR = 1.001; OR = 1.003), hematocrit (RR = 0.970; OR = 0.985), and bilirubin (RR = 1.181; OR = 2.021). Although these analyses, using two different statistical techniques on two different populations studied during 2 different years, are not identical, they are remarkably similar.

Peritoneal Dialysis and Hemodialysis

Table 4 summarizes the results from the Cox analysis of the combined treatment population. As expected, albumin, creatinine, age, and anion gap are the four variables most closely associated with death risk. Peritoneal dialysis patients experienced approximately 32% excess risk (*P* = 0.005) after adjustment for all other variables.

Figures 5 through 11 compare the risk ratios among patients grouped jointly by the type of dialysis and the respective concentrations of serum albumin, creatinine, anion gap, and cholesterol, lactate dehydrogenase, serum iron, and hematocrit. Hemodialysis patients with laboratory

Table 4. Case Mix and Laboratory Death Risk Predictors Among Hemodialysis and Peritoneal Dialysis Patients

Predictors	Risk Ratio	χ^2	*P*
Case mix			
Age (yrs)	1.026	182.9	0.0001
Sex (Ref = male)	0.671	67.3	0.0001
Diagnosis			
Chronic renal failure	2.243	5.8	0.0159
Chronic glomerulonephritis	0.813	5.0	0.0253
Multiple myeloma	1.637	4.9	0.0266
Race (Ref = nonwhite)	1.122	4.7	0.0308
Laboratory predictors			
Albumin (g/dL)	0.234	410.7	0.0001
Creatinine (mg/dL)	0.866	171.5	0.0001
Anion gap (mEq/L)	1.128	166.7	0.0001
Chloride (mEq/dL)	0.953	61.1	0.0001
Iron (mEq/dL)	0.991	57.4	0.0001
LDH (U/L)	1.001	43.5	0.0001
Ferritin (ng/nL)	1.000*	43.5	0.0001
WBC (1,000/μL)	1.054	34.2	0.0001
Bilirubin (mg/dL)	1.180	30.5	0.0001
Cholesterol (mg/dL)	0.997	28.7	0.0001
Protein (g/dL)	1.210	25.3	0.0001
SGPT (U/L)	1.003	24.3	0.0001
HCT (%)	0.969	22.5	0.0001
Platelet (1,000/μL)	0.999	9.5	0.0021
Uric acid (mg/dL)	1.058	6.8	0.0089
BUN (mg/dL)	0.996	5.8	0.0157
PO_4 (mg/dL)	0.960	5.8	0.0164
Peritoneal dialysis (Ref = hemodialysis)	1.322	7.8	0.0052

NOTE. n = 17,926; Cox Model.

Abbreviations: *P*, associated probability for accepting the null hypothesis; Ref, reference.

* 1.000167.

values in a particular range were chosen for the reference group in each analysis. The *P* values over the bars indicate the significance of the RR difference between the group and hemodialysis patients with values in the reference range. The row labeled "P" below the graph indicates the significance of the risk ratio difference between the peritoneal dialysis patients in the group and those with values in the reference range. The row labeled "H" below the bar shows the significance of the RR difference between hemodialysis and peritoneal dialysis patients with the laboratory values in the range for that pair of bars.

In general, the risk contours—the relationship of risk to laboratory value—implied by the heights of the bars are quite similar for peritoneal and hemodialysis patients. The exceptions to this

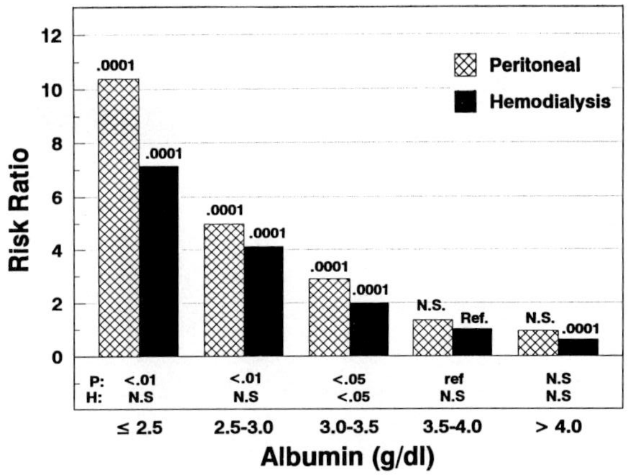

Fig 5. Risk profile for serum albumin concentration among peritoneal and hemodialysis patients. See text for explanation.

generality are serum cholesterol and serum iron concentration, for which no profile is apparent among peritoneal dialysis patients.

Figure 12 shows the evolution of the peritoneal dialysis risk ratio (compared with hemodialysis) as variables are added to a Cox model in the order implied by Table 4. Case mix–related variables were entered first according to their χ^2 value. Laboratory predictors were then added in order of their χ^2 value.

Before adding the first variable, the RR for peritoneal patients, compared with hemodialysis, was approximately 1.08, which was not significantly different from 1.00. Age was then added to the model. Peritoneal dialysis patients are sig-

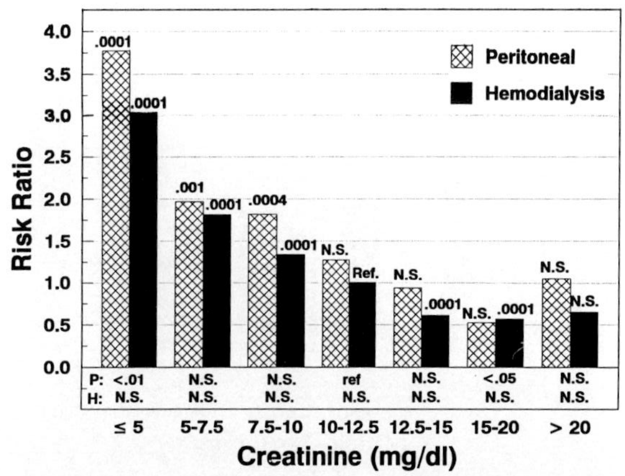

Fig 6. Risk profile for serum creatinine concentration among peritoneal and hemodialysis patients. See text for explanation.

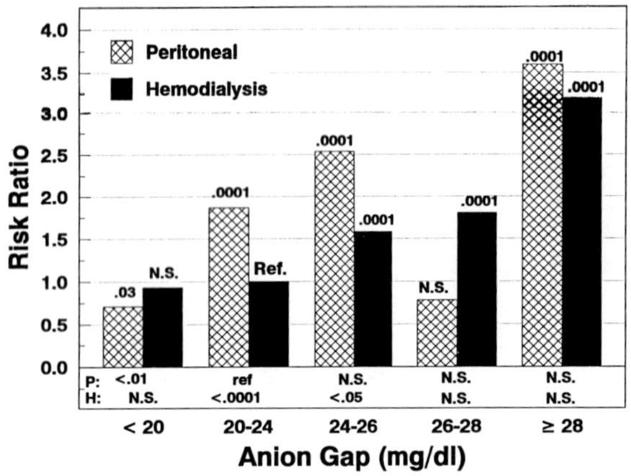

Fig 7. Risk profile for anion gap among peritoneal and hemodialysis patients. See text for explanation.

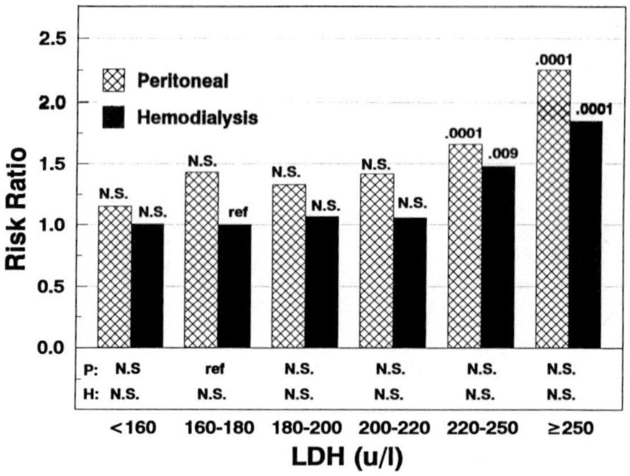

Fig 9. Risk profile for LDH among peritoneal and hemodialysis patients. See text for explanation.

nificantly younger than hemodialysis patients (Table 1), so correcting for age increases the relative risk associated with peritoneal dialysis to about 1.33. The RR did not change substantially after the addition of sex or the various renal diagnoses. The addition of race, however, reduced the ratio slightly to approximately 1.29. Although the relationship is weak, whites generally experience greater risk on dialysis than nonwhites,[3] and a greater fraction of peritoneal dialysis patients are white.

Adding serum albumin concentration to the model reduced the RR associated with peritoneal dialysis to approximately 0.6. Albumin concentration was substantially lower among peritoneal than hemodialysis patients and is strongly associated with death risk in both treatment populations. The observation suggests that peritoneal dialysis patients could benefit measurably if albumin concentrations were similar to patients receiving hemodialysis.

Anion gap among peritoneal dialysis patients is slightly lower than among hemodialysis patients. Adding anion gap to the model increased the peritoneal dialysis RR to approximately 1.0. Risk remained at that value, changing substantially only after cholesterol and other variables were sequentially added to the model. When all significant variables were added to the model, the RR associated with peritoneal dialysis was 1.32.

DISCUSSION

Recent analyses of hemodialysis patients have suggested two primary clinical dimensions that

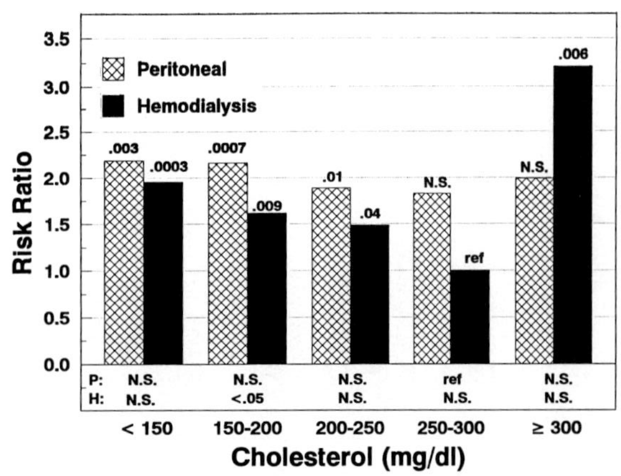

Fig 8. Risk profile for serum cholesterol concentration among peritoneal and hemodialysis patients. See text for explanation.

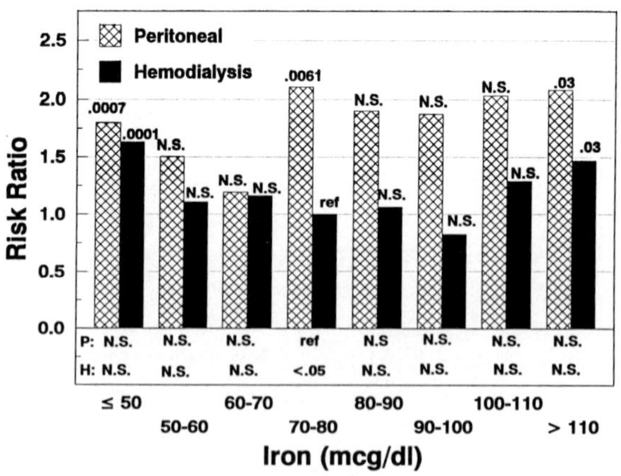

Fig 10. Risk profile for serum iron concentration among peritoneal and hemodialysis patients. See text for explanation.

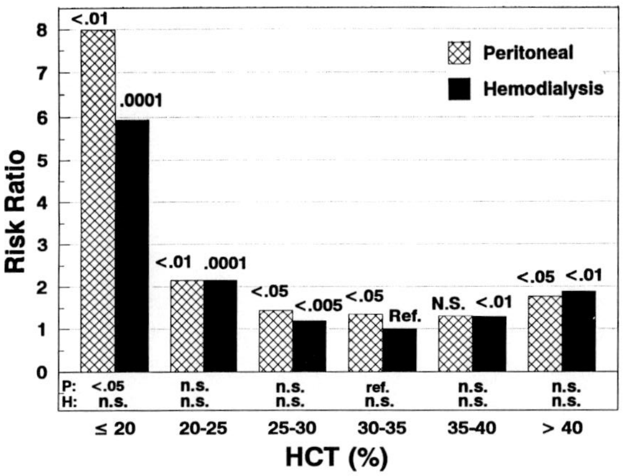

Fig 11. Risk profile for hematocrit among peritoneal and hemodialysis patients. See text for explanation.

contribute to most of the explainable death risk difference among patients and that also may be amenable to therapeutic manipulation. Those are dialysis exposure, as reflected by the urea reduction ratio (URR), and the nutritional status of patients.[3] Combined with the age of patients (one variable), dialysis exposure (one variable) and nutrition-related variables (four variables) contribute most of the explainable death odds differences among hemodialysis patients.[1,2] The more than 40 other variables in those analyses explained only 20% to 25% of the difference. Hence, relatively few parameters appear to be associated with major differences in death risk. Although little can be done about the age of patients, both dialysis exposure and the nutritional status of patients may be improved by appropriate medical manipulation.

The purpose of these analyses, however, is to provide clinical clues about how the results of therapies might be improved. Further, they should suggest practical strategies for implementing quality-enhancing therapeutic and disease prevention programs by the teams who provide the care.

Responding to technical memoranda distributed in 1992 and routine availability of a simple test (the URR), physicians and clinical staff changed prescriptive behaviors so that the median URR among patients treated in NMC-affiliated facilities increased from approximately 59% to current values exceeding 64%.[3] Furthermore, approximately 37% of patients were treated at URR < 55%. Today, fewer than 14% are treated

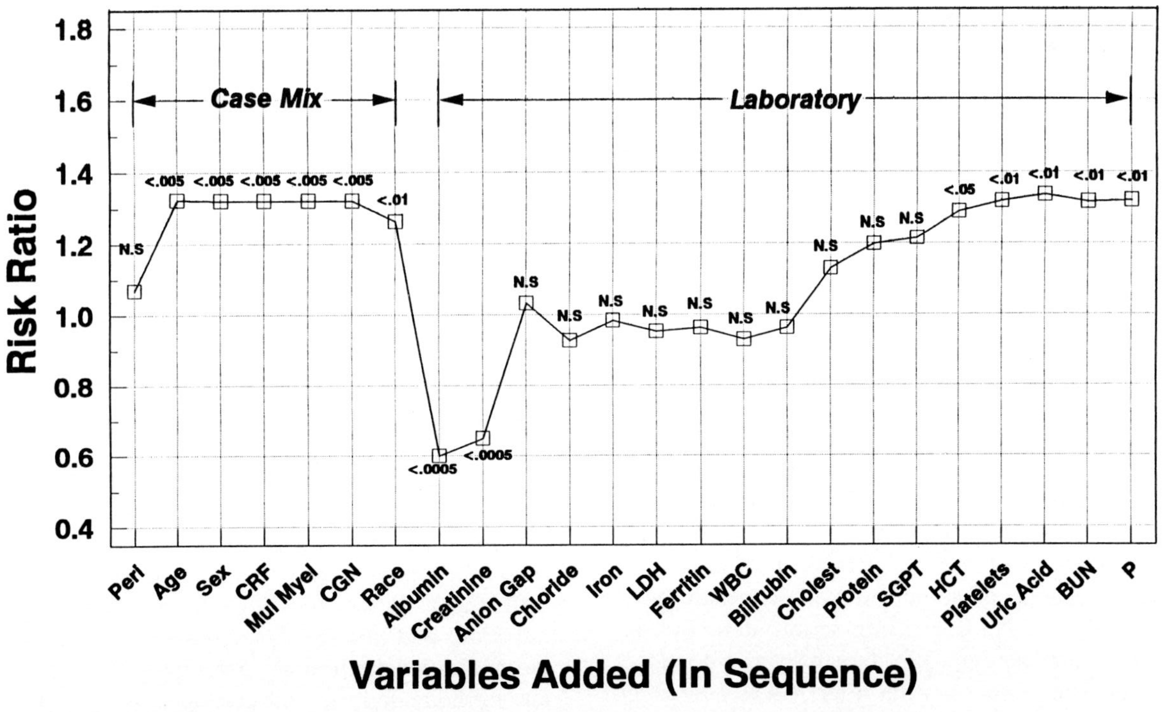

Fig 12. The evolution of relative risk associated with peritoneal dialysis as variables are added to a Cox model in the order shown by Table 4.

below that value. Hence, clinicians know how to manipulate the dialysis exposure dimension of clinical care. The strategies may have lead to improved survival among patients.[10]

The nutrition-related dimension is another matter. Methods to control nutritional status are not so well understood. Indeed, some have suggested that low albumin may simply be a harbinger of inevitable death about which little can be done. Chertow et al,[11] however, have recently shown that albumin concentration increases in response to intradialytic parenteral nutrition (IDPN) among patients in whom albumin concentration is low.[11] Further, treatment by IDPN was associated with reduced odds of death in groups of patients with low albumin. Hence, nutritional status may be manipulated among malnourished dialysis patients by therapeutic intervention. If so, clinicians may be able to develop strategies to prevent undernutrition rather than simply treat it once it has become severe.

Some have suggested that nutrition may be improved simply by increasing the dose of dialysis.[12] Those studies, however, generally involve the demonstration of statistical correlations between two variables (of three primary variables) in the mathematical model commonly used for urea kinetic calculations. All variables in the equation are mathematically linked and therefore depend mechanistically on each other. The use of correlation analysis in such cases may be risky. Harty et al[13] have entered random inputs into kinetic equations and found correlations between the outputs expressed in terms of protein catabolic rate and the ratio of the urea clearance-dialysis time product to the volume of urea distribution [Kt/V]. Hence, a mechanistic relationship producing artifacts may exist among the variables and inferring biologic associations from such analysis may be risky.

Correlation analysis between truly independent estimates of dialysis intensity (URR) and a nutrition indicator (serum albumin concentration) have repeatedly failed to show significant associations.[1-3] Furthermore, substantial increases or decreases in URR were not associated with change of serum albumin concentration.[3] Finally, neither decreasing serum albumin concentration before IDPN therapy was started nor increasing concentration after it was associated with changes in URR. Although dialysis dose within the usual ranges of dose used in this country may or may not contribute to change of nutritional status, it is unlikely that dialysis dose is the major factor contributing to change of nutritional status among patients.

Against this background we begin a comparative evaluation of peritoneal dialysis. The purpose is not to decide which is the better therapy but to discover clues permitting improved use of both treatments. Unfortunately, reliable estimators of dialysis intensity are not yet available for peritoneal dialysis. Furthermore, such values as serum creatinine concentration, blood urea nitrogen concentration, CO_2, and anion gap are directly comparable in hemodialysis and peritoneal dialysis patients only if one accepts the so-called peak concentration hypothesis.[14] The hypothesis states that it is the peak concentration of a substance or toxin rather than the average concentration that is associated with uremic toxicity. Nevertheless, evaluation of the associates of death risk among peritoneal dialysis patients and in a combined sample of patients receiving both therapies is instructive.

Examination of Tables 2 and 3 shows that albumin, age, creatinine, and anion gap are the variables most closely associated with death risk. The analyses are remarkably similar to those published earlier.[1-3] Furthermore, the risk profiles for most laboratory variables appear remarkably similar among hemodialysis and peritoneal dialysis patients. Even the U-shaped profile for hematocrit[2] is similar among patients treated by both therapies. The exceptions to this generality appear to be serum iron and cholesterol, which show no significant profile for patients treated by peritoneal dialysis.

Earlier studies[1-3] included URR, reflecting dialysis intensity, among the variables tested. That was not done here. Teehan et al,[15] however, have reported an association between intensity and survival among peritoneal dialysis patients. They also have observed the contribution of low albumin to mortal risk.

Whether the risk profile differences of iron and cholesterol reflect fundamental differences between therapy types or are due to a relatively small peritoneal dialysis sample is not clear. The differences notwithstanding, the importance of nutrition and related[1,2] acid-base status seem clear. Hence, the primary associates of survival among hemodialysis and peritoneal dialysis patients are likely similar. The primary dimensions of care are likely to be similar as well.

REFERENCES

1. Lowrie EG: Chronic dialysis treatment: Clinical outcome and related processes of care. Am J Kidney Dis 24:255-266, 1994

2. Lowrie EG, Huang WH, Lew NL, Liu Y: The relative contribution of measured variables to death risk among hemodialysis patients, in E. Friedman (ed): Death on Hemodialysis: Preventable or Inevitable?, chap 13. Hingham, MA, Kluwer Academic Publishers, 1994, pp 121-141

3. Owen WF Jr, Lew NL, Liu Y, Lowrie EG, Lazarus JM: The urea reduction ratio and serum albumin concentration as predictors of mortality in patients undergoing hemodialysis. N Engl J Med 329:1001-1006, 1993

4. Lowrie EG, Lew NL, Huang WH: Race and diabetes as death risk predictors in hemodialysis patients. Kidney Int 42:S-22-S-31, 1992 (Suppl 38)

5. Lowrie EG, Lew NL: Commonly measured laboratory variables in hemodialysis patients: Relationships among them and to death risk. Semin Nephrol 12:276-283, 1992

6. Lowrie EG, Lew NL: Death risk in hemodialysis patients: The predictive value of commonly measured variables and an evaluation of death rate differences between facilities. Am J Kidney Dis 15:458-482, 1990

7. Cox DR: Regression models and life tables. J R Stat Soc B34:187-220, 1972

8. SAS Institute Inc: SAS® Technical Report P-229, SAS/STAT® Software: Changes and Enhancements, Release 6.07, Cary, NC, SAS Institute Inc., 1992, 620 pp

9. Armitage P: Statistical Methods in Medical Research. New York, NY, Wiley and Sons, 1971, pp 138-140

10. Parker TF, Husni L, Huang W, Lew N, Lowrie EG: Survival of hemodialysis patients in the United States is improved with a greater quantity of dialysis. Am J Kidney Dis 23:670-680, 1994

11. Chertow GM, Ling J, Lew NL, Lazarus JM, Lowrie EG: The association of intradialytic parenteral nutrition administration with survival in hemodialysis patients. Am J Kidney Dis 24:912-920, 1994

12. Lindsay RM, Spanner E, Heidenheim RP, LeFebvre JM, Hodsman A, Bard J, Allison MEM: Which comes first, Kt/V or PCR: Chicken or egg? Kidney Int 42:S32-S36, 1992 (suppl 38)

13. Harty JC, Farragher B, Boulton H, Kirwell J, Heelis N, Uttley L, Venning MC, Gokal R: Is the correlation between the normalised protein catabolic rate (nPCR) and Kt/V the result of mathematical coupling? [Abstract]. Clin Sci 86:3C, 1994

14. Keshaviah P, Nolph K: The peak concentration hypothesis: A urea kinetic approach to comparing the adequacy of continuous ambulatory peritoneal dialysis (CAPD) and hemodialysis. Perit Dial Int 9:257-260, 1989

15. Teehan BP, Schleifer CR, Brown J: Adequacy of continuous ambulatory peritoneal dialysis: Morbidity and morality in continuous peritoneal dialysis. Am J Kidney Dis 24:990-1001, 1994

Why Are Dialysis Patients Malnourished?

Jonas Bergström, MD

● There are multiple causes of protein-energy malnutrtion in maintenance dialysis patients. The requirements of protein in dialysis patients are higher than in healthy individuals, and the intake of protein and energy in relation to the requirements is frequently low. Anorexia may be caused by uremia and underdialysis. There is experimental evidence that dialyzable uremic toxins accumulate in renal failure and suppress the appetite. In addition there are several psychosocial and comorbidity factors that may hamper adequate nutrition. There are also several factors in dialysis patients that may enhance protein catabolism and increase protein requirements, such as low energy intake, metabolic acidosis, dialytic loss of glucose, protein and amino acids and other catabolic effects of the dialytic procedures, as well as effects of infections and other comorbidity factors. The relative importance of the various factors that cause anorexia and stimulate protein catabolism is still not well understood.

INDEX WORDS: Anorexia; catabolism; malnutrition; energy; protein; hemodialysis; continuous ambulatory peritoneal dialysis.

PROTEIN-ENERGY malnutrition and wasting are present in a large proportion of patients with chronic renal failure. These findings may have many causes, including disturbances in protein and energy metabolism, hormonal derangement, as well as poor food intake because of anorexia, nausea, and vomiting, caused by uremic toxicity. Underlying diseases such as diabetes mellitus, rheumatoid arthritis, and vasculitis, plus superimposed illnesses, such as infections, pericarditis, congestive heart failure, and complications of therapy, in particular corticosteroid therapy, may result in a severely debilitated state with aggravation of malnutrition.

When dialysis therapy begins, the uremic symptoms are reduced, the diet is less restricted and some patients may show improved nutritional status. However, anorexia can persist in hemodialysis (HD) patients, and many of the catabolic factors found at the onset of therapy remain abnormal. The dialytic procedures may induce catabolism and increase protein requirements above those for nondialyzed uremic patients. These changes, in addition to the metabolic abnormalities of uremia, may further aggravate malnutrition and susceptibility to infection and increase the rates of hospitalization and mortality.

Protein-energy malnutrition in maintenance dialysis patients is very common. In various studies, signs of malnutrition have been observed in 10% to 70% of HD patients and 18% to 51% of continuous ambulatory peritoneal dialysis (CAPD) patients.[1] Several reports suggest that anthropometric and biochemical signs of malnutrition are risk factors for infection, morbidity, and mortality in HD and CAPD patients.[1]

PROTEIN AND ENERGY REQUIREMENTS

In normal adults, the average requirements for protein are about 0.6 g/kg body weight/day, which after correction for 25% variability to include 97.5% of the population of young adults, raises the safe level of intake (daily allowance) to 0.75 g/kg/day.[2] This variability is due to genetic differences, sex, age, physical activity, environment, chemical form of nutrients, and effects of other dietary constituents.[2]

The protein requirements in maintenance dialysis patients are not well defined. It may be assumed that the variation in requirements is much larger in dialysis patients than in healthy subjects, because there are additional sources of variability, such as endocrine and biochemical abnormalities, anemia, infections, cardiac disease, diabetes, corticosteroids and other drugs, and specific effects of the dialytic procedures. A few nitrogen balance studies in small groups of HD and CAPD patients and longitudinal studies of nutritional intakes and nutritional status in larger groups of patients suggest that the daily requirements for protein are considerably higher than in normal individuals.[1] On the basis of these results, an intake of 1.2 g protein/kg body weight/day is generally recommended for HD and CAPD patients.

Energy requirements depend on the level of physical activity, an intake of 35 to 40 kcal/kg of body weight/day being recommended for adult individuals not performing heavy physical exercise. There is no evidence that the energy requirements of maintenance dialysis patients differ from those of normal subjects.[3]

LOW NUTRITIONAL INTAKE AND ANOREXIA

Considering all the evidence that requirements for protein are increased in HD patients and that an adequate energy supply is mandatory for maintaining the energy stores and optimizing the utilization of ingested protein, low protein and energy intakes must be especially harmful in such patients. It may be difficult to fulfil the nutritional requirements, because some dialysis patients tend to lose their appetite and reduce protein and energy intakes spontaneously.

Recent data from the MDRD study in the United States[4] demonstrate that an adaptive reduction in the intake of protein may start early during progression of renal failure (glomerular filtration rate 25 mL/min or higher) with a further reduction in protein intake along with progression toward end-stage renal failure and an associated reduction in energy intake and various nutritional parameters (body weight, fat mass, serum albumin, and transferrin).

Nutritional surveys indicate that the mean intake of protein is less than 1 g/kg of body weight/day in a large proportion of patients on maintenance HD,[5-8] suggesting that the requirements for protein are not fulfilled. The energy intake, like the protein intake, is often low in groups of dialysis patients; the mean intake in HD has been reported to be 26 to 29 kcal/kg of body weight/day.[6-8] The total energy intake may also be low in CAPD patients, despite the continuous supply of energy by glucose absorbed from the dialysis fluid.[9,10]

Hylander et al[11] investigated hunger, "fullness," and food preferences in healthy controls, CAPD patients, and HD patients by serving a test meal placed on a hidden scale with computer registration of the eating process on-line. Mean total food intake was higher in healthy controls than in HD patients who, in turn, had a higher intake than the CAPD patients; both groups of dialysis patients had lower eating velocity than the controls. The reasons for low eating drive in the dialysis patients could not be explained, but it was speculated that gastric retention, insufficient dialysis, and metabolic effects of the dialysate might be of importance.

Some factors that contribute to a low intake of protein and energy are listed in Table 1. Anorexia may be due to unpalatable or inadequate diets, gastropathy and reduced intestinal motility (eg, in diabetic patients with autonomic neuropathy), peritonitis in CAPD patients, other forms of comorbidity, medications, and psychosocial and socioeconomic factors, such as loneliness, depression, ignorance and poverty, especially in elderly patients and those with alcohol and drug problems. Nausea and vomiting during and immediately after HD, which are frequently associated with cardiovascular instability and postdialysis fatigue, may lead to a reduction in food intake during the days on dialysis.

Table 1. Causes of Anorexia in Maintenance Dialysis Patients

Uremic toxicity (underdialysis)
Unpalatable or inadequate diets
Gastropathy (diabetic patients)
Other complicating illnesses
Inflammation, infection, sepsis
Medications
Psychosocial and socioeconomic factors
Loneliness
Depression
Ignorance
Poverty
Dental status
Alcohol and drug abuse
Effects of the HD procedure
Cardiovascular instability
Nausea, vomiting
Postdialysis fatigue
Effects of the PD procedures
Abdominal discomfort
Absorption of glucose and amino acids
Peritonitis

In CAPD, the presence of dialysate in the peritoneal cavity may interfere with gastric emptying and intestinal motility and cause discomfort or pain, as may the peritoneal catheter. It is also possible that glucose or amino acids absorbed from the dialysis fluid may exert an inhibiting effect on food consumption. Balaskas et al[12] studied the effect of intraperitoneal infusion of various volumes and concentrations of glucose and amino acid solutions on food intake in rabbits. They reported that large filling volumes (100 mL/kg body weight) and high osmolality solutions suppressed the appetite. They found no difference in effect between amino acid and glucose solutions at any of the concentrations studied, and they therefore concluded that the peritoneal uptake of these nutrients had no specific appetite-suppressing effect.

Our group has recently introduced a highly reproducible experimental model for the study of ingestive behavior[13,14] in free-moving, unstressed, male Wistar rats (300 to 350 g) with catheters channeled from the top of the skull to the oral cavity. After recovering from surgery, the rats are tested by intraoral infusions (1 mL/min) of nutritional solutions (1 mol/L sucrose or protein 9.7 g/L) with registration of the time (volume) of ingestion. Tests performed after intraperitoneal injection of up to 30 mL 0.9% NaCl showed no effect on carbohydrate or protein ingestion.[14] Injection of 30 mL peritoneal dialysis solutions containing 13.6%, 22.7%, and 36.1% of glucose induced a dose-dependent inhibition of sucrose intake but had no effect on protein intake, whereas injection of dialysis solutions containing 11 g/L, 18 g/L, and 31 g/L amino acids reduced the intake of both sucrose and protein in a dose-dependent manner.[14] Our results indicate that the inhibition of appetite caused by solutions containing glucose or amino acids is specific to each nutritional constituent and not simply an effect of hyperosmolality or large filling volumes.

Uremic Anorexia

Anorexia, nausea, and vomiting are signs of severe uremic intoxication. It is a common clinical experience that uremic patients who are anorectic regain appetite after the initiation of maintenance dialysis. This suggests that one or more uremic toxins causing anorexia has been removed by dialysis. Assuming that a dialyzable uremic toxin accumulates in severe renal failure and causes anorexia, it is conceivable that underdialysis may affect the appetite and thus cause malnutrition. There are several studies in HD and CAPD patients that report a correlation between the dose of dialysis for small molecule removal (Kt/V_{urea}) and the protein intake, especially in the lowest dose intervals.[10,15-20] Lindsay et al[15,21] also noted that the relationship between Kt/V_{urea} and protein intake, assessed by urea kinetics, varied with different hemodialysis membranes, so that it seemed to increase more markedly with increasing Kt/V_{urea} when a highly permeable, more biocompatible membrane (AN 69S) was used than with a cellulose acetate membrane (Fig 1).

It has been found that the relationship between Kt/V_{urea} and protein intake in CAPD patients, estimated from the urea appearance rate, differed from that in HD patients, most of whom were treated with low-flux membranes.[17,20] At the same low Kt/V_{urea} levels, the estimated protein intake was higher in the CAPD patients than in the HD patients and the protein intake increased more for the same increase in Kt/V_{urea} in the CAPD than in the HD patients (Fig 1). Observations in small groups of patients have shown that increasing the dose of dialysis prospectively results in a significant increase in the estimated protein intake.[21,22]

In most of the aforementioned studies, the intake of protein was assessed by urea kinetic modeling based on the concept that the amount of

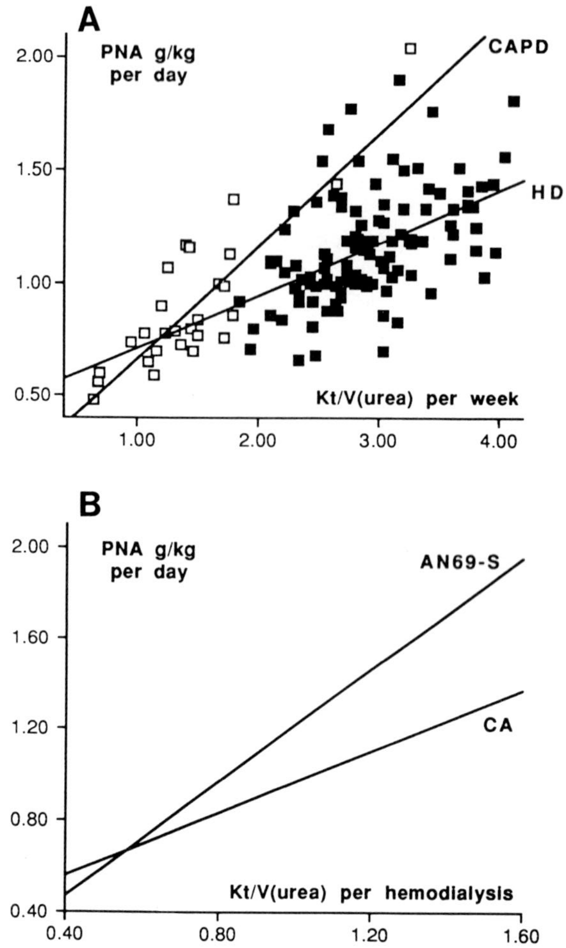

Fig 1. Relationship between Kt/V_{urea} and estimated protein intake (PNA = protein equivalent of nitrogen appearance calculated from urea appearance), (A) in HD and CAPD patients (used with permission from *Kidney International,* volume 43, page S-47, 1993[1]), (B) in patients treated by HD using a cellulose acetate (CA) and high flux (AN 69-S) membrane (modified and reprinted with permission[15]).

urea generated reflects the net amount of protein catabolized, which, in patients who are in a metabolic steady state (ie, not markedly catabolic or anabolic), gives an estimate of the protein intake.[23,24] It has been argued that the relationship between Kt/V_{urea} and protein intake (urea appearance) reflects a mathematical coupling rather than a biological relationship, because the two variables are to some extent dependent (both are normalized to body size, and both are dependent on urea determinations in plasma predialysis and postdialysis).[25] However, some data show a relationship between the dose of urea removal and protein intake, calculated from the dietary records and interviews, and also that in CAPD patients the relationship may be statistically significant, even when the dose of urea or creatinine removal (weekly clearances) is not normalized to body size.[10,20] Multiple regression analysis showed that the dominating factor in the correlation was the residual renal function, whereas the dose of peritoneal dialysis had no statistically significant influence. The impact of residual renal function on protein intake is also supported by longitudinal studies in CAPD patients, demonstrating that the estimated protein intake (urea appearance) decreases along with the loss of residual renal function,[26] and by an international cross-sectional multicenter study that demonstrated that loss of renal function is associated with anorexia and symptoms of severe malnutrition.[27]

It remains controversial whether the dose of dialysis has an impact on nutrition and whether the correction of underdialysis improves the nutritional status. In a retrospective analysis of laboratory data from more than 12,000 hemodialysis patients, Owen et al[28] reported a highly increased risk of death in patients with low serum albumin levels and also an increased mortality risk when the dose of dialysis, measured as the percent urea reduction ratio, was low. However, they found no correlation between the urea reduction ratio and the serum albumin concentration. They therefore concluded that underdialysis and malnutrition were two independent mortality risk factors for increased mortality in HD patients.

It should be emphasized that a low serum albumin concentration is not only and perhaps not mainly a marker of protein depletion. Several other factors may cause or contribute to hypoalbuminemia; these include advanced age, overhydration, infection, trauma, liver disease, intestinal disease, renal and peritoneal albumin losses and, unspecifically, as an effect of acute and chronic diseases. An association between hypoalbuminemia and increased morbidity and mortality is not unique for renal failure patients but is also found in the general population of patients admitted to hospital for acute illness.[29] Results in HD patients using ^{125}I-labeled human serum albumin suggests that hypoalbuminemia and reduced albumin synthesis results primarily from nonnutritional factors and at least partly from a (negative) acute-phase response.[30]

In CAPD patients, low serum albumin is also a strong risk factor for increased mortality.[31] Four studies show a correlation between the dose of dialysis assessed by Kt/V_{urea} and serum albumin,[20,32-35] whereas in another nine studies there was no correlation.[31] A retrospective analysis of data from an international cross-sectional multicenter study[35] demonstrated that severely malnourished patients by "subjective nutritional assessment" without residual renal function had significantly lower peritoneal urea clearance normalized to desireable body weight, and lower 24-hour dwell volumes than well-nourished patients without residual renal function. It was suggested that failure to compensate for loss of renal function by increasing the dose of dialysis can lead to malnutrition, whereas increasing the dose as residual renal function decreases can help to maintain good nutritional status.

Prospective studies with measurements of anthropometric and biochemical markers of nutritional status in addition to albumin obviously are needed before definitive conclusions can be drawn about the influence of the dose of dialysis on appetite and nutritional status in HD and CAPD patients.

ARE THERE ONE OR MORE DIALYZABLE UREMIC TOXINS CAUSING ANOREXIA?

An attractive hypothesis for explaining the difference in the relationship between Kt/V_{urea} and protein intake (estimated from urea appearance) in CAPD patients and HD patients may be that one or more of the factors causing anorexia are molecules of larger molecular size than urea—so-called middle molecules—which are more efficiently dialyzed by the peritoneal route than by the membranes in the artificial kidney. The hypothesis that middle molecule compounds cause anorexia is also in keeping with the observation by Lindsay and Spanner[15] that, with a high-flux membrane, the protein intake, estimated from the urea appearance, increases proportionally more with a given increase in Kt/V_{urea} than with a low-flux membrane (Fig 1). It has been reported that the plasma concentration of middle molecule fractions, isolated by gel permeation and ion exchange chromatography, are higher in HD patients than in CAPD patients.[36] However, the middle molecule hypothesis is still controversial, because as yet there are no middle molecule compounds identified with proven in vivo toxicity.

The peak concentration hypothesis, presented by Keshaviah et al,[37] affords an alternative explanation—namely, that the periodic predialysis peak concentrations of urea and other small-molecular uremic toxins in HD may have a better correlation to clinical outcome than the time average concentration. If this is relevant, the Kt/V_{urea} for HD should be higher than for CAPD to match the peak HD concentration to the steady-state CAPD concentration. On the basis of a theoretical analysis concerning the permeability characteristics of peritoneal and hemodialysis membranes, Keshaviah has argued at length against the possible clinical importance of middle molecules.[38]

Using the aforementioned experimental animal model to study ingestive behavior as a bioassay, our group has recently started to isolate and characterize factors in uremic plasma and normal urine that suppress appetite; the first results were recently reported.[13] We collected and pooled ultrafiltrate (UF) obtained from end-stage renal failure patients at the beginning of their first dialysis treatment. UF from pooled normal plasma and from pooled urine was obtained in vitro by filtration through the same type of dialyzer as used in the patients. Uremic UF and normal urine UF injected intraperitoneally in the rats inhibited the ingestion of both carbohydrate (sucrose) and protein, whereas UF from normal plasma had no effect. Fractions of the pooled ultrafiltrates of various molecular sizes (0.1 to 0.5, 0.5 to 1, 1 to 5, 5 to 10 kd) were isolated and concentrated by serial filtration, using membranes with known cutoffs. The 1 to 5-kd fraction (the middle molecule fraction) isolated from uremic UF and normal urine elicited a dose-dependent inhibition of carbohydrate and protein intakes, whereas the fractions with lower molecular weight had no effect. Our results suggest that toxic middle molecule fractions that are normally excreted in the urine accumulate in uremia and may suppress appetite. Our further aim is to identify and characterize the anorectic compound(s) and assess their clinical relevance.

PROTEIN CATABOLIC FACTORS IN MAINTENANCE DIALYSIS PATIENTS

The observation that HD and CAPD patients seem to have increased protein requirements and a diminished utilization of ingested protein, compared with normal individuals, indicates that metabolic factors, not fully corrected by dialysis treatment and by the treatment per se, may enhance net protein catabolism and impair the utilization of dietary protein (Table 2). Many patients on renal replacement therapy are physically inactive for various reasons, such as fatigue, anemia, skeletomuscular disease, and psychological factors. Physical inactivity may result in muscle wasting and a negative nitrogen balance.[39]

In maintenance HD patients, investigated by ^{13}C leucine kinetics immediately before a routine thrice-weekly HD treatment, the protein breakdown was the same as that in controls, but the protein oxidation rate was higher and the net protein synthesis was lower, which was thought to contribute to muscle wasting.[40] In contrast, kinetic leucine studies in CAPD patients showed that the protein turnover and the rate of protein oxidation were lower than in controls and that the balance between synthesis and breakdown was higher before the start of dialysis and after 3 months on CAPD, suggesting protein anabolism.[41]

Low Energy Intake

Metabolic studies in healthy individuals indicate that the nitrogen balance is greatly dependent on the energy intake, so that a low energy intake results in negative nitrogen balance, whereas a high energy intake has a protein-saving effect.[42] Slomowitz et al[43] demonstrated that this also applies to HD patients. In six patients on a constant protein intake, averaging 1.13 g/kg desirable body weight/day, the nitrogen balance,

Table 2. Protein Catabolic Factors in Hemodialysis Patients

General effects		
Physical inactivity		
Heart failure		
Low energy intake		
Endocrine abnormalities		
Corticosteroid therapy		
Inflammation, infection, sepsis		
Acidosis		
Amino acid abnormalities		
Catabolic effects of the dialytic procedures		
	Hemodialysis	CAPD
Loss of amino acids	9-13 g/dialysis (27-39 g/week)	2-4 g/day (14-28 g/week)
Loss of glucose	25 g/dialysis (glucose-free dialysate)	(uptake)
Loss of protein	Minor	5-15 g/day (higher with peritonitis)
Inflammatory stimuli	Blood-membrane contact	Low-grade inflammation ? (particles, chemicals)
	Complement activation	Peritonitis
	Endotoxin	
	Acetate	
	Cytokine release	Cytokine release

adjusted for unmeasured losses, was negative when the energy intake was 25 kcal/kg/day, but neutral or positive when the energy intake was 35 or 45 kcal/kg/day.

Our group performed 23 nitrogen balance studies in 11 CAPD patients, 12 of which were performed within 2 to 6 months after the start of CAPD (early studies) and 11 studies after 9 to 16 months on CAPD (late studies).[10] During the nitrogen balance periods, each patient received an individualized diet that was composed to resemble the patient's spontaneously chosen diet before the studies, as assessed in diaries and interviews. The influence of the dietary protein and energy intake on the nitrogen balance is shown in Fig 2. This demonstrates that in the early studies both dietary protein intake and total energy intake were significantly correlated to the nitrogen balance, whereas in the late studies the protein intake had no influence on the utilization of nitrogen, and the energy intake seemed to have an even stronger influence than in the early studies. The results indicate that energy deficiency is detrimental to the utilization of dietary protein in CAPD patients. Considering that many patients on maintenance dialysis ingest less than 35 kcal/kg/day, energy deficiency may be an important factor contributing to impaired utilization of dietary protein.

Metabolic Acidosis

It has become increasingly evident that metabolic acidosis is an important stimulus for net protein catabolism. In nondialyzed chronic uremic patients, the correction of metabolic acidosis improves the nitrogen balance and reduces urea appearance and muscle proteolysis.[44,45] Studies in normal subjects, using continuous infusion of ^{13}C-leucine, have demonstrated that total body protein breakdown as well as apparent leucine oxidation are higher during acidosis than during alkalosis.[46] In nondialyzed patients with chronic renal failure, the correction of acidosis reduced protein degradation and leucine oxidation.[47] However, in a study of HD patients the correction of acidosis was reported to have had no effect on protein degradation, but it tended to reduce protein synthesis and to increase leucine oxidation.[48]

In rats with chronic renal failure, acidosis, rather than uremia per se, appears to enhance protein catabolism.[49] This effect seems to be mediated by the stimulation of skeletal muscle branched-chain keto acid decarboxylation, which increases the catabolism of the branched-chain amino acids (valine, leucine, and isoleucine); these are mainly metabolized in muscle tissue.[50] Mitch et al recently reported that acidosis stimu-

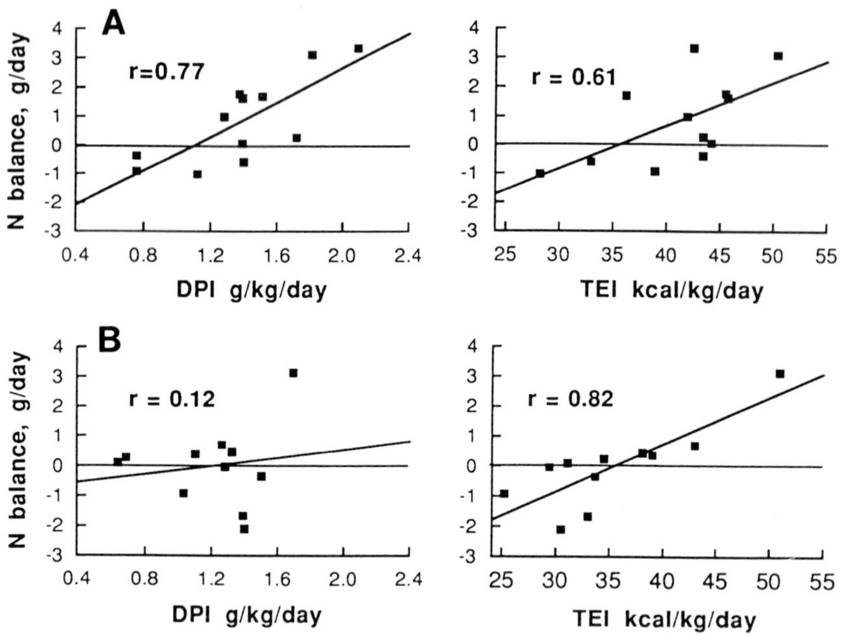

Fig 2. Relationships between nitrogen balance (NB) corrected for "unmeasured" nitrogen losses assumed to be 1.9 g/day (see reference 10) and dietary protein intake (DPI) and total energy intake (TEI), respectively, during studies performed within 2 to 6 months after start of CAPD ([A] early studies) and during studies performed after 9 to 16 months on CAPD ([B] Late studies). (Used with permission from *Kidney International,* volume 44, page 1052, 1993.[10])

lates proteolysis in muscle by inducing the transcription of genes encoding for enzymes participating in the adenosine-triphosphate–dependent cytosolic ubiquitin-proteasome proteolytic pathway and that cortisol is required for the activation to occur.[51,52]

Our group has reported that the intracellular concentration of valine (one of the branched-chain amino acids) is low in HD patients and correlates with the predialysis blood standard bicarbonate level, which varied between 18 and 24 mmol/L,[53] suggesting that even slight and intermittent acidosis may stimulate the catabolism of valine in muscle, resulting in a valine depletion that may potentially limit protein synthesis. We also reported that correction of acidosis in nine HD patients over a period of 6 months resulted in a significant increase in the muscle concentration of all three branched-chain amino acids.[54]

In our experience, acidosis is common in HD patients, despite the use of bicarbonate as the buffer in the dialysis fluid. In a group of 129 HD patients, we observed that 41% of the HD patients had predialysis plasma bicarbonate concentrations ≤21 mmol/L and 17% ≤19 mmol/L.[1] We therefore speculate whether the intermittent acidosis in HD patients with a nadir concentration of plasma bicarbonate before each dialysis may act as an intermittent stimulus for protein catabolism.

It should be pointed out that acidosis is today the only identified uremic "toxic" factor that induces catabolism and impairs nitrogen utilization. However, the clinical importance of uremic acidosis as a factor for the development of malnutrition has not been determined. Retrospective analysis of laboratory data and mortality in more than 12,000 HD patients showed that the death risk was significantly increased with metabolic acidosis, but only at total CO_2 levels in serum lower than 12.5 to 15 mmol/L.[55] No apparent association was noted between CO_2 levels and nutritional factors as assessed by serum albumin and cholesterol levels. Predialysis CO_2 levels above 20 mmol/L were also associaterd with a slightly increased risk of death. In support of Lowrie's data, we observed no correlation between standard bicarbonate and serum albumin levels in 133 HD patients (Fig 3).

The absence of an association between acid-base status and nutritional parameters is perhaps not surprising, considering that nonvolatile acids are mainly generated by protein breakdown and amino acid oxidation, implying that the tendency to metabolic acidosis increases when the protein intake is high, whereas it decreases with a low protein intake. Hence, it is conceivable that a high protein intake may stimulate protein synthesis to the extent that the negative effect of the increase in metabolic acidosis with an enhanced

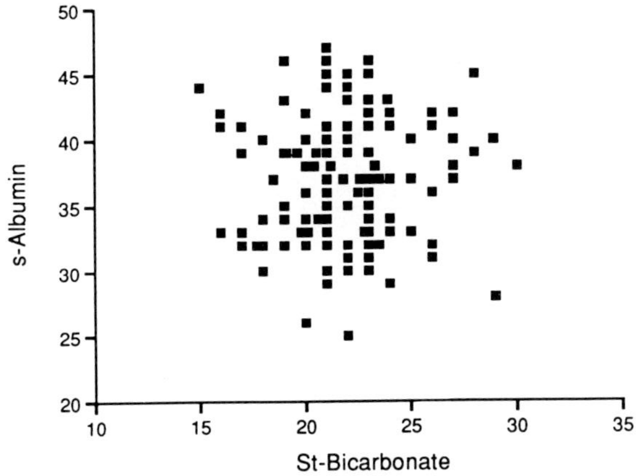

Fig 3. No correlation between blood standard bicarbonate and serum albumin in 133 HD patients.

activation of proteolysis is overcome. Relevant experimental studies of this problem are still lacking. Prospective, longitudinal clinical studies are also needed to determine whether the correction of acidosis in maintenance dialysis patients influences nutritional status and clinical outcome.

Loss of Metabolizing Renal Tissue

Normal kidneys actively take part in the metabolism of amino acids where, among other processes, phenylalanine hydroxylation to tyrosine[56,57] and glycine conversion to serine take place.[58] In patients with chronic renal failure, the concentration of free tyrosine is low and the phenylalanine/tyrosine ratio is increased in plasma and muscle, serine in plasma is low, and glycine increased.[59,60] We observed that HD patients suffer a more severe serine depletion with significantly lower intracellular levels in muscle than in controls, nondialyzed chronic uremic patients and CAPD patients.[60] A possible explanation is that the nondialyzed patients and CAPD patients still had some functioning renal tissue left, by means of which serine conversion could take place. The role of tyrosine and serine depletion as factors in the malnutrition of dialysis patients has not been determined.

DIALYSIS PROCEDURES AS STIMULI OF NET PROTEIN CATABOLISM

Some evidence suggests that the dialytic procedures per se induce net catabolism of protein. The mechanisms probably differ to some extent in HD and CAPD patients. In five HD patients investigated during 1 week on high protein intake and 1 week on low protein intake, Borah et al[61] observed that the nitrogen balance (corrected for changes in total body urea) was negative on the days when dialysis was given, but less negative (with a protein intake of 0.5 g/kg/day) or positive (with a protein intake of 1.4 g/kg/day) on the days between the dialyses. However, in these studies the energy intake (21 to 31 kcal/kg/day) was less than optimal for an efficient nitrogen balance. Farrell, Ward, and co-workers[62,63] reported that the urea appearance rate is 30% higher during the HD procedure than in the interdialytic period. These results suggest that the dialytic procedure is a strong intermittent stimulus for net protein catabolism.

An increase in the urea appearance rate or a decrease in nitrogen balance may be due to reduced protein synthesis, enhanced breakdown of protein or a combination of both. With regard to the catabolic effect of the HD procedure, the data suggest that both processes are involved. Löfberg et al[64] performed percutaneous muscle biopsies before and after routine HD with acetate and found that the size distribution of ribosomes in muscle changed with a relative decrease in polyribosomes, suggesting that the protein synthetic capacity had decreased. In healthy subjects the incorporation of ^{2}H-phenylalanine in muscle protein after a flooding dose was also reduced after HD.[64] Lim et al[65] studied leucine and alpha-ketoisocaproate kinetics by using stable isotopes before, during, and after cuprophane HD with bicarbonate. They concluded that HD is a catabolic event, characterized not by enhanced protein degradation but by reduction in protein synthesis, and suggested that the loss of amino acids might be a causative factor.[66] However, there is also evidence that proteolysis is enhanced as a result of blood dialyzer interaction (see section about biocompatibility and protein catabolism).

Loss of Glucose

When a glucose-free dialysis fluid is used for HD, 25 g glucose is removed during 3 to 4 hours of HD, whereas the addition of glucose (10 to 11 mmol/L) to the dialysis fluid results in a gain of about 25 g glucose by the patient.[67,68] To avoid symptomatic hypoglycemia, glucose removed from the extracellular fluid by dialysis must be replaced by ingested carbohydrate, by breakdown of liver glycogen or by gluconeogenesis from amino acids; the latter should result in an enhanced protein breakdown and urea synthesis. Observations by Wathen et al[67] showing that pyruvate decreased during glucose-free dialysis, but was unchanged during glucose dialysis, indicate that gluconeogenesis may be stimulated by glucose-free dialysis. However, in nonfasting HD patients the urea appearance rate, which was found to be stimulated by HD, was not different whether glucose was present in the dialysis fluid or not.[62,63] After an overnight fast, the efflux of amino acids from leg muscle and the loss of urea and amino acids in the dialysate were not different during HD, with or without glucose (10 mmol/L) in the dialysis fluid, indicating that the addition of glucose had no protein-sparing effect.[68]

CAPD patients are provided with glucose continuously by the peritoneal route, which is potentially beneficial by providing an additional energy supply. However, glucose uptake may also have negative metabolic effects, such as hyperglycemia, hyperinsulinemia, hyperlipidemia, and obesity.[1]

Loss of Amino Acids

During HD, the average loss of free amino acids in the dialysis fluid has been reported to be 5 to 8 g/dialysis, of which about one third are essential amino acids.[68-71] Moreover, 4 to 5 g peptide-bound amino acids are lost per dialysis[69]; thus, the total loss of amino acids is about 10 to 13 g/dialysis. Obviously, the loss of amino acids per se by dialysis is too small to account fully for the increased protein requirements in maintenance dialysis patients. The loss of free amino acids into the dialysate during CAPD is of the same magnitude (per week) or smaller than with HD.

Protein Losses During CAPD

Substantial loss of protein into the dialysate is a major drawback with peritoneal dialysis that is not present in HD. In CAPD, the average loss of protein into the dialysate reportedly ranges between 5 and 15 g in various studies with large interindividual differences. Thus, the loss of dialysate protein may vary between 20 and 140 g/week in different patients. In CAPD patients with mild peritonitis, the loss of dialysate protein increases by 50% to 100% to an average of 15.1 ± 3.6 g/day,[72] and remains elevated for several weeks.[73,74]

Biocompatibility and Protein Catabolism

The HD procedure may give rise to an inflammatory reaction, the intensity of which depends on the membrane material used, being more marked with cellulosic than with synthetic membranes.[75] Blood-membrane contact induces complement activation by the alternative pathway, with release of anaphylaxotoxins (C3a, C5a). Monocyte activation with an increased release of interleukin-I (IL-1), tumor necrosis factor (TNF), and other cytokines may result from direct membrane contact,[76] activated complement (C5a),[77] endotoxin fragments passing through the membrane,[78,79] and acetate in the dialysis fluid.[80] IL-1 and TNF may act in concert and result in *inter alia* lysosomal catabolism of muscle protein,[81] an effect that is mediated by the release of prostaglandin E_2.[82] More recently, it has been observed that IL-1, TNF, and endotoxin may cause a net catabolism of muscle protein by stimulating branched-chain keto acid dehydrogenase, which leads to an enhanced oxidation of branched-chain amino acids.[83]

Our group has conducted a series of experiments with sham-dialysis in normal subjects,[84,85] and reports that blood-membrane contact in a dialyzer with a cuprophane membrane elicited an enhanced release of amino acids from the leg tissue (mainly skeletal muscle), corresponding to an enhanced protein breakdown of 15 to 20 g. By giving indomethacin before and during the procedure, this catabolic response could be abolished, a finding that suggests that the catabolic effect is mediated by prostaglandins. However, with more biocompatible membranes (cellulose acetate, AN 69®, and polysulfone), no significant proteolysis occurred. These studies demonstrate that in vivo blood-membrane interaction in a dialyzer without dialysate stimulates net protein catabolism, especially when the membrane has low biocompatibility.

It was also observed that sham-dialysis with cuprophane, but not with more biocompatible membranes, elicited an increased release from the leg musculature and an elevation in the arterial plasma concentration of 3-methylhistidine.[85]

This amino acid is formed posttranslationally by the irreversible methylation of histidine in actinomyosin proteins and it cannot be reutilized after being released during protein degradation.[86] The increase in leg efflux and elevated arterial concentration of 3-methylhistidine after sham-hemodialysis using cuprophane dialyzers, therefore indicates that increased protein breakdown plays a part in the net catabolic process induced by blood-membrane contact.

The importance of blood-dialyzer contact during clinical dialysis as a factor in malnutrition remains a matter of speculation. It is conceivable that bacterial pyrogens (endotoxins) transmitted to the patients's blood from contaminated dialysis fluid may act independently or in concert with blood contact with bioincompatible dialysis membranes to activate monocyte production of cytokines that stimulate protein catabolism.[78,79,87] Cuprophane is now to an increasing extent replaced by modified cellulosic membranes or other more biocompatible membranes, which according to our results[84,85] have no discernible effect on leg muscle proteolysis.

Apparently the peritoneal dialysis procedure is not such a strong catabolic stimulus as HD, provided that the patient is free of peritonitis. However, there is a possibility that in CAPD the dialytic procedure per se elicits a low-grade infammatory response, induced by substances other than live bacteria, thereby stimulating protein catabolism. These substances could be microbial products (endotoxins), acetate, plastics, silicon, glucose, or other products from the system that elute into the peritoneal cavity.

CONCLUSION

There are multiple causes of malnutrtion in maintenance dialysis patients, some of which are unspecific and related to psychosocial and comorbidity factors and some more specifically related to the toxic and metabolic effects of renal failure and to the blood purification procedures. Low intake of protein and energy due to anorexia in underdialyzed patients as well as catabolic effects of acidosis, energy depletion, losses of glucose, protein and amino acid, and inflammatory responses to dialysis may to a varying extent be involved. In prevention and treatment of dialysis-associated malnutrition, the aim should be to to ensure an adequate protein and energy intake by reducing or eliminating factors that cause anorexia and increase protein catabolism.

REFERENCES

1. Bergström J, Lindholm B: Nutrition and adequacy of dialysis: How do hemodialysis and CAPD compare? Kidney Int 43:S39-50, 1993 (Suppl 40)

2. Young VR: Nutritional requirements of normal adults, in Mitch WE, Klahr S (eds): Nutrition and the Kidney, chap 1. Boston, MA, Little, Brown, 1993, pp 1-34

3. Slomovitz LA, Monteon FJ, Grosvenor M, Laidlaw SA, Kopple JD: Energy expenditure in patients with chronic renal failure. Kidney Int 35:704-711, 1989

4. Kopple JD, Chumlea WC, Gassman JJ, Hollinger DL, Maroni BJ, Merril D, Scherch LK, Schulman G, Zimmer GS: Relationship between GFR and nutritional status: Results from the MDRD study. J Am Soc Nephrol 5:325, 1994

5. Guarnieri G, Toigo G, Situlin R, Faccini L, Coli U, Lannini S, Bazzato G, Dardi F, Campanacci L: Muscle biopsy studies in chronically uremic patients: Evidence for malnutrition. Kidney Int 187-193, 1983 (Suppl 16)

6. Jacob V, Le Carpentier JE, Salzano S, Naylor V, Wilde G, Brown CB, El Nahas AM: IGF-1, a marker of undernutrition in hemodialysis patients. Am J Cin Nutr 52:39-44, 1990

7. Marckmann P: Nutritional status and mortality of patients on regular dialysis therapy. J Intern Med 226:429-432, 1989

8. Schoenfeld PY, Henry RR, Laird NM, Roxe DM: Assessment of nutritional status of the National Cooperative Study population. Kidney Int 80-88, 1983 (Suppl 13)

9. Von Baeyer H, Gahl GM, Riedinger H, Borowzak R, Averdunk R, Schurig R, Kessel M: Adaptation of CAPD patients to the continuous peritoneal energy uptake. Kidney Int 23:29-34, 1983

10. Bergström J, Fürst P, Alvestrand A, Lindholm B: Protein and energy intake, nitrogen balance and nitrogen losses in patients treated with continuous ambulatory peritoneal dialysis. Kidney Int 44:1048-1057, 1993

11. Hylander B, Barkeling B, Rössner S: Eating behavior in continuous ambulatory peritoneal dialysis and hemodialysis patients. Am J Kidney Dis 20:592-597, 1992

12. Balaskas EV, Rodela H, Oreopoulos DG: Effects of intraperitoneal infusion of dextrose and amino acids on the appetite of rabbits. Perit Dial Int 13:S490-498, 1993 (Suppl 2)

13. Bergström J, Mamoun AH, Anderstam B, Södersten P: Middle molecules (MM) isolated from uremic ultrafiltrate (UF) and normal urine induce dose-dependent inhibition of appetite in the rat. J Am Soc Nephrol 5:488, 1994

14. Mamoun AH, Anderstam B, Lindholm B, Södersten P, Bergström J: Peritoneal dialysis (PD) solutions with glucose and amino acids (AA) suppress appetite in the rat. J Am Soc Nephrol 5:498, 1994

15. Lindsay RM, Spanner E: A hypothesis: The protein catabolic rate is dependent upon the type and amount of treatment in dialyzed uremic patients. Am J Kidney Dis 13:382-389, 1989

16. Lysaght MJ, Pollock CA, Hallet MD, Ibels LS, Farrell PC: The relevance of urea kinetic modeling to CAPD. Trans Am Soc Artif Intern Organs 35:784-790, 1989

17. Bergström J, Alvestrand A, Lindholm B, Tranaeus A: Relationship between Kt/V and protein catabolic rate (PCR) is different in continuous peritoneal dialysis (CPD) and hemodialysis (HD) patients. J Am Soc Nephrol 2:358, 1991

18. Ronco C, Conz P, Agostini F, Bosch JP, Lew SQ, La Greca G: The concept of adequacy in peritoneal dialysis. Perit Dial Int 14:S93-98, 1994 (Suppl 3)

19. Goodship THJ, Passlick-Deetjen J, Ward MK, Wilkinson R: Adequacy of dialysis and nutritional status in CAPD. Nephrol Dial Transplant 8:1366-1371, 1993

20. Nolph KD, Moore HL, Prowant B, Meyer M, Twardowski ZJ, Khanna R, Ponferrada L, Keshaviah P: Cross-sectional assessment of weekly urea and creatinine clearances and indices of nutrition in continuous ambulatory peritoneal dialysis patients. Perit Dial Int 13:178-183, 1993

21. Lindsay RM, Spanner E, Heidenheim P, Kortas C, Blake PG: PCR, Kt/V and membrane. Kidney Int 43:S268-273, 1993 (Suppl 41)

22. Heimbürger O, Tranaeus A, Bergström J, Lindholm B: The effect of increased PD on Kt/V, protein catabolic rate (PCR) and serum albumin. Perit Dial Int 22:S19, 1992 (Suppl 2)

23. Borah MF, Schoenfeld PY, Gotch FA, Sargent JA, Wolfson M, Humphreys MH: Nitrogen balance during intermittent dialysis therapy of uremia. Kidney Int 14:491-500, 1978

24. Gotch FA, Sargent JA: A mechanistic analysis of the National Cooperative Dialysis Study. Kidney Int 28:526-534, 1985

25. Harty JC, Boulton H, Curwell J, Heelis N, Uttley L, Venning MC, Gokal R: The normalized protein catabolic rate is a flawed marker of nutrition in CAPD patients. Kidney Int 45:103-109, 1994

26. Lameire NH, Vanholder R, Veyt D, Lambert MC, Ringoir S: A longitudinal, five-year survey of urea kinetic parameters in CAPD patients. Kidney Int 42:426-432, 1992

27. Young GA, Kopple JD, Lindholm B, Vonesh EF, De Vecchi A, Scalamogna A, Castelnova G, Oreopoulos DG, Anderson GH, Bergström J, Di Chiro J, Gentile D, Nissenson A, Sanraki L, Brownjohn AM, Nolph KD, Prowant BF, Algrim CE, Martis L, Serkes KD: Nutritional assessment of continuous ambulatory peritoneal dialysis patients: An international study. Am J Kidney Dis 17:462-471, 1991

28. Owen WF, Lew NL, Liu Y, Lowrie EG, Lazarus JM: The urea reduction ratio and serum albumin concentration as predictors of mortality in patients undergoing hemodialysis. N Engl J Med 329:1001-1006, 1993

29. Herrmann FR, Safran C, Levkoff SE, Minaker KL: Serum albumin level on admission as a predictor of death, length of stay, and readmission. Arch Intern Med 152:125-130, 1992

30. Rathore V, Depner TA, Shearer GC, Kaysen GA: Hypoalbuminemia results from reduced albumin synthesis (AlbSyn) determined premiarly by non-nutritional factors in hemodialysis patients. J Am Soc Nephrol 5:502, 1994

31. Heimbürger O, Bergström J, Lindholm B: Albumin and amino acid levels as markers of adequacy in continuous ambulatory peritoneal dialysis. Perit Dial Int 14:S123-132, 1994 (suppl 3)

32. Teehan BP, Schleifer CR, Brown JM, Sigler MH, Raimondo J: Urea kinetic analysis and clinical out-come on CAPD: A five-year longitudinal study. Perit Dial Bull 6:181-185, 1990

33. Kumano K, Yokota S, Go M, Suyama K, Sakai T, Era S, Sogami M: Quantitative and qualitative changes of serum albumin in CAPD patients. Perit Dial Bull 8:127-130, 1992

34. Lee HB, Han DC, Cha HK, Chung SH, Lee SK, Hwang SD, Moon C: Kt/V and clinical out-come in CAPD. J Am Soc Nephrol 4:411, 1993

35. Jones MR: Etiology of severe malnutrition: Results of an international cross-sectional study in continuous ambulatory peritonel dialysis patients. Am J Kidney Dis 23:412-420, 1994

36. Bergström J, Asaba H, Fürst P, Lindholm B: Middle molecules in chronic uremic patients treated with peritoneal dialysis, in Advances in Peritoneal Dialysis, International Congress Series 567. Amsterdam, Excerpta Medica, 1981, pp 47-53

37. Keshaviah PR, Nolph KD, Van Stone JC: The peak concentration hypothesis: A urea kinetic approach to comparing the adequacy of continuous ambulatory peritoneal dialysis (CAPD) and hemodialysis. Perit Dial Int 9:257-260, 1989

38. Keshaviah PR: Urea kinetic and middle molecule approaches to assessing the adequacy of hemodialysis and CAPD. Kidney Int 43:S28-38, 1993 (Suppl 40)

39. Schoenheyder F, Heilskov NSC, Olsen K: Isotopic studies on the mechanism of negative nitrogen balance produced by immobilization. Scand J Clin Lab Invest 6:178-188, 1954

40. Berkelhammer CH, Baker JP, Leither LA, Uldall PR, Whittal R, Slater A, Wolman SL: Whole-body protein turnover in adult hemodialysis patients as measured by ^{13}C-leucine. Am J Clin Nutr 46:778-783, 1987

41. Goodship THJ, Lloyd S, Clague MB, Bartlett K, Ward MK, Wilkinson R: Whole body leucine turnover and nutritional status in continuous ambulatory peritoneal dialysis. Clin Sci 73:463-469, 1987

42. Kishi K, Miytani K, Inoue G: Requirement and utilization of egg protein by Japanese young men with marginal intakes of energy. J Nutr 198:658-669, 1978

43. Slomowitz LA, Monteon FJ, Grosvenor M, Laidlaw SA, Kopple JD: Effect of energy intake on nutritonal status in maintenance hemodialysis patients. Kidney Int 35:704-711, 1989

44. Papadoyannakis NJ, Stefanidis CJ, Mcgeown M: The effect of the correction of metabolic acidosis on nitrogen and potassium balance of patients with chronic renal failure. Am J Clin Nutr 40:623-627, 1984

45. Williams B, Hattersley J, Layward E, Walls J: Metabolic acidosis and skeletal muscle adaptation to low protein diets in chronic uremia. Kidney Int 40:779-786, 1991

46. Straumann E, Keller U, Küry D, Bloesch D, Thélin A, Arnaud MJ, Stauffacher W: Effect of acute acidosis and alkalosis on leucine kinetics in man. Clin Physiol 12:39-51, 1992

47. Reaich D, Channon SM, Scrimgeour CM, Daley SE, Wilkinson R, Goodship THJ: Correction of acidosis in humans with CRF decreases protein degradation and amino acid oxidation. Am J Physiol 265:E230-235, 1993

48. Lim VS, Bier DM Flanigan MJ, Sum-Ping ST: Acido-

sis increased amino acid oxidation in chronic renal failure (CRF) patients. J Am Soc Nephrol 4:252, 1993

49. Hara Y, May RC, Kelly RC, Mitch WE: Acidosis, not azotemia, stimulates branched-chain amino acid catabolism in uremic rats. Kidney Int 32:808-814, 1987

50. May RC, Hara Y, Kelly RA, Block KP, Buse M, Mitch WE: Branched-chain amino acid metabolism in rat muscle: Abnormal regulation in acidosis. Am J Physiol 252:E712-718, 1987

51. May RC, Masud T, Logue B, Bailey J, England BK: Metabolic acidosis accelerates whole body protein degradation and leucine oxidation by a glucocorticoid-dependent mechanism. Miner Electrolyte Metab 18:245-249, 1992

52. Mitch WE, Medina R, Grieber S, May RC, England BK, Russ Price S, Bailey JL, Goldberg A: Metabolic acidosis stimulates muscle protein degradation by activating the adenosine triphosphate-dependent pathway involving ubiquitin and proteasomes. J Clin Invest 93:2127-2133, 1994

53. Bergström J, Alvestrand A, Fürst P: Plasma and muscle free amino acids in maintenance hemodialysis patients without protein malnutrition. Kidney Int 38:108-114, 1990

54. Löfberg E, Wernerman J, Bergström J: Branched-chain amino acids in muscle increase during correction of metabolic acidosis in hemodialysis (HD) patients. J Am Soc Nephrol 4:363, 1993

55. Lowrie EG, Lew NL: Commonly measured laboratory variables in hemodialysis patients: Relationships among them and to death risk. Semin Nephrol 12:276-283, 1992

56. Tizianello A, Deferrari G, Garibotto G, Gurreri G, Robaudo C: Renal metabolism of amino acids and ammonia in subjects with normal renal function and in patients with chronic renal insufficiency. J Clin Invest 65:1162-1173, 1980

57. Fukuda S, Kopple JD: Uptake and release of amino acids by the kidney of dogs made chronicallly uremic with uranyl nitrate. Miner Electrolyte Metab 3:248-260, 1980

58. Pitts RF, Macleod MB: Synthesis of serine by the dog kidney in vivo. Am J Physiol 222:394-398, 1972

59. European Dialysis and Transplant Association-European Renal Association: EDTA/ERA Registry Report, Demography of Dialysis and Transplantation in Europe, 1984. Nephrol Dial Transplant 1:1-8, 1986

60. Excerpts from United States Renal Data System: 1991 Annual Data Report, V. Survival probabilities and causes of death. Am J Kidney Dis 18:49-60, 1991 (Suppl 2)

61. Borah MF, Schoenfeld PY, Gotch FA, Sargent JA, Wolfson M, Humphreys MH: Nitrogen balance during intermittent dialysis therapy of uremia. Kidney Int 14:491-500, 1978

62. Ward RA, Shirlow MJ, Hayes JM, Chapman GV, Farrell PC: Protein catabolism during hemodialysis. Am J Clin Nutr 32:243-249, 1979

63. Farrell PC, Hone PW: Dialysis-induced catabolism. Am J Clin Nutr 33:1417-1422, 1980

64. Löfberg E, Wernerman J, Garlick P, Bergström J: Hemodialysis decreases protein synthesis (PS) in healthy volunteers. J Am Soc Nephrol 4:364, 1993

65. Lim VS, Bier DM, Flanigan M, Symreng T: The effect of hemodialysis on protein metabolism. J Am Soc Nephrol 1:366, 1990

66. Lim VS, Bier DM, Flanigan MJ, Sum-Ping ST: The effect of hemodialysis on protein metabolism: A leucine kinetic study. J Clin Invest 91:2429-2436, 1993

67. Wathen RL, Keshaviah P, Hommeyer P, Cadwell K, Comty CM: The metabolic effects of hemodialysis with and without glucose in the dialysate. Am J Clin Nutr 31:1870-1875, 1978

68. Gutierrez A, Bergström J, Alvestrand A: Hemodialysis-associated protein catabolism with and without glucose in the dialysis fluid. Kidney Int 46:814-822, 1994

69. Kopple JD, Swendseid ME, Shinaberger JH, Umezawa CY: The free and bound amino acids removed by hemodialysis. Trans Am Soc Artif Intern Organs 19:309-313, 1973

70. Wolfson M, Jones MR, Kopple JD: Amino acid losses during hemodialysis with infusion of amino acids and glucose. Kidney Int 21:500-506, 1982

71. Tepper T, Hem GK, van der Klip HG, Donker AJM: Loss of amino acids during hemodialysis: Effect of oral essential amino acid supplementation. Nephron 29:25-29, 1981

72. Bannister DK, Acciardo SR, Moore LW, Kraus AP: Nutritional effects of peritonitis in continuous ambulatory peritoneal dialysis (CAPD) patients. J Am Diet Assoc 87:53-56, 1987

73. Williams P, Kay R, Harrison J, McNeil K, Petit J, Kellman B, Mendez M, Klein M, Ogilvie R, Khanna R, Carmichal D, Oreopoulos DG: Nutritional and anthropometric assessment of patients on CAPD over one year: Contrasting changes in total body nitrogen and potassium. Perit Dial Bull 1:82-87, 1981

74. Verger C, Larpent I, Dumontet M: Prognostic value of peritoneal equilibration curves (EC) in CAPD patients, in Maher JF, Winchester JF (eds): Frontiers in peritoneal dialysis. New York, NY, Field, Rich and Assoc, 1986, pp 88-93

75. Cheung AK: Biocompatibility of hemodialysis membranes. J Am Soc Nephrol 1:150-161, 1990

76. Betz M, Haensch GM, Rauterberg EW, Bommer J, Ritz E: Cuprammonium membranes stimulates interleukin-1 release and arachidonic acid metabolism in monocytes in the absence of complement. Kidney Int 34:67-73, 1988

77. Haeffner-Cavaillon N, Cavaillon MJ, Laude M, Kazatchkine MD: C3a/C3adesArg induces production and release of interleukin-1 (IL-1) by cultured human monocytes. J Immunol 139:794-799, 1987

78. Lonnemann G, Bingel M, Floege J, Koch KM, Shaldon S, Dinarello CA: Detection of endotoxin-like interleukin-1-inducing activity during in vitro dialysis. Kidney Int 33:29-35, 1988

79. Evans RC, Holmes CJ: In vitro study of the transfer of cytokine-inducing substances across selected high-flux hemodialysis membranes. Blood Purif 9:92-101, 1991

80. Bingel M, Lonnemann G, Koch KM, Dinarello CA, Shaldon S: Enhancement of in vitro human interleukin-1 production by sodium acetate. Lancet 1:14-16, 1987

81. Flores EA, Bistrian BR, Pomposelli JJ, Dinarello CA, Blackburn GL, Istfan NW: Infusion of tumor necrosis factor: Cachectin promotes muscle catabolism in the rat. J Clin Invest 83:1614-1622, 1989

82. Baracos V, Rodeman HP, Dinarello CA, Goldberg AL: Stimulation of muscle protein degradation and prostaglandin E_2 release by leukocytic pyrogen (interleukin-1). N Engl J Med 308:553-558, 1983

83. Nawabi MD, Block KP, Chakrabarti MC, Buse MG: Administration of endotoxin, tumor necrosis, or Interleukin 1 to rats activates skeletal muscle branched-chain alpha-keto acid dehydrogenase. J Clin Invest 85:256-263, 1990

84. Gutierrez A, Alvestrand A, Wahren J, Bergström J: Effect of in vivo contact between blood and dialysis membranes on protein catabolism in humans. Kidney Int 38:487-494, 1990

85. Gutierrez A, Bergström J, Alvestrand A: Protein catabolism in sham hemodialysis: The effect of different membranes. Clin Nephrol 38:20-29, 1992

86. Young VR, Munro HN: Methylhistidine and muscle protein turnover: An overview. Fed Proc 37:2291-2300, 1978

87. Schindler R, Lonnemann G, Shaldon S, Koch K-M, Dinarello CA: Transcription, not synthesis of interleukin-1 and tumor necrosis factor by complement. Kidney Int 37:85-93, 1990

Mechanisms Causing Muscle Loss in Chronic Renal Failure

D. Reaich, MD, S.R. Price, PhD, B.K. England, MD, and W.E. Mitch, MD

● The loss of lean body mass in uremia is associated with excessive morbidity and mortality. A potential mechanism causing protein catabolism is that uremia overcomes critical metabolic responses required to maintain protein balance whenever dietary protein is limited. These responses include reduced oxidation of essential amino acids, which improves the efficiency of protein utilization and a reduction in protein degradation. We find that metabolic acidosis stimulates both amino acid oxidation and protein degradation in muscle and thus could overcome the adaptive responses. The molecular mechanisms stimulating catabolism involve glucocorticoids and includes increased mRNAs of components of catabolic pathways. Studies in patients have confirmed that acidosis causes catabolism in chronic renal failure. Thus, we recommend that patients with metabolic acidosis receive an adequate diet and sufficient alkali to correct acidosis.

INDEX WORDS: Metabolic acidosis; protein degradation; amino acid catabolism.

IN HUMANS, there is a constant "turning over" (ie, synthesizing and degrading) of protein. Average values indicate that a normal 70-kg adult in neutral protein balance will synthesize and degrade approximately 280 g protein daily.[1] Consequently, even a slight decrease in protein synthesis or increase in protein degradation persisting over many weeks would lead to significant loss of protein and hence, lean body mass. Because there are large day-to-day variations in dietary protein and calories, robust metabolic responses must be activated to maintain protein balance. The responses must be precise so that when protein intake is limited (from anorexia, dietary fads to lose weight, or prescribed for therapy), there is no loss of muscle mass.

METABOLIC RESPONSES TO DIETARY RESTRICTION

Adaptive mechanisms activated by changes in the diet have been identified using the L-leucine turnover technique based on a constant infusion of L-leucine labeled in the carboxyl position with ^{13}C or ^{14}C. L-leucine is labeled at this position because the initial reaction in its irreversible degradation is a decarboxylation producing $^{13}CO_2$ or $^{14}CO_2$, which can be collected in expired air. The amount of labeled CO_2 collected is an index of essential amino acid (EAA) degradation. If the enrichment (or specific radioactivity) of plasma leucine is measured simultaneously, it can be used to estimate whole-body protein synthesis and protein degradation because the rate of infusion is known. The accuracy of leucine turnover measurements are improved if the enrichment (or specific radioactivity) of the ketoacid of leucine (α-ketoisocaproate) in plasma is used in calculating protein turnover because this compound more accurately reflects intracellular metabolic events.[2,3]

The major response to variation in protein intake (Fig 1) consists of changes in amino acid oxidation, which eliminates amino acids in excess of the amount required to maintain nitrogen balance.[1,4] The magnitude of the reduction in amino acid oxidation varies with the degree of dietary protein restriction, to ensure that a sufficient amount of EAA are available for synthesis of body protein. Note that amino acid oxidation reaches a minimum when the amount of dietary protein (and hence, the intake of EAA) is at the minimum daily requirement to maintain nitrogen balance (0.6 g/kg/day). At this level, a second adaptive response can be detected, a reduction in the degradation of body protein. There can also be an increase in the synthesis of body protein, but the magnitude and metabolic importance of protein synthesis appear to be small.[4] Importantly, the ability to limit protein degradation will be insufficient to maintain protein balance if dietary protein is too low, but this response does limit the magnitude of negative nitrogen balance.

In considering patients with chronic renal failure (CRF), the initial question is whether these adaptive, metabolic responses are impaired. The answer seems to be that the responses are intact at least as long as the patients are not acidotic. Goodship et al[2] provided the first examination of this question in a study of patients with moder-

Supported by National Institutes of Health, Bethesda, MD, grant no. DK37175. D.R. was supported by the Northern Counties Kidney Research Fund, Newcastle Upon Tyne, United Kingdom.

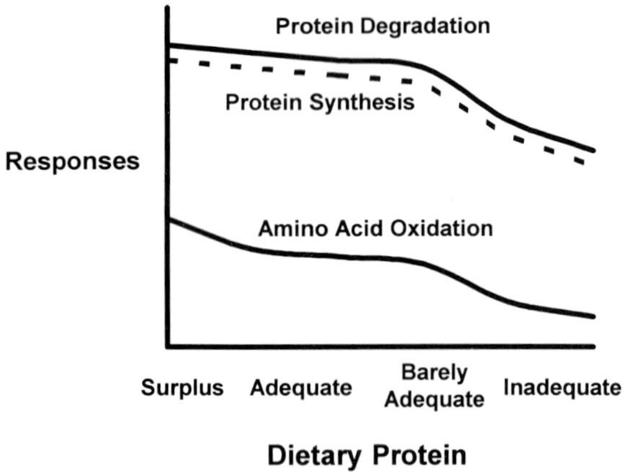

Fig 1. Adaptive metabolic responses to a reduction in dietary protein.

ately severe CRF but without metabolic acidosis. Their dietary protein was reduced from 1 g/kg/day to the minimum daily requirement, and the patients were studied at each level.[2] The adaptive responses of CRF and normal subjects were essentially identical: when dietary protein was at 0.6 g protein/kg/day, both groups had lower rates of amino acid oxidation and protein degradation. Masud et al[3] examined CRF patients fed an even more restricted diet (0.3 g protein/kg/day) supplemented with either EAA or their nitrogen-free analogs. With both supplements, amino acid oxidation was low, indicating improved efficiency of EAA utilization plus protein degradation was low.[4] Again, none of the patients had metabolic acidosis. Thus, if some condition stimulated EAA oxidation or protein degradation, the ability of a patient to adapt to a low-protein diet would be impaired. In fact, Williams et al[5] showed that CRF patients with metabolic acidosis were unable to adapt to a low-protein diet until their acidosis was corrected.[5]

BRANCHED-CHAIN AMINO ACID METABOLISM IN ACIDOSIS

Plasma levels of branched-chain amino acids (BCAAs) are low in uremia, valine having the greatest reduction.[6] Because low BCAA occurs even in CRF patients fed an adequate diet, excessive BCAA catabolism is the most likely cause. The catabolism of the BCAAs begins by transamination to their respective α-ketoacids, followed by irreversible oxidation by the branched-chain ketoacid dehydrogenase (BCKAD) complex.[7] Hara et al[8] found that plasma levels of all BCAAs and muscle levels of valine were lower in CRF rats compared with those in pair-fed, sham-operated rats. The lower BCAA levels were linked to increased oxidation in skeletal muscle and correction of the acidosis of CRF not only increased plasma and muscle BCAAs to levels measured in control rats, but also normalized the rates of BCAA oxidation in muscle. Clearly, the abnormal metabolism of BCAA was secondary to the acidosis of uremia.

In rats with normal kidneys as well, acidosis results in lower plasma and muscle BCAA levels than in pair-fed control rats, and the rates of BCAA transamination and decarboxylation in skeletal muscle are increased.[9] The mechanism for accelerated oxidation is that BCKAD activity is increased in muscle. Recently, England et al[10] found that stimulation of BCKAD is caused by two factors: there is a greater fraction of the enzyme in the activated form and there is an increase in the mRNA for E1α, E1β, and E2 subunits of BCKAD.[10] Interestingly, there was no increase in the enzyme measured by Western blotting. However, the increase in mRNA could prevent loss of BCKAD caused by acidosis-induced stimulation of protein degradation.

PROTEIN METABOLISM IN METABOLIC ACIDOSIS

Protein metabolism is abnormal in rats with CRF.[6] After subtotal nephrectomy, the degree of azotemia and acidosis will depend on the amount of protein eaten and with a high-protein diet, our model of CRF has a blood urea nitrogen averaging about 90 mg/dL and a serum bicarbonate concentration of 16 mmol/L.[11] Acidotic CRF rats were found to excrete 22% more nitrogen than pair-fed controls, and this was linked to a 90% increase in muscle protein degradation.[11] The stimulation of protein degradation was corrected by adding sodium bicarbonate to the diet to bring serum bicarbonate to 24 mmol/L.

To elucidate the mechanism for muscle proteolysis, rats were made chronically acidotic by feeding ammonium chloride (NH_4Cl). To eliminate the confounding effects of variation in dietary protein, an identical intake of calories, protein, and minerals was given to all rats by gavage feeding.[12] Acidotic rats had a blood pH of 7.15, impaired growth, abnormal nitrogen utilization, and increased muscle protein degradation. Others find that the urinary excretion of 3-methylhistidine is increased by acidosis, indicating that the catabolic response involves actin and myosin (the structural proteins of muscle).[13]

It is difficult, if not impossible, to isolate factors stimulating changes in protein metabolism in intact animals. Cultured cells offer the possibility of eliminating some factors (eg, hormones, cytokines) while measuring changes in protein turnover. We studied protein metabolism in the BC_3H1 myocyte.[14] When the media pH was reduced to 7.1, protein degradation increased sharply and protein synthesis fell slightly. Adding insulin-suppressed protein degradation regardless of the extracellular pH, but did not fully correct the catabolic effect of acidosis. In sharp contrast, when the pH of media of incubated LLC-PK_1 kidney cells is reduced, protein degradation is unchanged.[15] The reason for this difference in response is unknown.

PROTEOLYTIC PATHWAYS IN ACIDOSIS

Mammalian cells have several proteolytic pathways that serve distinct physiologic functions.[16] The bulk of muscle protein is degraded by an energy-dependant process known as the soluble, adenosine triphosphate (ATP)-dependent, ubiquitin-requiring proteolytic pathway. In this pathway, proteins destined for catabolism are conjugated to several ubiquitin molecules by an ATP-requiring mechanism. After ubiquitination, proteins are degraded by a large (1,500 kd) cytosolic, multifunctional proteolytic complex, known as the proteasome.[17]

We demonstrated that metabolic acidosis stimulates the ATP-dependent, ubiquitin-requiring pathway.[18] Protein degradation in isolated muscles from gavage-fed, acidotic, and control animals was compared. Using inhibitors of proteolytic pathways, it was found that the increase in muscle protein degradation stimulated by acidosis required ATP. Evidence for activation of the ATP-ubiquitin-proteasome–dependant pathway included a fourfold increase in ubiquitin mRNA in muscle plus increases in mRNA for the proteasome subunits C2 and C3. Thus, muscle proteolysis, like BCAA catabolism, involves an increase in the levels of mRNAs for key components of the degradative pathway. Interestingly, the mRNAs for ubiquitin and the E_2 subunit of BCKAD returned to control levels within 24 hours of switching rats to a standard diet; the change coincided with correction of the acidosis.

GLUCOCORTICOIDS AND THE PROTEOLYTIC RESPONSE TO ACIDOSIS

May et al[12] demonstrated that glucocorticoids were necessary for the increase in muscle protein degradation stimulated by acidosis. Urinary corticosterone was 87% higher in acidotic rats with accelerated muscle proteolysis but when acidotic rats were adrenalectomized, there was no increase in muscle protein degradation. Excessive proteolysis returned when acidotic, adrenalectomized rats were given dexamethasone at doses comparable to high physiologic glucocorticoid responses. Glucocorticoids are also necessary for the increase in ubiquitin and proteasome subunit mRNAs seen in acidotic rats.[19] When adrenalectomized rats were gavage-fed the NH_4Cl-containing diet, the effects of glucocorticoids could be separated from those of the low blood pH. Glucocorticoids were replaced by subcutaneous dexamethasone injections. Neither acidosis alone nor steroids alone changed mRNAs. But the combination of acidosis plus glucocorticoids increased levels of ubiquitin and the C2 and C9 proteasome subunit mRNAs (Fig 2). Thus, acidosis-induced stimulation of ATP-ubiquitin-proteasome pathway requires glucocorticoids.

ACIDOSIS AND CATABOLISM IN HUMANS

Metabolic acidosis is common in CRF and is present in almost 50% of hemodialysis patients.[20] The concept that acidosis has deleterious effects on lean body mass is not new. Sixty years ago, it was concluded that "on alkaline treatment clinical improvement was usual . . . and there was also improvement in the non-protein nitrogen."[20] The mechanism was not linked to decreased protein breakdown. Almost 50 years later, Papadoyannakis et al[21] concluded that giving sodium bicarbonate improved both nitrogen and potassium balance in CRF patients with acidosis. Other evidence for acidosis-induced catabolism is that adequately nourished children with renal tubular acidosis have impaired growth that is corrected when their acidosis is treated with sodium bicarbonate.[22] Finally, acidosis impairs the ability to adapt to a low-protein diet.[5]

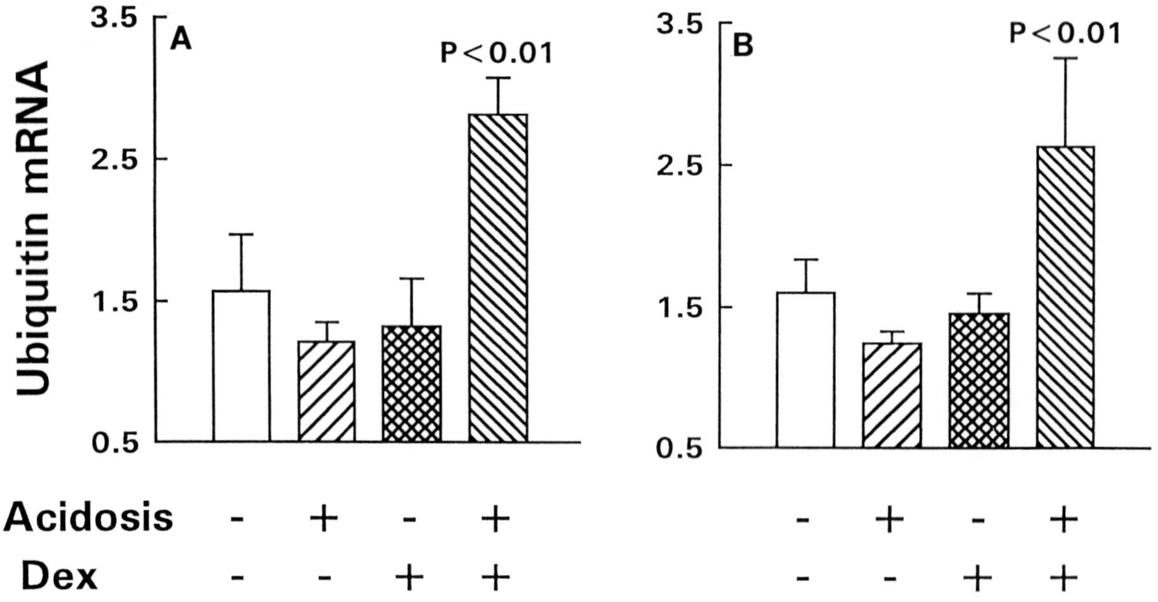

Fig 2. Acidosis plus glucocorticoids are required to increase ubiquitin mRNA in rat skeletal muscle. Adrenalectomized rats were fed a constant diet but groups were supplemented with NH_4Cl (acidosis) and/or dexamethasone (Dex). Ubiquitin mRNA in extensor digitorum longus (EDL) (A) and gastrocnemius (Gast) (B) muscles was measured by Northern hybridization and corrected for differences in loading by hybridizing with a cDNA for glyceraldehyde-3-phosphate dehydrogenase.

Regarding specific abnormalities in amino acid turnover, when normal subjects were fed NH_4Cl to induce chronic acidosis, leucine oxidation increased 25%.[23] In patients with CRF, there is a direct correlation between the concentrations of plasma bicarbonate and the ketoacid of leucine.[24] There also is a strong correlation in hemodialysis patients between the predialysis plasma bicarbonate concentration and the intracellular concentration of free valine measured in skeletal muscle biopsies.[25] Moreover, when acidosis in uremic subjects being treated with a low-protein diet (0.6 to 0.8 g/kg/day) is corrected, plasma BCAAs and branched-chain ketoacids increase and there is improvement in nitrogen balance.[26]

Protein metabolism is also abnormal in aci-

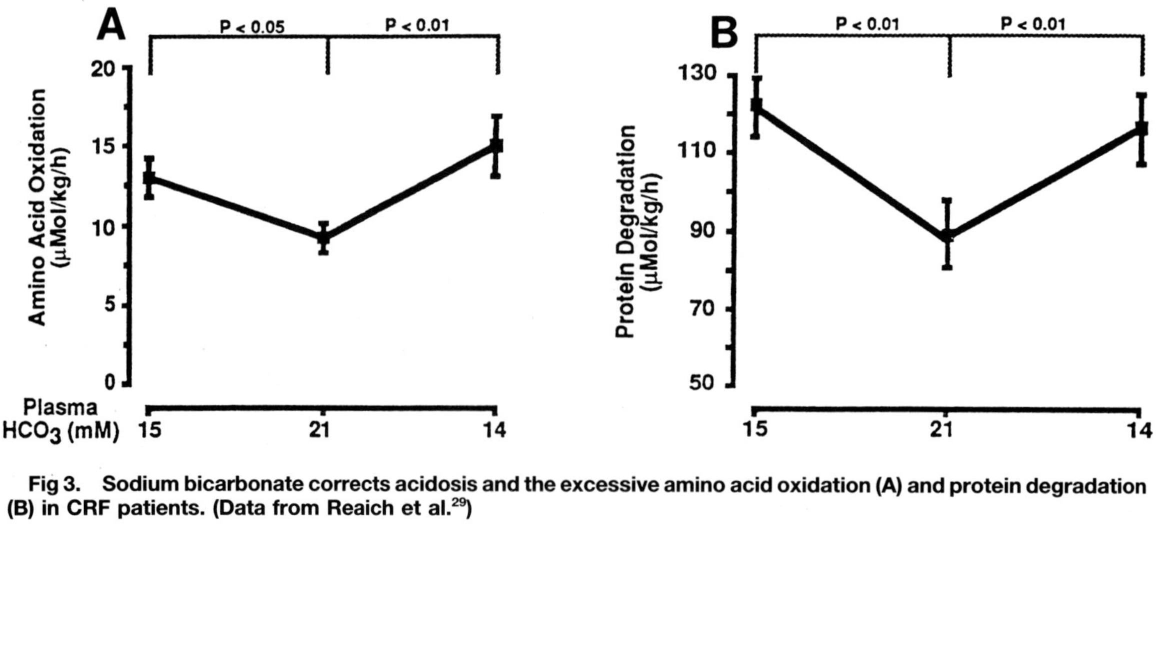

Fig 3. Sodium bicarbonate corrects acidosis and the excessive amino acid oxidation (A) and protein degradation (B) in CRF patients. (Data from Reaich et al.[29])

dotic patients. After 5 days of feeding NH_4Cl, the blood pH fell from 7.42 to 7.35 and there was increased degradation of protein.[23] Using a similar, NH_4Cl-feeding protocol, Ballmer et al[27] showed that acidosis limits albumin synthesis. This raises the important question of whether the increased mortality associated with hypoalbuminemia[28] may be related to acidosis.

Acidosis also causes abnormal protein metabolism in CRF. In CRF patients with a mean serum HCO_3 of 15 mmol/L, treatment with $NaHCO_3$ for 4 weeks increased their serum HCO_3 to 21 mmol/L and protein degradation fell 28% while leucine oxidation decreased 29%[29] (Fig 3). When given an equimolar amount of sodium chloride for 4 weeks, the mean serum HCO_3 was 14 mmol/L and protein degradation and leucine oxidation returned to the higher pretreatment levels. Thus, correction of the acidosis rather than giving sodium caused the changes in amino acid and protein metabolism.

The mechanism for this response can not be attributed solely to insulin resistance because excessive proteolysis persisted even during an insulin-clamp study.[30] The mechanism does involve glucocorticoids, as might be expected from our studies in rats.[12,19] Garibotto et al[31] infused labeled phenylalanine to measure whole body protein turnover and rates of protein synthesis and degradation in the forearms of CRF patients.[31] Whole-body protein breakdown was increased, whereas there was an increase in both protein breakdown and protein synthesis in the forearm. Although the balance (or net proteolysis) was the same as in controls, there was a significant inverse correlation between net proteolysis and plasma bicarbonate and a positive correlation between net proteolysis and plasma cortisol. In short, as plasma bicarbonate falls, or as serum cortisol increases, net proteolysis is higher.

In conclusion, there is abundant evidence that metabolic acidosis stimulates catabolism. Catabolism of BCAA involves activation of the rate-limiting enzyme for their oxidation and an increase in mRNAs for subunits of the enzyme. The proteolytic response occurs via stimulation of the ATP-ubiquitin-proteasome pathway and requires the presence of glucocorticoids. Based on these findings, we recommend that patients with metabolic acidosis receive a diet with an adequate amount of protein and sufficient sodium bicarbonate to correct the acidosis.

REFERENCES

1. Young VR: Some metabolic and nutritional considerations of dietary protein restriction, in Mitch WE (ed): Contemporary Issues in Nephrology: The Progressive Nature of Renal Disease. New York, NY, Churchill Livingstone, 1986, pp 263-283

2. Goodship THJ, Mitch WE, Hoerr RA, Wagner DA, Steinman TI, Young VR: Adaptation to low-protein diets in renal failure: Leucine turnover and nitrogen balance. J Am Soc Nephrol 1:66-75, 1990

3. Masud T, Young VR, Chapman T, Maroni BJ: Adaptive responses to very low protein diets: The first comparison of ketoacids to essential amino acids. Kidney Int 45:1182-1192, 1994

4. Motil KJ, Matthews DE, Bier DM, Burke JF, Munro HN, Young VR: Whole-body leucine and lysine metabolism: Response to dietary protein intake in young men. Am J Physiol 240:E712-E721, 1981

5. Williams B, Hattersley J, Layward E, Walls J: Metabolic acidosis and skeletal muscle adaptation to low protein diets in chronic uremia. Kidney Int 40:779-786, 1991

6. Mitch WE, Walser M: Nutritional therapy of the uremic patient, in Brenner BM, Rector FC (eds): The Kidney. New York, NY, Saunders, 1991, pp 2186-2222

7. Harper AE, Miller RH, Block KP: Branched-chain amino acid metabolism. Annu Rev Nutr 4:409-454, 1984

8. Hara Y, May RC, Kelly RA, Mitch WE: Acidosis, not azotemia, stimulates branched-chain amino acid catabolism in uremic rats. Kidney Int 32:808-814, 1987

9. May RC, Hara Y, Kelly RA, Block KP, Buse MG, Mitch WE: Branched-chain amino acid metabolism in rat muscle: Abnormal regulation in acidosis. Am J Physiol 252:E712-E718, 1987

10. England BK, Greiber S, Mitch WE, Bowers BA, Herring WJ, McKean MC, Price SR, Danner DJ: Rat muscle branched-chain ketoacid dehydrogenase activity and mRNAs increase with extracellular acidemia. Am J Physiol Cell (in press)

11. May RC, Kelly RA, Mitch WE: Mechanisms for defects in muscle protein metabolism in rats with chronic uremia: The influence of metabolic acidosis. J Clin Invest 79:1099-1103, 1987

12. May RC, Kelly RA, Mitch WE: Metabolic acidosis stimulates protein degradation in rat muscle by a glucocorticoid-dependent mechanism. J Clin Invest 77:614-621, 1986

13. Williams B, Layward E, Walls J: Skeletal muscle degradation and nitrogen wasting in rats with chronic metabolic acidosis. Clin Sci 80:457-462, 1991

14. England BE, Chastain J, Mitch WE: Extracellular acidification changes protein synthesis and degradation in BC3H-1 myocytes. Am J Physiol 260:C277-C282, 1991

15. Jurkovitz CT, England BK, Ebb RG, Mitch WE: Influence of ammonia and pH on protein and amino acid metabolism in LLC-PK1 cells. Kidney Int 42:595-601, 1992

16. Kettlehut IC, Wing SS, Goldberg AL: Endocrine regulation of protein breakdown in skeletal muscle. Diabetes Metab Rev 4:751-772, 1988

17. Hershko A, Ciechanover A: The ubiquitin system for protein degradation. Annu Rev Biochem 61:761-807, 1992

18. Mitch WE, Medina R, Greiber S, May RC, England

BK, Price SR, Bailey JL, Goldberg AL: Metabolic acidosis stimulates muscle protein degradation by activating the ATP-dependent pathway involving ubiquitin and proteasomes. J Clin Invest 93:2127-2133, 1994

19. Price SR, England BK, Bailey JL, Van Vreede K, Mitch WE: Acidosis and glucocorticoids concomitantly increase ubiquitin and proteasome subunit mRNAs in rat muscle. Am J Physiol 267:C955-C960, 1994

20. Price SR, Mitch WE: Metabolic acidosis and uremic toxicity: Protein and amino acid metabolism. Semin Nephrol 14:232-237, 1994

21. Papadoyannakis NJ, Stefanides CJ, McGeown M: The effect of the correction of metabolic acidosis on nitrogen and protein balance of patients with chronic renal failure. Am J Clin Nutr 40:623-627, 1984

22. McSherry E, Morris RC: Attainment of normal stature with alkali therapy in infants and children with classic renal tubular acidosis. J Clin Invest 61:509-514, 1978

23. Reaich D, Channon SM, Scrimgeour CM, Goodship THJ: Ammonium chloride-induced acidosis increases protein breakdown and amino acid oxidation in humans. Am J Physiol 263:E735-E739, 1992

24. Garibotto G, Paoletti E, Fiorini F, Russo R, Robaudo C, DeFerrari G, Tizianello A: Peripheral metabolism of branched-chain keto acids in patients with chronic renal failure. Miner Electrolyte Metab 19:25-31, 1993

25. Bergstrom J, Alvestrand A, Furst P: Plasma and muscle free amino acids in maintenance hemodialysis patients without protein malnutrition. Kidney Int 38:108-114, 1990

26. Mochizuki T: The effect of metabolic acidosis on amino and keto acid metabolism in chronic renal failure. Jpn J Nephrol 33:213-224, 1991

27. Ballmer PE, McNurlan MA, Hulter HN, Anderson SE, Garlick PJ, Krapf R: Chronic metabolic acidosis decreases albumin synthesis and induces negative nitrogen balance in humans. J Clin Invest 95:39-45, 1995

28. Lowrie EG, Lew NL: Death risk in hemodialysis patients: The predictive value of commonly measured variables and an evaluation of the death rate differences among facilities. Am J Kidney Dis 15:458-482, 1990

29. Reaich D, Channon SM, Scrimgeour CM, Daley SE, Wilkinson R, Goodship THJ: Correction of acidosis in humans with CRF decreases protein degradation and amino acid oxidation. Am J Physiol 265:E230-E235, 1993

30. Reaich D, Graham KA, Channon SM, Hetherington C, Scrimgeour CM, Wilkinson R, Goodship THJ: Insulin mediated changes in protein degradation and glucose utilization following correction of acidosis in humans with CRF. Am J Physiol 268:E121-E126, 1995

31. Garibotto G, Russo R, Sofia A, Sala MR, Robaudo C, Moscatelli P, DeFerrari G, Tizianello A: Skeletal muscle protein synthesis and degradation in patients with chronic renal failure. Kidney Int 45:1432-1439, 1994

Altered Physiology and Action of Insulin-like Growth Factor 1 in Skeletal Muscle in Chronic Renal Failure

Joel D. Kopple, MD, Hu Ding, MD, and Xiu-Lin Gao, MD

● Chronic renal failure is associated with abnormalities of skeletal muscle that include reduction in size, fibrosis, protein depletion, and functional disorders. These disorders may be caused by several factors, including protein-calorie malnutrition, acidemia, and superimposed illnesses. However, animal research suggests that these abnormalities may occur with chronic renal failure per se in the absence of the above complications. Insulin-like growth factor 1 (IGF-1) is an anabolic hormone that, in skeletal muscle, stimulates intracellular amino acid and glucose transport and protein synthesis, suppresses protein degradation, and causes hypertrophy. In chronic renal failure, there is evidence for inhibition of the actions of IGF-1. Studies in humans with chronic renal failure given a subcutaneous injection of recombinant human IGF-1 (rhIGF-1) indicate that the rhIGF-1 induced acute suppression of plasma amino acids, insulin, and C peptide is impaired. In skeletal muscle of rats with chronic renal failure, we observed reduced IGF-1 and IGF-1 mRNA levels, resistance to the rhIGF-1–induced suppression of protein degradation, and stimulation of protein synthesis, increased IGF-1 receptor mRNA and IGF-1 receptor number and impaired receptor tyrosine kinase activity. These findings suggest that in skeletal muscle in chronic renal failure there are several abnormalities in the physiology of IGF-1 and the sensitivity to IGF-1. It is possible that these alterations contribute to the disorders of skeletal muscle structure and function in chronic renal failure. Notwithstanding these abnormalities, repeated subcutaneous injections of rhIGF-1 in malnourished patients undergoing continuous ambulatory peritoneal dialysis led to strongly positive nitrogen balance that was sustained for the 20 days of study. These data suggest the possibility that rhIGF-1 may have a therapeutic role in malnourished patients with chronic renal failure.

INDEX WORDS: Insulin-like growth factor 1 (IGF-1); IGF-1 receptor; skeletal muscle; uremia; chronic renal failure; protein synthesis; protein degradation.

THERE IS substantial evidence that in chronic renal failure, the uremic milieu, independent of poor nutrient intake, intercurrent illnesses, or therapeutic maneuvers (eg, dialysis), adversely affects skeletal muscle metabolism. Disordered skeletal muscle structure and function in chronic renal failure has been described by many investigators.[1-3] In exercise-trained or erythropoietin-treated maintenance hemodialysis patients, hemodynamic and oxygen uptake studies suggest that the factor limiting exercise capacity in most individuals is not heart disease or blood oxygen carrying capacity (ie, anemia) but impaired skeletal muscle function. Skeletal muscle often is atrophied and has increased fibrous tissue and chronic inflammatory cells.[1,3,4] There is low skeletal muscle alkali soluble protein,[5,6] decreased skeletal muscle intracellular concentrations of several amino acids, and increased intracellular water,[6,7] increased or normal intracellular sodium and chloride, and normal[6] or reduced potassium and trace element levels.[6,7] Chronic renal failure rats grow less than sham-operated control rats, even when they are pair-fed.[8] Garber,[9] Harter et al,[10] and May et al[11] demonstrated increased net protein degradation in skeletal muscle from chronic renal failure rats as compared with sham-operated controls.

Holliday et al[12] reported that in young chronic renal failure rats, skeletal muscle protein synthesis was not reduced in the postabsorptive state, but it was diminished after 18 to 24 hours of fasting in comparison with control rats fasted for similar periods. Chronic renal failure rats that were fasted for 36 hours, except for glucose and water, had a more severe reduction in skeletal muscle protein synthesis and increased urea nitrogen appearance (net urea production) than did similarly fasted controls.[12] Li and Wassner[13] described normal skeletal muscle protein synthesis and degradation in the perfused hemicorpus from chronic renal failure rats, with or without insulin in the perfusate, but increased myofibrillar skeletal muscle degradation. When chronic renal failure rats were fasted, in comparison with pair-fed controls fasted for similar periods, the chronic renal failure rats displayed lower protein synthesis, higher protein degradation, greater net protein catabolism, and greater weight loss. These data suggest that when confronted with an inadequate protein-calorie intake or short-term starvation, common events in uremic patients, the chronic renal failure animal may not be able to conserve protein mass normally, either by maintaining skeletal muscle protein synthesis or reducing protein degradation. An inverse relation has been described between the magnitude of skeletal muscle protein degradation and body fat mass,[13] suggesting, as has previously been indicated,[14] that an adequate energy supply may be essential for maintaining protein mass.

MECHANISMS RESPONSIBLE FOR ALTERED SKELETAL MUSCLE PROTEIN METABOLISM IN UREMIA

The mechanisms responsible for altered skeletal muscle protein metabolism are still not well understood. In vitro dialysate of plasma from maintenance hemodialysis patients containing molecules with molecular weights less than 10,000 impair protein synthesis in a cell-free system.[15] Specific compounds identified in uremic sera decrease protein synthesis,[16] however, the concentrations that inhibit protein synthesis are greater than are found in uremic plasma. Insulin resistance may play a role. Harter et al[10] reported a decreased effect of insulin on the suppression of net skeletal muscle protein degradation in chronic renal failure rats fed high-protein diets; this reduced effect of insulin was not observed in chronic renal failure rats fed low-protein diets.[10] May et al[11] also observed a decreased effect of insulin on protein synthesis and degradation in chronic renal failure. In contrast, Garber[9] reported an increased effect of insulin in suppressing protein degradation in chronic renal failure rats. Insulin resistance to carbohydrate and adipocyte metabolism also occurs in chronic renal failure.[17,18]

Circulating inhibitors may play a role in the insulin resistance in uremia.[18] Garber described reduced suppression of net skeletal muscle protein degradation by epinephrine and serotonin in chronic renal failure as compared with control rats.[19] Interestingly, 25-hydroxycholecalciferol (25-OHD_3), but not 1,25$(OH)_2D_3$, or vitamin D_3, appears to stimulate adenosine triphosphate content and protein synthesis in vitamin D–deficient rats.[20]

In both normal rats and rats or patients with chronic renal failure, acidemia stunts growth and increases skeletal muscle protein breakdown and urea excretion.[21,22] Glucocorticoids may be necessary for the acidemia-induced skeletal muscle proteolysis[22] and may also promote skeletal muscle protein wasting independently of acidemia.[11,22,23] Mitch et al[24] have shown clearly that acidemia induces skeletal muscle protein degradation, and they have made major advances in our understanding of the mechanisms for this effect. Our observations indicate that chronic renal failure, independent of acidemia, enhances skeletal muscle protein degradation as well as suppresses protein synthesis.[25] The impaired insulin stimulation of skeletal muscle protein synthesis in chronic renal failure also appears to be independent of acidemia.[11]

Altered carnitine activity may affect skeletal muscle metabolism in chronic renal failure. Fatty acids normally are the major fuel substrate for skeletal muscle at rest and with low-intensity exercise.[26] Carnitine is essential for the normal transfer of long-chain ($\geq$ 10 carbons) fatty acyl groups into the mitochondria, where they are oxidized and may serve as a buffer or small reservoir for the mitochondrial pool of acyl-coenzyme A compounds.[27] Some but not all investigators report low plasma-free carnitine in maintenance hemodialysis patients; both low and normal skeletal muscle free and total carnitine have been reported.[28,29] However, plasma acylcarnitine is increased, and muscle acylcarnitine is low. Several investigators suggest that in chronic renal failure carnitine usually is not deficient, but increased levels of certain acylcarnitines may be toxic, possibly by competitively inhibiting the intramitochondrial transfer of more physiologically effective acylcarnitines.[28] Impaired fatty acid oxidation in skeletal muscle from uremic patients does not improve with carnitine supplements.[30] Thus, probably a number of factors, including acidemia and possibly abnormal carnitine levels, may alter skeletal muscle protein metabolism in chronic renal failure. We now review accumulating evidence that resistance to insulin-like growth factor-1 (IGF-1) is also present, that such resistance might contribute to skeletal muscle protein depletion in chronic renal failure, and that therapy with growth factors may promote anabolism.

INHIBITION OF IGF-I IN CHRONIC RENAL FAILURE

We and others have reported that chronic renal failure patients have circulating inhibitors to IGF-I.[31-33] These inhibitors are both large molecular weight compounds, at least some of which are IGF-1 binding proteins or binding protein fragments that are increased in uremic sera[32,33] and dialyzable compounds that are of smaller molecular weight (ie, 800 to 1,100 and possibly lower.[31] These small molecular weight inhibitors impair somatomedin (IGF-1) stimulated hypophysectomized rat costal cartilage uptake of sulfate, ^{3}H-uridine or ^{3}H-thymidine.[31] To our knowledge, no one has examined whether, in chronic renal failure, such inhibitors impair IGF-1–stimulated skeletal muscle cell glucose or amino acid transport and protein synthesis or IGF-1–induced reduction in protein degradation. Some children with chronic renal failure do not grow normally with recombinant DNA-synthesized human growth hormone (rhGH) therapy, and it is possible that this could be related to the presence of IGF-I inhibition.[33]

THEORETICAL BASIS FOR THERAPY OF DISORDERED SKELETAL MUSCLE METABOLISM IN CHRONIC RENAL FAILURE WITH GROWTH FACTORS INCLUDING IGF-1

As a result of the foregoing considerations, many researchers believe that the altered hormonal and metabolic milieu contributes to skeletal muscle protein wasting in chronic renal failure.[11-13,15-34] Hence, improving nutritional intake, which in itself can be difficult to achieve,[34] even with the use of erythropoietin therapy[35] or greater dialysis therapy[36] is often not sufficient to achieve or maintain normal protein mass in chronic renal failure patients.[14,34] This realization, which applies to many acute or chronic nonrenal diseases, has led a number of investigators to experiment with growth factors.[37] rhGH has been used to promote anabolism in patients with these conditions.[37] Chronic renal failure rats given rhGH grow more normally and display an increase in protein synthesis and mass.[38] In children with chronic renal failure, rhGH therapy is the only effective method for promoting catchup growth and maintaining normal growth.[33,34] We, Ziegler et al, and Shulman et al have shown that rhGH will reduce the urea nitrogen appearance in maintenance hemodialysis patients.[39-42] We have also shown that rhGH improves nitrogen balance, sometimes markedly, in these patients.[39-42]

Given the potential anabolic benefits of rhGH therapy, why evaluate the possible therapeutic benefits of IGF-I in chronic renal failure? Several considerations suggest that there are potentially unique therapeutic benefits to IGF-1 therapy: First, chronic renal failure patients commonly are poorly conditioned with markedly impaired skeletal muscle work capacity,[1,30,43,44] erythropoietin therapy may improve these disorders but does not normalize them.[1,43] Skeletal muscle atrophy and fibrosis often occur in chronic renal failure patients.[1,3] The endogenous elaboration of IGF-I appears to play an important role in skeletal muscle protein anabolism and growth.[45] rhIGF-I administration stimulates skeletal muscle protein synthesis and hypertrophy in nonuremic animals or skeletal muscle cell cultures,[46,47] and it is possible that such anabolic effects could promote skeletal muscle protein accrual and reduce atrophy and fibrosis in chronic renal failure patients. Second, as indicated above, there is evidence for resistance to IGF-I in chronic renal failure,[32-34] whether this resistance is due to alterations in the IGF-I molecule (eg, by binding), gene expression or transcription, or the signal transduction system and whether it suppresses anabolic processes in skeletal muscle protein or causes clinical sequelae are not known. Third, tissue and plasma IGF-I do not always increase in response to rhGH injections. Both low intake of protein or calories and severe sepsis in rats or humans[37,48,49] may impair the serum IGF-I response to rhGH therapy. Indeed, serum IGF-I may be a marker for nutritional status.[50] Some data suggest that reduced protein intake lowers serum IGF-I more than does low energy intake. Moreover, there are no data concerning the effects of nutritional status on skeletal muscle IGF-I levels or gene expression in either normal or chronic renal failure rats. We have observed an impaired response of serum IGF-I to rhGH in maintenance hemodialysis patients who were eating poorly or were septic.[37] Thus, the chronic renal failure patients who may be most in need of treatment with an anabolic hormone (ie, those who have the most difficulty in eating adequately or who are most catabolic from sepsis or trauma) are the individuals who may be least able to respond to rhGH therapy. It is for these reasons that some researchers suggest the use of rhIGF-I for the treatment of malnourished or sick catabolic patients.[37,38,48]

CHARACTERISTICS OF IGF-1 AND THE IGF TYPE I RECEPTOR

IGF-1 is a peptide hormone (molecular weight, 7,796) that is structurally and functionally similar to insulin.[51,52] rhIGF-1 has many anabolic effects in nonuremic animals and humans. It increases total body growth and particularly growth of certain organs,[53] stimulates erythropoiesis,[54] and reduces weight loss during starvation.[55] rhIGF-1 causes both cell hypertrophy and mitosis in the kidney,[56,57] promotes differentiation of certain cells, and stimulates renal tubular reabsorption of phosphorus.[58,59] Mice transgenic for the IGF-I gene undergo increased growth and organ hypertrophy.[60] IGF-1 lowers serum glucose, but this occurs primarily at higher doses.[59,61,62] On a molar basis in comparison with insulin, IGF-1 is only about 6% to 7% as potent as insulin in reducing blood glucose and about 1% as potent as an antilipotrophic agent. When rhIGF-1 is infused over several days, there is a decrease in plasma growth hormone, insulin, C-peptide, and IGF-2.[59] The hypoglycemic effects induced by IGF-1 are mediated by at least three mechanisms: selectively enhancing glucose uptake by tissues, suppressing hepatic glucose production, and accelerating tissue glycogen synthesis. IGF-1 has potent effects on protein metabolism, which include enhancing the intracellular transport of circulating amino acids, suppressing protein degradation, and increasing protein synthesis.[63-65] The main target organs for these effects of IGF-1 on glucose and protein metabolism include skeletal muscle, myocardium, liver, pancreas, and adipose tissue. Not only does IGF-1 have major structural homology with insulin, but the insulin receptor and the IGF-I receptor also have considerable homology in their protein sequence.[66,67] These receptors exhibit considerable similarities in their interaction with the two hormones. Insulin binds to the IGF-I receptor with approximately 100 to 1,000-fold lower affinity than it does to its own receptor, and the same holds true for IGF-I binding to the insulin receptor.[66,67] Both receptors are hormone-activated tyrosine-specific protein kinases.[68] Both receptors are also phosphorylated on serine and threonine residues,[68] and under basal conditions this phosphorylation predominates. We have now observed a defect in IGF-I receptor phosphorylation in epitrochlearis skeletal muscle from chronic renal failure rats (see below), perhaps similar to the postreceptor defect in the insulin response reported in chronic renal failure.[69]

The mechanisms of action of IGF-1 in skeletal muscle seem to be different from other organs. In liver and adipose tissue, for example, where the expression of the IGF-1 receptor is much less than the expression of the insulin receptor, the rapid insulin-like effects of IGF-1 on glucose and protein turnover appear largely mediated through the insulin receptor.[70-72] However, in skeletal muscle (and myocardium), most, if not all, of the anabolic effects of IGF-1 are mediated by its own receptor, the IGF type 1 receptor, which is abundantly expressed in this organ.[73,74] Because skeletal muscle accounts for the largest protein pool in the body, the anabolic effects of IGF-1 on protein turnover has been considered to be one of the most important regulators in body protein balance. In fact, abnormalities in the skeletal muscle IGF-1 system, both in the production of IGF-1 and its functions, has been reported to be involved in several clinical wasting illnesses, including chronic renal failure, malnutrition, sepsis, diabetes and growth retardation, and rhIGF-1 has been used to reverse the skeletal muscle protein wasting in these conditions.[26,69,75-78] In spite of the knowledge that we have obtained during the past several decades about skeletal muscle IGF-1, most of the mechanisms by which IGF-1 influences skeletal muscle protein turnover are largely unknown.

IGF-1 and IGF-2 bind to a family of specific IGF binding proteins (IGFBPs). In humans and rats, six structurally distinct forms of IGFBPs have been characterized, cloned, and designated as IGFBP-1 to IGFBP-6.[79-81] The IGFBPs are structurally related to each other but have different sizes. The IGF binding proteins appear to exert both inhibitory and facilitory actions on IGF-1. IGFBP-2 and IGFBP-3 have been identified in skeletal muscle, whereas all six IGFBPs are detected in various concentrations in serum, with the possible exception of IGFBP-5.

There are two published studies of the metabolic or nutritional response to rhIGF-1 treatment in chronic renal failure rats.[82,83] Subcutaneous injection of rhIGF-1 and a Des variant that binds less well to IGF-1 binding proteins increased growth, food utilization, nitrogen balance, and reduced the serum urea, insulin, and cholesterol. Urine N^{T}-methylhistidine excretion tended to decrease with both rhIGF-1 and the Des variant, but was significantly lower only with the latter compound; rhIGF-I may have exerted a greater anabolic effect at larger doses. These latter findings are consistent with the possibility that IGF binding proteins inhibit the actions of rhIGF-1 on skeletal muscle protein degradation in chronic renal failure. This inhibition could be due to an elevation in IGF binding protein concentrations.

EXPERIENCE WITH rhIGF-1 ON SKELETAL MUSCLE METABOLISM IN CHRONIC RENAL FAILURE

Skeletal muscle is the major endogenous compartment for protein and free amino acids. Because in chronic renal failure, skeletal muscle structure and function are abnormal and there are few data on the physiology of skeletal muscle IGF-1, we have begun to examine IGF-1 physiology and actions in skeletal muscle in rats with chronic renal failure.[25,69] Chronic renal failure rats were produced by ligation of two thirds of the left renal artery and contralateral nephrectomy. Sham-operated rats were pair-fed a regular chow diet to the chronic renal failure rats for 21 days. The chronic renal failure rats were given sodium bicarbonate daily to prevent acidemia. At the end of 3 weeks, the chronic renal failure and sham rats were then killed, and each pair of epitrochlearis muscles were incubated with either increasing concentrations of rhIGF-1 or vehicle. The dose-response relationship of the effects of IGF-1 on skeletal muscle protein synthesis and degradation was determined. As compared with sham-operated rats, chronic renal failure rats had enhanced protein degradation and reduced protein synthesis ($P < 0.001$). Incubation of epitrochlearis muscles from sham rats with increasing concentrations of IGF-1 resulted in increased protein synthesis and decreased protein degradation; the anabolic effects of IGF-1 on muscle protein turnover was significantly dose-dependent. However, when IGF-1 was added to the incubation medium for the epitrochlearis muscles from chronic renal failure rats, the same doses of IGF-1 induced only a slight reduction in muscle protein degradation and a slight increase in muscle protein synthesis ($P < 0.01$ *v* sham rats). The dose-dependent pattern of IGF-1–induced anabolic effects on skeletal muscle protein turnover in chronic renal failure rats was significantly less than in sham rats. These data indicate that there is resistance to the effects of IGF-1 on skeletal muscle protein synthesis and degradation in rats with chronic renal failure.

We then extended these studies to examine potential mechanisms for the skeletal muscle resistance to rhIGF-1 with the following findings: After 3 weeks of pair-feeding, we observed that in chronic renal failure as compared with sham-operated rats, serum and skeletal muscle IGF-1 were reduced. In skeletal muscle of chronic renal failure rats, IGF-1 mRNA was decreased, whereas IGF type 1 receptor mRNA was increased. We also observed increased total type 1 IGF receptor number with normal affinity in skeletal muscle of rats with chronic renal failure. However, the tyrosine kinase activity of the IGF-1 receptor was significantly reduced in chronic renal failure.[69,84]

These findings indicate that in skeletal muscle of chronic renal failure rats, as compared with sham-operated, pair-fed controls, there is (1) reduced IGF-1 and IGF-1 mRNA, (2) resistance to the suppressive actions of rhIGF-1 on protein degradation and stimulatory effects of rhIGF-1 on protein synthesis, (3) increased IGF type 1 receptor mRNA and receptor number with normal binding affinity, and (4) impaired receptor tyrosine kinase activity. Reduced IGF-1 synthesis and decreased IGF-1 receptor tyrosine kinase activity may be a cause of the atrophy and abnormal metabolism of skeletal muscle in chronic renal failure. We conclude from these studies that decreased IGF-1 receptor kinase activity might contribute to the resistance to IGF-1 in skeletal muscle of chronic renal failure rats and that resistance to IGF-1 may be a cause of skeletal muscle atrophy, altered physiology, and dysfunction in chronic renal failure.

Notwithstanding this evidence for resistance to IGF-1, our observations suggest that pharmacologic doses of rhIGF-1 induce an anabolic response in patients with chronic renal failure. We gave subcutaneous injections of rhIGF-1 to six patients with end-stage renal disease who had protein-calorie malnutrition and were undergoing continuous ambulatory peritoneal dialysis.[77] Patients received 100 μg rhIGF-1/kg body weight every 12 hours. rhIGF-1 induced strongly positive nitrogen balance that was sustained for the 20 days of rhIGF-1 treatment.

REFERENCES

1. Robertson HT, Haley NR, Gruthrie M, Cardenas D, Eschbach JW, Adamson JW: Recombinant erythropoietin im-

proves exercise capacity in anemic hemodialysis patients. Am J Kidney Dis 15:325-332, 1990

2. Lazaro RP, Kirshner HS: Proximal muscle weakness in uremia: Case reports and review of the literature. Arch Neurol 37:555-558, 1980

3. Ahonen RE: Light microscopic study of striated muscle in uremia. Acta Neuropathol (Berl) 49:51-55, 1980

4. Floyd M, Ayyar DR, Barwick DD, Weightman D: Myopathy in chronic renal failure. Q J Med XLIII 172:509-524, 1974

5. Guarnieri G, Toigo G, Situlin R, Faccini L, Coli U: Muscle biopsy studies in chronically uremic patients: Evidence for malnutrition. Kidney Int 16:S187-S193, 1983

6. Bergstrom J, Alvestrand A, Furst P, Hultman E: Muscle intracellular electrolytes in patients with chronic uremia. Kidney Int 16:S153-S160, 1983

7. Furst P, Alvestrand A, Berstrom J: Effects of nutrition and catabolic stress on intracellular amino acid pools in uremia. Am J Clin Nutr 33:1387-1395, 1980

8. Wang M, Vyhmeister I, Kopple JD, Swendseid ME: Effect of protein intake on weight gain and plasma amino acid levels in uremic rats. Am J Physiol 230:1455-1459, 1976

9. Garber AJ: Skeletal muscle protein and amino acid metabolism in experimental chronic uremia in the rat. J Clin Invest 62:623-632, 1978

10. Harter HR, Karl IE, Kipnis DM: Effects of reduced renal mass and dietary protein intake on amino acid release and glucose uptake by rat muscle in vitro. J Clin Invest 64:513-523, 1979

11. May RC, Kelly RA, Mitch WE: Mechanisms for defects in muscle protein metabolism in rats with chronic uremia. J Clin Invest 79:1099-1103, 1987

12. Holliday MA, Chantler C, MacDonnell R, Keitges J: Effect of uremia on nutritionally-induced variations in protein metabolism. Kidney Int 11:236-245, 1977

13. Li JB, Wassner SJ: Protein synthesis and degradation in skeletal muscle of chronically uremic rats. Kidney Int 29:1136-1143, 1986

14. Slomowitz LA, Monteon FJ, Grosvenor M, Laidlaw SA, Kopple JD: Effect of energy intake on nutritional status in maintenance hemodialysis patients. Kidney Int 35:704-711, 1989

15. Delaporte C, Gross F: In vitro inhibition of protein synthesis by dialysate of plasma from uraemic patients. Eur J Clin Invest 11:139-143, 1981

16. Clayton EM, Seligson D, Seligson H: Inhibition of protein synthesis by n-methyl-2-pyridine-5-formamidoacetic acid and other compounds isolated from uremic patients. Yale J Biol Med 38:273-281, 1965

17. Cecchin F, Ittoop O, Sinha MK, Caro JF: Insulin resistance in uremia: Insulin receptor kinase activity in liver and muscle from chronic uremic rats. Am J Physiol 254(Endocrinol Metab 17):E394-E401, 1988

18. Maloff BL, McCaleb ML, Lockwood DH: Cellular basis of insulin resistance in chronic uremia. Am J Physiol 245(Endocrinol Metab 8):E178-E184, 1983

19. Garber AJ: The regulation of skeletal muscle alanine and glutamine formation and release in experimental chronic uremia in the rat. J Clin Invest 62:633-641, 1978

20. Birge SJ, Haddad JG: 25-hydroxycholecalciferol stimulation of muscle metabolism. J Clin Invest 56:1100-1107, 1975

21. Papadoyannakis NJ, Stefanidis CJ, McGeown M: The effect of the correction of metabolic acidosis on nitrogen and potassium balance of patients with chronic renal failure. Am J Clin Nutr 40:623-627, 1984

22. May RC, Kelly RA, Mitch WE: Metabolic acidosis stimulates protein degradation in rat muscle by a glucocorticoid-dependent mechanism. J Clin Invest 77:614-621, 1986

23. Rannels SR, Jefferson LS: Effects of glucocorticoids on muscle protein turnover in perfused rat hemicorpus. Am J Physiol 238:E564-E572, 1980

24. Mitch WE, Medina R, Grieber S, May RC, England BK, Price SR, Bailey JK, Goldberg AL: Metabolic acidosis stimulates muscle protein degradation by activating the adenosine triphosphate-dependent pathway involving ubiquitin and proteasomes. J Clin Invest 93:2127-2133, 1994

25. Ding H, Gao XL, Kopple JD: Resistance to recombinant human IGF-1 in skeletal muscle of rats with chronic renal failure. J Am Soc Nephrol 4:768, 1993 (abstr)

26. Jones NL, Heigenhauser GJF, Kuksis A, Matsos CG, Sutton JR: Fat metabolism in heavy exercise. Clin Sci 59:469-478, 1980

27. Bieber LL, Emaus R, Valknerk K, Farrel S: Possible functions of short-chain and medium-chain carnitine acyltransferases. Fed Proc 41:2858-2862, 1982

28. Wanner C, Horl WH: Carnitine abnormalities in patients with renal insufficiency: Pathophysiological and therapeutical aspects. Nephron 50:89-102, 1988

29. Ahmad S, Robertson HT, Golper TA, Wolfson M, Kurtin P, Katz LA, Hirschberg R, Nicora R, Ashbrook DW, Kopple JD: Multicenter trial of L-carnitine in maintenance hemodialysis patients. II. Clinical and biochemical effects. Kidney Int 38:912-918, 1990

30. Siami G, Clinton ME, Mrak R, Griffis J, Stone W: Evaluation of the effect of intravenous L-carnitine therapy on function, structure and fatty acid metabolism of skeletal muscle in patients receiving chronic hemodialysis. Nephron 57:306-313, 1991

31. Phillips LS, Kopple JD: Circulating somatomedin activity and sulfate levels in adults with normal and impaired kidney function. Metabolism 30:1091-1095, 1981

32. Lee PD, Hintz RL, Sperry JB, Baxter RC, Powell DR: IGF binding proteins in growth retarded children with chronic renal failure. Pediatr Res 26:308-315, 1989

33. Blum WF, Ranke MB, Kietzmann K, Tonshoff B, Mehls O: Growth hormone resistance and inhibition of somatomedin activity by excess of insulin-like growth factor binding protein in uraemia. Pediatr Nephrol 5:539-544, 1991

34. For general review/citations see: Kopple JD, Schrier R, Gottschalk C (eds): Diseases of the Kidney (ed 4). Nutrition, Drugs, and the Kidney: Dietary Considerations in Patients with Advanced Chronic Renal Failure, Acute Renal Failure, and Transplantation. Boston, MA, Little Brown, 1992, pp 3167-3210

35. Ellis PW: EPO and renal nutrition: One year later. Evidence lacking in appetite improvement. Nephrology News and Issues, June: 26, 29, 38, 1990

36. Lindsay RM, Spanner E: A hypothesis: The protein catabolic rate is dependent upon the type and amount of treatment in dialyzed uremic patients. Am J Kidney Dis 13:382-389, 1989

37. Wilmore DW: Catabolic illness: Strategies for enhancing recovery. N Engl J Med 325:695-702, 1991

38. Mehls O, Ritz E, Hunziker E-B, Eggli P, Heinrich U: Improvement of growth and food utilization by human recombinant growth hormone in uremia. Kidney Int 33:45-52, 1988

39. Schulman G, Wingard RL, Hutchison RL, Lawrence R, Hakim RM: The effects of recombinant human growth hormone and intradialytic parenteral nutrition in malnourished hemodialysis patients. Am J Kidney Dis 21:527-534, 1993

40. Kopple JD, Leiserowitz M, Brunori G, Mattimore C: Treatment of malnourished maintenance hemodialysis (MHD) patients with recombinant human growth hormone. J Am Soc Nephrol 1:364, 1990

41. Kopple JD, Brunori G, Leiserowitz M, Mattimore C, Hirschberg R: Growth hormone treatment for patients with renal failure, in Hatano M (ed): Nephrology Proceedings of the XIth International Congress of Nephrology. Vol 1. Tokyo, Springer-Verlag, 1991, pp 379-388

42. Ziegler TR, Lazarus JM, Young LS, Hakim R, Wilmore DW: Effects of recombinant human growth hormone in adults receiving maintenance hemodialysis. J Am Soc Nephrol 2:1130-1135, 1991

43. Lim VS, DeGowin RL, Zavala D, Kirchner PT, Abels R: Recombinant human erythropoietin treatment in pre-dialysis patients: A double-blind placebo-controlled trial. J Ann Intern Med 110:108-114, 1989

44. Painter P: The importance of exercise training in rehabilitation of patients with end-stage renal disease. Am J Kidney Dis 24:S2-S9, 1994 (suppl 1)

45. DeVol DL, Rotwein P, Sadow JL, Novakofski J, Bechtel PJ: Activation of insulin-like growth factor gene expression during work-induced skeletal growth. Am J Physiol 259:(Endocrinol Metab 22):E89-E95, 1990

46. Roeder RA, Hossner KL, Sasser RG, Gunn JM: Regulation of protein turnover by recombinant human insulin-like growth factor-I in L6 myotube cultures. Horm Metabol Res 20:698-700, 1988

47. Tomas FM, Knowles SE, Owens PC, Read LC, Chandler CS, Gargosky SE, Ballard FJ: Effects of full-length and truncated insulin-like growth factor-I on nitrogen balance and muscle protein metabolism in nitrogen-restricted rats. J Endocrinol 128:97-105, 1991

48. Dahn MS, Lange MP, Jacobs LA: Insulin-like growth factor I production is inhibited in human sepsis. Arch Surg 123:1409-1414, 1988

49. Bier DM: Growth hormone and insulin-like growth factor I: Nutritional pathophysiology and therapeutic potential. Acta Pediatr Scand 374:119-128, 1991

50. Donahue SP, Phillips LS: Response of IGF-I to nutritional support in malnourished hospital patients: A possible indicator of short-term changes in nutritional status. Am J Clin Nutr 50:962-969, 1989

51. Adrian C: Herington: Insulin-like growth factors: Biochemistry and physiology. Baillieres Clin Endocrinol Metab 5:531-551, 1991

52. Guler HP: Insulin-like growth factor 1 and insulin: What is the difference? An overview of in-vivo studies, in Spencer EM (ed): Modern Concepts of Insulin-like Growth Factors. New York, NY, Elsevier, 1991, pp 583-590

53. Guler HP, Zapf J, Scheiwiller F, Froesch ER: Recombinant human insulin-like growth factor I stimulates growth and has distinct effects on organ size in hypophysectomized rats. Proc Natl Acad Sci USA 85:4889-4893, 1988

54. Froesch ER, Guler HP, Schmid C, Binz K, Zapf J: Trends in Endocrinology and Metabolism 1:254-260, 1990

55. O'Sullivan U, Glackman PD, Breier BH, Woodall S, Siddiqui R: Insulin-like growth factor-I (IGF-I) in mice reduces weight loss during starvation. Endocrinology 125: 2793-2794, 1989

56. Conti FG, Striker LS, Lesniak MA, MacKaey K, Roth J: Studies on binding and mitogenic effect of insulin-like growth factor I in glomerular mesangial cells. Endocrinology 122:2788-2795, 1988

57. Fagin JA, Melmed S: Relative increase in insulin-like growth factor I messenger ribonucleic acid levels in compensatory renal hypertrophy. Endocrinology 120:718-724, 1987

58. Hirschberg R, Brunori G, Kopple JD, Guler HP: Effects of insulin-like growth factor I on renal function in normal men. Kidney Int 43:387-397, 1993

59. Guler H-P, Schmid C, Zapf J, Froesch ER: Effects of recombinant insulin-like growth factor I on insulin secretion and renal function in normal human subjects. Proc Natl Acad Sci USA 86:2868-2872, 1989

60. Doi T, Striker LJ, Quaife C, Conti FG, Palmiter R: Progressive glomerulosclerosis develops in transgenic mice chronically expressing growth hormone and growth hormone releasing factor but not in those expressing insulin-like growth factor-I. Am J Pathol 131:398-403, 1988

61. Zapf J, Hauri C, Waldvogel M, Froesch ER: Acute metabolic effects and half-lives of intravenously administered insulin-like growth factors I and II in normal and hypophysectomized rats. J Clin Invest. 77:1768-1775, 1986

62. Guler HP, Zapf J, Froesch ER: Short-term metabolic effects of recombinant human insulin-like growth factor I in healthy adults. N Engl J Med 317:137-140, 1987

63. Ding H, Kopple JD, Cohen A, Hirschberg R: Recombinant human insulin-like growth factor-1 accelerates recovery and reduces catabolism in rats with ischemic acute renal failure. J Clin Invest 91:2281-2287, 1993

64. Hussain MA, Schmitz O, Mengel A, Keller A, Christiansen JS, Zapf J, Froesch ER: Insulin-like growth factor 1 stimulates lipid oxidation, reduces protein oxidation, and enhances insulin sensitivity in humans. J Clin Invest 92:2249-2256, 1993

65. Jacob R, Barrett E, Plewe G, Fagin KD, Sherwin RS: Acute effects of insulin-like growth factor 1 on glucose and amino acid metabolism in the awake fasted rat: Comparison with insulin. J Clin Invest 83:1717-1723, 1989

66. Massague J, Czech MP: The subunit structures of two distinct receptors for insulin-like growth factors I and II and their relationship to the insulin receptor. J Biol Chem 257:5038-5045, 1982

67. Rechler MM, Zapf J, Nissley SP, Froesch ER, Moses A: Interactions of insulin-like growth factors I and III and multiplication-stimulating activity with receptors and serum carrier proteins. Endocrinology 107:1451-1459, 1980

68. Yu K-T, Peters MA, Czech MP: Similar control mechanisms regulate the insulin and type I insulin-like growth factor receptor kinases: Affinity-purified insulin-like growth factor I receptor kinase is activated by tyrosine phosphorylation of its beta subunit. J Biol Chem 261:11341-11349, 1986

69. Ding H, Gao XL, Kopple JD: Mechanisms of resis-

tance to IGF-1 in skeletal muscles in rats with chronic renal failure. J Am Soc Nephrol 5:941, 1994 (abstr)

70. Hartmenn H, Schmitz R, Christ B, Jungermann K, Creutzfeldt W: Metabolic actions of insulin-like growth factor-1 in cultured hepatocytes from adult rats. Hepatology 12:1139-1143, 1990

71. Caro JR, Poulos J, Ittoop O, Pories WJ, Flickinger EG, Sinha MK: Insulin-like growth factor 1 binding in hepatocytes from human liver, human hepatoma, and normal, regenerating, and fetal rat liver. J Clin Invest 81:976-981, 1988

72. Verspohl EJ, Roth RA, Vigneri R, Goldfine ID: Dual regulation of glycogen metabolism by insulin and insulin-like growth factors in human hepatoma cells (HEP-G2): Analysis with an anti-receptor monoclonal antibody. J Clin Invest 74:1436-1443, 1984

73. Yu KT, Czech MP: The type I insulin-like growth factor receptor mediates the rapid effects of multiplication-stimulating activity on membrane transport system in rat soleus muscle. J Biol Chem 259:3090-3095, 1984

74. Dardevet D, Attaix SD, Baracos VE, Grizard J: Insulin-like growth factor-1 and insulin resistance in skeletal muscles of adult and old rats. Endocrinology 134:1474-1484, 1994

75. Fouque D, Peng S, Kopple JD: Impaired metabolic response to recombinant insulin-like growth factor 1 in dialysis patients. Kidney Int 47:876-883, 1995

76. Fouque D, Peng S, Kopple JD: IGF-1 treatment in chronic renal failure: Abnormal plasma kinetics. Kidney Int 47:869-875, 1995

77. Peng S, Fouque D, Kopple JD: Insulin-like growth factor 1 (IGF-1) causes anabolism in malnourished CAPD patients. JASN 4:414, 1993 (abstr)

78. Canalis E: Clinical reviews 35: Growth factors and their potential clinical value. J Clin Endocrinol Metab 75:1-4, 1992

79. Ballard FJ, Baxter RC, Binoux M, Clemmons DR, Drop SLS, Hall K, Hintz RL, Rechler MM, Rutanen EM, Schwander JC, Spencer EM, Zapf J: On the nomenclature of IGFBPs, in Spencer EM (ed): Modern Concepts of Insulin-like Growth Factors. New York, NY, Elsevier, 1991, pp 731-732

80. Gargosky SE, Walton PE, Owens PC, Wallace JC, Ballard FJ: Insulin-like growth factor-1 (IGF-1) and IGF-binding proteins both decline in the rat during late pregnancy. J Endocrinol 127:383-390, 1990

81. Oh Y, Muler HL, Lee DY, Fielder PJ, Rosenfeld RG. Characterization of the affinities of insulin-like growth factor (IGF)-binding proteins 1-4 for IGF-1, IGF-2, IGF-insulin hybrid, and IGF-1 analogues. Endocrinology 132:1337-1344, 1993

82. Martin AA, Tomas FM, Ballard FJ, Read LC: Insulin-like growth factor I and its variant, Des (1-3) IGF-I, improve nitrogen balance and food utilization in rats with renal failure, in Proceedings of the 6th International Congress on Renal Nutrition and Metabolism, Mineral and Electrolyte Metabolism 18:264-268, 1992

83. Hazel DJ, Gillespie CM, Moore RJ, Clark RG, Jureidini KF, Martin AA: Enhanced body growth in uremic rats treated with IGF-1 and growth hormone in combination. Kidney Int 46:58-68, 1994

84. Ding H, Gao XL, Hirschberg R, Kopple JD: Evidence for impaired activity of type 1 IGF receptor tyrosine kinase in skeletal muscle of rats with chronic renal failure. Endocrinology 1995 (abstr) (in press)

Interventions to Treat Malnutrition in Dialysis Patients: The Role of the Dose of Dialysis, Intradialytic Parenteral Nutrition, and Growth Hormone

T. Alp Ikizler, MD, Rebecca L. Wingard, RN, MSN, and Raymond M. Hakim, MD, PhD

● Protein and calorie malnutrition often starts before initiation of dialysis, and reflects the anorexia and the catabolic state of chronic renal failure. In the face of inadequate dialysis, which perpetuates the uremic state, malnutrition often worsens. Several studies, though not all, suggest that optimal dialysis improves nutritional status of dialysis patients. Such optimal dialysis now must include the use of biocompatible membranes to deliver Kt/V > 1.4 (urea reduction ratio > 65%). Additional interventions can include the use of enteral or intravenous hyperalimentation, and recombinant growth factors such as growth hormone or insulin-like growth factor-1. Importantly, studies to document the improvement in the morbidity and mortality of patients with these interventions are still needed and require large multicenter trials.

INDEX WORDS: Malnutrition; biocompatibility; dialysis dose; growth factors; intradialytic parenteral nutrition.

REDUCTION in anthropometric measurements,[1] low concentrations of visceral proteins such as serum albumin,[2] and abnormalities in plasma and muscle amino acid profiles[3] are some of the indices of malnutrition that have been identified in dialysis patients (Table 1). Using these indices, protein and calorie malnutrition has been found in a substantial proportion of dialysis patients.

RELATIONSHIP OF MALNUTRITION TO MORBIDITY AND MORTALITY

A number of reports have documented a high prevalence of malnutrition in both hemodialysis (HD) and continuous ambulatory peritoneal dialysis (CAPD) patients and have shown a relationship between the extent of malnutrition and increased morbidity and mortality in this patient population.[2,4-7] In the National Cooperative Dialysis Study (NCDS), low protein catabolic rate, a reflection of dietary protein intake in the stable HD patient, was strongly associated with treatment failure.[7] In a more recent study, Lowrie and Lew,[2] using data in more than 12,000 HD patients, have shown that low concentration of serum albumin, creatinine, and blood urea nitrogen (BUN) levels were all associated with increased death risk.[2] This study also showed a prevalence of 25% of patients with albumin concentrations less than 3.7 g/dL. These findings were later confirmed by 4-year prospective study by Goldwasser et al,[8] who also showed the importance of low serum albumin and cholesterol as indices of malnutrition associated with an increased risk for mortality. Finally, Acchiardo et al[4] demonstrated that malnutrition, determined by low protein intake, was associated with high morbidity and mortality in chronic HD patients.

The prevalence of malnutrition in CAPD patients is even greater. A recent international multicenter study found a prevalence of "moderate to severe" malnutrition in 40% of these patients.[5] Low serum albumin was again found to be associated with increased morbidity and mortality in this patient population.[9] Serum prealbumin level below 30 mg/dL was also reported to be a significant risk factor in CAPD patients in a subsequent study by Avram et al[10]; interestingly, prealbumin had a higher predictive power compared with albumin in this study, probably because of its shorter serum half-life. These findings strongly suggest that poor nutritional status contributes, along with other factors, to the high mortality and morbidity rates seen in dialysis-dependent patients.

PATHOGENESIS OF MALNUTRITION IN DIALYSIS-DEPENDENT PATIENTS

Predialysis Factors

Several factors that contribute to malnutrition are listed in Table 2. Anorexia and decreased nutrient intake are seen in uremic patients even before the initiation of dialysis and reflect the uremic state. Although the exact mechanism of

---

Supported in part by National Institutes of Health, Bethesda, MD, grant no. DK-45604-01 and Food and Drug Administration grant no. FD-R-000943-01. T.A. Ikizler, MD, is partly supported by an International Society of Nephrology/American Society of Nephrology Fellowship Training Award.

Table 1. Indices of Malnutrition in Dialysis Patients

Reduction in anthropometric measurements
Serum albumin <4.0 g/dL
Abnormal plasma and muscle amino acid profiles
Low percent ideal body weight (<85%)
Low insulin-like growth factor 1, transferrin, and prealbumin levels

this catabolic state is not clearly defined, there is evidence suggesting that at least in the pre–end-stage renal disease (ESRD) stage, spontaneous dietary protein as well as energy intake directly correlate with the glomerular filtration rate.[11] We have recently performed a prospective longitudinal study in which a marked spontaneous decrease in dietary protein intake occurred with progression of renal failure, and DPI was strongly correlated with CrCl, suggesting that chronic renal failure patients who have anorexia are already prone to poor nutritional status.[12]

In addition to decreased nutrient intake, metabolic acidosis,[13] which commonly accompanies progressive renal failure, as well as hormonal derangements, such as insulin resistance,[14] may further contribute to increased catabolism in dialysis patients.

Dialysis-Related Factors

Dialysis-related factors also have an impact on the nutritional status of the dialysis-dependent patient population. Increased protein and energy requirements, particularly on dialysis days, have been proposed for dialysis-dependent patients,[15] who already have a precarious dietary intake that may be well below their needs. The cause of this increased requirement is multifactorial and mostly attributed to the catabolic effects of HD.[16,17]

Several factors may explain this dialysis-induced catabolism: Losses of free and bound amino acids during both HD and CAPD are substantial and contribute to negative nitrogen balance during dialysis. Wolfson et al[18] have shown a loss of 5 to 8 g free amino acids during each HD session, using conventional low-flux dialyzers. In a more recent study, we documented further increase in amino acid losses with high-flux (HF) dialyzers compared with low-flux dialyzers.[19] These losses were not due to an intrinsic problem with HF membranes, but were ''pare passu'' effects of the larger surface area and higher blood flow used in HF membranes. In other words, they were inevitable consequences of higher clearance of urea with HF membranes. In addition, although HD resulted in a significant reduction in plasma levels of individual and total amino acids, these changes in plasma levels were much less than what can be measured from the total amino acid losses in the dialysate. This finding suggested that during each HD session there is a net release of amino acids from intracellular stores, and patients can lose net body protein equivalent to 25 to 30 g.

With regard to CAPD patients, several studies reported a loss of 5.5 to 11.8 g proteins into the dialysate daily.[20,21] A large amount of these losses consists of albumin, along with immunoglobulins as well as amino acids. During episodes of peritonitis, these losses increase substantially. Several studies reported free amino acid losses in a range of 1.7 to 3.4 g per day.[21,22] We recently measured these losses in stable CAPD patients and found them to be equivalent to 3.7 g total amino acids per day.

Passive dialysate losses of amino acids are not the only cause of abnormal plasma amino acid profiles. Several lines of evidence also suggest that the type of membrane used during HD may play a role/participate in protein catabolism.[23] Gutierrez et al[24] have shown increased amino acid release from peripheral muscle tissues in healthy subjects during sham dialysis (without dialysate flow and where no amino acids are lost during dialysis) with bioincompatible (cuprophane) membranes, but not with more biocompatible membranes. Recently, we have shown

Table 2. Factors Contributing to Malnutrition

Anorexia and decreased nutrient intake
Hormonal derangements (eg, insulin resistance)
Metabolic acidosis, contributing to increased catabolism
Frequent hospitalizations
Multiple medications
Socioeconomic status of the patient
Dialysis-related factors
Inadequate dialysis
Protein and amino acid losses in dialysate
Dialysis membrane bioincompatibility-induced catabolism

that the level of plasma amino acids during HD decreased less with cuprophane membranes when compared with biocompatible membranes, although the dialysate losses were comparable in both membranes, suggesting increased appearance in plasma.[19] This finding is in agreement with the results of Gutierrez et al of an increased release of amino acids from peripheral tissues during HD with the bioincompatible membranes.[25] There are as yet no data to show whether different peritoneal dialysate solutions may induce more or less protein or amino acid losses.

Several earlier studies have suggested that the energy requirements were not different in ESRD patients compared with normal subjects. Monteon et al[26] and Schneeweiss et al,[27] using indirect calorimetry with the cart technique, found no differences in energy expenditures in these patient groups compared with normal controls. We have recently conducted a study to further explore this issue in HD patients.[28] The patients resting energy expenditures during dialysis and nondialysis hours were measured in a metabolic chamber unit, which is a unique whole-room indirect calorimeter where dialysis can be performed and patient can be mobile. More recent and probably more precise measurements show significantly higher resting energy expenditure in HD patients compared with age-, sex-, and body mass index–matched normal controls, even during nondialysis hours. Resting energy expenditure was also significantly higher during HD compared with nondialysis hours. Although the cause of this phenomena needs further elucidation, it may in part explain the increased energy and protein requirements of dialysis patients.

The last, but certainly not the least, dialysis-related factor that may affect the nutritional status in dialysis patients is the adequacy of dialysis.[29] The NCDS was the first study to highlight the interrelationship between the dose of dialysis (using conventional cuprophane membrane), protein intake determined by protein catabolic rate (PCR), and morbidity in dialysis patients.[30] Thus, a trend for lower protein intake was observed in patients with higher time-average urea concentrations, and both were associated with higher hospitalization rates. More recently, Lindsay and Spanner[31] have hypothesized that PCR was dependent on the type and the dose of dialysis in uremic patients. In a study of 55 HD patients, they were able to show a significant linear relationship between Kt/V and PCR. Moreover, the attempts to increase DPI of these patients by dietary counseling were unsuccessful unless the dose of dialysis was first increased. Of note, their data further suggested that the type of dialysis membrane used also affected the nature of the relationship between the dose of dialysis and PCR. Specifically, lower dialysis doses were needed to obtain a specific PCR when a biocompatible membrane was used in comparison with a cellulosic membrane. In a more recent study by Burrowes et al,[32] a significant increase in serum albumin levels was observed in a cohort of chronic HD patients when they were dialyzed adequately. Serum albumin levels increased from 3.13 ± 0.24 g/dL to 3.51 ± 0.41 g/dL ($P < 0.001$) in 30 newly initiated HD patients when they were dialyzed with a Kt/V of 1.37 ± 0.17. Similar increases were seen in patients who were transferred from other units and in patients who received intradialytic parenteral nutrition. Likewise, Acchiardo et al[33] also reported an increase in serum albumin (3.2 ± 0.1 g/dL to 3.8 ± 0.1 g/dL) in conjunction with a decrease in mortality (12%) when the dialysis dose was increased in 416 patients (1.09 ± 0.1 to 1.44 ± 0.3).

Similar conclusions with regard to the dose of dialysis are reported in CAPD patients in several studies. In a cross-sectional analysis of an international multicenter study, a higher incidence of malnutrition was observed in patients who were treated with CAPD longer than 3 months compared with the patients who were treated less than 3 months, suggesting that as residual renal function decreased, the patients became more malnourished.[9] Keshaviah et al[34] and Teehan et al[35] also reported higher survival rates with higher Kt/V. Nevertheless, it must be said that there are several studies in CAPD patients that failed to show a significant correlation between either dialysis dose or PCR and serum albumin.

In summary, chronic dialysis patients are prone to develop malnutrition because of decreased intake, metabolic derangements, and several dialysis-related factors, such as low dose of dialysis, increased losses of amino acids and proteins, and higher energy expenditure.

INTERVENTIONS TO PREVENT OR TREAT MALNUTRITION IN DIALYSIS PATIENTS

In the presence of a high prevalence of malnutrition and its relationship to mortality and mor-

Table 3. Interventions to Prevent or Treat Malnutrition

Optimal dialysis prescriptions
Biocompatibility (of hemodialysis membranes and peritoneal dialysis solutions)
Nutritional counseling
Intradialytic parenteral & enteral nutritional supplements
Growth factors
Recombinant human growth hormone (rhGH)
Recombinant human insulin-like growth factor-1 (rhIGF-1)

bidity in dialysis patients, it is not surprising that multiple interventions have been tried to either prevent or to treat this diseased state. These interventions are summarized in Table 3.

Effects of Dialysis Dose and Membrane on Nutritional Parameters

A number of studies have suggested that dialysis dose is related to nutritional parameters and mortality and morbidity. In addition to their cross-sectional study where they established a linear relationship between dose of dialysis and PCR, Lindsay et al prospectively analyzed the effects of increasing the dialysis dose in a group of patients with PCR values < 1 g/kg/d.[36] Their results showed that PCR increased significantly in the group of patients whose Kt/V values was increased, whereas there was no change in PCR values in the group of patients whose Kt/V values remained the same. However, the study did not clarify whether improvement in dietary protein intake, as assessed by PCR, will improve nutritional parameters, such as serum albumin levels or anthropometric measurements. As mentioned earlier, studies by Burrowes et al[32] as well as those by Acchiardo et al[33] demonstrated significant increases in serum albumin levels in chronic HD patients when their dose of dialysis increased to adequate levels.

Our laboratory has performed a prospective study in which the dose of dialysis was increased intentionally in 130 patients treated in an affiliated chronic HD unit.[37] During a 4-year period, the dose of dialysis (measured by delivered Kt/V) was gradually increased to 1.33. Our results showed that the standardized mortality rates of the patients declined from 22.8% to 9.1% during the study period. When the data obtained from kinetic modeling were plotted for Kt/V and PCR, a strong positive correlation was observed between dose of dialysis and protein intake as defined by urea appearance (Fig 1). Moreover, when the nutritional parameters of patients with yearly average Kt/V values below 0.86 and above 1.21 were identified, statistically significant differences were found between serum albumin, transferrin, and PCR measurements.

In another retrospective study, Owen et al[38] proposed that mortality improved in HD patients with increasing urea reduction ratio, another index of dialysis adequacy, as well as by higher serum albumin levels. Conversely, they were unable to show a significant correlation between serum albumin levels and increasing the dialysis dose. This observation is puzzling and contradicts the other studies mentioned in which a relationship between the dose of dialysis and serum albumin concentration was observed. It is possible that the differences between the study by Owen and Lowrie and others relate to two additional issues that have been highlighted recently. One observation relates to the significant loss of albumin across high-flux membranes reused with bleach and formaldehyde. These losses of albumin increased to substantial amounts (up to 10 g/dialysis session) especially after the 15th reuse.[19,39] Indeed, when the reuse number was limited to 15, there was an increase of 0.22 ± 0.19 g/dL in serum albumin levels of the patients. The other observation relates to the finding that dialysis with biocompatible membranes leads to a higher weight gain, higher albumin concentrations, as well as higher insulin-like growth factor-1 levels.[40] Also, as suggested earlier, the biocompatible membranes may lead to a lesser amount of amino acid release from peripheral muscle tissues, compared with bioincompatible membranes.[19,24] Thus, the relationship between the dose of dialysis and nutritional status may be more complex than originally thought, and may depend on the membrane used as well as the reuse method.

With regard to the adequacy of CAPD, there are no prospective, randomized studies that correlate the dialysis dose to nutritional parameters or outcome in peritoneal dialysis patients. However, there are several retrospective studies[34,35,41] that show significant correlations between dialysis dose and nutritional parameters and, separately, morbidity and mortality.

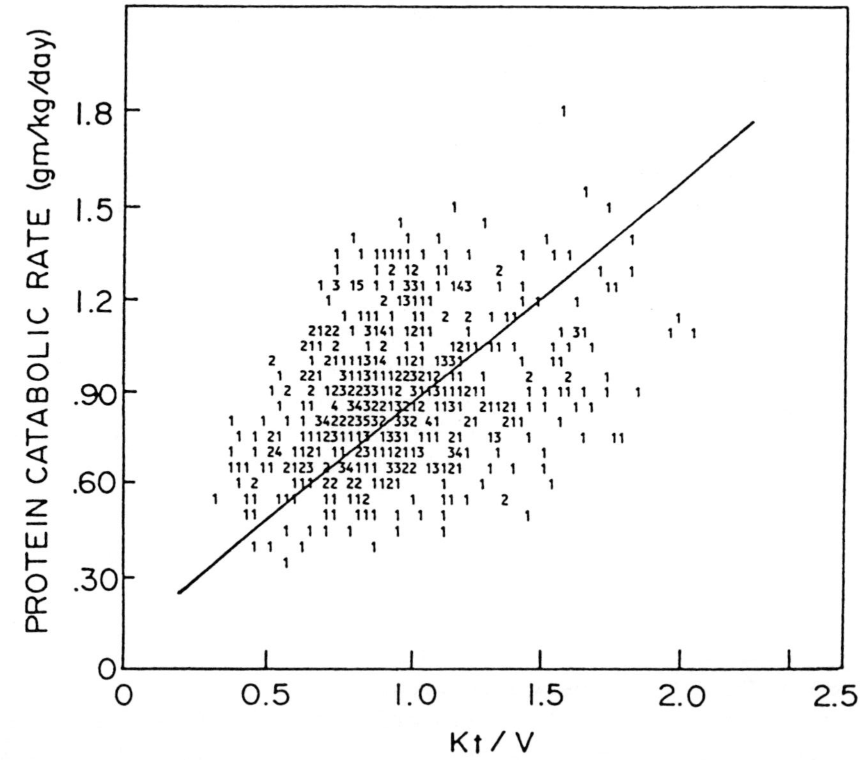

Fig 1. The relationship of the dose of dialysis (Kt/V) and interdialytic urea appearance (PCR) in hemodialysis patients. The numbers inside the figure refer to the number of data points at each point. The least square fit is best described by the equation PCR = 0.12 + 0.73 * (Kt/V). The relationship is statistically significant (*P* < 0.001) with a correlation coefficient of 0.838. (Reprinted with permission.[37])

In summary, although the cause and effect relationship between the dose of dialysis and nutritional parameters is not completely established, in view of the strong relationship between dialysis dose and mortality and morbidity, and separately, between malnutrition with morbidity and mortality, it is reasonable to assume that increasing the dialysis dose may improve nutritional status, at least in malnourished dialysis patients. Several prospective studies are underway to explore this issue, in both HD and CAPD patients.

Nutritional Interventions

Another component for treating malnutrition in dialysis patients is nutritional interventions. Dietetic counseling, oral supplementation, enteral feeding, and intradialytic parenteral nutrition are among the possible options. Unfortunately, attempts to treat malnutrition solely with dietetic counseling and oral supplementation have not been reported to be successful.[29,42] Similarly, there are limited data on the effectiveness of enteral feeding on dialysis patients.[29] Of note is that many studies of this issue have drawbacks in their design, such as patient selection, provision of variable, and difficult-to-quantitate energy and protein intake, lack of patient acceptance and problems with study design; the difficulties of conducting such a trial probably account for the fact that no complete study on the effects of oral supplementation on nutritional status or morbidity and mortality has been published.[43] Nevertheless, these options should be tried in all patients before more invasive interventions are attempted.

Intradialytic Parenteral Nutrition (IDPN)

Heidland and Kult[44] were the first to report an improvement in nutritional parameters in chronic HD patients with intradialytic infusion of essential amino acids. Although several subsequent studies using intradialytic infusion have been reported to be positive,[45,46] many of them had problems in their design, such as small number of patients, lack of control groups, and inappropriate length of time. Conversely, other studies were unable demonstrate any benefit with this treatment because of similar problems.[47,48] In a recent well-controlled study, Cano et al[49] reported improvements in several nutritional parameters, such as arm muscle circumference, albumin, prealbumin, and skin-test reactivity, in addition to increased appetite and weight gain. More recently, Capelli et al,[50] in a retrospective, nonrandomized study, showed reduced mortality rates in malnourished HD patients who were treated with IDPN compared with patients who were not treated. Similarly, Chertow et al[51] performed a retrospective study in which more than 1,500 patients who received IDPN were identified and analyzed for mortality risk factors by comparing with more than 20,000 patients who were not treated with IDPN. Their results showed that odds ratio of death decreased in patients in whom IDPN was used, particularly when serum albumin levels were below 3.5 g/dL and serum creatinine levels were below 8.0 mg/dL.

In summary, because of the limited number of studies done and the retrospective methodologies in most of these studies, it is not possible to definitively conclude whether IDPN therapy is effective in malnourished hemodialysis patients, and these conflicting results warrant further long-term controlled trials.

Amino acid dialysate (AAD) solutions are the counterpart of IDPN in CAPD patients. A number of studies have explored the effects of AAD in CAPD patients.[22,52,53] Although several of these studies had shortcomings in their study design, patient selection, and the composition of the solution, other well-controlled studies were able to demonstrate positive effects of AAD in CAPD patients, in both short term and long term. Serum transferrin and total protein levels increased and plasma amino acid profiles tended toward normal in CAPD patients who received one or two exchanges of AAD. Conversely, increases in BUN levels, associated with exacerbation of uremic symptoms as well as metabolic acidosis, continue to be a complication of AAD.[52-54] Nevertheless, the weight of evidence suggests that AAD may improve the nutritional parameters in malnourished CAPD patients, and long-term studies are warranted to see whether these effects will improve the excessive prevalence of malnutrition in this patient population.

Recombinant Human Growth Hormone (rhGH)

Another promising strategy to treat malnourished dialysis patients is use of pharmacologic doses of rhGH. rhGH is a hormone with well-established anabolic properties. It promotes protein synthesis, decreases protein degradation, enhances lipolysis, and increases food conversion ratio.[55-57] Although the exact mechanisms by which rhGH exerts its metabolic effects are not clear, it has been demonstrated that these properties are in part mediated through induction of the anabolic hormone insulin-like growth factor-1 (IGF-1)[58] (Table 4). rhGH has been employed in various catabolic states, such as severe burns, sepsis, and corticosteroid administration, which resulted in improvement in nitrogen balances.[59] Studies have shown that growth hormone levels in uremic patients are either normal or slightly increased, probably because of decreased metabolic clearance.[60] In spite of this finding, animal studies suggest that there is growth hormone resistance at cellular levels in uremia.[61] Accordingly, a number of studies have also been reported regarding the positive growth-promoting effects of rhGH in pediatric uremic patients using pharmacologic doses of rhGH.[62,63] In view of these encouraging results, several studies have been performed investigating the nutritional effects of rhGH in both HD and CAPD patients.

In a study by Ziegler et al,[64] administration of rhGH for 2 weeks to five well-nourished HD patients who were followed in a clinical research center resulted in a decrease of predialysis BUN levels by approximately 25% and a significant reduction in urea generation and PCR. In addition, there was a significant decrease in phosphorus levels. These changes returned to baseline when rhGH was discontinued. Based on these results, we performed a study in which the effects of IDPN, alone and combined with rhGH, were analyzed in seven malnourished HD patients.[65]

Table 4. Pathways of rhGH Action

Direct actions
Interactions with GH receptors in tissues (ie, adipocytes, chondrocytes, and fibroblast precursors)
Increase in cellular IGF-1 (autocrine effect)
Increase in tyrosine kinase activity
Indirect actions
Increased serum IGF-1 levels
Increased serum IGFBP-3 levels
Increased insulin resistance

Table 5. Biochemical and Urea Kinetic Parameters During Different rhGH Study Periods

	Baseline	Treatment With rhGH	Post-GH
BUN (mg/dL)	54 ± 15	40 ± 12*	55 ± 15†
Creatinine (mg/dL)	12.2 ± 5.7	12.9 ± 5.7*	12.0 ± 5.1
Potassium (mEq/L)	4.0 ± 0.4	3.6 ± 0.2*	4.0 ± 0.4†
Phosphorus (mg/dL)	4.8 ± 1.6	4.4 ± 1.8*	4.7 ± 1.9
DUN (g/day)	4.53 ± 1.23	3.44 ± 1.09*	4.16 ± 1.22*†
NUN (g/day)	5.69 ± 1.86	4.04 ± 1.13*	5.19 ± 2.07*†
PCR (g/kg/day)	0.82 ± 0.13	0.67 ± 0.09*	0.77 ± 0.14*†

NOTE. Values are expressed as mean ± SD.
* $P < 0.05$ *v* baseline.
† $P < 0.05$ *v* treatment.
Used with permission from *Kidney International,* volume 46, page 1180, 1994.[66]

Although the study was not controlled and limited to a small number of patients, our results indicated that IDPN alone was not sufficient to improve nutritional parameters, whereas combination of IDPN with rhGH resulted in significant improvements in serum albumin, transferrin and IGF-1 levels. These results suggested that rhGH potentiated the anabolic effects of IDPN.

We have recently evaluated the short-term effects and safety of rhGH on urea kinetics and commonly measured biochemical parameters in 10 stable CAPD patients in a prospective, crossover study.[66] The study consisted of three periods, namely, baseline, 7-day treatment, and follow-up periods. The results of the study are depicted in Table 5. As can be seen, BUN decreased significantly during the treatment period in conjunction with decreases in serum potassium and phosphorus levels. In addition, there was a small but statistically significant increase in serum creatinine levels. Urea kinetic parameters have also shown significant changes, with decreases in dialysate urea nitrogen (DUN) excretion, net urea nitrogen (NUN) excretion, and PCR. These findings suggested a favorable effect on protein turnover attributable to either increased anabolism or decreased catabolism of dietary or body proteins. Glycemic control was difficult in one insulin-dependent diabetic patient, but there was no other noted side effect.

Preliminary data from analysis of amino acid profiles in these patients suggested that this effect was caused by increased anabolism as evidenced by a significant decrease in essential amino acid levels in both plasma and dialysate during the treatment period.[67] Plasma and dialysate essential amino acids decreased from 935 ± 243 μmol/L to 801 ± 186 μmol/L, and from 625 ± 244 μmol/L to 415 ± 122 μmol/L, respectively. These findings are in accordance with the anabolic effects of rhGH in peripheral tissues. In addition, Kang et al[68] reported in abstract form the nutritional effects of rhGH on 10 CAPD patients after treatment for 12 weeks. They showed significant improvements in lean body mass and total body muscle measurements after the treatment period.

Another recombinant hormone, namely, rhIGF-1, has also been proposed as a nutritional support in malnourished dialysis patients.[69] Preliminary evidence suggest that rhIGF-1 also promotes significant improvements in nitrogen balances in CAPD patients.[70] Conversely, several studies on healthy subjects failed to show similar responses on protein metabolism with administration of rhIGF-1 alone, contrasted to the results of rhGH administration.[71] Moreover, a recent study on chronic renal failure patients suggested that the side-effect profile of rhIGF-1 was worse than that for rhGH.[72] Nevertheless, it seems that both of these new agents are promising, either alone or in combination, for treatment of malnutrition in dialysis patients. Whether improved nitrogen balances will result in improved nutritional indices and morbidity and mortality need to be defined by long-term studies.

In summary, it is clear that malnutrition is common in chronic dialysis patients and is associated with increased morbidity and mortality. Evidence is accumulating that several measures can be taken to improve the nutritional status of these patients. Early start of dialysis, increase in dialysis doses, use of biocompatible membranes or dialysis solutions, and intensive nutritional counseling should be applied when necessary. If these measures fail, additional interventions, such as parenteral or enteral nutritional supplements, rhGH, and rhIGF-1, alone or in combination, should be tried. Studies demonstrating the impact of these interventions on morbidity and mortality are lacking and are urgently needed.

REFERENCES

1. Nelson EE, Hong CD, Pesce AL, Peterson DW, Singh S, Pollak VE: Anthropometric norms for the dialysis population. Am J Kidney Dis 16:32-37, 1990

2. Lowrie EG, Lew NL: Death risk in hemodialysis patients: The predictive value of commonly measured variables and an evaluation of death rate differences between facilities. Am J Kidney Dis 15:458-482, 1990

3. Bergstrom J, Alvestrand A, Furst P: Plasma and muscle free amino acids in maintenance hemodialysis patients without protein malnutrition. Kidney Int 38:108-114, 1990

4. Acchiardo SR, Moore LW, Latour PA. Malnutrition as the main factor in morbidity and mortality of hemodialysis patients. Kidney Int 24:S199-S203, 1983 (suppl 16)

5. Young GA, Kopple JD, Lindholm B, Vonesh EF, DeVecchi A, Scalamogna A, Castelnova C, Oreopoulos DG, Anderson GH, Bergstrom J, DiChiro J, Gentile D, Nissenson A, Sakhrani L, Brownjohn AM, Nolph KD, Prowant BF, Algrim CE, Martis L, Serkes KD: Nutritional assessment of continuous ambulatory peritoneal dialysis patients: An international study. Am J Kidney Dis 17:462-471, 1991

6. Oksa H, Ahonen K, Pasternack A, Marnela KM: Malnutrition in hemodialysis patients. Scand J Urol Nephrol 25:157-161, 1991

7. Schoenfeld PY, Henry RR, Laird NM, Roxe DM: Assessment of nutritional status of the national cooperative dialysis study population. Kidney Int 23:80-88, 1983

8. Goldwasser P, Mittman M, Antignani A, Burrel D, Michel M-A, Collier T, Avram MM: Predictors of mortality on hemodialysis. J Am Soc Nephrol 3:1613-1622, 1993

9. Jones MR: Etiology of severe malnutrition: Results of an international cross-sectional study in continuous peritoneal dialysis patients. Am J Kidney Dis 23:412-420, 1994

10. Avram MM, Goldwasser P, Erroa M, Fein PA: Predictors of survival in continuous ambulatory peritoneal dialysis patients: The importance of prealbumin and other nutritional and metabolic markers. Am J Kidney Dis 23:91-98, 1994

11. MDRD Study Group (prepared by Kopple JD CW Gassman JJ, Hollinger DL, Maroni BJ, Merrill D, Scherch LK, Sculman G, Zimmer GS): Relationship between GFR and nutritional status: Results from the MDRD study. J Am Soc Nephrol 5:335, 1994 (Abstr)

12. Ikizler TA, Greene J, Wingard RL, Parker RA, Hakim RM: Effects of progression of chronic renal failure (CRF) on spontaneous dietary protein intake in CRF patients. J Am Soc Nephrol 5:332, 1994 (Abstr)

13. Mitch WE, May RC, Maroni BJ, Bruml W: Protein and amino acid metabolism in uremia: Influence of metabolic acidosis. Kidney Int 27:205-207, 1989

14. DeFronzo RA, Alvestrand A, Smith D, Hendler R, Hendler E, Wahren J: Insulin resistance in uremia. J Clin Invest 67:563-568, 1981

15. Alvestrand A. Nutritional requirements of hemodialysis patients, in Mitch WE, Klahr S (eds): Nutrition and the Kidney. Boston, MA, 1988, pp 180-197

16. Borah MF, Schoenfeld PY, Gotch FA, Sargent JA, Wolfson M, Humphreys MH: Nitrogen balance during intermittent dialysis therapy of uremia. Kidney Int 14:491-500, 1978

17. Lim VS, Flanigan MJ: The effect of interdialytic interval on protein metabolism: Evidence suggesting dialysis-induced catabolism. Am J Kidney Dis 14:96-101, 1989

18. Wolfson M, Jones MR, Kopple JD: Amino acid losses during hemodialysis with infusion of amino acids and glucose. Kidney Int 21:500-506, 1982

19. Ikizler TA, Flakoll PJ, Parker RA, Hakim RM: Amino acid and albumin losses during hemodialysis. Kidney Int 46:830-837, 1994

20. Blumenkrantz MJ, Kopple JD, Moran JK, Coburn JW: Metabolic balance studies and dietary protein requirements in patients undergoing continuous ambulatory peritoneal dialysis. Kidney Int 21:849-861, 1982

21. Teehan B, Brown J, Schleifer C: Kinetic modeling in peritoneal dialysis, in Nissenson A, Fine R, Gentile D (eds): Clinical Dialysis. London, Prentice-Hall International, 1990, pp 319-329

22. Kopple JD, Hirschberg R. Nutrition and peritoneal dialysis, in Mitch WE, Klahr S (eds): Nutrition and the Kidney. Boston, MA, Little, Brown, 1993, pp 290-313

23. Hakim R: Clinical implications of hemodialysis membrane biocompatibility. Kidney Int 44:484-494, 1993

24. Gutierrez A, Alvestrand A, Wahren J, Bergstrom J: Effect of in vivo contact between blood and dialysis membranes on protein catabolism in humans. Kidney Int 38:487-494, 1990

25. Gutierrez A, Bergstrom J, Alvestrand A: Hemodialysis-associated protein catabolism with and without glucose in the dialysis fluid. Kidney Int 46:814-822, 1994

26. Monteon FJ, Laidlaw SA, Shaib JK, Kopple JD: Energy expenditure in patients with chronic renal failure. Kidney Int 30:741-747, 1986

27. Schneeweiss B, Graninger W, Stokenhuber F, Druml W, Ferenci P, Eichinger S, Grimm G, Laggner AN, Lenz K: Energy metabolism in acute and chronic renal failure. Am J Clin Nutr 52:596-601, 1990

28. Ikizler TA, Wingard RL, Sun M, Hakim RM: Energy expenditure (EE) and respiratory quotient (RQ) during hemodialysis (HD) with different dialysis membranes. J Am Soc Nephrol 5:493, 1994 (Abstr)

29. Hakim R, Levin N: Malnutrition in hemodialysis patients. Am J Kidney Dis 21:125-137, 1993

30. Parker TF, Laird NM, Lowrie EG: Comparison of the study groups in the national cooperative dialysis study and a description of morbidity, mortality, and patient withdrawal. Kidney Int 23:42-49, 1983

31. Lindsay RM, Spanner E: A hypothesis: The protein catabolic rate is dependent upon the type and amount of treatment in dialyzed uremic patients. Am J Kidney Dis 132:382-389, 1989

32. Burrowes DD, Lyons TA, Kaufman AM, Levin NW: Improvement in serum albumin with adequate hemodialysis. J Renal Nutr 3:171-176, 1993

33. Acchiardo S, Fuller J, Dyson B, Hatten KW, Ellis K: Can we improve mortality rate in hemodialysis patients? J Am Soc Nephrol 5:430, 1994 (Abstr)

34. Keshaviah PR, Nolph KD, Prowant P, Moore H, Ponferrada L, Van Stone J, Twardowski ZJ, Khanna R: Defining adequacy of CAPD with urea kinetics. Adv Perit Dial 6:173-177, 1990

35. Teehan B, Schleifer C, Brown J: Urea kinetic modeling is an appropriate assessment of adequacy. Semin Dial 5:189-192, 1992

36. Lindsay R, Spanner E, Heidenheim P, LeFebure J, Hodsman A, Baird J, Allison M: Which comes first, Kt/V or PCR—Chicken or egg? Kidney Int 42:S32-S37, 1992 (Suppl 38)

37. Hakim RM, Breyer J, Ismail N, Schulman G: Effects of dose of dialysis on morbidity and mortality. Am J Kidney Dis 23:661-669, 1994

38. Owen W Jr, Lew N, Liu Y, Lowrie E, Lazarus J: The urea reduction ratio and serum albumin concentrations as predictors of mortality in patients undergoing hemodialysis. N Engl J Med 329:1001-1006, 1993

39. Graeber WC, Halley SE, Lapkin RA, Graeber CA, Kaplan AA: Protein losses with reused dialyzers. J Am Soc Nephrol 4:349, 1993 (Abstr)

40. Hakim RM, Wingard RL, Ikizler TA, Parker RA, Vanholder R, Husni L, Parker TF III: Effects of biocompatibility on nutritional status in chronic hemodialysis patients. J Am Soc Nephrol 5:451, 1994 (Abstr)

41. Lameire NH, Vanholder R, Veyt D, Lambert M-C, Ringoir S: A longitudinal, five year survey of kinetic parameters in CAPD patients. Kidney Int 42:426-432, 1992

42. Compher C, Mullen JL, Barker CF: Nutritional support in renal failure. Surg Clin North Am 71:597-608, 1991

43. Wolfson M: Use of nutritional supplements in dialysis patients. Semin Dial 5:285-290, 1992

44. Heidland A, Kult J: Long-term effects of essential amino acids supplementation in patients on regular dialysis treatment. Clin Nephrol 3:234-239, 1975

45. Guarnieri B, Faccini L, Lipartiti T, Ranieri F, Spangaro F, Giuntini D, Toigo G, Dardi F, Berquier-Vidali F, Raimondi A: Simple methods for nutritional assessment in hemodialyzed patients. Am J Clin Nutr 33:1598-1607, 1980

46. Piraino A, Tirpo J, Powers D: Prolonged hyperalimentation in catabolic chronic dialysis therapy patients. J Parenter Enteral Nutr 5:463-477, 1981

47. Foulkes CJ, Goldstein DJ, Kelly MP, Hunt JM: Indications for the use of intradialytic parenteral nutrition in the malnourished hemodialysis patient. J Renal Nutr 1:23-33, 1991

48. Thunberg B, Jain V, Patterson PG, Cestero RV, Swamy AP: Nutritional measurements and urea kinetics to guide intradialytic hyperalimentation. Proc Dial Transplant Forum 10:22-28, 1980

49. Cano N, Labastie-Coeyrehourq J, Lacombe P, Stroumza P, di Costanzo-Dufetel J, Durbec JP, Coudray-Lucas C, Cynober L: Perdialytic parenteral nutrition with lipids and amino acids in malnourished hemodialysis patients. Am J Clin Nutr 52:726-730, 1990

50. Capelli JP, Kushner H, Camiscioli TC, Chen S-M, Torres MA: Effect of intradialytic parenteral nutrition on mortality rates in end-stage renal disease care. Am J Kidney Dis 23:808-816, 1994

51. Chertow GM, Ling J, Lew NL, Lazarus JM, Lowrie EG: The association of intradialytic parenteral nutrition with survival in hemodialysis patients. Am J Kidney Dis 24:912-920, 1994

52. Bruno M, Bagnis C, Marangella M, Rovera L, Cantaluppi A, Linari F: CAPD with an amino acid dialysis solution: A long-term, cross-over study. Kidney Int 35:1189-1194, 1989

53. Young GA, Dibble JB, Hobson SM, Tompkins L, Gibson J, Turney JH, Brownjohn AM: The use of an amino-acid-based CAPD fluid over 12 weeks. Nephrol Dial Transplant 4:285-292, 1989

54. Arfeen S, Goodship TH, Kirkwood A, Ward MK: The nutritional/metabolic and hormonal effects of 8 weeks of continuous ambulatory peritoneal dialysis with 1% amino acid solution. Clin Nephrol 33:192-199, 1990

55. Davidson M. Effect of growth hormone on carbohydrate and lipid metabolism. Endocr Rev 8:115-131, 1987

56. Mehls O, Ritz E, Hunziker EB, Eggli P, Heinrich U, Zapf J: Improvement of growth and food utilization by human recombinant growth hormone in uremia. Kidney Int 33:45-52, 1988

57. Chwals W, Bistrian B: Role of exogenous growth hormone and insulin-like growth factor 1 in malnutrition and acute metabolic stress: A hypothesis. Crit Care Med 19:1317-1322, 1991

58. Clemmons D, Smith-Banks A, Underwood L: Reversal of diet-induced catabolism by infusion of recombinant insulin-like growth factor (IGF-1) in humans. J Clin Endocrinol Metab 75:234-238, 1992

59. Wilmore DW: Catabolic illness: Strategies for enhancing recovery. N Engl J Med 325:695, 1991

60. Veldhuis JD, Johnson ML, Wilkowski MJ, Iranmanesh A, Bolton WK: Neuroendocrine alterations in the somatotrophic axis in chronic renal failure. Acta Paediatr Scand 379:12-22, 1991

61. Chan W, Valerie K, Chan J: Expression of insulin-like growth factor-1 in uremic rats: Growth hormone resistance and nutritional intake. Kidney Int 43:790-795, 1993

62. Fine RN, Pyke-Grimm K, Nelson PA, Boechat MI, Lippe BM, Yadin O, Kamil E: Recombinant human growth hormone treatment of children with chronic renal failure: Long-term (1 to 3 year) outcome. Pediatr Nephrol 5:477-481, 1991

63. Tonshoff B, Haffner D, Mehls O, Dietz M, Ruder H, Blum W, Heinrich U, Stover B: Efficacy and safety of growth hormone treatment in short children with renal allografts: Three year experience. Kidney Int 44:199-207, 1993

64. Ziegler TR, Lazarus JM, Young LS, Hakim R, Wilmore DW: Effects of recombinant human growth hormone in adults receiving maintenance hemodialysis. J Am Soc Nephrol 2:1130-1135, 1991

65. Schulman G, Wingard RL, Hutchinson RL, Lawrence P, Hakim RM: The effects of recombinant human growth hormone and intradialytic parenteral nutrition in malnourished hemodialysis patients. Am J Kidney Dis 21:527-534, 1993

66. Ikizler TA, Wingard RL, Breyer JA, Schulman G, Parker RA, Hakim RM: Short-term effects of recombinant human growth hormone in CAPD patients. Kidney Int 46:1178-1183, 1994

67. Ikizler TA, Wingard RL, Flakoll PJ, Schulman G, Par-

ker RA, Hakim RM: Effects of recombinant human growth hormone (rhGH) on amino acid (AA) profiles in CAPD patients. J Am Soc Nephrol 5:493, 1994 (Abstr)

68. Kang DH, Lee SW, Kim HS, Choi KH, Lee HY, Han DS: Recombinant human growth hormone (rhGH) improves nutritional status of undernourished adult CAPD patients. J Am Soc Nephrol 5:494, 1994 (Abstr)

69. Kopple J: The rationale for the use of growth hormone or insulin-like growth factor-1 in adult patients with renal failure. Miner Electrolyte Metab 18:269-275, 1992

70. Peng S, Fouque D, Kopple J: Insulin-like growth factor-1 causes anabolism in malnourished CAPD patients. J Am Soc Nephrol 4:414, 1993

71. Mauras N, Horber F, Haymond M: Low dose recombinant human insulin-like growth factor-1 fails to affect protein anabolism but inhibits islet cell secretion in humans. J Clin Endocrinol Metab 75:1192-1197, 1992

72. Miller SB, Moulton M, O'Shea M, Hammermann MR: Effects of IGF-1 on renal function in end-stage chronic renal failure. Kidney Int 46:201-207, 1994

INDEX